Annual Update in Intensive Care
and Emergency Medicine

The series *Annual Update in Intensive Care and Emergency Medicine* is the continuation of the series entitled *Yearbook of Intensive Care Medicine* in Europe and *Intensive Care Medicine: Annual Update* in the United States.

Jean-Louis Vincent
Editor

Annual Update in Intensive Care and Emergency Medicine 2020

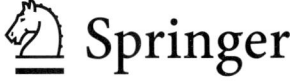 Springer

Editor
Jean-Louis Vincent
Department of Intensive Care
Erasme University Hospital
Université libre de Bruxelles
Brussels
Belgium
jlvincent@intensive.org

ISSN 2191-5709 ISSN 2191-5717 (electronic)
Annual Update in Intensive Care and Emergency Medicine
ISBN 978-3-030-37322-1 ISBN 978-3-030-37323-8 (eBook)
https://doi.org/10.1007/978-3-030-37323-8

© Springer Nature Switzerland AG 2020
This work is subject to copyright. All rights are reserved by the Publisher, whether the whole or part of the material is concerned, specifically the rights of translation, reprinting, reuse of illustrations, recitation, broadcasting, reproduction on microfilms or in any other physical way, and transmission or information storage and retrieval, electronic adaptation, computer software, or by similar or dissimilar methodology now known or hereafter developed.
The use of general descriptive names, registered names, trademarks, service marks, etc. in this publication does not imply, even in the absence of a specific statement, that such names are exempt from the relevant protective laws and regulations and therefore free for general use.
The publisher, the authors, and the editors are safe to assume that the advice and information in this book are believed to be true and accurate at the date of publication. Neither the publisher nor the authors or the editors give a warranty, expressed or implied, with respect to the material contained herein or for any errors or omissions that may have been made. The publisher remains neutral with regard to jurisdictional claims in published maps and institutional affiliations.

This Springer imprint is published by the registered company Springer Nature Switzerland AG
The registered company address is: Gewerbestrasse 11, 6330 Cham, Switzerland

Contents

Part I Respiratory Issues

1 **Physiology of the Respiratory Drive in ICU Patients: Implications for Diagnosis and Treatment** 3
A. H. Jonkman, H. J. de Vries, and L. M. A. Heunks

2 **Monitoring Patient Respiratory Effort During Mechanical Ventilation: Lung and Diaphragm-Protective Ventilation** 21
M. Bertoni, S. Spadaro, and E. C. Goligher

3 **Ten Reasons to Use Mechanical Power to Guide Ventilator Settings in Patients Without ARDS** 37
P. L. Silva, P. R. M. Rocco, and P. Pelosi

Part II Acute Respiratory Distress Syndrome

4 **Extracellular Vesicles in ARDS: New Insights into Pathogenesis with Novel Clinical Applications** 53
R. Y. Mahida, S. Matsumoto, and M. A. Matthay

5 **ARDS Subphenotypes: Understanding a Heterogeneous Syndrome** 67
J. G. Wilson and C. S. Calfee

6 **Assessment of VILI Risk During Spontaneous Breathing and Assisted Mechanical Ventilation** 81
G. Bellani and M. Teggia-Droghi

Part III Biomarkers

7 **The Future of ARDS Biomarkers: Where Are the Gaps in Implementation of Precision Medicine?** 91
P. Yang, A. M. Esper, and G. S. Martin

8 **Utility of Inflammatory Biomarkers for Predicting Organ Failure and Outcomes in Cardiac Arrest Patients** 101
H. Vuopio, P. Pekkarinen, and M. B. Skrifvars

9 Troponin Elevations after Cardiac Surgery: Just "Troponitis"? 113
  D. E. C. van Beek, I. C. C. van der Horst, and T. W. L. Scheeren

10 Biomarkers of Sepsis During Continuous Renal
   Replacement Therapy: Have We Found the Appropriate
   Biomarker to Use Under This Condition? 125
   P. M. Honore, S. Redant, and D. De Bels

Part IV Fluids

11 Do Intensivists Need to Care About the Revised
   Starling Principle? 137
   R. G. Hahn

12 Right Ventricular Dysfunction and Fluid
   Administration in Critically Ill Patients 145
   F. Gavelli, X. Monnet, and J.-L. Teboul

13 Intravenous Fluids: Do Not Drown in Confusion! 153
   J. N. Wilkinson, F. M. P. van Haren, and M. L. N. G. Malbrain

Part V Hemodynamic Management

14 Update on Right Ventricular Hemodynamic,
   Echocardiographic and Extra-Cardiac Ultrasound
   Monitoring.. 175
   E. J. Couture and A. Y. Denault

15 Management of Hypotension: Implications for
   Noncardiac Surgery and Intensive Care......................... 189
   E. Schneck, B. Saugel, and M. Sander

16 Heterogeneity of Cardiovascular Response to
   Standardized Sepsis Resuscitation 205
   F. Guarracino, P. Bertini, and M. R. Pinsky

Part VI The Microcirculation

17 Clinical Relevance of the Endothelial Glycocalyx
   in Critically Ill Patients 213
   D. Astapenko, J. Benes, and V. Cerny

18 Customized Monitoring of the Microcirculation
   in Patients with a Left Ventricular Assist Device 223
   S. Akin, O. I. Soliman, and C. Ince

19 Monitoring of the Sublingual Microcirculation at
   the Bedside: Yes, It Is Possible and Useful 235
   V. Tarazona, A. Harrois, and J. Duranteau

20 Microcirculation in Patients with Sepsis: From
    Physiology to Interventions 245
    B. Cantan and I. Martín-Loeches

Part VII Sepsis

21 Macrophage Activation Syndrome in Sepsis: Does
    It Exist and How to Recognize It? 261
    E. J. Giamarellos-Bourboulis and M. G. Netea

22 Is T Cell Exhaustion a Treatable Trait in Sepsis? 271
    M. Fish, C. M. Swanson, and M. Shankar-Hari

23 Cell-Free Hemoglobin: A New Therapeutic Target in Sepsis? 281
    L. B. Ware

24 Therapeutic Potential of the Gut Microbiota in
    the Management of Sepsis 293
    M. Bassetti, A. Bandera, and A. Gori

Part VIII Bleeding and Transfusion

25 Blood Transfusion Practice During Extracorporeal
    Membrane Oxygenation: Rationale and Modern
    Approaches to Management 307
    C. Agerstrand, B. Bromberger, and D. Brodie

26 The Use of Frozen Platelets for the Treatment of Bleeding 317
    D. J. B. Kleinveld, N. P. Juffermans, and F. Noorman

27 Viscoelastic Assay-Guided Hemostatic Therapy
    in Perioperative and Critical Care 331
    G. E. Iapichino, E. Costantini, and M. Cecconi

28 Extracorporeal Filter and Circuit Patency:
    A Personalized Approach to Anticoagulation 345
    S. Romagnoli, Z. Ricci, and C. Ronco

Part IX Prehospital Intervention

29 Prehospital Resuscitation with Low Titer O+ Whole
    Blood by Civilian EMS Teams: Rationale and
    Evolving Strategies for Use 365
    P. E. Pepe, J. P. Roach, and C. J. Winckler

30 Mobile Stroke Units: Taking the Emergency Room
    to the Patient 377
    T. Bhalla, C. Zammit, and P. Leroux

Part X Trauma

31 Evaluating Quality in Trauma Systems 397
A. J. Mahoney and M. C. Reade

**32 Vasopressors for Post-traumatic Hemorrhagic Shock:
Friends or Foe?** 413
J. Richards, T. Gauss, and P. Bouzat

33 Extracranial Tsunami After Traumatic Brain Injury 427
G. Bonatti, C. Robba, and G. Citerio

Part XI Neurological Aspects

**34 Ten False Beliefs About Mechanical Ventilation
in Patients with Brain Injury** 441
D. Battaglini, P. Pelosi, and C. Robba

35 Manifestations of Critical Illness Brain Injury 457
S. Williams Roberson, E. W. Ely, and J. E. Wilson

**36 Essential Noninvasive Multimodality Neuromonitoring
for the Critically Ill Patient** 469
F. A. Rasulo, T. Togni, and S. Romagnoli

Part XII Organ Donation

**37 Brain Death After Cardiac Arrest: Pathophysiology,
Prevalence, and Potential for Organ Donation** 491
C. Sandroni, M. Scarpino, and M. Antonelli

**38 Organ Recovery Procedure in Donation After Controlled
Circulatory Death with Normothermic Regional Perfusion:
State of the Art** 503
R. Badenes, B. Monleón, and I. Martín-Loeches

Part XIII Oncology

**39 Admitting Adult Critically Ill Patients with
Hematological Malignancies to the ICU: A Sisyphean
Task or Work in Progress?** 521
E. N. van der Zee, E. J. O. Kompanje, and J. Bakker

**40 Onco-Nephrology: Acute Kidney Injury in Critically Ill
Cancer Patients** 531
N. Seylanova, J. Zhang, and M. Ostermann

Part XIV Severe Complications

41 A Clinician's Guide to Management of Intra-abdominal Hypertension and Abdominal Compartment Syndrome in Critically Ill Patients 543
I. E. De laet, M. L. N. G. Malbrain, and J. J. De Waele

42 Update on the Management of Iatrogenic Gas Embolism 559
N. Heming, M.-A. Melone, and D. Annane

43 Alcohol Withdrawal Syndrome in the ICU: Preventing Rather than Treating? 569
M. Geslain and O. Huet

Part XV Prolonged Critical Illness

44 Muscle Dysfunction in Critically Ill Children 583
T. Schepens and H. Mtaweh

45 Respiratory Muscle Rehabilitation in Patients with Prolonged Mechanical Ventilation: A Targeted Approach 595
B. Bissett, R. Gosselink, and F. M. P. van Haren

46 Post-Intensive Care Syndrome and Chronic Critical Illness: A Tale of Two Syndromes 611
H. Bailey and L. J. Kaplan

Part XVI Organizational and Ethical Aspects

47 Sepsis as Organ and Health System Failure 623
P. Dickmann and M. Bauer

48 Burnout and Joy in the Profession of Critical Care Medicine 633
M. P. Kerlin, J. McPeake, and M. E. Mikkelsen

49 Advance Directives in the United Kingdom: Ethical, Legal, and Practical Considerations 643
V. Metaxa

Part XVII Future Aspects

50 Mobile Devices for Hemodynamic Monitoring 655
L. Briesenick, F. Michard, and B. Saugel

51 Artificial Intelligence in the Intensive Care Unit 667
G. Gutierrez

Index 683

Abbreviations

AKI	Acute kidney injury
ARDS	Acute respiratory distress syndrome
COPD	Chronic obstructive pulmonary disease
CPB	Cardiopulmonary bypass
CPR	Cardiopulmonary resuscitation
CRRT	Continuous renal replacement therapy
CT	Computed tomography
CVP	Central venous pressure
ECMO	Extracorporeal membrane oxygenation
EEG	Electroencephalogram
EKG	Electrocardiogram
GCS	Glasgow Coma Scale
ICU	Intensive care unit
IL	Interleukin
LV	Left ventricular
MAP	Mean arterial pressure
PCT	Procalcitonin
PEEP	Positive end-expiratory pressure
RBC	Red blood cell
RCT	Randomized controlled trial
RRT	Renal replacement therapy
RV	Right ventricular
$ScvO_2$	Central venous oxygen saturation
SvO_2	Mixed venous oxygen saturation
TBI	Traumatic brain injury
TNF	Tumor necrosis factor
VAP	Ventilator-associated pneumonia
VILI	Ventilator-induced lung injury

Part I
Respiratory Issues

Physiology of the Respiratory Drive in ICU Patients: Implications for Diagnosis and Treatment

A. H. Jonkman, H. J. de Vries, and L. M. A. Heunks

1.1 Introduction

The primary goal of the respiratory system is gas exchange, especially the uptake of oxygen and elimination of carbon dioxide. The latter plays an important role in maintaining acid-base homeostasis. This requires tight control of ventilation by the respiratory centers in the brain stem. The respiratory drive is the intensity of the output of the respiratory centers, and determines the mechanical output of the respiratory muscles (also known as breathing effort) [1, 2].

Detrimental respiratory drive is an important contributor to inadequate mechanical output of the respiratory muscles, and may therefore contribute to the onset, duration, and recovery from acute respiratory failure. Studies in mechanically ventilated patients have demonstrated detrimental effects of both high and low breathing effort, including patient self-inflicted lung injury (P-SILI), critical illness-associated diaphragm weakness, hemodynamic compromise, and poor patient-ventilator interaction [3, 4]. Strategies that prevent the detrimental effects of both high and low respiratory drive might therefore improve patient outcome [5].

Such strategies require a thorough understanding of the physiology of respiratory drive. The aim of this chapter is to discuss the (patho)physiology of respiratory drive, as relevant to critically ill ventilated patients. We discuss the clinical consequences of high and low respiratory drive and evaluate techniques that can be used to assess respiratory drive at the bedside. Finally, we propose optimal ranges for respiratory drive and breathing effort, and discuss interventions that can be used to modulate a patient's respiratory drive.

A. H. Jonkman and H. J. de Vries contributed equally.

A. H. Jonkman · H. J. de Vries · L. M. A. Heunks (✉)
Department of Intensive Care Medicine, Amsterdam UMC, Location VUmc, Amsterdam, The Netherlands

Amsterdam Cardiovascular Sciences Research Institute, Amsterdam UMC, Amsterdam, The Netherlands
e-mail: L.Heunks@amsterdamumc.nl

1.2 Definition of Respiratory Drive

The term "respiratory drive" is frequently used, but is rarely precisely defined. It is important to stress that the activity of the respiratory centers cannot be measured directly, and therefore the physiological consequences are used to quantify respiratory drive. Most authors define respiratory drive as the intensity of the output of the respiratory centers [3], using the amplitude of a physiological signal as a measure for intensity. Alternatively, we consider the respiratory centers to act as oscillatory neuronal networks that generate rhythmic, wave-like signals. The intensity of such a signal depends on several components, including the amplitude and frequency of the signal. Accordingly, we propose a more precise but clinically useful definition of respiratory drive: the time integral of the neuronal network output of the respiratory centers, derived from estimates of breathing effort. As such, a high respiratory drive may mean that the output of the respiratory centers has a higher amplitude, a higher frequency, or both.

The respiratory drive directly determines breathing effort when neuromuscular transmission and respiratory muscle function are intact. We define breathing effort as the mechanical output of the respiratory muscles, including both the magnitude and the frequency of respiratory muscle contraction [1].

1.3 What Determines the Respiratory Drive?

1.3.1 Neuroanatomy and Physiology of the Respiratory Control Centers

The respiratory drive originates from clusters of interneurons (respiratory centers) located in the brain stem (Fig. 1.1) [2]. These centers receive continuous information from sources sensitive to chemical, mechanical, behavioral, and emotional stimuli. The respiratory centers integrate this information and generate a neural signal. The amplitude of this signal determines the mechanical output of the respiratory muscles (and thus tidal volume). The frequency and timing of the neural pattern

Fig. 1.1 Schematic representation of the anatomy and physiology of respiratory drive. The respiratory centers are located in the medulla and the pons and consist of groups of interneurons that receive information from sources sensitive to chemical, mechanical, behavioral, and emotional stimuli. Important central chemoreceptors are located near the ventral parafacial nucleus (pF_V) and are sensitive to direct changes in pH of the cerebrospinal fluid. Peripheral chemoreceptors in the carotid bodies are the primary site sensitive to changes in PaO_2, and moderately sensitive to changes in pH and $PaCO_2$. Mechano and irritant receptors are located in the chest wall, airway, lungs, and respiratory muscles. Emotional and behavioral feedback originate in the cerebral cortex and hypothalamus. The pre-Bötzinger complex (preBötC) is the main control center of inspiration, located between the ventral respiratory group (VRG) and the Bötzinger complex (BötC). The post-inspiratory complex (PiCo) is located near the Bötzinger complex. The lateral parafacial nucleus (pF_L) controls expiratory activity and has continuous interaction with the pre-Bötzinger complex, to prevent inefficient concomitant activation of inspiratory and expiratory muscle groups: lung inflation depresses inspiratory activity and enhances expiratory activity, which ultimately results in lung deflation. Lung deflation has the opposite effect on these centers

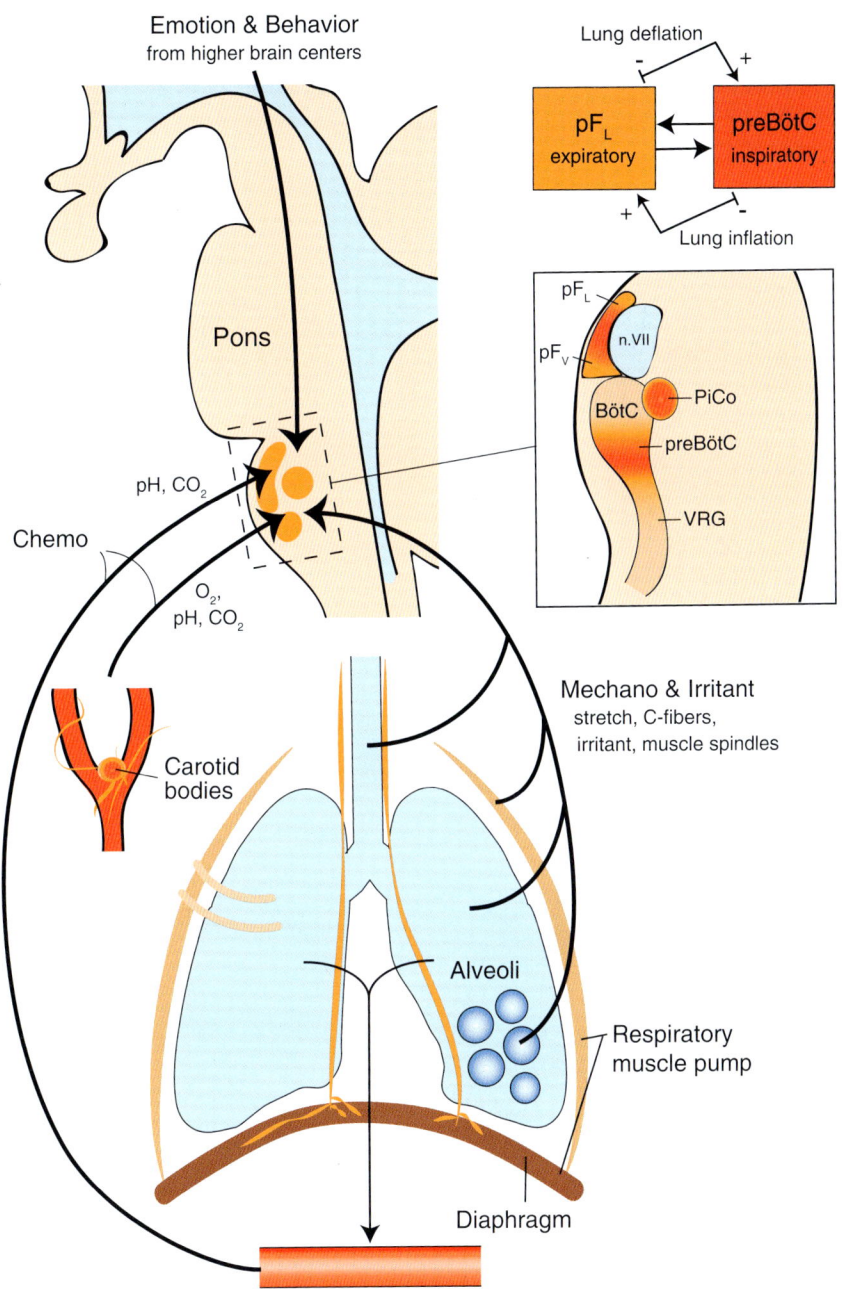

relates to the breathing frequency and the duration of the different phases of the breathing cycle. Three phases can be distinguished in the human breathing cycle: inspiration, post-inspiration, and expiration (Fig. 1.2). Each phase is predominately controlled by a specific respiratory center (Fig. 1.1) [2].

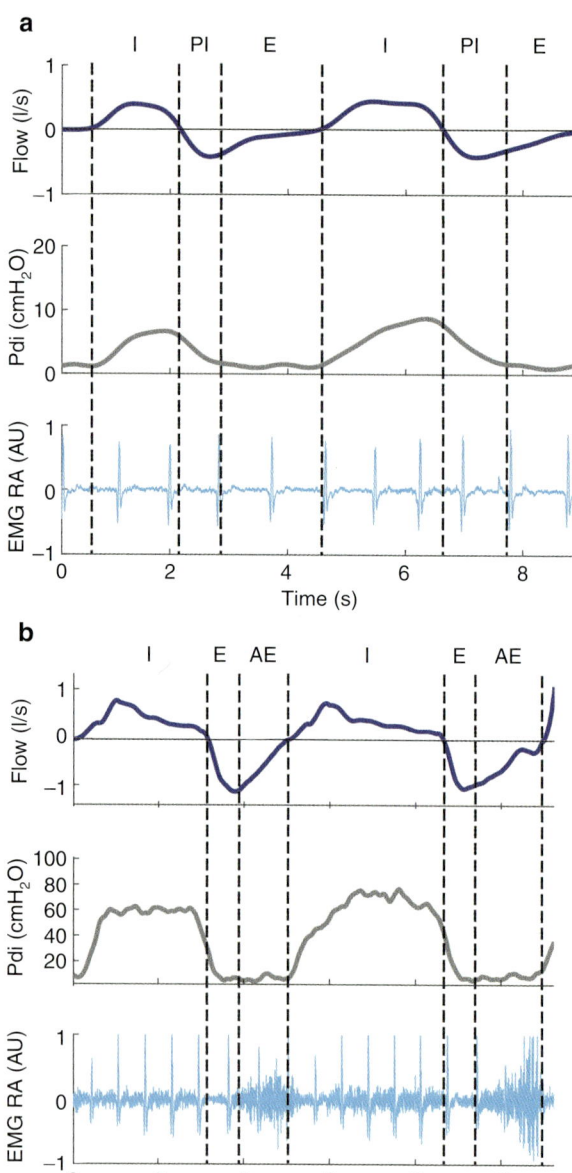

Fig. 1.2 Breathing phases. Flow, transdiaphragmatic pressure (P_{di}) and electromyography of the rectus abdominal muscle (EMG RA, in arbitrary units; note that this signal is disturbed with electrocardiogram [EKG] artifacts) during tidal breathing at rest (**a**) and during high resistive loading (**b**) in one healthy subject. Vertical dashed lines mark the onset of the different breathing phases. Inspiration (I) is characterized by a steady increase in P_{di} and positive flow, and is present during both tidal breathing and high loading. The gradual decrease in P_{di} during expiratory flow in (**a**) is consistent with post-inspiration (PI). Note that the rate of decline in P_{di} is much more rapid during high loading. During tidal breathing (**a**), expiration (E) is characterized by the absence of P_{di} and EMG RA activity and occurs after post-inspiration. High loading (**b**) leads to expiration (AE), which can be recognized by the increase in EMG RA activity. Also, expiration directly follows the inspiratory phase

1.3.1.1 Inspiration
Inspiration is an active process that requires neural activation and subsequent contraction (and energy expenditure) of the inspiratory muscles. The pre-Bötzinger complex, a group of interneurons positioned between the ventral respiratory group and the Bötzinger complex in the brain stem (Fig. 1.1), is the main control center of inspiration [2]. The output from the pre-Bötzinger complex increases gradually during inspiration and rapidly declines when expiration commences. Axons of the pre-Bötzinger complex project to premotor and motor neurons that drive the inspiratory muscles and the muscles of the upper airways. The pre-Bötzinger complex has multiple connections to the other respiratory centers, which is thought to ensure a smooth transition between the different breathing phases and to prevent concomitant activation of opposing muscle groups [6].

1.3.1.2 Post-inspiration
The aptly named post-inspiratory complex controls the transitional phase between inspiration and expiration by reducing expiratory flow. This is achieved by gradually reducing the excitation (and thus contraction) of the inspiratory muscles, which leads to active lengthening (i.e., eccentric contractions) of the diaphragm [2, 7]. Additionally, the post-inspiratory center controls the upper airway muscles. Contraction of the upper airway muscles increases expiratory flow resistance, effectively reducing expiratory flow. Post-inspiratory activity increases the time before the respiratory system reaches end-expiratory lung volume. This can lead to a more laminar expiratory flow and might prevent alveolar collapse, while also increasing the duration of gas exchange in the alveoli [2]. Post-inspiration is a common part of the breathing cycle in healthy subjects at rest, but disappears rapidly when respiratory demands increase, to favor faster expiration [8] (Fig. 1.2).

The importance of the post-inspiratory phase in mechanically ventilated patients remains unclear, as the onset and duration of inspiratory and expiratory flow depend predominantly on the interplay between ventilator settings (e.g., cycle criteria, breathing frequency, ventilator mode) and the respiratory mechanics of the patient. Additionally, the endotracheal tube bypasses the actions of the upper airway muscles. Experimental data in piglets suggest that post-inspiratory activity of the diaphragm prevents atelectasis and possibly cyclic alveolar recruitment [9], although studies in patients weaning from the ventilator did not find clear evidence for post-inspiratory activity [10]. Clearly, this field requires further research.

1.3.1.3 Expiration
Expiration is generally a passive event during tidal breathing. The elastic recoil pressure of the lungs and chest wall will drive expiratory flow until the lung and chest wall recoil pressures are in equilibrium at functional residual capacity, or at the level of positive end-expiratory pressure (PEEP) in mechanically ventilated

patients. In passive conditions, expiratory flow depends solely on the time-constant (i.e., the product of compliance and resistance) of the respiratory system. The expiratory muscles are recruited with high metabolic demands, low inspiratory muscle capacity, increased end-expiratory lung volume, and/or increased expiratory resistance [11].

The lateral parafacial nucleus controls the expiratory phase of breathing. An increased respiratory drive leads to late-expiratory bursts, and consequent recruitment of the expiratory muscles (extensively reviewed in reference [11]). Several inhibitory connections exist between the inspiratory pre-Bötzinger complex and the expiratory lateral parafacial nucleus, which prevent concomitant activation of inspiratory and expiratory muscle groups (Fig. 1.1) [2, 6].

1.3.2 Feedback to the Respiratory Control Centers

1.3.2.1 Central Chemoreceptors

The most important chemoreceptors in the central nervous system are positioned on the ventral surface of the medulla and near the ventral parafacial nucleus (also referred to as the retrotrapezoid nucleus). These receptors are sensitive to the hydrogen proton concentration ([H$^+$]) of the cerebrospinal fluid (CSF), commonly known as pH [12]. Because CO_2 can rapidly diffuse across the blood-brain barrier, changes in $PaCO_2$ quickly affect the pH of the CSF. A set point exists in the control centers, which keeps pH (and $PaCO_2$) within a relatively tight range. A slight increase in $PaCO_2$ above this set point provides a powerful stimulus to breathe: a change in $PaCO_2$ of 5 mmHg can already double minute ventilation in healthy subjects. When $PaCO_2$ decreases only a few mmHg below the set point, the respiratory drive lowers gradually [13] and can abruptly disappear causing apnea, especially during sleep. In contrast, metabolic changes in pH are sensed less rapidly because it takes several hours before the electrolyte composition of the CSF is affected by changes in metabolic acid-base conditions.

1.3.2.2 Peripheral Chemoreceptors

The carotid bodies are positioned close to the carotid bifurcation and are the primary sites sensitive to PO_2, PCO_2, and pH of the arterial blood. The aortic bodies contribute to respiratory drive in infants, but their importance in adults is probably minor [14]. The output of the carotid bodies in healthy subjects remains relatively stable over a wide range of PaO_2 values; their output increases gradually below a PaO_2 of 80 mmHg and then rises steeply when PaO_2 falls below 60 mmHg [15]. Their contribution to respiratory drive in healthy subjects is therefore probably modest. However, concomitant hypercapnia and acidosis have a synergistic effect on the response of the carotid bodies, meaning their output is increased by more than the sum of the individual parts. This makes the carotid bodies in theory more relevant in ventilated patients in whom hypoxemia, hypercapnia, and acidosis are more common.

1.3.2.3 Thoracic Receptors

Several receptors have been identified in the chest wall, lungs, respiratory muscles, and airways that provide sensory feedback to the respiratory centers on mechanical and chemical conditions. Slowly adapting stretch receptors and muscle spindles are located in the chest wall, respiratory muscles, upper airways, and terminal bronchioles, and provide information on stretch and volume of the respiratory system, through vagal fibers [2]. These receptors are well known for their contribution to the Hering-Breuer reflexes, which terminate inspiration and facilitate expiration at high tidal volumes (Fig. 1.1). Irritant receptors line the epithelium of the proximal airways, and are sensitive to irritant gases and local inflammation. These sensors promote mucus production, coughing, and expiration. C-fibers are found inside the lung tissue and might be activated by local congestion causing dyspnea, rapid breathing, and coughing [16].

The relative contribution of these receptors to the respiratory drive of critically ill patients is uncertain. Feedback from these sensors may explain the hyperventilation observed in pulmonary fibrosis, pulmonary edema, interstitial lung disease, and pulmonary embolism, which persists even in the absence of hypoxemia or hypercapnia. Further research into the contribution of these sensors during mechanical ventilation is warranted.

1.3.2.4 Cortical and Emotional Feedback

Stimuli based on emotional and behavioral feedback, originating in the cerebral cortex and hypothalamus, modulate the respiratory drive. Pain, agitation, delirium, and fear are common in mechanically ventilated patients and can increase respiratory drive [17]. The role of the cortex and hypothalamus in the respiratory drive of critically ill patients has rarely been studied and requires more attention before recommendations can be made.

There is some evidence that the cerebral cortex has an inhibitory influence on breathing. Damage to the cortex might dampen this inhibitory effect, which could explain the hyperventilation sometimes observed in patients with severe neurotrauma [18].

1.4 What Is the Effect of Non-physiological Respiratory Drive on My Patients?

1.4.1 Consequences of Excessive Respiratory Drive

1.4.1.1 Patient Self-Inflicted Lung Injury

Excessive respiratory drive could promote lung injury through several mechanisms. In the absence of (severe) respiratory muscle weakness, high respiratory drive leads to vigorous inspiratory efforts, resulting in injurious lung distending pressures. Recent experimental studies demonstrate that this may worsen lung injury, especially when the underlying injury is more severe [19, 20]. Particularly in patients with acute respiratory failure, large inspiratory efforts could result in global and regional over-distention of alveoli and cyclic recruitment of collapsed lung areas, due to an inhomogeneous and transient transmission of stress and strain (so-called P-SILI) [3, 21]. Large efforts may cause "pendelluft": air redistributes from non-dependent to dependent lung regions, even before the start of mechanical insufflation, and hence without a change in tidal volume [20]. Excessive respiratory drive may overwhelm lung-protective reflexes (e.g., Hering-Breuer inflation-inhibition reflex), which in turn leads to high tidal volumes and promotes further lung injury and inflammation [3]. In addition, large inspiratory efforts could result in negative pressure pulmonary edema, especially in patients with lung injury and/or capillary leaks [21]. As such, a high respiratory drive is potentially harmful in spontaneously breathing mechanically ventilated patients with lung injury. Applying and maintaining a lung-protective ventilation strategy (i.e., low tidal volumes and low plateau pressures) is challenging in these patients and may often lead to the development of patient-ventilator dyssynchronies, such as double-triggering and breath stacking, again leading to high tidal volumes and increased lung stress. Furthermore, maintaining low plateau pressures and low tidal volumes does not guarantee lung-protective ventilation in patients with high respiratory drive.

1.4.1.2 Diaphragm Load-Induced Injury

In non-ventilated patients, excessive inspiratory loading can result in diaphragm fatigue and injury as demonstrated by sarcomere disruption in diaphragm biopsies [5]. Whether this occurs in critically ill ventilated patients is less clear, although we have reported evidence of diaphragm injury, including sarcomere disruption [22]. The concept of load-induced diaphragm injury may explain recent ultrasound findings demonstrating increased diaphragm thickness during the course of mechanical ventilation in patients with high inspiratory efforts [23]. In addition to high breathing effort, patient-ventilator dyssynchronies, especially eccentric (lengthening) contractions, may promote load-induced diaphragm injury [24]. Whether eccentric contractions are sufficiently severe and frequent to contribute to diaphragm injury in intensive care unit (ICU) patients is not yet known.

1.4.1.3 Weaning and Extubation Failure

During ventilator weaning, high ventilatory demands with high respiratory drive increase dyspnea, which is associated with anxiety and impacts weaning outcome [25]. "Air hunger" is probably the most distressing form of dyspnea sensation, which occurs in particular when inspiratory flow rate is insufficient ("flow starvation"), or when tidal volumes are decreased under mechanical ventilation while the $PaCO_2$ level is held constant [25]. In patients with decreased respiratory muscle strength and excessive respiratory drive, the muscle's ability to respond to neural demands is insufficient; dyspnea is then characteristically experienced as a form of excessive breathing effort. Activation of accessory respiratory muscles was found to be strongly related to the intensity of dyspnea [26], and can lead to weaning and/or extubation failure [10]. In addition, dyspnea impacts ICU outcome and may contribute to ICU-related post-traumatic stress disorders.

1.4.2 Consequences of Low Respiratory Drive

In ventilated patients, a low respiratory drive due to excessive ventilator assistance and/or sedation is a critical contributor to diaphragm weakness. The effects of diaphragm inactivity have been demonstrated both *in vivo* and *in vitro* in the form of myofibrillar atrophy and contractile force reduction [22, 27]. Diaphragm weakness is associated with prolonged ventilator weaning and increased risks of ICU readmission, hospital readmission, and mortality [28]. In addition, low respiratory drive can lead to patient-ventilator dyssynchronies, such as ineffective efforts, central apneas, auto-triggering, and reverse triggering [29]. Excessive ventilator assistance may result in dynamic hyperinflation, particularly in patients with obstructive airway diseases. Dynamic hyperinflation reduces respiratory drive and promotes ineffective efforts (i.e., a patient's effort becomes insufficient to overcome intrinsic PEEP). Although asynchronies have been associated with worse outcome, whether this is a causal relationship requires further investigation.

1.5 How Can We Assess Respiratory Drive?

Because respiratory center output cannot be measured directly, several indirect measurements have been described to assess respiratory drive. It follows that the more proximal these parameters are to the respiratory centers in the respiratory feedback loop, the better they reflect respiratory drive. This includes, from proximal to distal: diaphragm electromyography, mechanical output of the respiratory muscles, and clinical evaluation.

1.5.1 Clinical Signs and Breathing Frequency

Clinical signs, such as dyspnea and activation of accessory respiratory muscles, strongly support the presence of high respiratory drive, but do not allow for quantification. Although respiratory drive comprises a frequency component, respiratory rate alone is a rather insensitive parameter for the assessment of respiratory drive; respiratory rate varies within and between subjects, depends on respiratory mechanics, and can be influenced by several factors independent of the status of respiratory drive, such as opioids [30] or the level of pressure support ventilation. We therefore need to evaluate more sensitive parameters of respiratory drive.

1.5.2 Diaphragm Electrical Activity

Diaphragm electrical activity (EA_{di}) reflects the strength of the electrical field produced by the diaphragm and, hence, the relative change in discharge of motor neurons over time. Provided that the neuromuscular transmission and muscle fiber membrane excitability are intact, EA_{di} is a valid measure of phrenic nerve output and thus the most precise estimation of respiratory drive [7, 31]. Real-time recording of the EA_{di} signal is readily available on a specific type of ICU ventilator (Servo-I/U, Maquet, Solna, Sweden). The EA_{di} signal is acquired using a dedicated nasogastric (feeding) catheter with nine ring-shaped electrodes positioned at the level of the diaphragm [31]. Computer algorithms within the ventilator software continuously select the electrode pair that is closest to the diaphragm, and correct for disturbances such as motion artifacts, esophageal peristalsis, and interference from the electrocardiogram or other nearby muscles. EA_{di} reflects crural diaphragm activity and is representative of activity from the costal parts of the diaphragm (and thus the whole diaphragm). In addition, the EA_{di} signal remains reliable at different lung volumes and was found to correlate well with transdiaphragmatic pressure (P_{di}) in healthy individuals and ICU patients [32, 33]. As respiratory drive comprises both an amplitude and duration component, the inspiratory EA_{di} integral may better reflect respiratory drive than EA_{di} amplitude alone.

1.5.2.1 Reference Values
Normal values for EA_{di} are not yet known, but it is proposed that an amplitude of at least 5 μV per breath in ICU patients is likely sufficient to prevent development of diaphragmatic disuse atrophy [1].

1.5.2.2 Limitations
As EA_{di} amplitude varies considerably between individuals and normal values are unknown, recordings are mainly used to evaluate changes in respiratory drive in the same patient. EA_{di} during tidal breathing is often standardized to respiratory muscle pressure (i.e., neuromechanical efficiency index) [34] or to that observed during a maximum inspiratory contraction (i.e., $EA_{di\%max}$) [7]. Although the latter was shown to correlate with the intensity of breathlessness in non-ventilated patients with chronic obstructive pulmonary disease (COPD) [35], it is generally not feasible to perform maximum inspiratory maneuvers in ICU patients. In addition, recruitment of accessory respiratory muscles is not reflected in the EA_{di} signal. Finally, suboptimal filtering of the raw electromyography signal may affect validity to quantify drive with EA_{di} [34].

1.5.3 Airway Occlusion Pressure

The airway occlusion pressure at 100 ms ($P_{0.1}$) is a readily accessible and noninvasive measurement that reflects output of the respiratory centers. The $P_{0.1}$ is the static pressure generated by all inspiratory muscles against an occluded airway at 0.1 s after the onset of inspiration. The $P_{0.1}$ was described over 40 years ago as an indirect measurement of drive that increases proportionally to an increase in inspiratory CO_2 and directly depends on neural stimulus (i.e., diaphragm electromyography or phrenic nerve activity) [36]. Advantages of $P_{0.1}$ are that short and unexpected occlusions are performed at irregular intervals such that there is no unconscious reaction (normal reaction time is >0.15 s) [36]. Second, the maneuver itself is relatively independent of respiratory mechanics, for the following reasons: (1) $P_{0.1}$ starts from end-expiratory lung volume, meaning that the drop in airway pressure is independent of the recoil pressures of the lung or chest wall; (2) since there is no flow during the maneuver, $P_{0.1}$ is not affected by flow resistance; and (3) lung volume during an occlusion does not change (with the exception of a small change due to gas decompression), which makes it unlikely that vagal volume-related reflexes or force-velocity relations of the respiratory muscles influence the measured pressure [7, 36]. In addition, the maneuver remains reliable in patients with respiratory muscle weakness [37], and in patients with various levels of intrinsic PEEP and dynamic hyperinflation [38]. Although the latter patient category shows an important delay between the onset of inspiratory activity at the alveolar level (estimated by esophageal pressure [P_{es}]) and the drop in airway pressure during an end-expiratory occlusion, Conti et al. proved good correlation and clinically acceptable agreement between $P_{0.1}$ measured at the mouth and the drop in P_{es} at the first 0.1 s of the inspiratory effort ($r = 0.92$, bias 0.3 ± 0.5 cmH$_2$O) [38]. The $P_{0.1}$ can therefore be considered as a valuable index for the estimation of respiratory drive.

1.5.3.1 Reference Values

During tidal breathing in healthy subjects, $P_{0.1}$ varies between 0.5 and 1.5 cmH$_2$O with an intrasubject breath-to-breath variability of 50%. Due to this variation, it is recommended to use an average of three or four $P_{0.1}$ measures for a reliable estimation of respiratory drive. In stable, non-intubated patients with COPD, $P_{0.1}$ values between 2.4 and 5 cmH$_2$O have been reported [7], and from 3 to 6 cmH$_2$O in patients with acute respiratory distress syndrome (ARDS) receiving mechanical ventilation [39]. An optimal upper threshold for $P_{0.1}$ was 3.5 cmH$_2$O in mechanically ventilated patients; a $P_{0.1}$ above this level is associated with increased respiratory muscle effort (i.e., esophageal pressure-time product [PTP] > 200 cmH$_2$O·s/min [40]).

1.5.3.2 Limitations

Although the $P_{0.1}$ is readily available on most modern mechanical ventilators, each ventilator type has a different algorithm to calculate $P_{0.1}$; some require manual activation of the maneuver, others continuously display an estimated value based on the ventilator trigger phase (i.e., the measured pressure decrease before the ventilator is triggered, extrapolated to 0.1 s), whether or not averaged over a few consecutive breaths. Considering that the trigger phase is often shorter than 0.05 s, $P_{0.1}$ is likely to underestimate true respiratory drive, especially in patients with high drive [39]. The accuracy of the different calculation methods remains to be investigated.

In addition, extra caution is required when interpreting the $P_{0.1}$ in patients with expiratory muscle activity; since recruitment of expiratory muscles results in an end-expiratory lung volume that may fall below functional residual capacity, the initial decrease in $P_{0.1}$ during the next inspiration may not reflect inspiratory muscle activity solely, but comprises the relaxation of the expiratory muscles and recoil of the chest wall as well [7].

1.5.4 Inspiratory Effort

Respiratory drive may also be inferred from inspiratory effort measured with esophageal and gastric pressure sensors. The derivative of P_{di} (dP_{di}/dt) reflects respiratory drive only if both the neural transmission and diaphragm muscle function are intact. As such, high dP_{di}/dt values reflect high respiratory drive. In healthy subjects, dP_{di}/dt values of 5 cmH$_2$O/s are observed during quiet breathing [4]. dP_{di}/dt is often normalized to the maximum P_{di}, but maximum inspiratory maneuvers are rarely feasible in ventilated ICU patients. A limitation of using P_{di}-derived parameters is that P_{di} is specific to the diaphragm and therefore does not include accessory inspiratory muscles, which are often recruited when respiratory drive is high. Calculating the pressure developed by all inspiratory muscles (P_{mus}) may overcome this. P_{mus} is defined as the difference between P_{es} (i.e., surrogate of pleural pressure) and the estimated pressure gradient over the chest wall. Other measurements of inspiratory effort are the work of breathing (WOB), and the PTP, which have been shown to correlate closely with $P_{0.1}$ [41, 42]. However, all the above measurements require esophageal manometry, a technique that demands expertise in positioning of the esophageal catheter and interpretation of waveforms, making it less suitable for daily clinical practice. Another major limitation is the risk of underestimating respiratory drive in patients with respiratory muscle weakness; despite a high neural drive, inspiratory effort might be low.

A noninvasive estimate of inspiratory effort can be derived with diaphragm ultrasound. Diaphragm thickening during inspiration (i.e., thickening fraction) has shown fair correlation with the diaphragmatic PTP [43]. However, diaphragm ultrasound does not account for recruitment of accessory inspiratory and expiratory muscles, and the determinants of diaphragm thickening fraction require further investigation. Nonetheless, diaphragm ultrasound is readily available at the bedside, relatively low cost and noninvasive, and may therefore be a potential promising technique for the evaluation of respiratory drive.

1.6 Strategies to Modulate Respiratory Drive

Targeting physiological levels of respiratory drive or breathing effort may limit the impact of inadequate respiratory drive on the lungs, diaphragm, dyspnea sensation, and patient outcome. However, optimal targets and upper safe limits for respiratory drive and inspiratory effort may vary among patients, depending on factors such as the severity and type of lung injury (e.g., inhomogeneity of lung injury), the patient's maximum diaphragm strength, and the presence and degree of systemic inflammation [3, 19]. In this section, we discuss the role of ventilator support, medication, and extracorporeal CO$_2$ removal (ECCO$_2$R) as potential clinical strategies for modulation of respiratory drive.

1.6.1 Modulation of Ventilator Support

Mechanical ventilation provides a unique opportunity to modulate respiratory drive by changing the level of inspiratory assist and PEEP. Ventilator settings directly influence PaO_2, $PaCO_2$, and mechanical deformation of the lungs and thorax, which are the main determinants of respiratory drive. Titrating the level of inspiratory support to obtain adequate respiratory drive and breathing effort might thus be an effective method to prevent the negative consequences of both high and low breathing effort on the lungs and diaphragm [44], although more research is required to determine optimal targets and the impact of such a strategy on patient outcomes.

Several studies have evaluated the effect of different ventilator support levels on respiratory drive during partially supported mechanical ventilation [45, 46]. Increasing inspiratory support reduces respiratory drive, most evidently seen as reduction in EA_{di} amplitude (Fig. 1.3) or the force exerted by the respiratory muscles per breath. With high inspiratory assistance the patient's respiratory effort may even decrease to virtually zero. The respiratory rate seems much less affected by modulation of ventilatory support [4].

If changing inspiratory support level has little to no influence on the patient's respiratory drive, a clinician should consider whether the elevated respiratory drive originates from irritant receptors in the thorax, agitation, pain, or intracerebral pathologies, and treat accordingly.

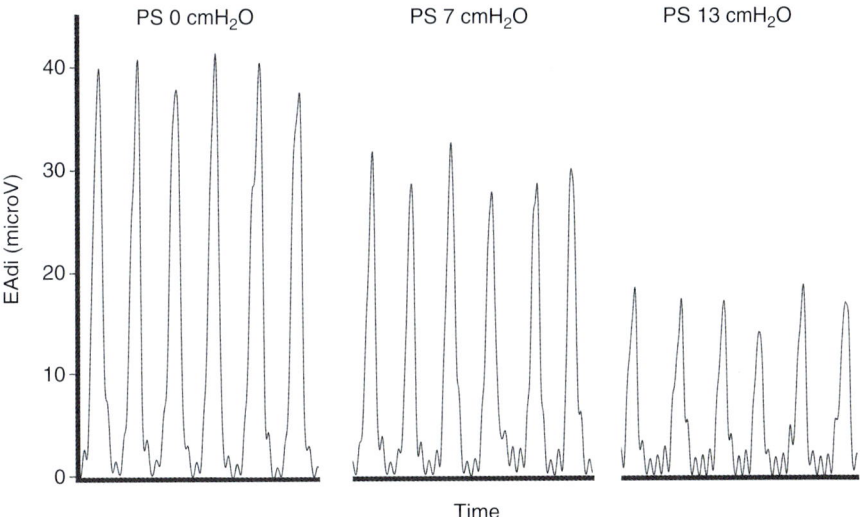

Fig. 1.3 Influence of inspiratory support levels on electrical activity of the diaphragm. Example of a representative patient showing a decrease in electrical activity of the diaphragm (EA_{di}, in micro volts) in response to increasing levels of inspiratory pressure support (PS)

1.6.2 Medication

Drugs can affect the respiratory centers directly, or act by modulating the afferent signals that contribute to respiratory drive [2]. Opioids such as remifentanil act on the μ-receptors in the pre-Bötzinger complex. Remifentanil was shown to reduce the respiratory rate, while having little effect on the amplitude of the respiratory drive [30]. The effect of propofol and benzodiazepines is likely mediated by gamma-aminobutyric acid (GABA) receptors, which are widely distributed in the central nervous system. In contrast to opioids, these drugs reduce the amplitude of the respiratory drive while having little effect on respiratory rate [47].

Neuromuscular blocking agents (NMBAs) block the signal transmission at the neuromuscular junction. These agents do not control drive *per se*, but can be used to reduce the mechanical output of the respiratory muscles. High doses of NMBAs completely prevent breathing effort, which might protect against the effects of detrimentally high breathing effort, but could also contribute to diaphragm atrophy [5]. A strategy using low dose NMBA to induce partial neuromuscular blockade allows for effective unloading of the respiratory muscles without causing muscle inactivity. Short-term partial neuromuscular blockade is feasible in ventilated patients [48]. The feasibility and safety of prolonged (24 h) partial neuromuscular blockade and the effects of this strategy on respiratory drive and diaphragm function are currently under investigation (ClinicalTrials.gov Identifier: NCT03646266).

1.6.3 Extracorporeal CO_2 Removal

$ECCO_2R$ (also known as low-flow extracorporeal membrane oxygenation) can be applied to facilitate lung-protective ventilation in patients with hypoxemic failure and respiratory acidosis due to low tidal volumes [49]. $ECCO_2R$ has been shown to reduce respiratory drive (EA_{di} and P_{mus}) in patients with ARDS and in patients with acute exacerbation of COPD [49, 50]. The feasibility, safety, and effectiveness of awake $ECCO_2R$ in patients with acute respiratory failure in order to limit excessive respiratory drive need further investigation. An $ECCO_2R$ strategy is probably more complex in this group, as the control of drive may be partly independent of $PaCO_2$ (e.g., if the Hering-Breuer reflex is overwhelmed), and other organ dysfunctions and sepsis may complicate the clinical picture [49, 50].

1.7 Conclusion

Respiratory drive is the intensity of the output by the respiratory centers and determines the effort of the respiratory muscles. A combination of chemical, mechanical, behavioral, and emotional factors contributes to respiratory drive. High and low respiratory drive in patients under mechanical ventilation may worsen or even cause lung injury and diaphragm injury, and should thus be prevented. Several techniques and interventions are available to monitor and modulate respiratory drive in critically ill patients. The impact of preventing detrimental respiratory drive requires further evaluation, but might be crucial to improve ICU outcomes.

References

1. De Vries H, Jonkman A, Shi ZH, Spoelstra-De Man A, Heunks L. Assessing breathing effort in mechanical ventilation: physiology and clinical implications. Ann Transl Med. 2018;6:387.
2. Del Negro CA, Funk GD, Feldman JL. Breathing matters. Nat Rev Neurosci. 2018;19:351–67.
3. Telias I, Brochard L, Goligher EC. Is my patient's respiratory drive (too) high? Intensive Care Med. 2018;44:1936–9.
4. Vaporidi K, Akoumianaka E, Telias I, Goligher EC, Brochard L, Georgopoulos D. Respiratory drive in critically ill patients: pathophysiology and clinical implications. Am J Respir Crit Care Med. 22 Aug 2019; https://doi.org/10.1164/rccm.201903-0596SO.
5. Dres M, Goligher EC, Heunks LMA, Brochard LJ. Critical illness-associated diaphragm weakness. Intensive Care Med. 2017;43:1441–52.
6. Feldman JL, Del Negro CA. Looking for inspiration: new perspectives on respiratory rhythm. Nat Rev Neurosci. 2006;7:232–42.
7. Tobin M, Gardner W. Monitoring the control of breathing. In: Tobin M, editor. Principles and practice of intensive care monitoring. New York: McGraw-Hill; 1998. p. 415–64.
8. Petit JM, Milic-Emili J, Delhez L. Role of the diaphragm in breathing in conscious normal man: an electromyographic study. J Appl Physiol (1985). 1969;15:1101–6.
9. Pellegrini M, Hedenstierna G, Roneus A, Segelsjö M, Larsson A, Perchiazzi G. The diaphragm acts as a brake during expiration to prevent lung collapse. Am J Respir Crit Care Med. 2017;195:1608–16.
10. Doorduin J, Roesthuis LH, Jansen D, Van Der Hoeven JG, Van Hees HWH, Heunks LMA. Respiratory muscle effort during expiration in successful and failed weaning from mechanical ventilation. Anesthesiology. 2018;129:490–501.
11. Shi ZH, Jonkman A, De Vries H, et al. Expiratory muscle dysfunction in critically ill patients: towards improved understanding. Intensive Care Med. 2019;45:1061–71.
12. Coates EL, Li A, Nattie EE. Widespread sites of brain stem ventilatory chemoreceptors. J Appl Physiol (1985). 1993;75:5–14.
13. Nielsen M, Smith H. Studies on the regulation of respiration in acute hypoxia: preliminary report. Acta Physiol Scand. 1951;22:44–6.
14. Prabhakar NR, Peng YJ. Peripheral chemoreceptors in health and disease. J Appl Physiol (1985). 2004;96:359–66.
15. Biscoe TJ, Purves MJ, Sampson SR. Frequency of nerve impulses in single carotid body chemoreceptor afferent fibres recorded in vivo with intact circulation. J Physiol. 1970;208:121–31.
16. Coleridge JCG, Coleridge HM. Afferent vagal c fibre innervation of the lungs and airways and its functional significance. Rev Physiol Biochem Pharmacol. 1984;99:2–110.
17. Tipton MJ, Harper A, Paton JFR, Costello JT. The human ventilatory response to stress: rate or depth? J Physiol. 2017;595:5729–52.
18. Leitch AG, Mclennan JE, Balkenhol S, Mclaurin RL, Loudon RG. Ventilatory response to transient hyperoxia in head injury hyperventilation. J Appl Physiol (1985). 1980;49:52–8.
19. Yoshida T, Nakahashi S, Nakamura MAM, et al. Volume-controlled ventilation does not prevent injurious inflation during spontaneous effort. Am J Respir Crit Care Med. 2017;196:590–601.
20. Yoshida T, Torsani V, Gomes S, et al. Spontaneous effort causes occult pendelluft during mechanical ventilation. Am J Respir Crit Care Med. 2013;188:1420–7.
21. Brochard L, Slutsky A, Pesenti A. Mechanical ventilation to minimize progression of lung injury in acute respiratory failure. Am J Respir Crit Care Med. 2017;195:438–42.
22. Hooijman PE, Beishuizen A, Witt CC, et al. Diaphragm muscle fiber weakness and ubiquitin-proteasome activation in critically ill patients. Am J Respir Crit Care Med. 2015;191:1126–38.

23. Goligher EC, Fan E, Herridge MS, et al. Evolution of diaphragm thickness during mechanical ventilation. Impact of inspiratory effort. Am J Respir Crit Care Med. 2015;192:1080–8.
24. Gea J, Zhu E, Gáldiz JB, et al. Functional consequences of eccentric contractions of the diaphragm. Arch Bronconeumol. 2008;45:68–74.
25. Schmidt M, Banzett RB, Raux M, et al. Unrecognized suffering in the ICU: addressing dyspnea in mechanically ventilated patients. Intensive Care Med. 2014;40:1–10.
26. Schmidt M, Kindler F, Gottfried SB, et al. Dyspnea and surface inspiratory electromyograms in mechanically ventilated patients. Intensive Care Med. 2013;39:1368–76.
27. Demoule A, Jung B, Prodanovic H, et al. Diaphragm dysfunction on admission to the intensive care unit. Prevalence, risk factors, and prognostic impact—a prospective study. Am J Respir Crit Care Med. 2013;188:213–9.
28. Goligher EC, Dres M, Fan E, et al. Mechanical ventilation-induced diaphragm atrophy strongly impacts clinical outcomes. Am J Respir Crit Care Med. 2018;197:204–13.
29. Epstein SK. How often does patient-ventilator asynchrony occur and what are the consequences? Respir Care. 2011;56:25–38.
30. Costa R, Navalesi P, Cammarota G, et al. Remifentanil effects on respiratory drive and timing during pressure support ventilation and neurally adjusted ventilatory assist. Respir Physiol Neurobiol. 2017;244:10–6.
31. Sinderby C, Navalesi P, Beck J, et al. Neural control of mechanical ventilation in respiratory failure. Nat Med. 1999;5:1433–6.
32. Sinderby C, Beck J, Spahija J, Weinberg J, Grassino AE. Voluntary activation of the human diaphragm in health and disease. J Appl Physiol. 1998;86:2146–58.
33. Beck J, Sinderby C, Lindstrom LH, Grassino AE. Influence of bipolar esophageal electrode positioning on measurements of human crural diaphragm electromyogram. J Appl Physiol. 1996;81:1434–49.
34. Jansen D, Jonkman AH, Roesthuis L, et al. Estimation of the diaphragm neuromuscular efficiency index in mechanically ventilated critically ill patients. Crit Care. 2018;22:238.
35. Jolley CJ, Luo YM, Steier J, Rafferty GF, Polkey MI, Moxham J. Neural respiratory drive and breathlessness in COPD. Eur Respir J. 2015;45:301–4.
36. Whitelaw WA, Derenne J-P, Milic-Emili J. Occlusion pressure as a measure of respiratory center output in conscious man. Respir Physiol. 1975;23:181–99.
37. Holle R, Schoene R, Pavlin E. Effect of respiratory muscle weakness on p0.1 induced by partial curarization. J Appl Physiol. 1984;57:1150–7.
38. Conti G, Cinnella G, Barboni E, Lemaire F, Harf A, Brochard L. Estimation of occlusion pressure during assisted ventilation in patients with intrinsic PEEP. Am J Respir Crit Care Med. 1996;154:907–12.
39. Telias I, Damiani F, Brochard L. The airway occlusion pressure (p0.1) to monitor respiratory drive during mechanical ventilation: increasing awareness of a not-so-new problem. Intensive Care Med. 2018;44:1532–5.
40. Rittayamai N, Beloncle F, Goligher EC, et al. Effect of inspiratory synchronization during pressure-controlled ventilation on lung distension and inspiratory effort. Ann Intensive Care. 2017;7:100.
41. Alberti A, Gallo F, Fongaro A, Valenti S, Rossi A. P0.1 is a useful parameter in setting the level of pressure support ventilation. Intensive Care Med. 1995;21:547–53.
42. Mancebo J, Albaladejo P, Touchard D, et al. Airway occlusion pressure to titrate positive end-expiratory pressure in patients with dynamic hyperinflation. Anesthesiology. 2000;93:81–90.
43. Vivier E, Mekontso Dessap A, Dimassi S, et al. Diaphragm ultrasonography to estimate the work of breathing during non-invasive ventilation. Intensive Care Med. 2012;38:796–803.
44. Heunks L, Ottenheijm C. Diaphragm-protective mechanical ventilation to improve outcomes in ICU patients? Am J Respir Crit Care Med. 2018;197:150–2.
45. Carteaux G, Cordoba-Izquierdo A, Lyazidi A, Heunks L, Thille AW, Brochard L. Comparison between neurally adjusted ventilatory assist and pressure support ventilation levels in terms of respiratory effort. Crit Care Med. 2016;44:503–11.

46. Doorduin J, Sinderby C, Beck J, Van Der Hoeven JG, Heunks L. Assisted ventilation in patients with acute respiratory distress syndrome. Anesthesiology. 2015;123:181–90.
47. Vaschetto R, Cammarota G, Colombo D, et al. Effects of propofol on patient-ventilator synchrony and interaction during pressure support ventilation and neurally adjusted ventilatory assist. Crit Care Med. 2014;42:74–82.
48. Doorduin J, Nollet JL, Roesthuis LH, et al. Partial neuromuscular blockade during partial ventilatory support in sedated patients with high tidal volumes. Am J Respir Crit Care Med. 2017;195:1033–42.
49. Karagiannidis C, Hesselmann F, Fan E. Physiological and technical considerations of extracorporeal CO_2 removal. Crit Care. 2019;23:75.
50. Crotti S, Bottino N, Spinelli E. Spontaneous breathing during veno-venous extracorporeal membrane oxygenation. J Thorac Dis. 2018;10(Suppl 5):S661–S9.

Monitoring Patient Respiratory Effort During Mechanical Ventilation: Lung and Diaphragm-Protective Ventilation

M. Bertoni, S. Spadaro, and E. C. Goligher

2.1 Introduction

At some point during mechanical ventilation, spontaneous breathing must commence. Spontaneous breathing presents a clinically important risk of injury to the lung and diaphragm. While clinicians are primarily focused on monitoring lung function to prevent ventilator-induced lung injury (VILI) during passive mechanical ventilation, less attention may be paid to the risk of VILI during assisted mechanical ventilation. Vigorous spontaneous inspiratory effort can cause both lung injury (patient self-inflicted lung injury [P-SILI]) [1, 2] and diaphragm injury (myotrauma) [3, 4]. These injuries lead to prolonged ventilation, difficult weaning, and increased morbidity and mortality [5–7]. Safe spontaneous breathing presents a complex challenge because one must aim to minimize the volume and transpulmonary pressure (P_L) to avoid P-SILI while also maintaining an appropriate level of patient respiratory effort to avoid diaphragm atrophy. To this end, respiratory monitoring is key. Several practical methods are available for monitoring patient respiratory effort during assisted mechanical ventilation; this review describes their use in clinical practice.

M. Bertoni
Department of Anesthesia, Critical Care and Emergency, Spedali Civili University Hospital, Brescia, Italy

S. Spadaro
Department of Morphology, Surgery and Experimental Medicine, Intensive Care Unit, University of Ferrara, Sant'Anna Hospital, Ferrara, Italy

E. C. Goligher (✉)
Interdepartmental Division of Critical Care Medicine, University of Toronto, Toronto, Canada

Division of Respirology, Department of Medicine, University Health Network, Toronto, Canada

Toronto General Hospital Research Institute, Toronto, Canada
e-mail: ewan.goligher@utoronto.ca

2.2 Mechanics of Spontaneous Breathing

During assisted mechanical ventilation, each breath results from a negative deflection in pleural pressure (P_{pl}) (arising from patient respiratory effort) combined with a positive airway pressure (P_{aw}) delivered by the ventilator. The P_{aw} increases to the support level set on the ventilator, whereas P_{pl} deflects proportionally to patient effort. P_L corresponds to the difference between P_{aw} and P_{pl} ($P_L = P_{aw} - P_{pl}$); this pressure reflects the stress applied to the lung by the combined effects of ventilator and patient effort. Although in passive mechanical ventilation P_{aw} is a reasonable surrogate for P_L [8], during assisted mechanical ventilation, vigorous inspiratory efforts can increase the P_L above a "safe limit." Such excessive pressures are "unseen" when relying on the ventilator P_{aw} waveform; at the same airway pressure value, transpulmonary pressure could be much higher in assisted than in controlled mechanical ventilation (Fig. 2.1).

2.3 Lung Injury During Spontaneous Breathing: Patient Self-Inflicted Lung Injury

During spontaneous breathing, vigorous patient respiratory efforts can cause lung injury (P-SILI) through different mechanisms (Fig. 2.2).

- *Excessive global lung stress.* As already discussed, patient respiratory efforts can increase tidal volume and P_L above safe limits when respiratory drive is elevated.
- *Excessive regional lung stress.* In the injured lung, collapsed and consolidated lung introduces parenchymal mechanical heterogeneities [9], increasing the risk of volutrauma through regional stress amplification. Mechanical stress and strain is not evenly redistributed during inflation. Consequently, inspiratory efforts generate large P_L swings in dorsal consolidated regions, resulting in the movement of air from nondependent to dependent regions (pendelluft). While this recruits collapsed lung and improves ventilation-perfusion mismatch, this phenomenon increases the overstretch of dependent lung area. In this case, the rise in P_L detected by esophageal manometry may not be a reliable measure of the local stress [10].
- *Transvascular pressure and pulmonary edema.* During spontaneous breathing, the negative P_{pl} generated by respiratory effort raises transvascular pressure (the pressure gradient driving fluid migration across pulmonary vessels), increasing total lung water and pulmonary edema [9, 10] and further impairing respiratory function.
- *Asynchronies.* Ventilator asynchronies, including double triggering (double mechanical breaths from a single inspiratory effort) and reverse triggering (diaphragm contractions induced by passive thoracic insufflation in passively ventilated patients) [11] can increase tidal volume and P_L and generate pendelluft, leading to lung injury.

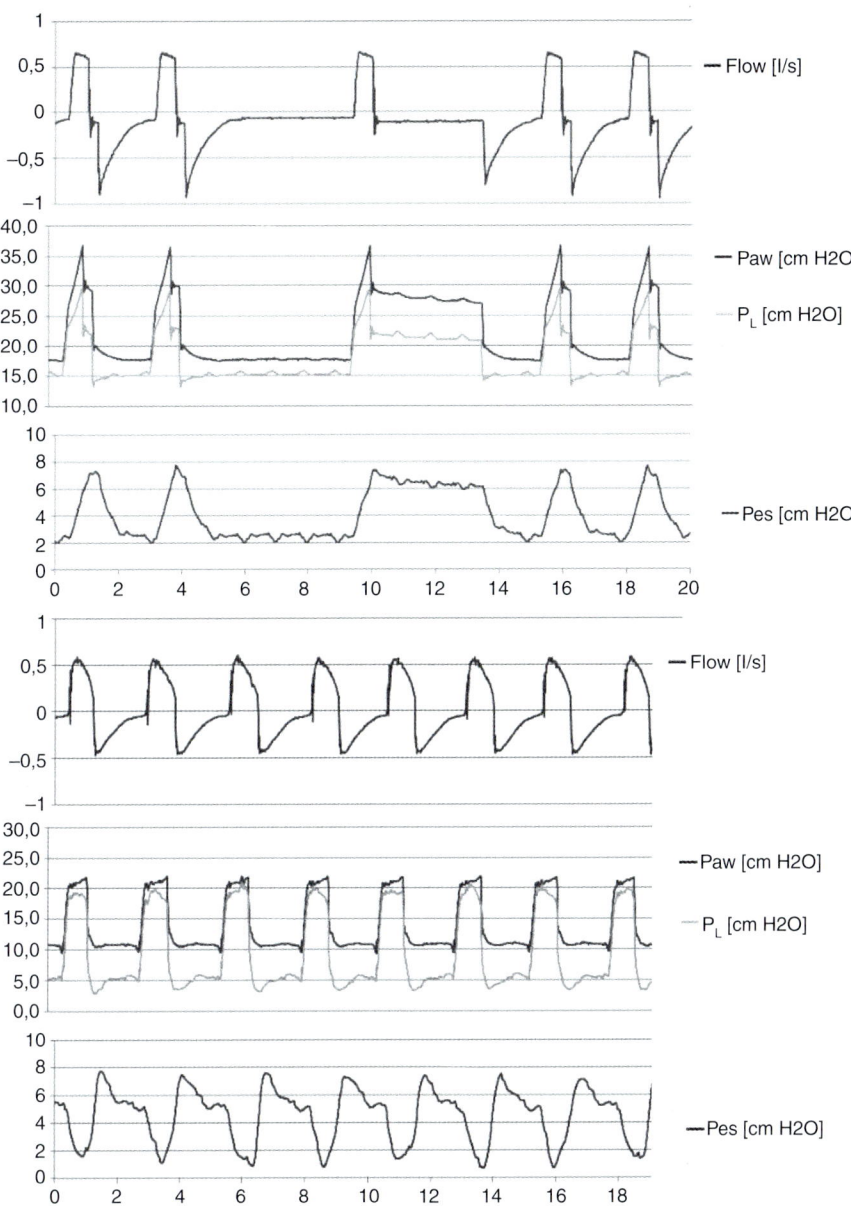

Fig. 2.1 Transpulmonary pressure (P_L) is generated differently in passive mechanical ventilation (upper panel) and assisted mechanical ventilation (lower panel). During passive ventilation, the pleural pressure swing is positive and transpulmonary pressure is therefore lower than airway pressure (P_{aw}). During assisted ventilation a vigorous inspiratory effort generates a negative swing in pleural pressure resulting in an additive increase in transpulmonary pressure; transpulmonary pressure may therefore be much higher than airway pressure. P_{es} esophageal pressure

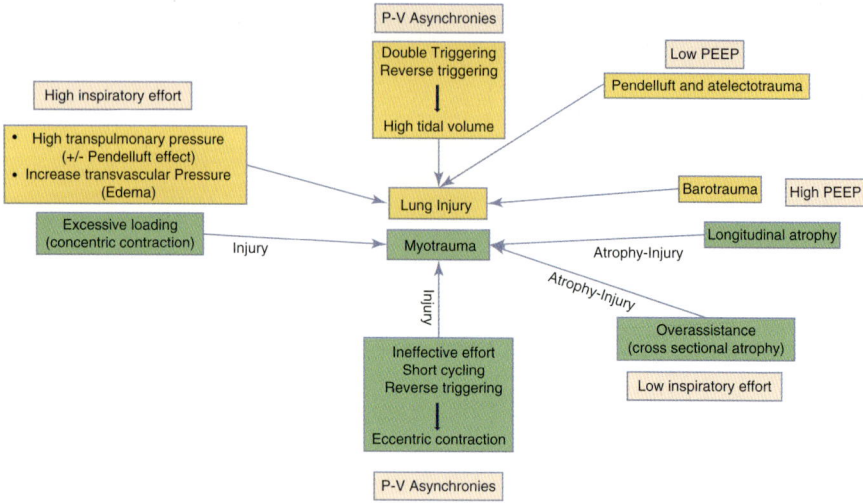

Fig. 2.2 Mechanisms of lung-diaphragm injury in spontaneous breathing patients under assisted mechanical ventilation. Note that some of these mechanisms also apply under controlled mechanical ventilation (e.g., reverse triggering). *PEEP* positive end-expiratory pressure

Close monitoring of patient respiratory effort during assisted mechanical ventilation to detect and mitigate these potential injury mechanisms is therefore imperative.

2.4 Diaphragm Injury During Spontaneous Breathing: Myotrauma

The inappropriate use of mechanical ventilation can injure not only the lung (barotrauma and volutrauma) but also respiratory muscles (myotrauma). Mechanical ventilation causes myotrauma by various mechanisms, leading to a final common pathway of VIDD [5].

Mechanisms of myotrauma are summarized in Fig. 2.2:

- *Excessive unloading.* Over-assistance from mechanical ventilation and suppression of respiratory drive from sedation leads to acute disuse atrophy and diaphragm weakness [12]. Diaphragmatic unloading caused by over-assisted ventilation (both in control or assisted mode) is frequent during mechanical ventilation, in particular during the first 48 h. Of note, the low level of respiratory effort required to trigger the ventilator is not sufficient to avoid disuse atrophy [3], such that diaphragm atrophy can occur under pressure support ventilation.
- *Excessive concentric loading.* The diaphragm is sensitive to excessive respiratory load. Higher inspiratory patient effort, dyssynchronies, and under-assistance

due to an insufficient level of support are frequent in assisted mechanical ventilation. Vigorous concentric contractions provoke high muscular tension resulting in muscle inflammation, proteolysis, myofibrillar damage, and sarcolemma disarray [13, 14]. In critically ill patients, systemic inflammation renders muscle myofibrils more vulnerable to mechanical injury ([10, 15]).

- *Eccentric loading.* Eccentric contractions occur when a muscle generates contractile tension while it is lengthening (rather than shortening); such contractions are much more injurious than concentric (shortening) contractions [16]. When a low positive end-expiratory pressure (PEEP) and excessive reduction in end-expiratory lung volume are present, the diaphragm contracts even as it lengthens during the expiratory ("post-inspiratory") phase to avoid atelectasis ("expiratory braking" phenomenon) [17]. Specific forms of dyssynchrony (reverse triggering, short cycling, ineffective effort) can generate eccentric contractions because the diaphragm is activated during the expiratory phase.
- *Excessive PEEP.* Preliminary experimental evidence suggests that maintaining the diaphragm at a shorter length with the use of excessive PEEP may cause sarcomeres to "drop out" of the muscle and shorten its length (longitudinal atrophy) [18]. This could theoretically disadvantage the length-tension characteristics of the muscle once PEEP is reduced, impairing diaphragm performance.

The first three of these injury mechanisms can be detected by monitoring respiratory effort, emphasizing the potential for such monitoring to help clinicians ensure safe spontaneous breathing during mechanical ventilation. We now proceed to review a range of monitoring techniques to achieve this goal.

2.5 Monitoring Spontaneous Breathing Using Esophageal Pressure

The use of esophageal pressure (P_{es}) monitoring is well-described in patients with acute respiratory distress syndrome (ARDS) under passive mechanical ventilation [19]. This technique is also the gold standard to assess respiratory effort and work of breathing but its use remains uncommon, perhaps because the utility of the information derived from P_{es} has been under-appreciated. When used to monitor the safety of spontaneous breathing, P_{es} monitoring permits several different relevant quantities to be estimated.

2.5.1 Transpulmonary Pressure

P_{es} can be used as a surrogate measure of P_{pl}, bearing in mind regional variations [20]. It can therefore be used to measure P_L ($P_{aw} - P_{pl}$), by substituting P_{pl} with P_{es}. As shown in Fig. 2.1, P_L can easily reach an injuriously high value during assisted mechanical ventilation (where both patient and ventilator distend the lung). An acceptable upper limit for P_L has not yet been defined; a "precautionary" peak inspiratory value of 20 cmH$_2$O in a lung-injured patient is a reasonable target to limit the risk of injury [2, 21].

Of note, in the presence of regional ventilation heterogeneity and pendelluft, the measured value of P_L will underestimate lung stress in the dependent lung areas. While the quasi-static plateau P_L obtained during an end-inspiratory occlusion reflects lung stress during passive ventilation, the dynamic swing in P_L (ΔP_L) may perhaps be more reflective of injury risk during spontaneous breathing because of the pendelluft phenomenon [22]. ΔP_L likely reflects the upper limit of mechanical stress experienced in dorsal regions of the lung under dynamic conditions [23]. Moreover, various lines of evidence suggest that the dynamic (tidal increase) in lung stress is a more important driver of lung injury than the global (peak) lung stress [24–26].

2.5.2 Respiratory Muscle Pressure

P_{es} permits measurement of inspiratory effort. The inspiratory muscle pressure (P_{mus}) corresponds to the global force generated by the inspiratory muscles. Although the diaphragm is the most important respiratory muscle, accessory inspiratory muscles (rib cage, sternomastoid, and scalene muscles) contribute significantly during vigorous effort, especially when diaphragm function is impaired. As shown in Fig. 2.3, P_{mus} is computed from the difference between P_{es} and the additional pressure required to overcome the chest wall elastic recoil (P_{cw}) ($P_{mus} = P_{cw} - P_{es}$).

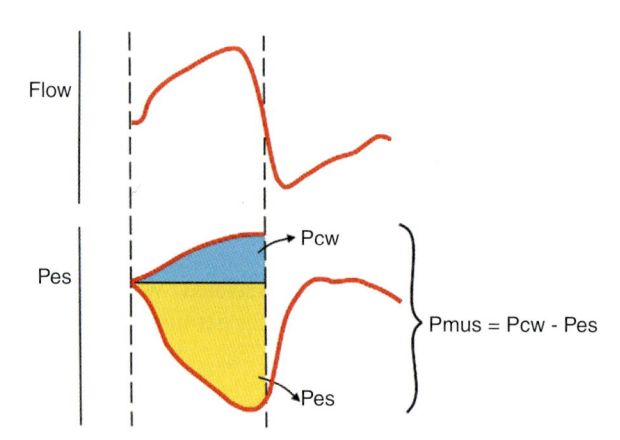

Fig. 2.3 Computing inspiratory muscle pressure (P_{mus}) from the esophageal pressure (P_{es}) swing. P_{mus} derives from the difference between P_{es} and the added muscle pressure generated to overcome the chest wall elastic recoil (P_{cw}). P_{cw} represents the elastic recoil of relaxed chest wall; it can be computed as the product of tidal volume and chest wall elastance (E_{cw}). The P_{mus} area over time constitutes the pressure-time product (PTP) (yellow and blue area together)

Optimal levels of P_{mus} during assisted mechanical ventilation are uncertain; recent data suggest that P_{mus} values similar to those of healthy subjects breathing at rest may be safe and may prevent diaphragm atrophy (5–10 cmH$_2$O) [4, 27]. In routine clinical practice, one can generally disregard the correction for P_{cw} because chest wall elastance is usually relatively low (even when pleural pressures are elevated). Hence, a target ΔP_{es} of around 3–8 cmH$_2$O can be considered reasonably comparable to a normal P_{mus} of 5–10 cmH$_2$O.

The gold standard measurement of respiratory effort is the integral of P_{mus} over the duration of inspiration (pressure-time product [PTP]) (Fig. 2.3). PTP is closely correlated to inspiratory muscle energy expenditure. PTP values between 50 and 100 cmH$_2$O/s/min probably reflect appropriate oxygen consumption and acceptable respiratory effort [28].

In routine clinical practice, the magnitude and frequency of the swing in ΔP_{es} are probably sufficient to monitor respiratory effort.

2.5.3 Transdiaphragmatic Pressure

A double balloon catheter can be used to monitor inspiratory swings in P_{es} and gastric pressure (P_{ga}) to specifically quantify the pressure generated by the diaphragm (transdiaphragmatic pressure [P_{di}]). During an inspiratory effort (depending on the pattern of thoracoabdominal motion), the diaphragm's contractile effort moves the abdominal organs downwards, increasing abdominal pressure (positive swing in P_{ga}) and expanding thoracic cavity (negative swing in P_{es}). Even when thoracoabdominal motion is such that the diaphragm moves upward during inspiration (i.e., P_{ga} decreases), the contractile effort of the diaphragm is reflected by the fact that P_{ga} declines less than P_{es} (and thus P_{di} increases). This technique is used mainly in research rather than clinical practice.

2.6 Monitoring Spontaneous Breathing by Occlusion Maneuvers

Expiratory and inspiratory occlusions represent easy, noninvasive, and reasonably reliable maneuvers to evaluate the safety of spontaneous breathing in assisted mechanical ventilation.

2.6.1 Inspiratory Occlusion Maneuver

Brief end-inspiratory occlusion maneuvers are widely used to measure plateau pressure (P_{plat}) in passive mechanical ventilation. Driving pressure (ΔP), calculated as the difference between PEEP and P_{pl}, reflects dynamic lung stress and lung injury risk and closely correlates to mortality in patients with ARDS [25]. Bellani et al.

[29] suggested that a brief inspiratory occlusion maneuver can enable reliable measurements of P_{plat} even in assisted mechanical ventilation. During an inspiratory occlusion in assisted mechanical ventilation, patients relax the contracting inspiratory muscles at end-inspiration, resulting in an increase in ΔP_{aw}, easily detectable on the ventilator waveform. When the patient is over-assisted and respiratory effort is low, P_{aw} drops during the occlusion (Fig. 2.4). A high P_{plat} and ΔP measured in this way raises concern for hyperdistention and lung injury. Bellani and colleagues [29] recently reported that ΔP and compliance measured by end-inspiratory occlusion maneuvers during assisted mechanical ventilation predict mortality, supporting the validity and relevance of these measures.

The measurement technique has some limitations. First, because the pressure is obtained under quasi-static conditions this measurement may underestimate the risk of regional lung injury due to the pendelluft mechanism of P-SILI [23]. Second, clinicians need to carefully evaluate the stability and pattern of the P_{aw} tracing during the occlusion to determine whether the measurement is confounded by the action of the abdominal muscles which may rapidly increase P_{aw} at the onset of neural expiration during the occlusion.

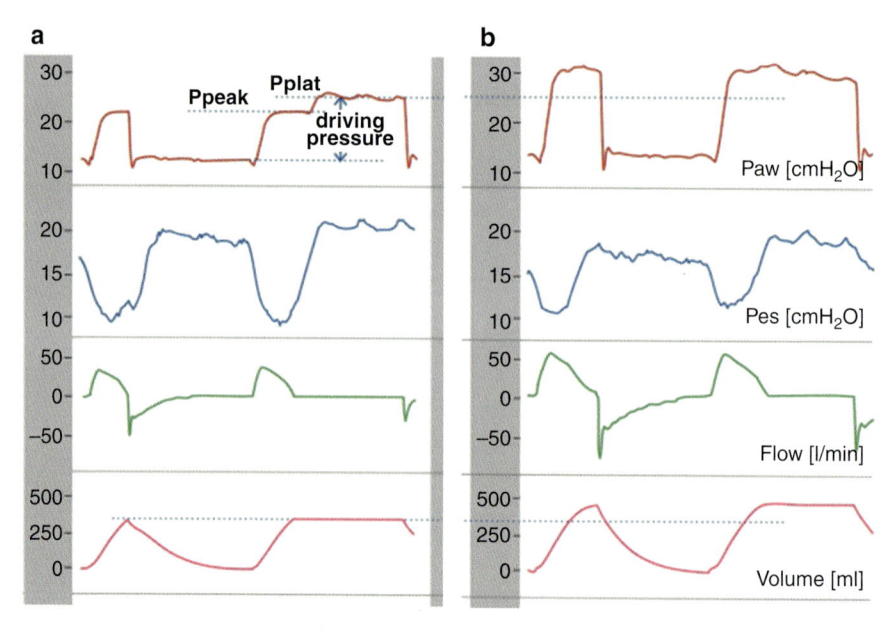

Fig. 2.4 Measuring plateau pressure (P_{plat}) during assisted mechanical ventilation (AMV). A brief inspiratory hold permits a reliable measure of P_{plat} in AMV, provided the patient relaxes with no immediate expiratory efforts. The difference between P_{plat} and positive end-expiratory pressure (PEEP) results in the driving pressure ΔP_{aw}. In panel (**a**), the patient's inspiratory effort is vigorous (greater esophageal swing): during inspiratory hold, the airflow stops and P_{plat} rises above P_{peak}; the previous activated respiratory muscles relaxes and expires, causing P_{aw} to increase. In panel (**b**), the patient's inspiratory effort is low: the difference between P_{peak} and P_{plat} is minimal, indicating minimal respiratory muscle effort during the current breath. This technique enables respiratory muscle activity to be assessed by measuring P_{plat}. (Modified from [29] with permission)

2.6.2 Expiratory Occlusion Maneuver

Expiratory occlusions are ordinarily employed to measure intrinsic PEEP in passively ventilated patients or to measure maximal inspiratory pressure in spontaneously breathing patients during maximal volitional inspiratory efforts. However, the airway pressure swing during a brief, randomly applied end-expiratory occlusion maneuver (duration equal to one respiratory cycle) may actually be used to assess inspiratory effort. Under occluded conditions, the swing in airway pressure is exactly correlated to the swing in pleural pressure. Consequently, the airway pressure swing during the occlusion (ΔP_{occ}) can be used to assess the presence and magnitude of pleural pressure swings due to patient respiratory effort (taking into account differences in pleural pressure swing between occluded and dynamic conditions). On this basis, ΔP_{occ} can be used to predict ΔP_{es}, P_{mus}, and ΔP_L during the respiratory cycle so long as the patient's respiratory drive during the tidal breath is unchanged by a single, brief, and unexpected end-expiratory occlusion [30, 31]. A transient end-expiratory occlusion maneuver is a practical and noninvasive method to routinely detect insufficient or excessive respiratory effort and P_L during assisted mechanical ventilation [32, 33].

2.6.3 Airway Occlusion Pressure

The $P_{0.1}$ (airway pressure generated in the first 100 ms of inspiration against an expiratory occlusion) provides a measure of the patient's respiratory drive (Fig. 2.5) [34]. Whitelaw et al. [35] demonstrated that an occlusion does not modify cortical respiratory output until it is prolonged beyond 200 ms. Additionally, during the first 100 ms, respiratory pressure generation is independent of pulmonary mechanics or diaphragm function [35, 36]. Although the reliability of $P_{0.1}$ has been confirmed only in small studies, a value between 1.5 and 3.5 cmH$_2$O [37, 38] seems to be an easy method to guide clinicians to adjust ventilation during assisted mechanical ventilation [34, 39–41]. $P_{0.1}$ values less than 1.5 cmH$_2$O might suggest that respiratory effort is inadequate [42], and values greater than 3.5 cmH$_2$O suggest high respiratory drive [37].

$P_{0.1}$ has several advantages: it is easy and practical to obtain, and most modern ventilators have a function for measuring it. A method for setting the pressure support level based on the $P_{0.1}$ value has been described [43]. $P_{0.1}$ may have substantial intra-patient variability and several repeated measurements are required to estimate a stable mean value. Moreover, in hyperinflated patients, the intrinsic PEEP causes a delay in the fall in P_{aw}, which might give rise to underestimation of $P_{0.1}$. Conti et al. demonstrated that in this condition, commencing the 100 ms for the $P_{0.1}$ measure when expiratory flow is equal to zero overcomes this problem [44].

Fig. 2.5 Airway occlusion pressure ($P_{0.1}$) is the airway pressure (P_{aw}) generated in the first 100 ms of inspiration against an expiratory occlusion. Importantly, the 100 ms time for $P_{0.1}$ calculation should start at the point where the expiratory flow trace reaches zero (dashed line) to correct for potential intrinsic positive end-expiratory pressure (PEEP). *PS* pressure support level. (From [34] with permission)

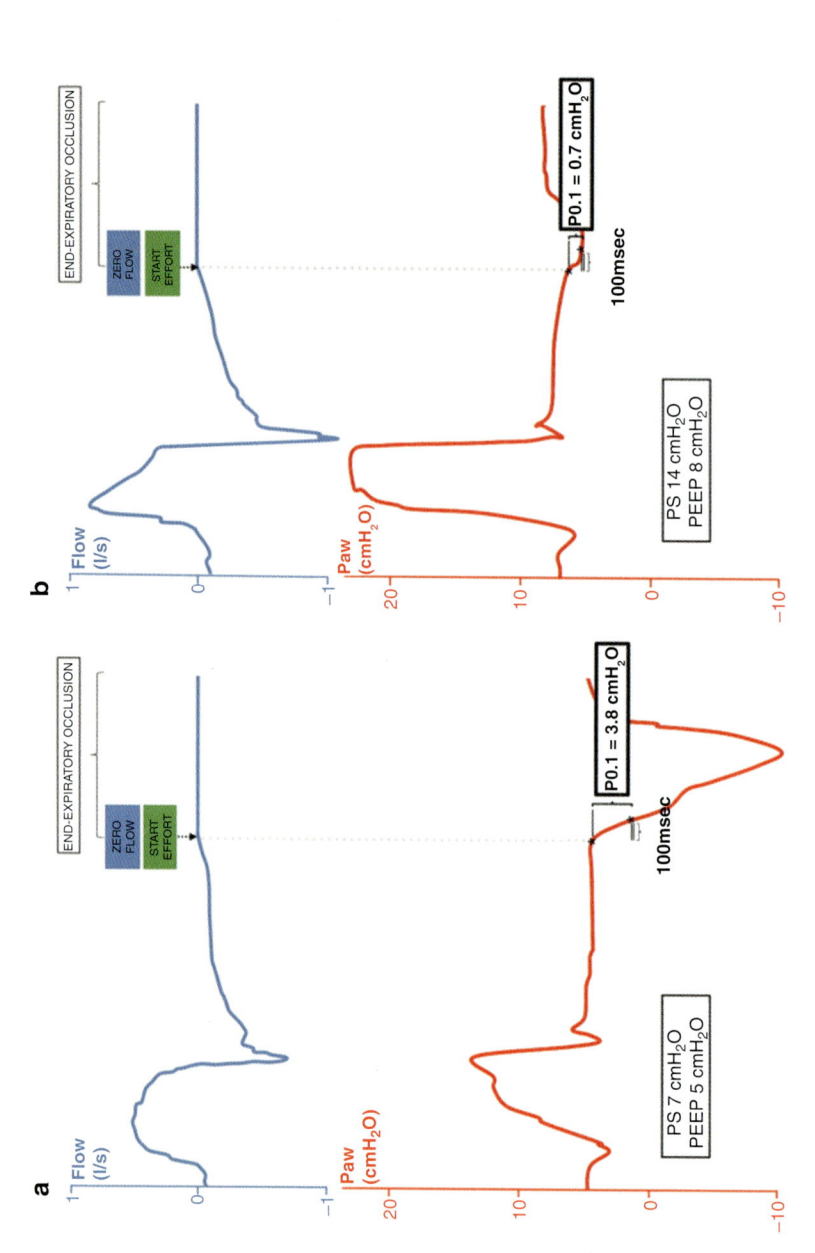

2.7 Monitoring Spontaneous Breathing by Diaphragm Electrical Activity

The use of a dedicated catheter fitted with electromyography electrodes permits continuous monitoring of the electrical activity of the diaphragm (EA_{di}) [45]. EA_{di} has been demonstrated to be comparable to the transdiaphragmatic pressure, and is more practical than surface electromyography (EMG) [46].

When ventilation is driven by EA_{di} (during neurally adjusted ventilatory assist [NAVA]), patient-ventilator interaction improves [47, 48]; EA_{di} also helps clinicians to recognize different asynchronies [47, 49]. As demonstrated by Barwing et al. [50], the EA_{di} trend can be used to detect weaning failure at an early stage [51, 52]: it progressively increases in patients who ultimately fail their spontaneous breathing trial whereas diaphragm activity remains stable in patients who pass the trial. EA_{di} alterations appeared before signs of fatigue [50].

As an electrical signal, EA_{di} is an expression of respiratory motor output (the central nervous system activation of the diaphragm) and not of diaphragmatic force generation (effort). During resting breathing in healthy subjects, EA_{di} varies anywhere between 5 and 30 µV [53]. Because of this wide variation, it is difficult to specify a target EA_{di} to achieve during mechanical ventilation. Alternatively, EA_{di} can be used to estimate P_{mus} under different conditions of ventilator assistance [54]. By considering coupling between electrical activity and pressure generation constant during the time (neuro-mechanical coupling = P_{mus}/EA_{di} obtained during expiratory occlusion), EA_{di} could permit a breath-by-breath assessment of P_{mus} during the normal breathing cycle.

2.8 Monitoring Spontaneous Breathing by Diaphragm Ultrasound

The diaphragm ultrasound technique is noninvasive, easy to perform, and reproducible. Variation in diaphragm thickness during the respiratory cycle (thickening fraction, TF_{di}) is correlated to respiratory pressure generation and EA_{di} [55] and can be used to detect diaphragm weakness [55]. TF_{di} values less than 30% during a maximal inspiratory effort detect diaphragm weakness with a high sensitivity [55]. Daily measurement of end-expiratory diaphragm thickness can detect structural changes in the respiratory muscles. In mechanically ventilated patients, a progressive increase in diaphragm thickness over time was correlated to excessive effort and may represent under-assistance myotrauma [3]. TF_{di} of 15–30% during tidal ventilation was associated with stable diaphragm thickness and the shortest duration of ventilation [4]. Ultrasound is best used for intermittent patient assessments, as it is not well suited for continuous monitoring.

Table 2.1 Potential target values for safe spontaneous breathing

Technique	Parameter	Possible target range of values for safe spontaneous breathing
Esophageal pressure	Peak end-inspiratory transpulmonary pressure (P_L)	≤20 cmH$_2$O
	Swing in transpulmonary pressure (ΔP_L)	≤15 cmH$_2$O
	Peak inspiratory muscle pressure (P_{mus})	5–10 cmH$_2$O
	Esophageal pressure swing (ΔP_{es})	3–8 cmH$_2$O
	Transdiaphragmatic pressure swing (ΔP_{di})	5–10 cmH$_2$O
	Pressure time product (PTP)	50–100 cmH$_2$O/s/min
Occlusion maneuvers	Inspiratory occlusion for plateau airway pressure (P_{plat})	≤30 cmH$_2$O
	Inspiratory occlusion for driving pressure ($\Delta P_{aw} = P_{plat} - $ PEEP)	≤15 cmH$_2$O
	Expiratory occlusion for estimated P_{mus}	5–10 cmH$_2$O
	Airway occlusion pressure ($P_{0.1}$)	1.5–3.5 cmH$_2$O
Electromyography	Diaphragm electrical activity (EA$_{di}$)	Uncertain

PEEP positive end-expiratory pressure

2.9 Conclusion: Targets for Lung and Diaphragm-Protective Ventilation

Table 2.1 summarizes the different methods available to monitor inspiratory effort and respiratory drive in assisted mechanical ventilation, along with possible targets for safe spontaneous breathing as discussed throughout this chapter. The interpretation and application of measurements must always be guided by the clinical context. Different forms and phases of acute respiratory failure require somewhat different priorities: in early ARDS, close attention must be taken to avoid high inspiratory effort to limit VILI and P-SILI. Adjustments to ventilation and sedation to obtain a low level of inspiratory effort should be implemented as early as possible to avoid myotrauma.

It remains uncertain whether it is possible to achieve an acceptable level of respiratory effort during the acute phase of illness and this remains a key area for clinical investigation. For the present, clinicians should strive to be aware of patient respiratory effort and appreciate the potential benefits and harms of manipulating respiratory effort during acute respiratory failure.

References

1. Yoshida T, Uchiyama A, Matsuura N, et al. Spontaneous breathing during lung-protective ventilation in an experimental acute lung injury model: high transpulmonary pressure associated with strong spontaneous breathing effort may worsen lung injury. Crit Care Med. 2012;40:1578–85.
2. Yoshida T, Torsani V, Gomes S, et al. Spontaneous effort causes occult pendelluft during mechanical ventilation. Am J Respir Crit Care Med. 2013;188:1420–7.
3. Goligher EC, Fan E, Herridge MS, et al. Evolution of diaphragm thickness during mechanical ventilation: impact of inspiratory effort. Am J Respir Crit Care Med. 2015;192:1080–8.

4. Goligher EC, Dres M, Fan E, et al. Mechanical ventilation-induced diaphragm atrophy strongly impacts clinical outcomes. Am J Respir Crit Care Med. 2018;197:204–13.
5. Goligher EC, Brochard LJ, Reid WD, et al. Diaphragmatic myotrauma: a mediator of prolonged ventilation and poor patient outcomes in acute respiratory failure. Lancet Respir Med. 2019;7:90–8.
6. Dres M, Dubé BP, Mayaux J, et al. Coexistence and impact of limb muscle and diaphragm weakness at time of liberation from mechanical ventilation in medical intensive care unit patients. Am J Respir Crit Care Med. 2017;195:57–66.
7. Brochard L, Slutsky A, Pesenti A. Mechanical ventilation to minimize progression of lung injury in acute respiratory failure. Am J Respir Crit Care Med. 2017;195:438–42.
8. Chiu L-C, Hu HC, Hung CY, et al. Dynamic driving pressure associated mortality in acute respiratory distress syndrome with extracorporeal membrane oxygenation. Ann Intensive Care. 2017;7:12.
9. Yoshida T, Fujino Y, Amato MBP, et al. Fifty years of research in ards. Spontaneous breathing during mechanical ventilation. Risks, mechanisms, and management. Am J Respir Crit Care Med. 2017;195:985–92.
10. Yoshida T, Roldan R, Beraldo MA, et al. Spontaneous effort during mechanical ventilation: maximal injury with less positive end-expiratory pressure. Crit Care Med. 2016;44:e678–88.
11. Akoumianaki E, Lyazidi A, Rey N, et al. Mechanical ventilation-induced reverse-triggered breaths a frequently unrecognized form of neuromechanical coupling. Chest. 2013;143:927–38.
12. Jung B, Moury PH, Mahul M, et al. Diaphragmatic dysfunction in patients with ICU-acquired weakness and its impact on extubation failure. Intensive Care Med. 2016;42:853–61.
13. Orozco-Levi M, Lloreta J, Minguella J, et al. Injury of the human diaphragm associated with exertion and chronic obstructive pulmonary disease. Am J Respir Crit Care Med. 2001;164:1734–9.
14. Jiang TX, Reid WD, Belcastro A, et al. Load dependence of secondary diaphragm inflammation and injury after acute inspiratory loading. Am J Respir Crit Care Med. 1998;157:230–6.
15. Lin MC, Ebihara S, Dwairi QEL, et al. Diaphragm sarcolemmal injury is induced by sepsis and alleviated by nitric oxide synthase inhibition. Am J Respir Crit Care Med. 1998;158:1656–63.
16. Proske U, Morgan DL. Muscle damage from eccentric exercise: mechanism, mechanical signs, adaptation and clinical applications. J Physiol. 2001;537:333–45.
17. Pellegrini M, Hedenstierna G, Roneus A, et al. The diaphragm acts as a brake during expiration to prevent lung collapse. Am J Respir Crit Care Med. 2017;195:1608–16.
18. Lindqvist J, van den Berg M, van der Pijl R, et al. Positive end-expiratory pressure ventilation induces longitudinal atrophy in diaphragm fibers. Am J Respir Crit Care Med. 2018;198:472–85.
19. Fish E, Novack V, Banner-Goodspeed VM, et al. The esophageal pressure-guided ventilation 2 (EPVent2) trial protocol: a multicentre, randomised clinical trial of mechanical ventilation guided by transpulmonary pressure. BMJ Open. 2014;4:e006356.
20. Luca Grieco D, Chen L, Brochard L. Transpulmonary pressure: importance and limits. Ann Transl Med. 2017;5:285.
21. Baedorf Kassis E, Loring SH, Talmor D. Mortality and pulmonary mechanics in relation to respiratory system and transpulmonary driving pressures in ARDS. Intensive Care Med. 2016;42:1206–13.
22. Yoshida T, Amato MBP, Grieco DL, et al. Esophageal manometry and regional transpulmonary pressure in lung injury. Am J Respir Crit Care Med. 2018;197:1018–26.
23. Yoshida T, Amato MBP, Kavanagh BP. Understanding spontaneous vs. ventilator breaths: impact and monitoring. Intensive Care Med. 2018;44:2235–8.
24. Protti A, Andreis DT, Monti M, et al. Lung stress and strain during mechanical ventilation: any difference between statics and dynamics? Crit Care Med. 2013;41:1046–55.
25. Amato MBP, Meade MO, Slutsky AS, et al. Driving pressure and survival in the acute respiratory distress syndrome. N Engl J Med. 2015;372:747–55.
26. Chiumello D, Carlesso E, Cadringher P, et al. Lung stress and strain during mechanical ventilation for acute respiratory distress syndrome. Am J Respir Crit Care Med. 2008;178:346–55.

27. Carteaux G, Mancebo J, Mercat A, et al. Bedside adjustment of proportional assist ventilation to target a predefined range of respiratory effort. Crit Care Med. 2013;41:2125–32.
28. Mauri T, Yoshida T, Bellani G, et al. Esophageal and transpulmonary pressure in the clinical setting: meaning, usefulness and perspectives. Intensive Care Med. 2016;42:1360–73.
29. Bellani G, Grassi A, Sosio S, et al. Plateau and driving pressure in the presence of spontaneous breathing. Intensive Care Med. 2019;45:97–8.
30. Goldman MD, Grassino A, Mead J, et al. Mechanics of the human diaphragm during voluntary contraction: dynamics. J Appl Physiol. 1978;44:840–8.
31. Grassino A, Goldman MD, Mead J, et al. Mechanics of the human diaphragm during voluntary contraction: statics. J Appl Physiol. 1978;44:829–39.
32. Spadaro S, Marangoni E, Ragazzi R, et al. A methodological approach for determination of maximal inspiratory pressure in patients undergoing invasive mechanical ventilation. Minerva Anestesiol. 2015;81:33–8.
33. Bertoni M, Telias I, Urner M, et al. A novel non-invasive method to detect excessively high respiratory effort and dynamic transpulmonary driving pressure during mechanical ventilation. Crit Care. 2019;23:346.
34. Telias I, Damiani F, Brochard L. The airway occlusion pressure (P0.1) to monitor respiratory drive during mechanical ventilation: increasing awareness of a not-so-new problem. Intensive Care Med. 2018;44:1532–5.
35. Whitelaw WA, Derenne JP, Milic-Emili J. Occlusion pressure as a measure of respiratory center output in conscious man. Respir Physiol. 1975;23:181–99.
36. Holle RH, Schoene RB, Pavlin EJ. Effect of respiratory muscle weakness on P0.1 induced by partial curarization. J Appl Physiol. 1984;57:1150–7.
37. Rittayamai N, Beloncle F, Goligher EC, et al. Effect of inspiratory synchronization during pressure-controlled ventilation on lung distension and inspiratory effort. Ann Intensive Care. 2017;7:100.
38. Vargas F, Boyer A, Bui HN, et al. Respiratory failure in chronic obstructive pulmonary disease after extubation: value of expiratory flow limitation and airway occlusion pressure after 0.1 second (P0.1). J Crit Care. 2008;23:577–84.
39. Kera T, Aihara A, Inomata T. Reliability of airway occlusion pressure as an index of respiratory motor output. Respir Care. 2013;58:845–9.
40. Alberti A, Gallo F, Fongaro A, et al. P0.1 is a useful parameter in setting the level of pressure support ventilation. Intensive Care Med. 1995;21:547–53.
41. Mauri T, Grasselli G, Suriano G, et al. Control of respiratory drive and effort in extracorporeal membrane oxygenation patients recovering from severe acute respiratory distress syndrome. Anesthesiology. 2016;125:159–67.
42. Pletsch-Assuncao R, Caleffi Pereira M, Ferreira JG, et al. Accuracy of invasive and noninvasive parameters for diagnosing ventilatory overassistance during pressure support ventilation. Crit Care Med. 2018;46:411–7.
43. Iotti GA, Brunner JX, Braschi A, et al. Closed-loop control of airway occlusion pressure at 0.1 second (P0.1) applied to pressure-support ventilation: algorithm and application in intubated patients [Internet]. Crit Care Med. 1996;24:771–9.
44. Conti G, Cinnella G, Barboni E, et al. Estimation of occlusion pressure during assisted ventilation in patients with intrinsic PEEP. Am J Respir Crit Care Med. 1996;154:907–12.
45. Sinderby C, Navalesi P, Beck J, et al. Neural control of mechanical ventilation in respiratory failure. Nat Med. 1999;5:1433–6.
46. Kim MJ, Druz WS, Danon J, et al. Effects of lung volume and electrode position on the esophageal diaphragmatic EMG. J Appl Physiol. 1978;45:392–8.
47. Beloncle F, Piquilloud L, Rittayamai N, et al. A diaphragmatic electrical activity-based optimization strategy during pressure support ventilation improves synchronization but does not impact work of breathing. Crit Care. 2017;21:21.
48. Sinderby C, Liu S, Colombo D, et al. An automated and standardized neural index to quantify patient-ventilator interaction. Crit Care. 2013;17:R239.

49. Di Mussi R, Spadaro S, Mirabella L, et al. Impact of prolonged assisted ventilation on diaphragmatic efficiency: NAVA versus PSV. Crit Care. 2016;20:1.
50. Barwing J, Pedroni C, Olgemöller U, et al. Electrical activity of the diaphragm (EAdi) as a monitoring parameter in difficult weaning from respirator: a pilot study. Crit Care. 2013;17:R182.
51. Gross D, Grassino A, Ross WR, et al. Electromyogram pattern of diaphragmatic fatigue. J Appl Physiol. 1979;46:1–7.
52. Dres M, Schmidt M, Ferre A, et al. Diaphragm electromyographic activity as a predictor of weaning failure. Intensive Care Med. 2012;38:2017–25.
53. Piquilloud L, Beloncle F, Richard JC, Mancebo J, Mercat A, Brochard L. Information conveyed by electrical diaphragmatic activity during unstressed, stressed and assisted spontaneous breathing: a physiological study [Internet]. Ann Intensive Care. 2019;9:89.
54. Bellani G, Mauri T, Coppadoro A, et al. Estimation of patient's inspiratory effort from the electrical activity of the diaphragm. Crit Care Med. 2013;41:1483–91.
55. Goligher EC, Laghi F, Detsky ME, et al. Measuring diaphragm thickness with ultrasound in mechanically ventilated patients: feasibility, reproducibility and validity. Intensive Care Med. 2015;41:642–9.

Ten Reasons to Use Mechanical Power to Guide Ventilator Settings in Patients Without ARDS

P. L. Silva, P. R. M. Rocco, and P. Pelosi

3.1 Introduction

Mechanical ventilation is frequently used in patients without acute respiratory distress syndrome (ARDS): during surgery, in the intensive care unit (ICU; e.g., to support breathing in respiratory and neurological failure), and for artificial respiration in cardiac arrest. Even though mechanical ventilation is a life-saving strategy, it may cause ventilator-induced lung injury (VILI). Analyses of the main factors involved in VILI have focused on separate evaluation of static parameters—such as tidal volume; peak (P_{peak}), plateau (P_{plat}), and driving (ΔP) pressures; and positive end-expiratory pressure (PEEP)—and of dynamic ones—airflow, inspiratory time, and respiratory rate. However, in the real-world setting, these factors interact with each other. Thus, combining these factors into a single parameter—the "mechanical power" imparted to the lung by the ventilator—may be a more suitable strategy for both research and clinical purposes.

Although early implementation of protective ventilation in patients without ARDS has been associated with better prognosis [1], optimization of mechanical ventilation settings is considered less important in daily clinical practice. In this chapter, we will discuss ten questions regarding the importance of the sole single ventilator parameter that has been associated with mortality in patients without ARDS: mechanical power. This parameter will then be discussed, focusing on the use of different formulas for its calculation and on the evidence of its impact on lung damage from preclinical and clinical studies.

P. L. Silva · P. R. M. Rocco
Laboratory of Pulmonary Investigation, Carlos Chagas Filho Institute of Biophysics, Federal University of Rio de Janeiro, Rio de Janeiro, Brazil

P. Pelosi (✉)
Department of Surgical Sciences and Integrated Diagnostics (DISC), University of Genoa, Genoa, Italy

IRCCS for Oncology and Neurosciences, San Martino Policlinico Hospital, Genoa, Italy
e-mail: paolo.pelosi@unige.it

3.2 Is Tidal Volume Associated with Mortality in Patients Without ARDS? No

The tidal volumes that are used in mechanically ventilated patients without ARDS have progressively been decreasing; however, the evidence for benefits of low tidal volumes remains scarce. A systematic review evaluated the change in tidal volume during a 39-year period (from 1975 to 2014) [2] and showed that tidal volumes have decreased significantly in the ICU (annual decrease of 0.16 ml/kg) and in the operating room (annual decrease of 0.09 ml/kg). In the PReVENT study [1], tidal volume was around 8 ml/kg predicted body weight (PBW) and did not differ between surviving patients and those who died. In a secondary analysis of the PRoVENT, tidal volume was not identified as a potential parameter associated with survival in patients without ARDS [3], which could be attributed to the fact that most patients were protectively ventilated. In the PReVENT trial, low tidal volume and intermediate tidal volume strategies were compared in patients without ARDS, focusing on the number of ventilator-free days and mortality rate at 28 days [1]. The low-tidal-volume group started at 6 ml/kg PBW, with decrements of 1 ml/kg PBW every hour to a minimum of 4 ml/kg PBW, whereas the intermediate-tidal-volume group started at 10 ml/kg PBW. P_{plat} was maintained at less than 25 cmH$_2$O; if it exceeded this threshold, tidal volume was progressively reduced by 1 ml/kg PBW. Ventilator-free days and mortality rate at 28 days did not differ between the low-tidal-volume (mean = 7.3 ml/kg PBW) and intermediate-tidal-volume (mean = 9.1 ml/kg PBW) groups. The intermediate-tidal-volume group showed higher P_{plat} and ΔP in the first 3 days of the study, but still within a protective range for patients without ARDS. Additionally, use of the low-tidal-volume strategy was associated with CO_2 retention and respiratory acidosis, perhaps related to less efficient alveolar ventilation. Furthermore, the use of oversedation to maintain low tidal volume may be associated with increased delirium, ventilator asynchrony, and the possibility of effort-induced lung injury. To date, there are no clinical trial data showing benefit or harm of low-tidal-volume ventilation in patients without ARDS. Since ARDS is only very rarely recognized at its onset, the safest approach is to use protective ventilation with tidal volume <8 ml/kg PBW.

3.3 Is Driving Pressure Associated with Mortality in Patients Without ARDS? No

The driving pressure of the respiratory system ($\Delta P,_{RS}$) can be easily calculated at the bedside as P_{plat} minus pressure at end-expiratory occlusion (PEEP + intrinsic PEEP). The $\Delta P,_{RS}$ represents the tidal volume normalized by the respiratory system compliance. Since the compliance of the respiratory system is proportional to the volume of aerated lung, $\Delta P,_{RS}$ is the tidal volume corrected for the end-expiratory lung volume, thus estimating the strain during tidal breath. In other words, if tidal volume remains constant, if the compliance of the respiratory system is low, the $\Delta P,_{RS}$ will proportionally increase; conversely, if the compliance of the respiratory system is high, the $\Delta P,_{RS}$ will proportionally decrease. Furthermore, under constant respiratory system compliance, $\Delta P_{,RS}$ will increase at higher tidal volumes. Finally, $\Delta P_{,RS}$ might be affected by the effects of PEEP on non-aerated lung areas. At a constant tidal volume, if PEEP increases lung volume by recruitment of previously collapsed alveoli, $\Delta P_{,RS}$ will decrease; if PEEP increases lung volume by overdistension of previously aerated alveoli, $\Delta P_{,RS}$ will increase. In patients without ARDS, the lung volume at end-expiration and the compliance of the respiratory system are either within normal ranges or moderately reduced, and low PEEP levels are usually applied, thus avoiding alveolar overdistension. In a retrospective study, $\Delta P_{,RS}$ on day 1 was not associated with hospital mortality in patients without ARDS [4]. A secondary analysis of the PRoVENT trial [3] showed no association between $\Delta P_{,RS}$ (≤ 12 vs. >12 cmH$_2$O) and hospital mortality. However, caution is warranted, given the relatively small sample size of the study. Therefore, to date there is no indication to guide ventilatory strategy on the basis of $\Delta P_{,RS}$ alone in patients without ARDS.

3.4 Is P_{peak} Associated with Mortality in Patients Without ARDS? Yes

P_{peak} is determined by the inspiratory flow and the position where pressure is measured along the respiratory circuit. In fact, it represents the total pressure gradient, at a fixed flow, to overcome the elastic, resistive, and viscoelastic properties of the respiratory system, the artificial airways, and the ventilator circuit. P_{peak} is one of the easiest respiratory variables to monitor at the bedside during mechanical ventilation. In patients with increased airway resistance, under volume-controlled ventilation, after occluding the airways at end-inspiration, the difference between P_{peak} and P_{plat} represents the resistive properties (patient and ventilator circuit), whereas during pressure-controlled ventilation, P_{peak} is close to P_{plat}, since flow at expiration is almost zero. In patients without increased airway resistance and/or ventilator circuit obstruction, P_{peak} is approximately equal to P_{plat}. A secondary analysis of PRoVENT reported a significant association between $P_{peak} > 18$ cmH$_2$O and inhospital mortality in patients without ARDS [3]. In conclusion, we suggest using a P_{peak} pressure < 30 cmH$_2$O and a $P_{plat} < 25$ cmH$_2$O in mechanically ventilated patients without ARDS in volume- and pressure-controlled ventilation.

3.5 Is PEEP Associated with Mortality in Patients Without ARDS? Yes

PEEP has been proposed to prevent or at least minimize atelectrauma during controlled mechanical ventilation. However, PEEP can also lead to lung injury due to overdistension (so-called volutrauma) and impair right ventricular function and hemodynamics. In a systematic review [5] of preclinical studies in small and large mammals, "high PEEP" (versus lower PEEP) or "PEEP" (versus no PEEP) was associated with improved respiratory system compliance and better oxygenation. However, "high PEEP" and "PEEP" were also associated with occurrence of hypotension, a reduction in cardiac output or development of hyperlactatemia, with no differences in mortality. Based on the findings of this systematic review in experimental settings, it is uncertain whether PEEP at any level truly prevents lung injury, and most trials suggested potential harmful effects on the systemic circulation. Patients without ARDS who have less atelectasis and better compliance of the respiratory system seem to have a better balance between benefit and harm in favor of lower PEEP levels. Nevertheless, whether higher PEEP levels can be associated with clinical improvement over time is unknown. A meta-analysis of clinical trials [6] compared lower (2.0 ± 2.8 cmH$_2$O) vs. higher (9.7 ± 4.0 cmH$_2$O) levels of PEEP and found no benefits in terms of mortality and duration of invasive ventilation in surgical or medical ICU patients. In addition, pooling all data in a recent cohort [3] of patients without ARDS, high PEEP levels (>5 cmH$_2$O) were associated with higher hospital mortality. A prospective randomized controlled trial in patients without ARDS to test the effects of low PEEP (lowest possible PEEP between 0 and 5 cmH$_2$O) and high PEEP (PEEP of 8 cmH$_2$O) on the number of ventilator-free days and survival at day 28 is ongoing [7]. To date, the evidence suggests that PEEP should not exceed 5 cmH$_2$O in patients without ARDS.

3.6 Is Respiratory Rate Associated with Mortality in Patients Without ARDS? No

Respiratory rate is one of the easiest variables to measure at the bedside. It may be controlled by the ventilator, by the patient, or both. Usually, respiratory rate is set to keep an adequate level of arterial partial pressure of carbon dioxide (PaCO$_2$) and arterial pH. Experimental studies have shown that increased respiratory rate may be associated with VILI [8, 9]. From a physiological standpoint, the respiratory rate can reflect the number of cycles of injured stress and strain in the lung parenchyma. In the PReVENT trial [1], respiratory rate was higher in volume-controlled compared to pressure-support ventilation groups, regardless of tidal volume. Conversely, PaCO$_2$ was higher in the low-tidal-volume compared to intermediate-tidal-volume group during volume-controlled ventilation, but not in pressure-support ventilation, suggesting that the increased spontaneous breathing decreased the dead space, thus improving gas exchange. In conclusion, we suggest using assisted mechanical ventilation modes in patients without ARDS, thus allowing selection of an appropriate respiratory rate for the patient.

3.7 Mechanical Energy and Power Calculations: Should We Abandon More Complex Formulas in Favor of Simplified Ones? Yes

The contribution of the energy and power applied to the lung parenchyma during mechanical ventilation, resulting in VILI, is known as ergotrauma. Work is force × distance and, in the case of the lungs, since pressure is force/area and volume is length × area, the product of pressure and volume is force × length, which is the work done during lung inflation. Work of breathing and energy are expressed in the same unit (J). Energy has been calculated as tidal volume (ml) × ΔP (cmH$_2$O), which gives a unit of ml/cmH$_2$O. (To convert from ml/cmH$_2$O to joules, all variables should be transformed to SI units.) Power is the rate of energy expenditure (Energy × Respiratory rate) [10, 11].

Different equations are available to calculate mechanical power. Since resistive properties are included, it should be mentioned that mechanical power calculation depends on the site of airway pressure measurement, i.e., whether at the end of the tracheal tube or at a transducer within the mechanical ventilator. In the first condition, only the resistance of the endotracheal tube is added to the airway resistance of the patient, while in the second condition, the total resistance encompasses the whole of the mechanical ventilator circuit, including the endotracheal tube. To correctly calculate mechanical power, the resistances of both the tracheal tube and mechanical ventilator should be subtracted or otherwise accounted for.

The complex equation initially described by Gattinoni et al. [12] is:

$$\text{Mechanical power}(J/\min) = 0.098 \times \text{Respiratory rate}$$
$$\times \left\{ \begin{array}{l} (\text{Tidal volume})^2 \times \left[\frac{1}{2} \cdot E_{rs} + \text{Respiratory rate} \times \left[(1 + I:E)/60 \times I:E \right] \times R_{aw} \right] \\ + \text{Tidal volume} \times \text{PEEP} \end{array} \right\}$$

where 0.098 is the conversion factor for units, E_{rs} is the respiratory system elastance, $I{:}E$ is the ratio between inspiratory and expiratory time, and R_{aw} is the airway resistance.

One important benefit of using this more complex formula is that it enables quantification of the relative contribution of each component (tidal volume, respiratory rate, $\Delta P_{,RS}$, PEEP, $I{:}E$, and airflow). This has been done previously by changing one parameter at a time and observing the overall effect on mechanical power [12]. Therefore, this formula takes into account the resistive properties and PEEP (and, consequently, lung volume changes caused by PEEP). The main disadvantages of this formula are that it is laborious to calculate and may be conditioned to perfect calibration of the mechanical ventilator, since more variables are used to calculate the mechanical power.

Furthermore, there are controversies regarding the computation of mechanical energy in a static condition, since there is no cyclic movement of the respiratory system after sole application of PEEP [10]. Therefore, when PEEP is included and lung volume is changed by PEEP application, both the static and dynamic components of mechanical energy should be calculated.

The static component of mechanical energy, which takes into account elastic mechanical power (MP$_{ELAST}$), can be calculated using the following formula:

$$\text{MP}_{ELAST} = 0.098 \times \text{Respiratory rate} \times \left[\text{Tidal volume} \times (P_{plat} - \text{PEEP}) \right]/2$$

The dynamic component of mechanical energy, which takes into account resistive mechanical power (MP$_{RES}$), can be calculated using the following formula:

$$\text{MP}_{RES} = 0.098 \times \text{Tidal volume} \times \text{Respiratory rate}$$
$$\times (P_{peak} \times \Delta P_{,RS} - 2 \times \text{PEEP} - \Delta P_{RS})/2$$

The simplest formula, which includes both elastic and resistive properties and is intended for use in critically ill patients [13], is composed of tidal volume, P_{peak}, respiratory rate, and ΔP [12]:

$$\text{Mechanical power}(J/\min) = 0.098 \times \text{Tidal volume} \times \text{Respiratory rate}$$
$$\times \left(P_{peak} - \tfrac{1}{2} \times \Delta P_{RS}\right)$$

Serpa Neto et al. [13] tested the hypothesis that mechanical power would be independently associated with patient-centered outcomes in mechanically ventilated critically ill patients for 48 h. This study was performed in two large cohorts of ICU patients whose data were prospectively collected in two databases. Mechanical power was independently associated with higher inhospital mortality, higher ICU mortality, fewer ventilator-free days, and longer ICU and hospital stays. One of the most important findings of this post hoc analysis was that, even at low tidal volume and low $\Delta P_{,RS}$, high mechanical power was associated with worse outcomes in critically ill patients. The combination of potential respiratory variables related to lung injury into a single parameter, instead of using only one respiratory variable, may have high predictive value for worse outcomes in the critically ill.

The concept of intensity, which is the distribution of mechanical power per unit of lung surface area [11, 14] or static compliance of the respiratory system (C_{RS} = Tidal volume/$\Delta P_{,RS}$), has also been proposed.

For the aforementioned formula, intensity (J/min) is given as = 0.098 × Tidal volume × Respiratory rate × (P_{peak} − ½ × $\Delta P_{,RS}$)/Tidal volume/$\Delta P_{,RS}$.

$$\text{After simplification, Intensity}(J/\min) = \text{Respiratory rate} \times \Delta P_{,RS}^2 / 2$$

If PEEP and resistive properties are added to the mechanical power formula, the intensity would be stated as:

$$\text{Intensity}(J/\min) = 0.098 \times \text{Respiratory rate} \times \left[P_{peak} - \left(\Delta P_{,RS}/2\right)\right] \times \Delta P_{,RS}$$

A recent study investigated whether mechanical power normalized for predicted body weight (norMP) could be a better marker of mortality compared to other ventilator variables [15]. NorMP (AUC = 0.751) showed good predictive value for mortality compared to non-normalized mechanical power (AUC = 0.747). Mechanical power normalized by respiratory system compliance (a surrogate of intensity) was an even better predictor of mortality (AUC = 0.753).

3.8 Does Use of a Simple Formula Enable Calculation of Mechanical Power in Volume-Controlled Ventilation? Yes: Simply Change the Variables and Observe the Consequences

Usually, changing a single respiratory variable may not promote lung protection if this change is not followed by significant changes in lung mechanics [16]. This phenomenon can be observed in different clinical scenarios. However, calculation of mechanical power using the simplest formula, which takes into account tidal volume, respiratory rate, P_{peak}, and $\Delta P,_{RS}$, can help understand why lung protection may not occur after changing only one respiratory variable.

The effects of different tidal volumes on mechanical power during volume-controlled ventilation have been simulated in a hypothetical patient with a PBW equal to 64 kg (the average body weight reported in patients without ARDS) [3]. The inspiratory:expiratory ratio was kept constant at 1:2. Three different respiratory system compliance values—0.02 l/cmH$_2$O (low), 0.04 l/cmH$_2$O (intermediate), and 0.06 l/cmH$_2$O (high)—were tested, with tidal volume reduced from 10 to 6 ml/kg PBW, total minute ventilation kept constant (9.6 l/min), and PEEP = 5 cmH$_2$O. To maintain minute ventilation constant, respiratory rate was increased from 15 to 25 bpm. As shown in Fig. 3.1, together with the increment in

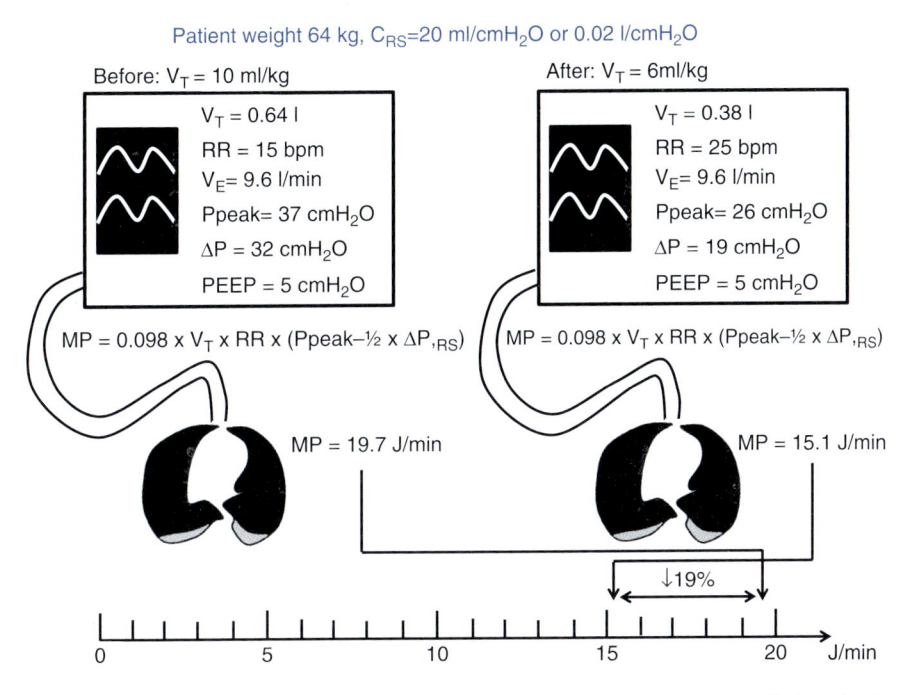

Fig. 3.1 Simulation of the effects of mechanical power (MP) during volume-controlled mechanical ventilation in a patient with a predicted body weight of 64 kg (the average body weight of patients without ARDS). Inspiratory:expiratory ratio kept constant at 1:2. Three different respiratory system compliance (C_{RS}) values—0.02 l/cmH$_2$O (low), 0.04 l/cmH$_2$O (intermediate), and 0.06 l/cmH$_2$O (high)—were tested, with tidal volume (V_T) reductions from 10 ml/kg predicted body weight (PBW) to 6 ml/kg PBW, while keeping total minute ventilation (V_E) constant (9.6 l/min) at positive end-expiratory pressure (PEEP) = 5 cmH$_2$O. To maintain constant minute ventilation, respiratory rate (RR) was increased from 15 to 25 bpm. A decrease in inspiratory time (from 1.3 to 0.8 s) and concomitant increase in airflow (from 0.36 to 0.59 l/s) are expected to follow, increasing the resistive pressure. Assuming a patient with constant airway resistance (4 cmH$_2$O/l/s), the increase in airflow would increase the resistive pressure by about 1.5 cmH$_2$O, with an impact in P_{peak} (one of the components of the mechanical power calculation). Reductions in V_T were associated with lower mechanical power in all conditions. Furthermore, the percent decrease in mechanical power after the reduction in V_T was greater at low compared to intermediate or higher respiratory system compliances (19% vs. 11% vs. 9%, respectively)

Patient weight 64 kg, C_{RS}=40 ml/cmH$_2$O or 0.04 l/cmH$_2$O

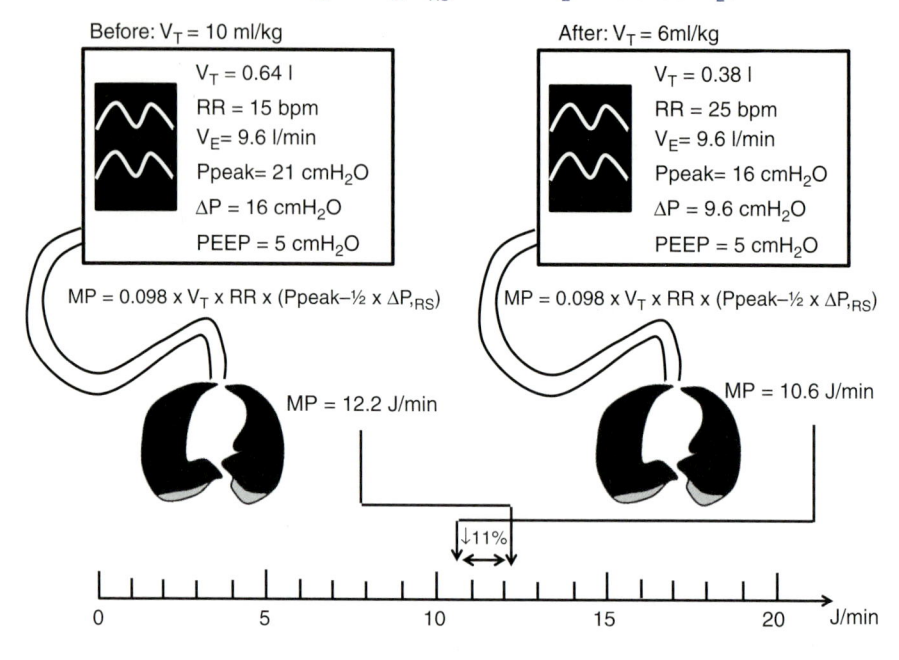

Before: V_T = 10 ml/kg

V_T = 0.64 l
RR = 15 bpm
V_E = 9.6 l/min
Ppeak = 21 cmH$_2$O
ΔP = 16 cmH$_2$O
PEEP = 5 cmH$_2$O

MP = 0.098 x V_T x RR x (Ppeak – ½ x $\Delta P_{,RS}$)

MP = 12.2 J/min

After: V_T = 6 ml/kg

V_T = 0.38 l
RR = 25 bpm
V_E = 9.6 l/min
Ppeak = 16 cmH$_2$O
ΔP = 9.6 cmH$_2$O
PEEP = 5 cmH$_2$O

MP = 0.098 x V_T x RR x (Ppeak – ½ x $\Delta P_{,RS}$)

MP = 10.6 J/min

↓11%

0   5   10   15   20   J/min

Patient weight 64 kg, C_{RS}=60 ml/cmH$_2$O or 0.06 l/H$_2$O

Before: V_T = 10 ml/kg

V_T = 0.64 l
RR = 15 bpm
V_E = 9.6 l/min
Ppeak = 16 cmH$_2$O
ΔP = 11 cmH$_2$O
PEEP = 5 cmH$_2$O

MP = 0.098 x V_T x RR x (Ppeak – ½ x $\Delta P_{,RS}$)

MP = 9.7 J/min

After: V_T = 6 ml/kg

V_T = 0.38 l
RR = 25 bpm
V_E = 9.6 l/min
Ppeak = 13 cmH$_2$O
ΔP = 6 cmH$_2$O
PEEP = 5 cmH$_2$O

MP = 0.098 x V_T x RR x (Ppeak – ½ x $\Delta P_{,RS}$)

MP = 9.1 J/min

↓9%

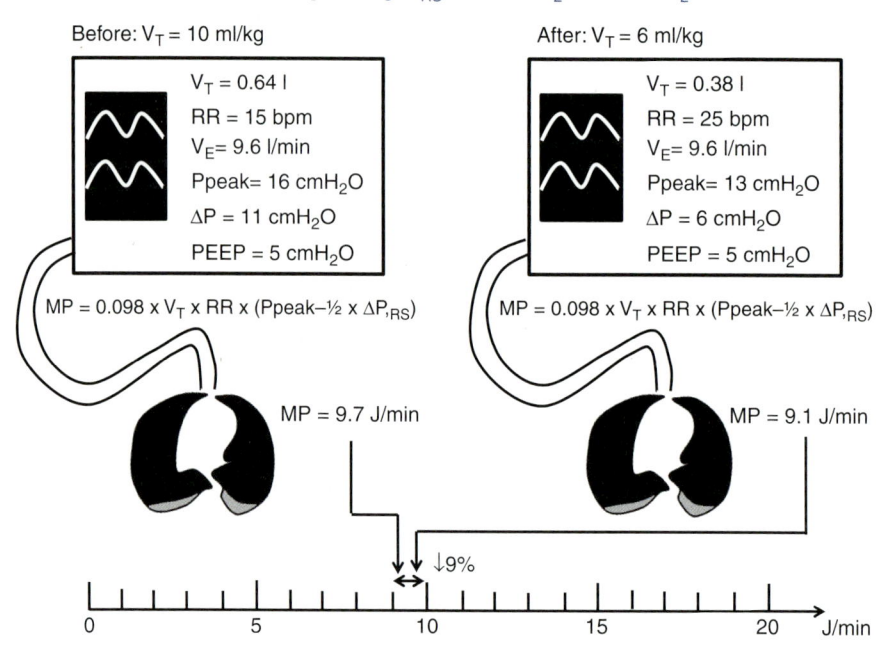

0   5   10   15   20   J/min

Fig. 3.1 (continued)

respiratory rate from 15 to 25 bpm, a decrease in inspiratory time (from 1.3 to 0.8 s) is expected, as well as a concomitant increase in airflow (from 0.36 to 0.59 l/s), which would increase the resistive pressure. Considering a patient with constant airway resistance (4 cmH$_2$O/l/s), the increase in airflow would increase the resistive pressure to approximately 1.5 cmH$_2$O, which would have an impact on P_{peak}. Reduction in tidal volume was associated with lower mechanical power in all conditions. Furthermore, the percentage of decrease in mechanical power after the reduction in tidal volume was greater at low compared to intermediate or higher compliances of the respiratory system (19% vs. 11% vs. 9%, respectively). This suggests that the effects of tidal volume reduction on mechanical power are greater at low respiratory system compliance.

Becher et al. [17], in a retrospective analysis of two previous studies, proposed two power equations for pressure-controlled ventilation (MP$_{PCV}$): a simplified formula,

$$MP_{PCV} = 0.098 \times \text{Respiratory rate} \times \text{Tidal volume} \times (\Delta P_{insp} + PEEP)$$

and a comprehensive equation,

$$MP_{PCV(slope)}$$
$$= 0.098 \times \text{Respiratory rate} \times \begin{bmatrix} (\Delta P_{insp} + PEEP) \times \text{Tidal volume} - \Delta P^2_{insp} \times C \\ \times \left(0.5 - R \times C / T_{slope} + (R \times C / T_{slope})^2 \times (1 - e^{-T slope / R \times C})\right) \end{bmatrix}$$

where R is resistance and C is compliance. Both formulas were compared to reference values obtained through integration of pressure-volume loops from the mechanical ventilator. The authors found that the simplified equation estimated mechanical power for pressure-controlled ventilation with a small bias, which resulted from not taking T_{slope} into account. On the other hand, the comprehensive equation was able to correct this bias, but requires knowledge of T_{slope}, resistance, and compliance. The formula proposed by Becher et al. was tested in a recent small validation study by van der Meijden et al. [18], in which the authors proposed a different equation:

$$MP_{PCV} = 0.098 \times \text{Respiratory rate} \times \text{Tidal volume} \times [PEEP + \Delta P_{insp} \times (1 - e^{-Tinsp/R \times C})]$$

These authors found that, for higher mechanical power values, the method proposed by Becher et al. [17] was somewhat inaccurate, although testing in larger samples was still warranted. Meanwhile, Becher et al. tested the equation proposed by van der Meijden et al. using a dataset of 301 pressure-volume loops obtained from 42 patients [19]. The authors found that on average, the equation proposed by van der Meijden et al. led to underestimation of mechanical power, with a bias of −0.56 J/min and a correlation coefficient of $r^2 = 0.937$, which is inferior to both the "simplified" and "comprehensive" equations originally proposed by Becher et al. ($r^2 = 0.981$ and $r^2 = 0.985$, respectively). In addition, the difference could be related to the assumption that, during pressure-controlled ventilation, end-inspiratory flow and pressure rise time are zero. In those respiratory cycles with end-inspiratory flow above zero, the formula will thus lead to underestimation of mechanical power, while pressure rise times above zero will lead to overestimation of mechanical power. The exchange of letters between these two groups of authors, with equation proposals and reanalysis of a larger dataset, is a step towards better understanding of mechanical power calculation during pressure-controlled ventilation [20].

3.9 Can Mechanical Power Be Computed During Assisted Ventilation? Yes

Mechanical energy and power, by definition, represent the total energy transferred from the mechanical ventilator in association with the respiratory muscles. To date, clinical studies have focused on relaxed respiratory muscles; therefore, only the mechanical power provided by the ventilator is computed [12, 21]. Nevertheless, the mechanical power generated by the respiratory muscles was calculated using an esophageal catheter in two pediatric studies [22, 23]. In an experimental study, mechanical power was calculated during pressure-support ventilation in rats. However, the authors chose to calculate only the portion attributable to the mechanical ventilator, which was reduced in pressure-support ventilation compared to pressure-controlled ventilation [24]. The calculation of lung mechanical power was done using the trapezoidal rule, as the integral of the inspiratory transpulmonary pressure versus the inspired tidal volume curve by numeric integration. A similar calculation was done in controlled mechanical ventilation [12].

There are further challenges to be overcome regarding calculation of respiratory system mechanical power during spontaneous breathing: (1) adjustment for chest wall movement; (2) distribution of mechanical power across the lung surface, which may not follow the same distribution determined by lung inhomogeneity [10]; and (3) the proper contribution of respiratory muscle activity to overall mechanical power under assisted mechanical ventilation.

3.10 Is Mechanical Power Associated with Lung Injury in Experimental Models? Yes

Recent studies have described the impact of mechanical power on VILI [25, 26, 29, 30]. In one such investigation, lung edema was observed when transpulmonary mechanical power was higher than 12.1 J/min [25]. Several analyses have been done to evaluate the relative contribution of tidal volume and respiratory rate to mechanical power [12]. An experimental study [26] investigated the impact of high and low mechanical power, obtained as combinations of low and high tidal volume and respiratory rate, on VILI. Mechanical power was calculated using different formulas [12, 27, 28]. Even when combined with high tidal volume, low mechanical power resulted in greater lung damage, thus suggesting the importance of using protective low tidal volume in ARDS [26]. PEEP is also an important parameter to calculate mechanical power. In this line, Collino et al. investigated the effects of increasing PEEP values on mechanical power in healthy lungs [30]. For this purpose, piglets were ventilated by a tidal volume (14.9 ml/kg) similar to functional residual capacity (FRC), which gives an overall strain close to 1, and increasing levels of PEEP were tested (0, 4, 7, 11, 14, and 18 cmH$_2$O) for 50 h. Mechanical power was calculated by the formula proposed by Gattinoni et al. [12], which takes into account the PEEP × ΔV related to PEEP.

The authors showed that mechanical power was constant from 0 up to 7 cmH$_2$O, which could be reflected by improvement of lung elastance within this range. On the other hand, increasing PEEP from 7 up to 18 cmH$_2$O was associated with greater damage and relevant hemodynamic instability. This experimental study emphasizes that PEEP may be a major determining factor of damage in certain settings, while in others, the driving pressure, respiratory rate, and tidal volume may be more important. More recently, Felix et al. [31] tested the hypothesis that the impact of an abrupt increase in tidal volume would be attenuated if tidal volume were increased slowly enough to reduce alveolar mechanical heterogeneity and VILI. Although the primary focus was not related to mechanical power itself, the authors showed that extending the adaptation period increased cumulative power and induced VILI, since animals were exposed to injurious strain earlier and for a longer time [32]. Therefore, the rapid recognition of high mechanical power mitigates lung damage.

3.11 Is Mechanical Power Associated with Mortality in Patients Without ARDS? Yes

In their dual-dataset study, Serpa Neto et al. [13] observed an association between increased risk of death and mechanical power higher than 17.0 J/min (Fig. 3.2). The most important result of this post hoc analysis was that even at low tidal volume and low ΔP, high mechanical power was associated with fewer ventilator-free days, longer ICU stays, and higher inhospital mortality. Similar findings were found in a secondary analysis of 1705 mechanically ventilated patients without ARDS [33]. By using the same formula described by Serpa Neto et al. [13], the authors found that ΔP, P_{plat}, and mechanical power were associated with inhospital mortality.

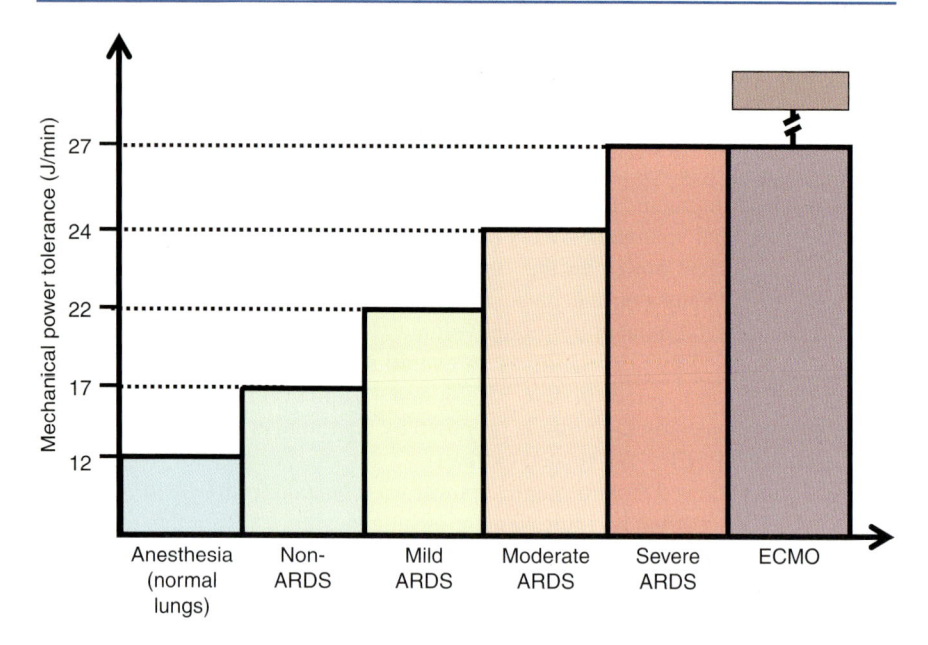

Fig. 3.2 Mechanical power tolerance. For anesthesia in a patient with normal lungs, the reported values are within very low limits, around 12 J/min. In critically ill patients without acute respiratory distress syndrome (non-ARDS), the threshold value of mechanical power to prevent ARDS is <17 J/min. In ARDS, regardless of severity, values are higher than in non-ARDS. For mild, moderate, and severe ARDS, the tolerated values are 22, 24, and 27 J/min. If mechanical power exceeds 27 J/min, extracorporeal membrane oxygenation (ECMO) should be considered

3.12 Conclusion

In patients without ARDS, ventilatory management has been associated with mortality. Commonly targeted ventilator parameters, such as tidal volume and ΔP, are not associated with mortality in patients without ARDS, while respiratory rate—which has been comparatively neglected in clinical trials—is gaining attention. Mechanical power, which pools these variables to reflect the amount of energy transferred from the mechanical ventilator to the lung parenchyma over time, can be easily calculated at the bedside. Experimental and clinical data show it is associated with VILI and outcomes. In short, mechanical power might be considered as a potential tool to optimize ventilation settings in patients without ARDS and should be validated for this purpose in prospective observational and interventional studies.

References

1. Simonis FD, Serpa Neto A, Binnekade JM, et al. Effect of a low vs intermediate tidal volume strategy on ventilator-free days in intensive care unit patients without ARDS: a randomized clinical trial. JAMA. 2018;320:1872–80.
2. Schaefer MS, Serpa Neto A, Pelosi P, et al. Temporal changes in ventilator settings in patients with uninjured lungs: a systematic review. Anesth Analg. 2019;129:129–40.

3. Simonis FD, Barbas CSV, Artigas-Raventos A, et al. Potentially modifiable respiratory variables contributing to outcome in ICU patients without ARDS: a secondary analysis of PRoVENT. Ann Intensive Care. 2018;8:39.
4. Schmidt MFS, Amaral A, Fan E, et al. Driving pressure and hospital mortality in patients without ARDS: a cohort study. Chest. 2018;153:46–54.
5. Algera AG, Pisani L, Chaves RCF, et al. Effects of PEEP on lung injury, pulmonary function, systemic circulation and mortality in animals with uninjured lungs-a systematic review. Ann Transl Med. 2018;6:25.
6. Serpa Neto A, Filho RR, Cherpanath T, et al. Associations between positive end-expiratory pressure and outcome of patients without ARDS at onset of ventilation: a systematic review and meta-analysis of randomized controlled trials. Ann Intensive Care. 2016;6:109.
7. Algera AG, Pisani L, Bergmans DCJ, et al. RELAx—REstricted versus Liberal positive end-expiratory pressure in patients without ARDS: protocol for a randomized controlled trial. Trials. 2018;19:272.
8. Vaporidi K, Voloudakis G, Priniannakis G, et al. Effects of respiratory rate on ventilator-induced lung injury at a constant $PaCO_2$ in a mouse model of normal lung. Crit Care Med. 2008;36:1277–83.
9. Grasso S, Stripoli T, Mazzone P, et al. Low respiratory rate plus minimally invasive extracorporeal CO_2 removal decreases systemic and pulmonary inflammatory mediators in experimental acute respiratory distress syndrome. Crit Care Med. 2014;42:e451–60.
10. Huhle R, Serpa Neto A, Schultz MJ, et al. Is mechanical power the final word on ventilator-induced lung injury?—no. Ann Transl Med. 2018;6:394.
11. Silva PL, Ball L, Rocco PRM, Pelosi P. Power to mechanical power to minimize ventilator-induced lung injury? Intensive Care Med Exp. 2019;7(Suppl 1):38.
12. Gattinoni L, Tonetti T, Cressoni M, et al. Ventilator-related causes of lung injury: the mechanical power. Intensive Care Med. 2016;42:1567–75.
13. Serpa Neto A, Deliberato RO, Johnson AEW, et al. Mechanical power of ventilation is associated with mortality in critically ill patients: an analysis of patients in two observational cohorts. Intensive Care Med. 2018;44:1914–22.
14. Guldner A, Braune A, Ball L, et al. The authors reply. Crit Care Med. 2017;45:e328–e9.
15. Zhang Z, Zheng B, Liu N, et al. Mechanical power normalized to predicted body weight as a predictor of mortality in patients with acute respiratory distress syndrome. Intensive Care Med. 2019;45:856–64.
16. Gattinoni L, Tonetti T, Quintel M. Intensive care medicine in 2050: ventilator-induced lung injury. Intensive Care Med. 2018;44:76–8.
17. Becher T, van der Staay M, Schadler D, Frerichs I, Weiler N. Calculation of mechanical power for pressure-controlled ventilation. Intensive Care Med. 2019;45:1321–3.
18. van der Meijden S, Molenaar M, Somhorst P, Schoe A. Calculating mechanical power for pressure-controlled ventilation. Intensive Care Med. 2019;45:1495–7.
19. Becher T, van der Staay M. Calculation of mechanical power for pressure-controlled ventilation: author's reply. Intensive Care Med. 2019;45:1498–9.
20. Esteban A, Frutos-Vivar F, Muriel A, et al. Evolution of mortality over time in patients receiving mechanical ventilation. Am J Respir Crit Care Med. 2013;188:220–30.
21. van der Staay M, Chatburn RL. Advanced modes of mechanical ventilation and optimal targeting schemes. Intensive Care Med Exp. 2018;6:30.
22. Wolfson MR, Bhutani VK, Shaffer TH, Bowen FW Jr. Mechanics and energetics of breathing helium in infants with bronchopulmonary dysplasia. J Pediatr. 1984;104:752–7.
23. Kao LC, Durand DJ, Nickerson BG. Improving pulmonary function does not decrease oxygen consumption in infants with bronchopulmonary dysplasia. J Pediatr. 1988;112:616–21.
24. Magalhaes PAF, Padilha GA, Moraes L, et al. Effects of pressure support ventilation on ventilator-induced lung injury in mild acute respiratory distress syndrome depend on level of positive end-expiratory pressure: a randomised animal study. Eur J Anaesthesiol. 2018;35:298–306.
25. Cressoni M, Gotti M, Chiurazzi C, et al. Mechanical power and development of ventilator-induced lung injury. Anesthesiology. 2016;124:1100–8.

26. Santos RS, Maia LA, Oliveira MV, et al. Biologic impact of mechanical power at high and low tidal volumes in experimental mild acute respiratory distress syndrome. Anesthesiology. 2018;128:1193–206.
27. Guerin C, Papazian L, Reignier J, et al. Effect of driving pressure on mortality in ARDS patients during lung protective mechanical ventilation in two randomized controlled trials. Crit Care. 2016;20:384.
28. Marini JJ, Jaber S. Dynamic predictors of VILI risk: beyond the driving pressure. Intensive Care Med. 2016;42:1597–600.
29. Moraes L, Silva PL, Thompson A, et al. Impact of different tidal volume levels at low mechanical power on ventilator-induced lung injury in rats. Front Physiol. 2018;9:318.
30. Collino F, Rapetti F, Vasques F, et al. Positive end-expiratory pressure and mechanical power. Anesthesiology. 2019;130:119–30.
31. Felix NS, Samary CS, Cruz FF, et al. Gradually increasing tidal volume may mitigate experimental lung injury in rats. Anesthesiology. 2019;130:767–77.
32. Marini JJ. Evolving concepts for safer ventilation. Crit Care. 2019;23(Suppl 1):114.
33. Fuller BM, Page D, Stephens RJ, et al. Pulmonary mechanics and mortality in mechanically ventilated patients without acute respiratory distress syndrome: a cohort study. Shock. 2018;49:311–6.

Part II

Acute Respiratory Distress Syndrome

Extracellular Vesicles in ARDS: New Insights into Pathogenesis with Novel Clinical Applications

4

R. Y. Mahida, S. Matsumoto, and M. A. Matthay

4.1 Introduction

Acute respiratory distress syndrome (ARDS) is an inflammatory disorder of the lungs that can develop following various insults, the commonest being pneumonia. Patients develop acute hypoxemic respiratory failure following inflammatory injury to the alveolar epithelium and endothelium [1]. The precipitating injury can be direct (e.g., pneumonia, aspiration) or indirect (e.g., peritonitis, pancreatitis, shock). Our understanding of ARDS pathogenesis has increased in the 50 years since this syndrome was first described; however, there are many aspects which continue to elude us [1]. Following the same insult, why do some patients develop ARDS and others do not? How can we predict which critically ill patients are at higher risk of developing ARDS? Advances in ventilation strategies [2] and fluid management have helped to reduce mortality; however, this still remains unacceptably high at 35–45% [3].

R. Y. Mahida
Cardiovascular Research Institute, University of California-San Francisco, San Francisco, CA, USA

Birmingham Acute Care Research Group, Institute of Inflammation and Ageing, University of Birmingham, Birmingham, UK

S. Matsumoto
Cardiovascular Research Institute, University of California-San Francisco, San Francisco, CA, USA

Department of Intensive Care Medicine, Tokyo Medical and Dental University, Tokyo, Japan

M. A. Matthay (✉)
Cardiovascular Research Institute, University of California-San Francisco, San Francisco, CA, USA

Department of Medicine, University of California-San Francisco, San Francisco, CA, USA

Department of Anesthesia, University of California-San Francisco, San Francisco, CA, USA
e-mail: Michael.matthay@ucsf.edu

Despite numerous clinical trials, there is still no effective pharmacotherapy available for ARDS patients. However, the rapidly developing field of extracellular vesicles may provide a major new opportunity for an improved understanding of ARDS pathogenesis, valuable biomarkers of injury, and targets for new therapies.

Extracellular vesicles are anuclear structures released by cells and bounded by a phospholipid bilayer membrane. Cells can release extracellular vesicles during states of health, injury/activation, and apoptosis. Extracellular vesicles can contain diverse cargo, including messenger RNA (mRNA), micro RNA (miR), cytokines, and mitochondria. Surface markers on extracellular vesicles can indicate the parent cell from which they were derived, and also determine which cells can incorporate specific extracellular vesicles. We are now beginning to appreciate the role extracellular vesicles play in intercellular communication in health and disease states, facilitating transfer of genetic material, proteins, and organelles between cell types. Distinctions between the two main subtypes of extracellular vesicles are based on size and origin: exosomes are smaller (<150 nm diameter) and may have an endosomal origin. Microvesicles are larger (up to 1 μm diameter) and derived from the cell membrane.

In this chapter, we highlight recent translational and clinical studies that have deepened our understanding of the role extracellular vesicles play in both mediating and attenuating inflammatory lung injury in ARDS. We discuss what future directions can be taken to utilize extracellular vesicles as diagnostic or prognostic biomarkers, as targets for novel therapeutics, or as therapeutic agents in their own right (Fig. 4.1).

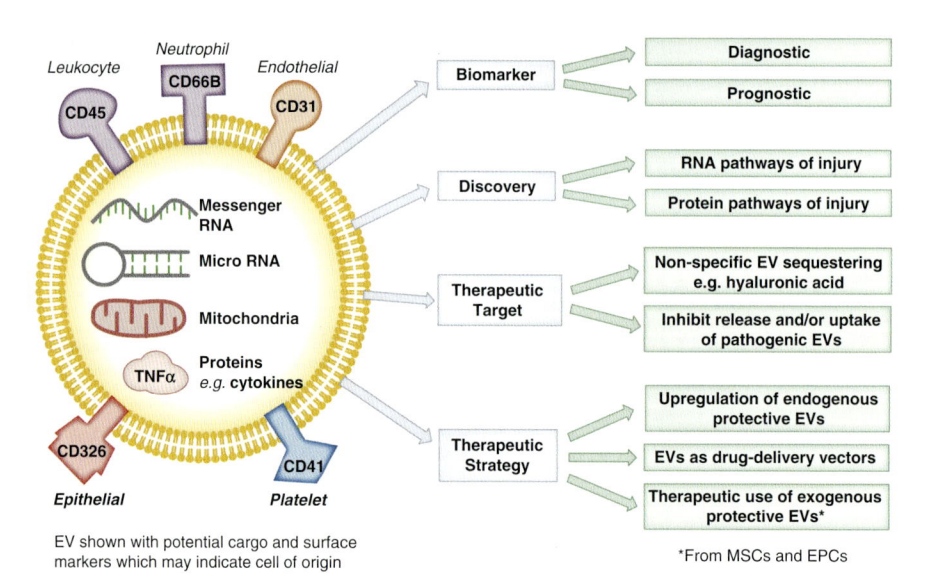

Fig. 4.1 Clinical relevance and applications of extracellular vesicles in acute respiratory distress syndrome (ARDS). Representative extracellular vesicle (EV) shown with phospholipid bilayer, surface markers, and cargo. Surface markers indicate cell of origin (e.g., CD45$^+$/CD66b$^+$ indicates a neutrophil-derived extracellular vesicle, CD31$^+$ endothelial-derived, CD41$^+$ platelet-derived, and CD326$^+$ epithelial-derived). Surface markers from different cell types shown for illustrative purposes; extracellular vesicles will not concurrently express all surface markers shown. Extracellular vesicle cargo can include micro RNA, messenger RNA, mitochondria, and protein (e.g., cytokines). *EPC* endothelial progenitor cell, *MSC* mesenchymal stem cell, *TNF-α* tumor necrosis factor-α

4.2 Contribution of Extracellular Vesicles to the Pathogenesis of ARDS

Preclinical models of ARDS have shown that extracellular vesicles released following lung injury can mediate inflammation and have an injurious effect. Endothelial injury is often the earliest pathological event leading to the development of ARDS [4]. Circulating endothelial and leukocyte-derived extracellular vesicles are elevated in the intratracheal lipopolysaccharide (LPS) rat model of lung injury [5]. Human endothelial cells also release extracellular vesicles following stimulation with plasminogen-activated inhibitor-1 [6]. Several studies have reported that intravenous administration of endothelial extracellular vesicles in rodents induced lung injury with alveolar neutrophilic infiltration, pulmonary edema, elevated inflammatory cytokines (myeloperoxidase [MPO], interleukin [IL]-1β and tumor necrosis factor [TNF]-α), and increased lung endothelial permeability [6–8]. These changes were similar to those observed following intratracheal LPS injury. Endothelial extracellular vesicle treatment of murine or human arterioles impaired nitric oxide release and vasodilation, which partly explains the *in vivo* findings [6]. Endothelial extracellular vesicles administered concurrently with LPS (intratracheal or intravenous) caused a greater increase in alveolar endothelial permeability and inflammatory cytokine release than either LPS or extracellular vesicles alone [6, 7]. However, when endothelial extracellular vesicles were administered 6 h prior to intravenous LPS, the resulting circulating and alveolar inflammatory cytokine release was significantly greater than with concurrent administration of extracellular vesicles and LPS. An initial endothelial injury triggered release of endothelial extracellular vesicles, which then primed the lung for a greater inflammatory response when exposed to a subsequent infectious insult.

Following LPS treatment, human endothelial cells release extracellular vesicles containing nitrated sphingosine-1-phosphate receptor-3 (S1PR3) [9]. Elevated circulating S1PR3 concentrations are associated with mortality in critically ill sepsis patients, with or without ARDS. Endothelial extracellular vesicles could therefore represent a potential biomarker and/or offer a novel therapeutic target for ARDS. Simvastatin treatment given concurrently with intravenous LPS in mice reduced endothelial extracellular vesicle release and lung endothelial permeability [10]. This is a particularly interesting finding, since a secondary analysis of an ARDS trial showed that simvastatin reduced mortality in patients with a hyperinflammatory endotype, suggesting that statin therapy was working in part by inhibiting extracellular vesicle release and lung injury [11]. Therefore, therapies aimed at reducing or blocking endothelial extracellular vesicles may attenuate lung injury.

Recently, the results of studies in the *ex vivo* perfused human lung model have provided compelling new evidence for the potential role of extracellular vesicles in mediating lung injury in ARDS. In an *ex vivo* perfused human lung model of Gram negative pneumonia, injury with intrabronchial *Escherichia coli* led to release of extracellular vesicles by lung tissue into the perfusate [12]; these extracellular vesicles were predominantly endothelial- and platelet-derived. Administration of *E. coli*-induced extracellular vesicles either into the perfusate or into the air spaces in naïve, uninjured human lungs induced injury similar to the degree of lung injury with *E. coli* pneumonia: pulmonary edema, impaired alveolar fluid clearance, neutrophilic infiltration, and elevated bronchoalveolar lavage fluid (BALF) TNF-α. E. coli-induced extracellular vesicles contained high levels of TNF-α and IL-6 mRNA, which explained at least part of their pro-inflammatory effects. Monocyte uptake of E. coli-induced extracellular vesicles resulted in increased secretion of TNF-α and IL-6. High molecular weight hyaluronic acid bound CD44 on the surface of E. coli-induced extracellular vesicles, thus preventing their uptake by monocytes. Intravenous administration of high molecular weight hyaluronic acid to ex vivo human lungs injured with E. coli or E. coli-induced extracellular vesicles attenuated lung injury, pulmonary edema, BALF TNF-α levels, and histologic evidence of lung injury. This important study showed that following infectious injury, human lung tissue releases pathogenic extracellular vesicles, which can mediate more severe inflammatory lung injury. The results suggest that strategies to sequester extracellular vesicles could prevent their uptake and biologic cargo delivery to target cells, thereby reducing subsequent inflammatory injury; extracellular vesicle sequestration may therefore offer a therapeutic strategy in ARDS.

ARDS patients have a higher total concentration of alveolar extracellular vesicles, compared to control patients with hydrostatic edema [13]. A significant proportion of alveolar extracellular vesicles in ARDS patients are derived from alveolar epithelial cells; these extracellular vesicles contain higher concentrations of tissue factor and exert a pro-coagulant effect. Alveolar epithelial cell-derived extracellular vesicles may therefore also contribute to the increased pro-coagulant activity observed in ARDS and thereby represent a therapeutic target.

Different alveolar cell types release extracellular vesicles in sequential order following murine intratracheal LPS lung injury [14]. Alveolar macrophage-derived extracellular vesicles are rapidly released first, followed by endothelial extracellular vesicles and then neutrophil extracellular vesicles. This temporal difference in BALF extracellular vesicles release by different alveolar cell types may give insight into the pathological mechanisms underpinning ARDS. Alveolar macrophage-derived extracellular vesicle release may subsequently trigger pro-inflammatory extracellular vesicle release by epithelial cells and neutrophils. The alveolar macrophage extracellular vesicles can deliver high concentrations of TNF-α cargo to alveolar epithelial cells, resulting in increased production of the neutrophil chemotactic factor keratinocyte-derived cytokine (KC) and expression of intercellular adhesion molecule-1 (ICAM-1). BALF extracellular vesicles generated from intratracheal LPS treated mice resulted in lung injury when they were administered intratracheally to naïve mice, with increased alveolar neutrophil infiltration, alveolar protein permeability, and elevated BALF KC levels. Administration of these pathogenic BALF extracellular vesicles caused lung injury similar to LPS treatment. Alveolar macrophage extracellular vesicles containing TNF-α may play a significant role in instigating the inflammatory cascade in early ARDS; therefore alveolar macrophage extracellular vesicles should be considered as potential novel biomarkers and/or therapeutic targets.

Different modalities of lung injury can induce release of extracellular vesicles from different cell types. One group found that following sterile lung injury, most BALF extracellular vesicles were derived from type 1 alveolar epithelial cells [15]. However, following infectious lung injury, most BALF extracellular vesicles were derived from alveolar macrophages. BALF extracellular vesicles generated from both sterile and infectious lung injury models promoted the recruitment of macrophages to the alveolar space. Sterile lung injury BALF extracellular vesicles (predominantly alveolar epithelial cell-derived) upregulated Toll-like receptor (TLR)2 and downregulated TLR8 expression in macrophages. Infectious lung injury BALF extracellular vesicles (predominantly alveolar macrophage-derived) upregulated TLR6 on macrophages. Differential effects on cytokine release were also observed with BALF extracellular vesicles: sterile injury extracellular vesicles upregulated alveolar macrophage release of IL-6 and TNF-α, whereas infectious injury extracellular vesicles upregulated IL-1β and IL-10 release by alveolar macrophages. BALF extracellular vesicles generated following different modalities of lung injury promote inflammation via different pathways.

Remarkably, mouse models have indicated that release of extracellular vesicles following distant injury, e.g., traumatic brain injury [16] or trauma and hemorrhagic shock [17], can mediate lung injury. Following trauma and hemorrhagic shock, gut-derived extracellular vesicles were released into the mesenteric lymphatic system. Intravenous administration of these extracellular vesicles to naïve mice caused lung injury via macrophage TLR4 activation, including increased alveolar vascular permeability and inflammatory cell infiltration [17]. These findings indicate that similar mechanisms may be present in patients who develop ARDS following similar distant (indirect) insults. This pathway might explain in part the development of neurogenic pulmonary edema as well as lung injury following shock and ischemia-reperfusion.

Following lung injury, pro-inflammatory miRNAs can be transported between cells by extracellular vesicles. One group found that miR-17-5p was upregulated in BALF extracellular vesicles from patients with influenza A-induced ARDS; these extracellular vesicles were likely alveolar epithelial cell-derived. When influenza A infected alveolar epithelial cells were transfected with miR-17-5p, this downregulated expression of the antiviral factor MX1 and increased viral replication [18]. Other investigators found that BALF extracellular vesicles contained high concentrations of miR-466 in intratracheal-LPS mice [19]. Transfection of macrophages with miR-466 was found to upregulate the nucleotide-binding oligomerization like receptor 3 (NLRP3) inflammasome, and stimulate increased release of IL-1β following LPS stimulation.

By learning how endogenous extracellular vesicles mediate inflammation and increase endothelial and epithelial permeability, it will be possible to gain greater insight into the protein and RNA pathways involved in the pathogenesis of ARDS. These pathogenic extracellular vesicles can be utilized as diagnostic/prognostic biomarkers, or as targets for novel therapeutic strategies.

4.3 Potential Endogenous Protective Effects of Extracellular Vesicles in ARDS

In the prior section, we discussed the evidence for how extracellular vesicles may contribute to ARDS pathogenesis; these harmful extracellular vesicles are predominantly derived from specific cell types (endothelium, alveolar epithelial cells, and alveolar macrophages). There is also evidence to suggest that extracellular vesicles from other cell types may have a protective, anti-inflammatory role in the context of ARDS. Clinical studies investigating harmful and protective extracellular vesicles in ARDS patients are summarized in Table 4.1.

The data suggest that extracellular vesicles within a given biofluid cannot be considered as a homogenous entity; the origin and cargo of extracellular vesicles from different cell types at different stages of ARDS are likely to have divergent effects. Heterogeneity in cellular function and transcriptome has been shown to impact on patient outcomes in sepsis-related ARDS [20]. It is therefore likely that heterogeneity in extracellular vesicle profiles will similarly impact on patient outcome.

Table 4.1 Clinical studies investigating protective and pathological extracellular vesicles in patients with acute respiratory syndrome (ARDS)

Author [Ref.]	Cell origin	Biofluid	Patient cohort	Extracellular vesicle effect
Pathological extracellular vesicles				
Bastarache et al. [13]	Epithelial	BALF	11 ARDS patients and 13 hydrostatic edema patients	Epithelial extracellular vesicles are present at higher concentrations in ARDS patient BALF. Epithelial extracellular vesicles are enriched for tissue factor and likely contribute to increased pro-coagulant activity
Sun et al. [9]	Endothelial	Plasma	23 sepsis-related ARDS, 24 sepsis without ARDS and 19 non-sepsis patients	Elevated concentrations of endothelial extracellular vesicles containing S1PR3 are associated with increased mortality in ARDS patients
Scheller et al. [18]	Epithelial	BALF	6 Influenza A H1N1-induced ARDS patients	Influenza A induced ARDS patients have elevated concentrations of epithelial extracellular vesicles containing miR-17-5p. This miR increases viral replication within alveolar epithelial cells
Protective extracellular vesicles				
Guervilly et al. [21]	Leukocyte Neutrophil Endothelial Platelet	BALF Plasma	52 ARDS patients, 10 non-ARDS ventilated ICU patients and 12 spontaneously breathing patients	Leukocyte and neutrophil extracellular vesicle concentrations were elevated in ARDS patient BALF. In early ARDS, elevated BALF and plasma concentrations of leukocyte extracellular vesicles were associated with increased survival and VFDs
Neudecker et al. [26]	Neutrophil	BALF	55 ARDS patients	Neutrophil extracellular vesicles transfer miR-223 to alveolar epithelial cells, reducing permeability and inflammatory cytokine release
Shaver et al. [22]	All	Plasma	280 ICU patients at risk of ARDS. Of these 90 developed ARDS	Elevated plasma extracellular vesicle concentrations on ICU admission were associated with a lower risk of developing ARDS

BALF bronchoalveolar lavage fluid, *ICU* intensive care unit, *miR* micro ribonucleic acid, *S1PR3* sphingosine-1-phosphate receptor-3, *VFDs* ventilator-free days

Some clinical studies have reported that total leukocyte extracellular vesicle numbers are associated with a better prognosis in ARDS patients. An observational study characterized BALF and circulating extracellular vesicles from 52 ventilated patients with ARDS; control groups included ventilated patients without ARDS, and non-ventilated patients undergoing outpatient bronchoscopy [21]. The majority (90%) of ARDS patients had direct lung injury; 73% had pneumonia. The BALF from ARDS patients contained elevated leukocyte- and neutrophil-derived extracellular vesicles compared to controls. In early ARDS, elevated BALF and plasma concentrations of leukocyte extracellular vesicles were associated with increased survival and ventilator-free days, thus suggesting a potential role for BALF and serum leukocyte extracellular vesicles as prognostic biomarkers in early ARDS. In a separate study, total plasma extracellular vesicle concentrations were measured in 280 critically ill patients on intensive care unit (ICU) admission; 90 of these patients subsequently developed ARDS [22]. Elevated plasma extracellular vesicle concentrations were associated with a lower risk of developing ARDS; this association was seen most strongly in patients admitted to ICU with sepsis. Another group of investigators [23] found that a subset of circulating leukocyte extracellular vesicles expressing α2-macroglobulin (A2MG) were associated with survival in ICU patients with sepsis secondary to pneumonia, but not in patients with sepsis secondary to fecal peritonitis. A2MG-EV treatment *in vitro* reduced endothelial cell permeability and increased bacterial phagocytosis by neutrophils.

Several studies have revealed a protective role for neutrophil extracellular vesicles in lung injury. Binding of neutrophil extracellular vesicles to Mer tyrosine kinase (MerTK) receptors on macrophages increased secretion of the pro-repair factor TGFβ and decreased secretion of pro-inflammatory cytokines TNF-α and IL-8 [24, 25]. Therefore, neutrophil extracellular vesicles have an anti-inflammatory effect on macrophages. Neutrophil extracellular vesicles containing miR-223 were found to have an anti-inflammatory effect on alveolar epithelial cells, via suppression of poly(adenosine diphosphate-ribose) polymerase-1 [26]. In murine staphylococcal or ventilator-induced lung injury (VILI), intratracheal delivery of extracellular vesicles containing miR-223 reduces inflammatory cytokine release, alveolar protein permeability, and lung injury. Infiltration of neutrophils into the alveolar space is a hallmark of ARDS pathogenesis, and their pro-inflammatory role is established [27]. However, this evidence suggests that neutrophils may also have a concurrent anti-inflammatory role, via release of extracellular vesicles that modulate alveolar macrophage and alveolar epithelial cell functions.

Innate mechanisms that inhibit release or promote clearance of pro-inflammatory extracellular vesicles may be present in ARDS patients. Alveolar macrophages can phagocytose inflammatory BALF extracellular vesicles via MerTK binding, to prevent their uptake by alveolar epithelial cells [28]. The inflammatory BALF extracellular vesicles have a more injurious effect on alveolar epithelial cells compared to alveolar macrophages. As discussed in the previous section, LPS-stimulated macrophages release extracellular vesicles containing TNF-α, which can initiate an inflammatory cascade. LPS-stimulated alveolar epithelial cells can release IL-25, which acts on macrophages to suppress release of inflammatory extracellular vesicles containing TNF-α [29]. Strategies to enhance IL-25 signaling or alveolar macrophage phagocytosis of extracellular vesicles may have therapeutic benefit in ARDS.

Subsets of leukocyte-derived extracellular vesicles appear to have a protective role in ARDS, which may be related to delivery of anti-inflammatory miRNAs. Mechanisms also exist to either inhibit inflammatory extracellular vesicle release or prevent their uptake by susceptible cell types. Therapeutic strategies to upregulate innate protective extracellular vesicles or enhance existing protective mechanisms may attenuate inflammation in ARDS.

4.4 Benefits of Extracellular Vesicles Derived from Mesenchymal Stromal Cells and Endothelial Progenitor Cells in ARDS Models

Extracellular vesicles derived from non-pulmonary cell types can have a protective effect in some models of ARDS. Mesenchymal stromal cells (MSCs) can attenuate inflammation and lung injury in preclinical models of ARDS, due to their intrinsic anti-inflammatory abilities [30]. Mesenchymal stromal cells mediate their effects via cell-cell contact and via release of paracrine factors; administration of mesenchymal stromal cell conditioned media was previously shown to attenuate lung injury in intratracheal-LPS injured mice [31]. Mesenchymal stromal cell-derived extracellular vesicles isolated from conditioned media attenuated inflammation and lung injury in both intratracheal-LPS and *E. coli* pneumonia models of murine lung injury [32, 33]. Prophylactic treatment with mesenchymal stromal cell extracellular vesicles increased survival in rats undergoing traumatic lung injury; inflammatory cytokines, infiltrating leukocytes, and pulmonary edema were all reduced [34]. These effects were in part due to mesenchymal stromal cell extracellular vesicle transfer of miR-124 [34]. In a pig model of influenza-induced lung injury, administration of mesenchymal stromal cell extracellular vesicles similarly reduced lung injury, alveolar protein permeability, and inflammatory cytokine release. Mesenchymal stromal cell extracellular vesicle treatment of alveolar epithelial cells reduced viral replication and virus-induced apoptosis. In addition, an experimental model of infant respiratory distress syndrome and bronchopulmonary dysplasia in newborn mice showed a therapeutic effect of extracellular vesicles isolated from mesenchymal stromal cells in reducing lung injury and restoring lung function, in part through induction of anti-inflammatory and pro-resolving macrophages [35].

Mesenchymal stromal cell extracellular vesicles can transfer mitochondria to alveolar macrophages, inducing a modified M2 (pro-resolving) phenotype [36]. Mesenchymal stromal cells stimulated with IL-1β release extracellular vesicles containing miR-146a, which also induces an M2 macrophage phenotype [37]. These mesenchymal stromal cell extracellular vesicle modified alveolar macrophages have pro-resolving characteristics (increased secretion of anti-inflammatory cytokine IL-10, reduced secretion of inflammatory cytokines TNF-α and IL-8), but also increased phagocytic activity against bacteria [31, 36, 38, 39]. Mesenchymal stromal cell extracellular vesicles modulate alveolar macrophages to clear bacteria more effectively, while minimizing surrounding tissue injury.

Mesenchymal stromal cell extracellular vesicles also contain mRNA for keratinocyte growth factor (KGF) and angiopoetin-1, which can be transferred to alveolar epithelial cells and endothelial cells [32, 40], thereby increasing the integrity of the alveolar-capillary barrier. These findings explain the ability of mesenchymal stromal cell extracellular vesicles to restore alveolar fluid clearance in *ex vivo* human lungs [41]. In an *E. coli* pneumonia model using *ex vivo* human lungs, administration of mesenchymal stromal cell extracellular vesicles reduced bacterial load within the alveolar space, reduced protein permeability, and increased alveolar fluid clearance [42]. Mouse studies indicated that mesenchymal stromal cell extracellular vesicle transfer of miR-145 to macrophages was responsible for the increased bacterial phagocytosis [43].

Endothelial progenitor cells (EPCs) also release extracellular vesicles that have a protective role in lung injury. Endothelial progenitor cells release extracellular vesicles containing miR-126, which are taken up by endothelial cells [44], resulting in enhanced endothelial cell proliferation, migration, angiogenesis, and transepithelial electrical resistance. Administration of endothelial progenitor cell extracellular vesicles decreased lung injury, hypoxia, alveolar cell count, protein permeability, pulmonary edema, and inflammatory cytokines in the murine intratracheal-LPS model [44, 45]. Work in human small airway epithelial cells found that miR-126 could increase expression of tight junction proteins [45]. Therefore, endothelial progenitor cell extracellular vesicles containing miR-126 have a protective effect on both the epithelium and endothelium in models of ARDS.

Mesenchymal stromal cells and endothelial progenitor cells mediate their anti-inflammatory and pro-repair effects in part by release of extracellular vesicles, which deliver miRNA, mRNA, and mitochondrial cargo to different alveolar cell types. Administration of mesenchymal stromal cell extracellular vesicles or endothelial progenitor cell extracellular vesicles may therefore offer a novel therapeutic strategy for ARDS patients.

4.5 Clinical Applications for Extracellular Vesicles in ARDS

As summarized in Fig. 4.1, extracellular vesicles have wide-ranging potential clinical applications in ARDS. Extracellular vesicles from specific cell types could be used as diagnostic or prognostic biomarkers. Human endothelial extracellular vesicles can induce lung injury in mice [6], and a subset of endothelial extracellular vesicles has been associated with mortality in ARDS patients [9]. Therefore, endothelial extracellular vesicles could be used as diagnostic and prognostic biomarkers in ARDS. By understanding how extracellular vesicles mediate intercellular transfer of genetic material, organelles, and proteins between different cell types in the alveolar space, it will be possible to learn how the RNA and protein pathways of injury are involved in ARDS pathogenesis.

Circulating and BALF pathogenic extracellular vesicles offer therapeutic targets in ARDS. Studies have thus far identified endothelial- and alveolar macrophage-derived extracellular vesicles as having the ability to induce lung injury [6, 14]. Therapeutic targeting of pathogenic extracellular vesicles could prevent transfer of pro-inflammatory genetic material and proteins to target cells. Nonspecific extracellular vesicle sequestering with hyaluronic acid [46] would target all extracellular vesicles expressing CD44 (a widely expressed glycoprotein), but has a potential disadvantage of sequestering both pathogenic and beneficial extracellular vesicles.

Alveolar macrophages can phagocytose pathogenic extracellular vesicles via MerTK receptors, thereby preventing extracellular vesicle uptake by alveolar epithelial cells and subsequent inflammatory injury [28]. Therapeutic strategies to upregulate MerTK expression on alveolar macrophages may aid uptake of pathogenic extracellular vesicles and attenuate inflammation in ARDS. Strategies to inhibit pathogenic extracellular vesicle release also require consideration: alveolar epithelial cells can release IL-25 to inhibit the release of pathogenic alveolar macrophage extracellular vesicles [29]. Simvastatin can inhibit the release of pathogenic endothelial extracellular vesicles in murine models of lung injury [10] and this may be relevant in the setting of ARDS [11]. Surprisingly, neutrophil extracellular vesicles have been shown to have an anti-inflammatory role in sepsis and ARDS [25, 26]. Therefore, strategies to stimulate extracellular vesicle release by neutrophils *in vivo* or administration of neutrophil extracellular vesicles generated *ex vivo* could be considered.

Extracellular vesicles derived from exogenous mesenchymal stromal cells and endothelial progenitor cells mediate the anti-inflammatory actions of the parent cell by delivery of mitochondria, genetic material, and proteins to injured alveolar cells. As described above, therapeutic use of mesenchymal stromal cell extracellular vesicles has shown efficacy at reducing lung injury in several preclinical models. In mouse models of lung injury, mesenchymal stromal cell extracellular vesicles have similar efficacy to mesenchymal stromal cells themselves. Finally, exogenous extracellular vesicles could be modified to package custom drugs or protective RNA cargo, which could be delivered to specific cell types as determined by the extracellular vesicle surface markers [47].

4.6 Future Directions

Several studies that have investigated the role of extracellular vesicles in acute lung injury and ARDS have been done in animal and *in vitro* models, although one recent study was done in the *ex vivo* perfused human lung [12], and there are a few clinical studies as well [13, 18, 21–23]. Future studies will need to characterize BALF and circulating extracellular vesicles from ARDS patients with regard to the cell of origin, cargo assessment (RNA, protein, organelle content), and their biological effect on human cells and human tissues. Standardized methods of biologic fluid collections and RNA isolation from extracellular vesicles are now possible, so that the data will be comparable and generalizable [48]. Extracellular vesicle profiles from ARDS patients will need to be compared with those from animal models and *ex vivo* human lung models in order to determine how well the extracellular vesicles released in these models correlate with those observed in the clinical setting of ARDS. Clinical studies to test the utility of extracellular vesicles as diagnostic and prognostic biomarkers in ARDS patients will be needed. Clinical trials of mesenchymal stromal cell extracellular vesicles are needed to determine therapeutic utility in patients with ARDS as well as infant respiratory distress syndrome and bronchopulmonary dysplasia.

4.7 Conclusions

Extracellular vesicles constitute an important intercellular communication mechanism, which allows targeted transfer of biologic cargo including RNA, micro RNA, proteins, and mitochondria between different cell types. New evidence indicates that extracellular vesicles are likely to be critical to the induction and resolution of injury in ARDS. Consequently, it is likely that there will be a wide range of clinical applications for extracellular vesicles, ranging from use as biomarkers to therapeutic agents for ARDS.

References

1. Matthay MA, Zemans RL, Zimmerman GA, et al. Acute respiratory distress syndrome. Nat Rev Dis Primers. 2019;5:18.
2. Chiumello D, Brochard L, Marini JJ, et al. Respiratory support in patients with acute respiratory distress syndrome: an expert opinion. Crit Care. 2017;21:240.
3. Bellani G, Laffey JG, Pham T, et al. Epidemiology, patterns of care, and mortality for patients with acute respiratory distress syndrome in intensive care units in 50 countries. JAMA. 2016;315:788–800.
4. Matthay MA, Zemans RL. The acute respiratory distress syndrome: pathogenesis and treatment. Annu Rev Pathol. 2011;6:147–63.
5. Li H, Meng X, Gao Y, Cai S. Isolation and phenotypic characteristics of microparticles in acute respiratory distress syndrome. Int J Clin Exp Pathol. 2015;8:1640–8.
6. Densmore JC, Signorino PR, Ou J, et al. Endothelium-derived microparticles induce endothelial dysfunction and acute lung injury. Shock. 2006;26:464–71.
7. Buesing KL, Densmore JC, Kaul S, et al. Endothelial microparticles induce inflammation in acute lung injury. J Surg Res. 2011;166:32–9.
8. Li H, Meng X, Liang X, Gao Y, Cai S. Administration of microparticles from blood of the lipopolysaccharide-treated rats serves to induce pathologic changes of acute respiratory distress syndrome. Exp Biol Med (Maywood). 2015;240:1735–41.
9. Sun X, Singleton PA, Letsiou E, et al. Sphingosine-1-phosphate receptor-3 is a novel biomarker in acute lung injury. Am J Respir Cell Mol Biol. 2012;47:628–36.
10. Yu Y, Jing L, Zhang X, Gao C. Simvastatin attenuates acute lung injury via regulating CDC42-PAK4 and endothelial microparticles. Shock. 2017;47:378–84.
11. Calfee CS, Delucchi KL, Sinha P, et al. Acute respiratory distress syndrome subphenotypes and differential response to simvastatin: secondary analysis of a randomised controlled trial. Lancet Respir Med. 2018;6:691–8.
12. Liu A, Park JH, Zhang X, et al. Therapeutic effects of hyaluronic acid in bacterial pneumonia in the ex vivo perfused human lungs. Am J Respir Crit Care Med. 2019;200:1234–45.

13. Bastarache JA, Fremont RD, Kropski JA, Bossert FR, Ware LB. Procoagulant alveolar microparticles in the lungs of patients with acute respiratory distress syndrome. Am J Physiol Lung Cell Mol Physiol. 2009;297:L1035–41.
14. Soni S, Wilson MR, O'Dea KP, et al. Alveolar macrophage-derived microvesicles mediate acute lung injury. Thorax. 2016;71:1020–9.
15. Lee H, Zhang D, Laskin DL, Jin Y. Functional evidence of pulmonary extracellular vesicles in infectious and noninfectious lung inflammation. J Immunol. 2018;201:1500–9.
16. Kerr NA, de Rivero Vaccari JP, Abbassi S, et al. Traumatic brain injury-induced acute lung injury: evidence for activation and inhibition of a neural-respiratory-inflammasome axis. J Neurotrauma. 2018;35:2067–76.
17. Kojima M, Gimenes-Junior JA, Chan TW, et al. Exosomes in postshock mesenteric lymph are key mediators of acute lung injury triggering the macrophage activation via Toll-like receptor 4. FASEB J. 2018;32:97–110.
18. Scheller N, Herold S, Kellner R, et al. Proviral microRNAs detected in extracellular vesicles from bronchoalveolar lavage fluid of patients with influenza virus-induced acute respiratory distress syndrome. J Infect Dis. 2019;219:540–3.
19. Shikano S, Gon Y, Maruoka S, et al. Increased extracellular vesicle miRNA-466 family in the bronchoalveolar lavage fluid as a precipitating factor of ARDS. BMC Pulm Med. 2019;19:110.
20. Leligdowicz A, Matthay MA. Heterogeneity in sepsis: new biological evidence with clinical applications. Crit Care. 2019;23:80.
21. Guervilly C, Lacroix R, Forel JM, et al. High levels of circulating leukocyte microparticles are associated with better outcome in acute respiratory distress syndrome. Crit Care. 2011;15:R31.
22. Shaver CM, Woods J, Clune JK, et al. Circulating microparticle levels are reduced in patients with ARDS. Crit Care. 2017;21:120.
23. Lashin HMS, Nadkarni S, Oggero S, et al. Microvesicle subsets in sepsis due to community acquired pneumonia compared to faecal peritonitis. Shock. 2018;49:393–401.
24. Eken C, Martin PJ, Sadallah S, Treves S, Schaller M, Schifferli JA. Ectosomes released by polymorphonuclear neutrophils induce a MerTK-dependent anti-inflammatory pathway in macrophages. J Biol Chem. 2010;285:39914–21.
25. Gasser O, Schifferli JA. Activated polymorphonuclear neutrophils disseminate anti-inflammatory microparticles by ectocytosis. Blood. 2004;104:2543–8.
26. Neudecker V, Brodsky KS, Clambey ET, et al. Neutrophil transfer of miR-223 to lung epithelial cells dampens acute lung injury in mice. Sci Transl Med. 2017;9:eaah5360.
27. Mikacenic C, Moore R, Dmyterko V, et al. Neutrophil extracellular traps (NETs) are increased in the alveolar spaces of patients with ventilator-associated pneumonia. Crit Care. 2018;22:358.
28. Mohning MP, Thomas SM, Barthel L, et al. Phagocytosis of microparticles by alveolar macrophages during acute lung injury requires MerTK. Am J Physiol Lung Cell Mol Physiol. 2018;314:L69–82.
29. Li ZG, Scott MJ, Brzoska T, et al. Lung epithelial cell-derived IL-25 negatively regulates LPS-induced exosome release from macrophages. Mil Med Res. 2018;5:24.
30. Laffey JG, Matthay MA. Fifty years of research in ARDS. Cell-based therapy for acute respiratory distress syndrome. Biology and potential therapeutic value. Am J Respir Crit Care Med. 2017;196:266–73.
31. Ionescu L, Byrne RN, van Haaften T, et al. Stem cell conditioned medium improves acute lung injury in mice: in vivo evidence for stem cell paracrine action. Am J Physiol Lung Cell Mol Physiol. 2012;303:L967–77.
32. Zhu YG, Feng XM, Abbott J, et al. Human mesenchymal stem cell microvesicles for treatment of Escherichia coli endotoxin-induced acute lung injury in mice. Stem Cells. 2014;32:116–25.
33. Monsel A, Zhu YG, Gennai S, et al. Therapeutic effects of human mesenchymal stem cell-derived microvesicles in severe pneumonia in mice. Am J Respir Crit Care Med. 2015;192:324–36.
34. Li QC, Liang Y, Su ZB. Prophylactic treatment with MSC-derived exosomes attenuates traumatic acute lung injury in rats. Am J Physiol Lung Cell Mol Physiol. 2019;316:L1107–17.

35. Willis GR, Fernandez-Gonzalez A, Anastas J, et al. Mesenchymal stromal cell exosomes ameliorate experimental bronchopulmonary dysplasia and restore lung function through macrophage immunomodulation. Am J Respir Crit Care Med. 2018;197:104–16.
36. Morrison TJ, Jackson MV, Cunningham EK, et al. Mesenchymal stromal cells modulate macrophages in clinically relevant lung injury models by extracellular vesicle mitochondrial transfer. Am J Respir Crit Care Med. 2017;196:1275–86.
37. Song Y, Dou H, Li X, et al. Exosomal miR-146a contributes to the enhanced therapeutic efficacy of interleukin-1beta-primed mesenchymal stem cells against sepsis. Stem Cells. 2017;35:1208–21.
38. Kim J, Hematti P. Mesenchymal stem cell-educated macrophages: a novel type of alternatively activated macrophages. Exp Hematol. 2009;37:1445–53.
39. Krasnodembskaya A, Samarani G, Song Y, et al. Human mesenchymal stem cells reduce mortality and bacteremia in gram-negative sepsis in mice in part by enhancing the phagocytic activity of blood monocytes. Am J Physiol Lung Cell Mol Physiol. 2012;302:L1003–13.
40. Tang XD, Shi L, Monsel A, et al. Mesenchymal stem cell microvesicles attenuate acute lung injury in mice partly mediated by Ang-1 mRNA. Stem Cells. 2017;35:1849–59.
41. Gennai S, Monsel A, Hao Q, Park J, Matthay MA, Lee JW. Microvesicles derived from human mesenchymal stem cells restore alveolar fluid clearance in human lungs rejected for transplantation. Am J Transplant. 2015;15:2404–12.
42. Park J, Kim S, Lim H, et al. Therapeutic effects of human mesenchymal stem cell microvesicles in an ex vivo perfused human lung injured with severe E. coli pneumonia. Thorax. 2019;74:43–50.
43. Hao Q, Gudapati V, Monsel A, et al. Mesenchymal stem cell-derived extracellular vesicles decrease lung injury in mice. J Immunol. 2019;203:1961–72.
44. Wu X, Liu Z, Hu L, Gu W, Zhu L. Exosomes derived from endothelial progenitor cells ameliorate acute lung injury by transferring miR-126. Exp Cell Res. 2018;370:13–23.
45. Zhou Y, Li P, Goodwin AJ, et al. Exosomes from endothelial progenitor cells improve outcomes of the lipopolysaccharide-induced acute lung injury. Crit Care. 2019;23:44.
46. Lesley J, Hascall VC, Tammi M, Hyman R. Hyaluronan binding by cell surface CD44. J Biol Chem. 2000;275:26967–75.
47. Ju Z, Ma J, Wang C, Yu J, Qiao Y, Hei F. Exosomes from iPSCs delivering siRNA attenuate intracellular adhesion molecule-1 expression and neutrophils adhesion in pulmonary microvascular endothelial cells. Inflammation. 2017;40:486–96.
48. Srinivasan S, Yeri A, Cheah PS, et al. Small RNA sequencing across diverse biofluids identifies optimal methods for exRNA isolation. Cell. 2019;177:446–62.e16.

ARDS Subphenotypes: Understanding a Heterogeneous Syndrome

J. G. Wilson and C. S. Calfee

5.1 Introduction

The acute respiratory distress syndrome (ARDS) is a clinical syndrome defined by acute onset hypoxemia (PaO_2:FiO_2 ratio < 300) and bilateral pulmonary opacities not fully explained by cardiac failure or volume overload [1]. The Berlin consensus definition of ARDS, like the American-European Consensus definition that preceded it, has enabled clinicians and researchers alike to prospectively identify patients with ARDS, implement lung protective ventilation strategies, and enroll patients in clinical trials. ARDS remains under-recognized clinically, however; therapies are limited, and mortality remains high [2]. Under-recognition of ARDS may stem in part from the considerable clinical heterogeneity observed among patients who meet standard ARDS criteria. The syndrome may be triggered, for example, by pulmonary or extrapulmonary sepsis, aspiration, trauma, blood product transfusion, or pancreatitis. Pulmonary infiltrates can be focal or diffuse. Hypoxemia can range from mild to severe, and duration of respiratory failure can be brief or prolonged. Many of these clinical variations may reflect underlying biological differences between ARDS patients that are now recognized as important drivers of treatment response and ultimate outcomes.

Substantial heterogeneity within the general ARDS population has likely contributed to the failure of experimental therapies for ARDS in recent large clinical trials, despite promising preclinical data [3]. Identifying subphenotypes of ARDS—more homogeneous groups within the general ARDS population—is one approach

---

J. G. Wilson
Department of Emergency Medicine, Stanford University, Palo Alto, CA, USA

C. S. Calfee (✉)
Department of Medicine, University of California, San Francisco, San Francisco, CA, USA

Department of Anesthesia, University of California, San Francisco, San Francisco, CA, USA
e-mail: carolyn.calfee@ucsf.edu

Table 5.1 Examples of factors used for identifying subphenotypes of the acute respiratory distress syndrome (ARDS)

Physiologic	Clinical	Biologic
$PaO_2:FiO_2$	Trauma vs. medical	Genomic
Dead space fraction	Direct vs. indirect	Transcriptomic
Driving pressure	Focal vs. diffuse	Proteomic
	±Acute kidney injury	Metabolomic

to untangling the clinical and biological complexity that many believe is a barrier to discovery of successful new treatments. By identifying meaningful but currently unrecognized subgroups encompassed by the broad consensus definition of ARDS, interventions can potentially be tested more efficiently in targeted cohorts. Selecting subphenotypes of patients at higher risk for poor outcomes for enrollment in clinical trials is called prognostic enrichment [4]. Selecting for patients more likely to respond to a given therapy due to the mechanism of benefit is called predictive enrichment [4]. Both enrichment strategies are recommended by the Food and Drug Administration to increase the efficiency of clinical trials across all fields, either by increasing the rate of the outcome of interest (prognostic enrichment) or by amplifying the effect size (predictive enrichment). These approaches may allow researchers to detect treatment effects in smaller cohorts, which is especially important in heterogeneous syndromes like ARDS. Ultimately, however, the discovery of ARDS subphenotypes may enrich more than clinical trial populations: within the next decade, these innovations could help us move from a one-size-fits-all approach to ARDS treatment to more effective, tailored therapies based on the clinical and biologic profile of each patient.

This chapter summarizes the state of the science of subphenotyping of ARDS patients, exploring the physiologic, clinical, and biologic characteristics that have been found to identify more homogeneous subgroups within this heterogeneous syndrome (Table 5.1), and the potential implications of these advances for practicing clinicians in the intensive care unit (ICU) and the emergency department.

5.2 ARDS Subphenotypes and Prognostic Enrichment

Prognostic enrichment in ARDS research involves selecting patients with a higher likelihood of having a particular disease-related endpoint, such as fewer ventilator-free days or higher mortality. Beyond increasing research efficiency, identifying subphenotypes of ARDS patients at highest risk for poor outcomes may also lead to improved risk stratification at the bedside, allowing clinicians to select patients more likely to benefit from inter-facility transfer for higher level of care, or early consideration of aggressive therapies such as extracorporeal membrane oxygenation (ECMO).

5.2.1 Physiologic Phenotyping for Prognostic Enrichment

Risk stratification of ARDS patients is not a new strategy. The Berlin definition itself stratifies ARDS into three subgroups (Table 5.2) according to the degree of

5 ARDS Subphenotypes: Understanding a Heterogeneous Syndrome

Table 5.2 The Berlin Definition of ARDS categorizes patients according to the severity of their oxygenation deficit; increasing severity is associated with increased mortality [1]

Severity	PaO$_2$:FiO$_2$ ratio (mmHg)	Patients (%)	Mortality (%)
Mild	201–300	22	27
Moderate	101–200	50	32
Severe	≤100	28	45

hypoxemia (mild, moderate, and severe), and mortality increases as the PaO$_2$:FiO$_2$ ratio decreases [1]. The advantage of this approach is that the PaO$_2$:FiO$_2$ ratio is available in all patients with ARDS and does not require expert interpretation or subjective clinical assessment. Multiple large clinical ARDS trials have used the PaO$_2$:FiO$_2$ ratio for prognostic enrichment. For example, the ACURASYS trial of early continuous neuromuscular blockade [5], the PROSEVA trial of prone positioning [6], and the ROSE trial reevaluating early continuous neuromuscular blockade [7] all targeted patients with moderate-to-severe ARDS (PaO$_2$:FiO$_2$ ratio < 150 mmHg). All three of these trials had mortality endpoints, and all three had mortality rates in the control arms that exceeded 40%.

In addition to the PaO$_2$:FiO$_2$ ratio, several other physiologic variables are known to predict poor outcomes in ARDS. Dead space fraction [8], ventilatory ratio (a simple bedside index of impaired ventilation) [9], and driving pressure (a measurement of respiratory system compliance) are all independently associated with poor outcomes in ARDS [10] and more routine measurement of these variables could improve prognostic enrichment in clinical trials and risk prediction in clinical practice.

One limitation of using these physiologic measurements, however, is that these variables can rapidly change. The application of higher positive end-expiratory pressure (PEEP), for example, could rapidly move a patient from one subgroup of ARDS severity to another, or a patient who aspirates at the time of intubation may develop severe hypoxemia that improves within hours. Perhaps more fundamentally, common physiologic characteristics in most cases do not capture important differences in biology between ARDS patients. A patient with transfusion-associated ARDS may have the same PaO$_2$:FiO$_2$ ratio or driving pressure as a patient with ARDS from H1N1 influenza, but their underlying pathophysiology may be very different, and they do not have the same risk of poor outcomes. Indeed, the Berlin definition of ARDS is far from perfect as a predictor of mortality, with an area under the curve of only 0.577 [1].

5.2.2 Clinical Phenotyping for Prognostic Enrichment

Recognizing the limitations of a purely physiologic approach to subphenotyping ARDS patients, investigators have also examined various clinical variables to enhance prognostic enrichment (Table 5.1). For example, patients with ARDS following trauma have been found to be at lower risk of death than non-trauma patients with ARDS (odds ratio 0.44) [11]. Luo et al. found that despite overall similar mortality rates, predictors of mortality differ between direct (pulmonary trigger) and indirect (extrapulmonary trigger) ARDS [12]. ARDS patients with acute kidney injury (AKI) have been shown to have significantly higher mortality than patients without AKI in several cohorts [13, 14]. Thus, when attempting to identify high-risk ARDS patients, non-trauma patients and patients with significant AKI are a higher-risk subset, but predictors of mortality differ depending on whether the lung injury is direct or indirect.

Beyond baseline clinical characteristics, the time-course of ARDS is another factor that can identify patients at greater risk of poor outcomes. Both time of onset and duration of disease appear to hold prognostic value. Several studies have shown that ARDS onset >48 h after ICU admission is associated with higher mortality [15, 16]. Not surprisingly, rapidly improving ARDS (ARDS that resolves within 1 day) has a better prognosis than persistent ARDS. More interesting, however, is the finding that most (63%) patients with rapidly improving ARDS present with moderate or severe hypoxemia [17], highlighting the limitations of using the $PaO_2:FiO_2$ ratio alone to identify patients for enrollment in clinical trials. Recognizing this issue, the PROSEVA trial of prone positioning only enrolled patients if they continued to meet inclusion criteria ($PaO_2:FiO_2$ ratio < 150 mmHg) after 12–24 h of stabilization [7].

Radiographic patterns of pulmonary infiltrates have also been used to sort ARDS patients into more homogeneous subgroups and identify those at highest risk of death, either alone or in combination with other physiologic and clinical variables. One small prospective study found that ARDS patients with non-focal infiltrates had higher mortality compared to patients with focal radiographic findings [18]. The CESAR trial of ECMO for severe ARDS required a Murray Lung Score (which incorporates chest radiography) of >3 for eligibility (or a pH < 7.20) [19, 20]. More recently, the RALE score—developed to systematically quantify the extent and density of alveolar infiltrates on chest radiograph—has been shown to predict 28-day mortality with an area under the curve of 0.82 [21].

An apparent drawback to relying exclusively on clinical characteristics for phenotyping, however, is the potential for misclassification. In a recent trial of mechanical ventilation personalized according to the presence of focal vs. diffuse infiltrates in ARDS (discussed further later), 21% of the radiographic subphenotypes assigned at the time of randomization were misclassified [22]. Similarly, investigators have found it difficult to classify patients as having direct or indirect ARDS, with 37% of cases deemed unclassifiable in one trial [23]. Pragmatic and reliable approaches to classification are needed to overcome the challenges inherent to clinical phenotyping.

5.2.3 Biologic Phenotyping for Prognostic Enrichment

It follows that there has been growing interest in identifying biologic subphenotypes of ARDS patients. Biologic markers are considered proximal to the clinical expression of ARDS, and potentially less prone to problems with misclassification that make clinical phenotyping so challenging. Moreover, our understanding of ARDS biology has advanced greatly in the past decade. We now better understand how an initial insult causes an inflammatory cascade that results in further injury to the alveolus and its microvasculature (Fig. 5.1) [3]. Measuring plasma biomarkers in ARDS can help find subgroups of patients that share important host-response features and/or that have worse clinical outcomes. Numerous genomic, transcriptomic, proteomic, and metabolomic factors have been studied for this purpose, with the

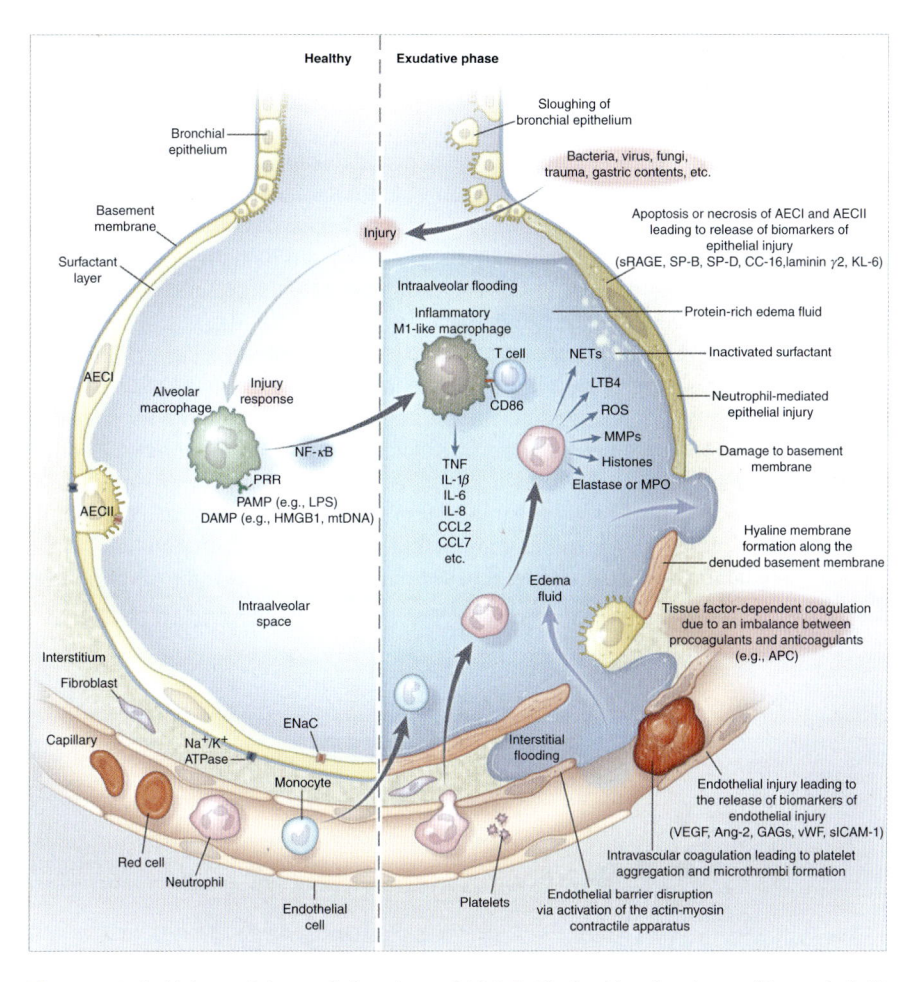

Fig. 5.1 Pathobiology of the exudative phase of ARDS. The healthy alveolar-capillary unit (left) and the exudative phase of ARDS (right). *AECI* type I alveolar epithelial cell, *AECII* type II alveolar epithelial cell, *Ang-2* angiopoietin-2, *APC* activated protein C, *CC-16* club cell (formerly Clara cell) secretory protein 16, *CCL* chemokine (CC motif) ligand, *DAMP* damage-associated molecular pattern, *ENaC* epithelial sodium channel, *GAG* glycosaminoglycan, *HMGB1* high-mobility group box 1 protein, *KL-6* Krebs von den Lungen 6, *LPS* lipopolysaccharide, *LTB4* leukotriene B4, *MMP* matrix metalloproteinase, *MPO* myeloperoxidase, *mtDNA* mitochondrial DNA, Na^+/K^+ *ATPase* sodium-potassium ATPase pump, *NF-κB* nuclear factor kappa light-chain enhancer of activated B cells, *NET* neutrophil extracellular trap, *PAMP* pathogen-associated molecular pattern, *PRR* pattern recognition receptor, *ROS* reactive oxygen species, *sICAM* soluble intercellular adhesion molecule, *SP* surfactant protein, *sRAGE* soluble receptor for advanced glycation end products, *TNF* tumor necrosis factor, *VEGF* vascular endothelial growth factor, *vWF* von Willebrand factor. (Reused from [3] with permission)

greatest depth of research focused on plasma protein biomarkers of ARDS. These include markers of systemic inflammation (interleukin [IL]-6, IL-8, soluble tumor necrosis factor [TNF] receptor-1, IL-18), epithelial injury (angiopoietin-2, intercellular adhesion molecule-1), endothelial injury (soluble receptor for advanced glycation end products [sRAGE], surfactant protein-D), and disordered coagulation (plasminogen activator inhibitor-1, protein C), all of which have been shown to hold prognostic value [24]. Baseline levels of sRAGE, for example, independently predicted 90-day mortality in one meta-analysis [25]. More recently, Rogers et al. found that elevations in baseline plasma IL-18 levels and rising IL-18 levels were both associated with increased mortality in sepsis-induced ARDS [26].

Using an approach to identify subgroups within a heterogeneous population called latent class analysis (LCA), two distinct subphenotypes of ARDS were identified based on combined clinical and biologic data from patients enrolled in two large clinical trial cohorts [27]. The "hyperinflammatory" subphenotype was characterized by enhanced inflammation, fewer ventilator-free days, and increased mortality compared to the "hypoinflammatory" subphenotype (Fig. 5.2). These two subphenotypes have been found in subsequent independent analyses of multiple other ARDS trial cohorts, and the poor prognosis associated with the hyperinflammatory phenotype persists [28, 29]. Using a different approach, called hierarchical clustering, to analyze a panel of plasma biomarkers from ARDS patients, Bos et al. identified two similar subphenotypes: a "reactive" subphenotype characterized by greater inflammation and increased mortality and an "uninflamed" subphenotype associated with better outcomes [30]. Taken together, these

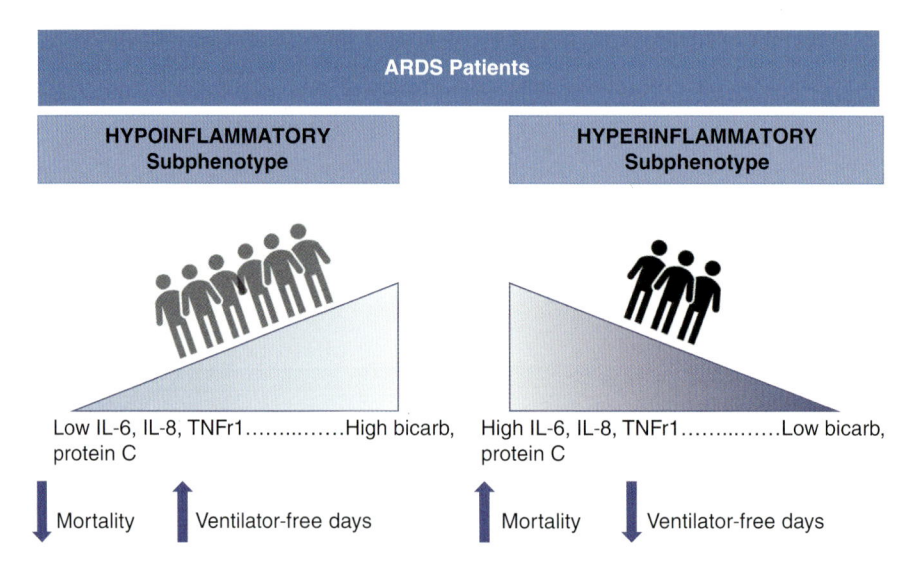

Fig. 5.2 The hypoinflammatory and hyperinflammatory subphenotypes of ARDS are associated with different biomarkers and outcomes. These two distinct subphenotypes have been identified by Calfee et al. in multiple previous ARDS clinical trial cohorts [27, 29, 40, 41]. *IL* interleukin, *bicarb* bicarbonate, *TNFr1* tumor necrosis factor receptor 1

findings support the idea that ARDS patients can be stratified according to markers of inflammation for prognostic enrichment.

The focus on proteomic profiling of ARDS patients has been paralleled by interest in genomic, transcriptomic, and metabolomic subphenotypes of ARDS, but less progress has been made in terms of prognostic enrichment with these strategies. Meyer et al. identified an *IL-1RN* coding variant that increased risk of developing ARDS in sepsis [31], and Zhu et al. found certain micro-RNAs to be risk biomarkers for ARDS among critically ill adults [32], but genomic and transcriptomic subphenotyping of patients with established ARDS remains largely unexplored. In a small cohort of patients with ARDS, Rogers et al. found a subset of patients with a distinct metabolic profile with higher levels of numerous metabolites in undiluted pulmonary edema fluid [33]. This "high metabolite" subphenotype was associated with higher mortality but, in part because of the challenges associated with analyzing pulmonary edema fluid, these findings have yet to be reproduced in a larger cohort.

Indeed, measurement of protein biomarkers and "-omics" data in ARDS patients is not currently available outside of the research setting. Furthermore, the impact of identifying biologic subphenotype on downstream outcomes in ARDS patients has not been prospectively evaluated. Investigators have recently identified a "parsimonious" model that classifies ARDS patients as "hypo-" or "hyperinflammatory" using only three plasma biomarkers (IL-8, bicarbonate and protein C) [34], and rapid analysis of biomarkers for identification of ARDS subphenotype at the point of care is now being piloted. Development of rapid assays is a critical step in leveraging the identification of ARDS subphenotypes for prognostic enrichment in future clinical trials, and ultimately bringing these discoveries to the bedside.

5.3 ARDS Subphenotypes and Predictive Enrichment

In parallel with these different strategies for identifying subgroups and phenotypes for prognostic enrichment in ARDS, investigators have also studied how treatment effects vary by subphenotype. By finding a subphenotype-specific treatment response retrospectively or targeting treatment based on mechanism and biologic features, researchers can then go on to prospectively test new interventions in patients who are more likely to respond. This approach provides predictive enrichment: by amplifying treatment response, the power to detect a benefit from experimental therapies increases, and discovery becomes more efficient. Just as biologic phenotyping of other diseases, such as breast cancer or asthma, has led to important improvements in patient outcomes, the eventual goal is to deploy targeted therapies for ARDS according to patient characteristics, moving the field from protocolized care to precision medicine.

5.3.1 Physiologic Phenotyping for Predictive Enrichment

While many view physiologic parameters such as $PaO_2:FiO_2$ ratio as purely prognostic indicators, they may provide predictive enrichment as well. As Prescott et al. note in their discussion of ARDS clinical trial strategies, a lower PaO_2:FiO_2 ratio not only identifies patients at higher risk of death, but also reflects patients with greater lung weight who may be more likely to benefit from recruitment maneuvers, higher PEEP or prone positioning [35]. Similarly, one could hypothesize that among patients with severe ARDS, those who have a plateau pressure >30 cmH_2O or an unfavorable driving pressure despite adherence to a lung-protective ventilation strategy may be more likely to benefit from "lung rest" with ultra-low tidal volumes on ECMO.

5.3.2 Clinical Phenotyping for Predictive Enrichment

As discussed above, difficulty classifying patients is a pragmatic challenge inherent to clinical phenotyping of ARDS patients, and a major drawback to the use of clinical phenotyping in both research and practice. Nonetheless, different clinical subphenotypes of ARDS may reflect different underlying biology, and in some cases have been shown to respond differently to treatment. For example, patients with direct ARDS have higher levels of biomarkers of epithelial injury than patients with indirect ARDS [36], and there is low-level evidence that patients with direct ARDS may respond differently to recruitment maneuvers and glucocorticoids than indirect lung injury patients [22, 37–39]. A recent, highly innovative randomized controlled trial compared a personalized mechanical ventilation strategy selected according to radiographic subphenotype (focal vs. non-focal) to standard low tidal volume ventilation in 400 patients with moderate-to-severe ARDS (LIVE trial) [22]. The intention-to-treat analysis found no difference in outcomes between groups, but in a post hoc analysis that excluded misclassified patients (21% of total patients), there was a mortality benefit to the personalized mechanical ventilation intervention. These results highlight both the promise and the peril of using subphenotype (in this case radiographic subphenotype) to guide therapy: on the one hand, if patients are appropriately classified, there may be a benefit of personalized care over protocolized care; on the other hand, the significant misclassification that occurs even in the relatively controlled setting of a clinical trial can completely offset the potential benefit. Regardless of this complexity, the LIVE trial was a first step in the direction of what many view as the future of ARDS research: leveraging subphenotype to personalize therapy and directly comparing outcomes to standard protocolized care.

5.3.3 Biologic Phenotyping for Predictive Enrichment

No trials have yet used biologic phenotyping pre-randomization, because bedside testing of biomarkers is not widely available. There is, however, mounting evidence that biologic phenotype predicts treatment response. In retrospective analyses, the hypo- and hyperinflammatory phenotypes discussed above have been observed to have differential treatment responses to several different interventions, including PEEP and fluid management strategies (Table 5.3) [27, 29]. Subphenotypic differences in response to simvastatin were also observed in reanalysis of one clinical trial (HARP-2 trial) [40], but not in a similar reanalysis of a separate trial of rosuvastatin

5 ARDS Subphenotypes: Understanding a Heterogeneous Syndrome

Table 5.3 Subphenotype-specific treatment response in the reanalyses of outcomes in four different clinical ARDS trials

Intervention/trial cohort analyzed	Outcome	Hypoinflammatory subphenotype response		Hyperinflammatory subphenotype response	
		Intervention	Control	Intervention	Control
High vs. low PEEP/ALVEOLI* [27]	90-day mortality	24% high PEEP	16% low PEEP	42% high PEEP	51% low PEEP
Conservative vs. liberal fluid strategy/FACCT* [29]	90-day mortality	18% conservative fluid strategy	26% liberal fluid strategy	50% conservative fluid strategy	40% liberal fluid strategy
Simvastatin/HARP-2 [40]	28-day survival	No difference		Improved survival with simvastatin ($p = 0.008$)	
Rosuvastatin/SAILS [41]	90-day mortality	No difference		No difference	

PEEP positive end-expiratory pressure; *p value <0.05 for interaction between treatment and subphenotype

for ARDS (SAILS trial) [41]. While it is possible this discrepancy reflects differences in trial design (and the particular statin that was tested), it also highlights the uncertainty that remains when differential treatment response has been observed only retrospectively.

The use of metabolomics, transcriptomics, and genomics for ARDS phenotyping and predictive enrichment is in even earlier stages than proteomic phenotyping. Bos et al. used the "uninflamed" and "reactive" subphenotypes they had previously identified based on plasma protein biomarkers to test whether there were differences in blood leukocyte gene expression between groups, and found that approximately one-third of genes were differentially expressed. Specifically, there was upregulation of oxidative phosphorylation genes in the "reactive" subphenotype, leading the authors to suggest that for patients in this group, interventions focused on this pathway should be explored [42]. While these data certainly merits further investigation, translating biologic associations into effective treatments based on mechanism is by no means straightforward. For example, a retrospective analysis of a previous negative clinical trial of recombinant IL-1 receptor antagonist for sepsis found a treatment benefit in the subset of patients with *higher* levels of baseline IL-1 receptor antagonist, arguably a completely counterintuitive result [43].

The benefit of biologically tailored precision therapies for ARDS remains theoretical. The translation of the insights gained from studying subphenotypes of ARDS into targeted therapies based on mechanism—and comparison of this precision approach to standard protocolized management—is the next frontier in ARDS research.

5.4 Beyond ARDS: Subphenotypes in Other Heterogeneous Syndromes

As mentioned earlier, the search for subphenotypes in ARDS is motivated in part by improvements in the treatment of other heterogeneous diseases gained by using a similar approach. Oncologic therapies in particular are increasingly guided by molecular phenotype, and this strategy has improved survival substantially even in patients with advanced disease. Survival with metastatic melanoma, for example, has improved significantly since the advent of checkpoint inhibitors and therapies targeting the BRAF V600 mutation [44]. Asthma therapy has also been changed by the identification of clinically significant subphenotypes: patients with severe, uncontrolled eosinophilic asthma have been found to have fewer exacerbations with monoclonal antibodies aimed at reducing eosinophil activation [45].

Subphenotypes have also been identified in sepsis, another heterogeneous syndrome in the critically ill that has historically been treated with a protocolized approach. Wong et al. have developed a biomarker-based mortality risk model for pediatric sepsis, as well as gene-expression-based subphenotypes of pediatric septic shock. In a retrospective analysis of a cohort of pediatric patients with septic shock, they found that among intermediate- and high-risk patients, corticosteroids were associated with a more than tenfold reduction in the risk of a complicated course in one subphenotype but not the other [46]. Similar subphenotyping of adult sepsis is an area of active study. Gårdlund et al. used latent class analysis to identify six distinct subphenotypes of septic shock using clinical data from a previous large clinical trial cohort [47]. Seymour et al. used a different approach (machine learning applied to electronic health record data) and identified four subphenotypes with different genetic and inflammatory markers and markedly different mortality rates [48].

Finally, there is a small but growing body of evidence that there are meaningful subphenotypes within the heterogeneous post-cardiac arrest syndrome, beyond type of arrest and initial post-resuscitation neurologic status. For example, Bro-Jeppesen et al. have reported that IL-6, a marker of systemic inflammation, is correlated with poor prognosis in comatose patients resuscitated from out-of-hospital cardiac arrest [49]. Anderson et al. found that patients with post-resuscitation shock who had a preserved left ventricular ejection fraction (LVEF) had less favorable neurologic outcomes, increased organ failure, and higher mortality compared to patients with depressed LVEF [50]. In addition, patients in the preserved LVEF group exhibited a subtype-specific response to early fluid resuscitation, with lower mortality and improved neurologic outcomes associated with larger volume fluid resuscitation that was not observed in the group with depressed LVEF. These findings suggest that there are identifiable subphenotypes in post-cardiac arrest syndrome, and that subphenotypes may be important drivers of variable treatment response.

5.5 Conclusion

The armamentarium of therapies for patients with ARDS remains limited and mortality remains high. While negative results in several large randomized controlled trials of new treatments for ARDS have frustrated many, they have also motivated multiple novel approaches to understanding the clinical and biologic heterogeneity among ARDS patients. The identification of meaningful ARDS subphenotypes—and the ways in which their outcomes and treatment responses differ—promises prognostic and predictive enrichment for future trials. Prospective evaluation of methods for reliable phenotyping at the point of care is a crucial next step in translating these discoveries into new personalized therapies for ARDS. Ultimately, identification of ARDS subphenotypes may help fulfill the aspiration of precision critical care for ARDS: replacing blunt interventions aimed at all patients who meet diagnostic criteria with therapies tailored to the clinical and biologic profile of each patient.

References

1. ARDS Definition Task Force, Ranieri VM, Rubenfeld GD, et al. Acute respiratory distress syndrome: the Berlin definition. JAMA. 2012;307:2526–33.
2. Bellani G, Laffey JG, Pham T, et al., LUNG SAFE Investigators, ESICM Trials Group. Epidemiology, patterns of care, and mortality for patients with acute respiratory distress syndrome in intensive care units in 50 countries. JAMA. 2016;315:788–800.
3. Thompson BT, Chambers RC, Liu KD. Acute respiratory distress syndrome. N Engl J Med. 2017;377:562–72.
4. FDA. Draft guidance: enrichment strategies for clinical trials to support approval of human drugs and biological products. Available from https://www.fda.gov/media/121320/download. Accessed 27 Aug 2019.
5. Papazian L, Forel JM, Gacouin A, et al., ACURASYS Study Investigators. Neuromuscular blockers in early acute respiratory distress syndrome. N Engl J Med. 2010;363:1107–16.
6. Guerin C, Reignier J, Richard JC, et al., PROSEVA Study Group. Prone positioning in severe acute respiratory distress syndrome. N Engl J Med. 2013;368:2159–68.
7. Moss M, Huang DT, Brower RG, et al. Early neuromuscular blockade in the acute respiratory distress syndrome. N Engl J Med. 2019;380:1997–2008.
8. Nuckton TJ, Alonso JA, Kallet RH, et al. Pulmonary dead-space fraction as a risk factor for death in the acute respiratory distress syndrome. N Engl J Med. 2002;346:1281–6.
9. Sinha P, Calfee CS, Beitler JR, et al. Physiological analysis and clinical performance of the ventilatory ratio in acute respiratory distress syndrome. Am J Respir Crit Care Med. 2019;199:333–41.
10. Amato MB, Meade MO, Slutsky AS, et al. Driving pressure and survival in the acute respiratory distress syndrome. N Engl J Med. 2015;372:747–55.
11. Calfee CS, Eisner MD, Ware LB, et al., Acute Respiratory Distress Syndrome Network, National Heart, Lung, and Blood Institute. Trauma-associated lung injury differs clinically and biologically from acute lung injury due to other clinical disorders. Crit Care Med. 2007;35:2243–50.
12. Luo L, Shaver CM, Zhao Z, et al. Clinical predictors of hospital mortality differ between direct and indirect ARDS. Chest. 2017;151:755–63.
13. Liu KD, Glidden DV, Eisner MD, et al. Predictive and pathogenetic value of plasma biomarkers for acute kidney injury in patients with acute lung injury. Crit Care Med. 2007;35(12):2755–61.
14. McNicholas BA, Rezoagli E, Pham T, et al. Impact of early acute kidney injury on management and outcome in patients with acute respiratory distress syndrome: a secondary analysis of a multicenter observational study. Crit Care Med. 2019;47:1216–25.
15. Liao KM, Chen CW, Hsiue TR, Lin WC. Timing of acute respiratory distress syndrome onset is related to patient outcome. J Formos Med Assoc. 2009;108:694–703.
16. Zhang R, Wang Z, Tejera P, et al. Late-onset moderate to severe acute respiratory distress syndrome is associated with shorter survival and higher mortality: a two-stage association study. Intensive Care Med. 2017;43:399–407.
17. Schenck EJ, Oromendia C, Torres LK, Berlin DA, Choi AMK, Siempos II. Rapidly improving ARDS in therapeutic randomized controlled trials. Chest. 2019;155:474–82.

18. Mrozek S, Jabaudon M, Jaber S, et al., Azurea Network. Elevated plasma levels of sRAGE are associated with nonfocal CT-based lung imaging in patients with ARDS: a prospective multicenter study. Chest. 2016;150:998–1007.
19. Murray JF, Matthay MA, Luce JM, Flick MR. An expanded definition of the adult respiratory distress syndrome. Am Rev Respir Dis. 1988;138:720–3.
20. Peek GJ, Mugford M, Tiruvoipati R, et al. Efficacy and economic assessment of conventional ventilatory support versus extracorporeal membrane oxygenation for severe adult respiratory failure (CESAR): a multicentre randomised controlled trial. Lancet. 2009;374:1351–63.
21. Warren MA, Zhao Z, Koyama T, et al. Severity scoring of lung oedema on the chest radiograph is associated with clinical outcomes in ARDS. Thorax. 2018;73:840–6.
22. Constantin JM, Jabaudon M, Lefrant JY, et al. Personalised mechanical ventilation tailored to lung morphology versus low positive end-expiratory pressure for patients with acute respiratory distress syndrome in France (the LIVE study): a multicentre, single-blind, randomised controlled trial. Lancet Respir Med. 2019;7:870–80.
23. Thille AW, Richard JC, Maggiore SM, et al. Alveolar recruitment in pulmonary and extrapulmonary acute respiratory distress syndrome: comparison using pressure-volume curve or static compliance. Anesthesiology. 2007;106:212–7.
24. Walter JM, Wilson J, Ware LB. Biomarkers in acute respiratory distress syndrome: from pathobiology to improving patient care. Expert Rev Respir Med. 2014;8:573–86.
25. Jabaudon M, Blondonnet R, Pereira B, et al. Plasma sRAGE is independently associated with increased mortality in ARDS: a meta-analysis of individual patient data. Intensive Care Med. 2018;44:1388–99.
26. Rogers AJ, Guan J, Trtchounian A, et al. Association of elevated plasma interleukin-18 level with increased mortality in a clinical trial of statin treatment for acute respiratory distress syndrome. Crit Care Med. 2019;47:1089–96.
27. Calfee CS, Delucchi K, Parsons PE, et al., NHLBI ARDS Network. Subphenotypes in acute respiratory distress syndrome: latent class analysis of data from two randomised controlled trials. Lancet Respir Med. 2014;2:611–20.
28. Delucchi K, Famous KR, Ware LB, et al. Stability of ARDS subphenotypes over time in two randomised controlled trials. Thorax. 2018;73:439–45.
29. Famous KR, Delucchi K, Ware LB, et al., ARDS Network. Acute respiratory distress syndrome subphenotypes respond differently to randomized fluid management strategy. Am J Respir Crit Care Med. 2017;195:331–8.
30. Bos LD, Schouten LR, van Vught LA, et al., MARS Consortium. Identification and validation of distinct biological phenotypes in patients with acute respiratory distress syndrome by cluster analysis. Thorax. 2017;72:876–83.
31. Meyer NJ, Feng R, Li M, et al. IL1RN coding variant is associated with lower risk of acute respiratory distress syndrome and increased plasma IL-1 receptor antagonist. Am J Respir Crit Care Med. 2013;187:950–9.
32. Zhu Z, Liang L, Zhang R, et al. Whole blood microRNA markers are associated with acute respiratory distress syndrome. Intensive Care Med Exp. 2017;5:38–50.
33. Rogers AJ, Contrepois K, Wu M, et al. Profiling of ARDS pulmonary edema fluid identifies a metabolically distinct subset. Am J Physiol Lung Cell Mol Physiol. 2017;312:L703–9.
34. Sinha P, Delucchi KL, McAuley DF, O'Kane CM, Matthay MA, Calfee CS. Development and validation of parsimonious algorithms to classify ARDS phenotypes. Lancet Respir Med. 2020. https://doi.org/10.1016/S2213-2600(19)30369-8 [Epub ahead of print].
35. Prescott HC, Calfee CS, Thompson BT, Angus DC, Liu VX. Toward smarter lumping and smarter splitting: rethinking strategies for sepsis and acute respiratory distress syndrome clinical trial design. Am J Respir Crit Care Med. 2016;194:147–55.
36. Calfee CS, Janz DR, Bernard GR, et al. Distinct molecular phenotypes of direct vs indirect ARDS in single-center and multicenter studies. Chest. 2015;147:1539–48.
37. Gattinoni L, Pelosi P, Suter PM, et al. Acute respiratory distress syndrome caused by pulmonary and extrapulmonary disease. Different syndromes? Am J Respir Crit Care Med. 1998;158:3–11.

38. Riva DR, Oliveira MB, Rzezinski AF, et al. Recruitment maneuver in pulmonary and extrapulmonary experimental acute lung injury. Crit Care Med. 2008;36:1900–8.
39. Leite-Junior JH, Garcia CS, Souza-Fernandes AB, et al. Methylprednisolone improves lung mechanics and reduces the inflammatory response in pulmonary but not in extrapulmonary mild acute lung injury in mice. Crit Care Med. 2008;36:2621–8.
40. Calfee CS, Delucchi KL, Sinha P, et al., Irish Critical Care Trials Group. Acute respiratory distress syndrome subphenotypes and differential response to simvastatin: secondary analysis of a randomised controlled trial. Lancet Respir Med. 2018;6:691–8.
41. Sinha P, Delucchi KL, Thompson BT, et al., NHLBI ARDS Network. Latent class analysis of ARDS subphenotypes: a secondary analysis of the statins for acutely injured lungs from sepsis (SAILS) study. Intensive Care Med. 2018;44:1859–69.
42. Bos LDJ, Scicluna BP, Ong DSY, et al., MARS Consortium. Understanding heterogeneity in biological phenotypes of acute respiratory distress syndrome by leukocyte expression profiles. Am J Respir Crit Care Med. 2019;200:42–50.
43. Meyer NJ, Reilly JP, Anderson BJ, et al. Mortality benefit of recombinant human interleukin-1 receptor antagonist for sepsis varies by initial interleukin-1 receptor antagonist plasma concentration. Crit Care Med. 2018;46:21–8.
44. Silva IP, Long GV. Systemic therapy in advanced melanoma: integrating targeted therapy and immunotherapy into clinical practice. Curr Opin Oncol. 2017;29:484–92.
45. FitzGerald JM, Bleecker ER, Nair P, et al. Benralizumab, an antiinterleukin-5 receptor alpha monoclonal antibody, as add-on treatment for patients with severe, uncontrolled, eosinophilic asthma (CALIMA): a randomised, double-blind, placebo-controlled phase 3 trial. Lancet. 2016;388:2128–41.
46. Wong HR, Atkinson SJ, Cvijanovich NZ, et al. Combining prognostic and predictive enrichment strategies to identify children with septic shock responsive to corticosteroids. Crit Care Med. 2016;44:e1000–3.
47. Gårdlund B, Dmitrieva NO, Pieper CF, Finfer S, Marshall JC, Thompson BT. Six subphenotypes in septic shock: latent class analysis of the PROWESS shock study. J Crit Care. 2018;47:70–9.
48. Seymour CW, Kennedy JN, Wang S, et al. Derivation, validation, and potential treatment implications of novel clinical phenotypes for sepsis. JAMA. 2019;321:2003–17.
49. Bro-Jeppesen J, Kjaergaard J, Wanscher M, et al. Systemic inflammatory response and potential prognostic implications after out-of-hospital cardiac arrest: a substudy of the Target Temperature Management Trial. Crit Care Med. 2015;43:1223–32.
50. Anderson RJ, Jinadasa SP, Hsu L, et al. Shock subtypes by left ventricular ejection fraction following out-of-hospital cardiac arrest. Crit Care. 2018;22:162.

Assessment of VILI Risk During Spontaneous Breathing and Assisted Mechanical Ventilation

G. Bellani and M. Teggia-Droghi

6.1 Introduction

Mechanical ventilation is a lifesaving procedure, applied in many critically ill patients to replace or support respiratory muscle function. However, since the first application during polio epidemic, it was immediately evident that this practice could carry several complications, even impacting patient survival [1]. The study of the complications of mechanical ventilation has proceeded at the same pace as the development of the technology, unveiling the need to personalize ventilatory settings based on the pathophysiology of different lung diseases. These complications can be classified depending on the mechanism of injury: direct injury on the lung (barotrauma, volutrauma and atelectauma), hemodynamic alteration, and oxygen toxicity.

6.2 Mechanical Ventilation and Mechanisms of VILI

Classically, four mechanisms of ventilator-induced lung injury (VILI) have been described: barotrauma, volutrauma, atelectauma, and biotrauma.

Barotrauma and volutrauma occur when high pressure in the former case and high volume in the latter are used to ventilate a patient. These conditions are related and lead to the same clinical manifestations: alveolar rupture, pneumothorax, pneumomediastinum, or/and subcutaneous emphysema. Even when "macroscopic

---

G. Bellani (✉)
Department of Anesthesia and Critical Care, San Gerardo Hospital, Monza, Italy

University of Milano Bicocca, Milan, Italy
e-mail: giacomo.bellani1@unimib.it

M. Teggia-Droghi
University of Milano Bicocca, Milan, Italy

injuries" are not detected, barotrauma and volutrauma can still lead to alveolar wall rupture, increased edema, hemorrhage, and inflammatory infiltrates. It is not the airway pressure *per se* that is harmful to the lung, but the pressure across the whole lung, called transpulmonary pressure. Transpulmonary pressure is calculated as airway pressure minus pleural pressure, this last evaluated using esophageal pressure as a surrogate.

This concept was elegantly demonstrated in a classical study by Dreyfuss and Saumon, when the authors, by stiffening the chest wall, showed that high airway pressures were not injurious as long as transpulmonary pressure was low [2]. However, in addition to cases of impaired chest wall mechanics, transpulmonary pressure also has great relevance during assisted ventilation in a spontaneously breathing patient. For example, one patient can be completely supported by the ventilator with a given amount of pressure and another can generate the same pressure using the respiratory muscles: the two patients will have the same tidal volume because they generate the same transpulmonary pressure, even though the airway pressure is profoundly different [3].

Atelectrauma is caused by the repetitive opening and closing (or collapse/recruitment) of the alveoli during the respiratory cycle. In a healthy lung, this phenomenon is not present, but in the presence of edema and inflammation, such as during the acute respiratory distress syndrome (ARDS), the physiologic forces that keep the alveoli open are impaired by the weight of the inflamed parenchyma and surfactant depletion.

During any inflammatory process in the body, there is activation of pro-inflammatory cytokines. In the lungs, this process is magnified by mechanical ventilation, which promotes injury by physically damaging the alveolar structure, increasing the weight of the parenchyma, and spreading the disease even to healthy lung parenchyma and distal organs [4].

Apart from the classic mechanism of VILI, other factors can contribute to damage the lung during mechanical ventilation. Based on computed tomography (CT) scans, ARDS lungs are divided into aerated, poorly aerated and non-aerated zones, suggesting that an inhomogeneous grade of illness characterizes this syndrome. For this reason, the mechanical dependence of the respiratory unit in sick lung will develop local forces that can stretch the parenchyma and contribute to VILI, due to differences in density and inflammation. VILI is not only responsible for damage in an already inflamed lung but is also responsible for initiating an inflammatory process even in healthy lungs [5].

6.3 How to Minimize the Risk?

It has been shown that a ventilatory strategy called "protective ventilation" aimed to minimize the injury caused by ventilation can decrease mortality. Hence, the goals of mechanical ventilation do not only include support of the respiratory muscles (borrowing time for the lungs to recover) but also restoring homogeneous ventilation without increasing the lung injury. Lung distension can be minimized by using a low tidal volume, low plateau pressure strategy. A significant reduction in mortality was demonstrated using 6 ml/kg instead of 12 ml/kg tidal volume [6].

Because of the inflammation and pulmonary edema, a higher level of positive end-expiratory pressure (PEEP) can keep the alveoli open and prevent the opening/closing phenomenon during the respiratory cycle. These guidelines [7] must be integrated with the measures of respiratory mechanics that describe the modification, from a physiopathological point of view, of the patient's respiratory system to the ongoing ventilatory strategy. Various safety thresholds have been defined in order to decrease the risk of VILI. Therefore, respiratory mechanics have to be monitored, on a daily basis, in particular compliance and resistance to evaluate the grade of disease and the healing process. Plateau pressure, measured using an inspiratory hold, is considered an acceptable surrogate of alveolar pressure, and the safe threshold to exclude overdistension is <30 cmH$_2$O.

6.4   Spontaneous Breathing and VILI

During mechanical ventilation, there are several advantages to switching the ventilatory mode from fully controlled to assisted, regardless of the support strategy. Allowing the use of a patient's respiratory muscles primarily counteracts muscular atrophy [8] that can contribute to difficult weaning and, likely, to long-term sequelae. Moreover, use of the diaphragm enables better ventilation of the dorsal area of the lung, coupling ventilation/perfusion match and improving respiratory gas exchange.

However, several mechanisms can further aggravate the risk of VILI due to the active contribution of the patient's breathing activity [9].

1. *Uncontrolled tidal volume*: In a spontaneously breathing patient, it is mandatory to set the support of the ventilator, but respiratory rate and tidal volume are more difficult to control. As an example, one of the ancillary studies of the LUNG SAFE [10] showed a decreasing trend in the PaCO$_2$ with increasing severity of the disease during noninvasive ventilation (NIV). This lower PaCO$_2$ was likely obtained, by the patients, with an extremely high minute ventilation. Similarly, Carteaux et al. demonstrated that a higher tidal volume is associated with an increased risk of NIV failure [11].
2. *Inhomogeneous transpulmonary pressure*: Even in a healthy lung, the pressure across the lung—transpulmonary pressure—is not evenly distributed, due to gravity. Furthermore, in an inflamed lung there are local inhomogeneities caused by different weights of the parenchyma and the inflammation process, that could generate stretch forces between the respiratory units [12]. Activation of the diaphragm can enable recruitment of the dorsal zone, but can magnify the local stress on the alveoli, in particular when there is still considerable lung disease. Unfortunately, these local alterations may not be reflected in a change in the overall transpulmonary pressure, making this phenomenon unmeasurable and often underestimated.

3. *Pulmonary edema*: The development of pulmonary edema in healthy lungs has been described after strenuous activation of the respiratory muscles. Similarly, in spontaneously breathing patients, because of hypoxia and parenchymal inhomogeneity, strong diaphragm activation can bring the alveolar pressure below the end expiratory pressure, favoring the development of pulmonary edema [13]. This phenomenon is worsened by the capillary leak, common in ARDS patients. Finally, the negative intrathoracic pressure generated by patient effort causes an increase in transmural pressure (and hence afterload) of the left ventricle favoring the development of cardiogenic pulmonary edema [14].
4. *Pendelluft*: In the normal lung, the negative pleural pressure generated during inspiration allows the gas to flow into the alveoli. The pressure distribution across the lung is influenced only by gravity forces. However, in the inflamed lung, the distribution of forces is not uniform. It is possible that gas flow migrates between alveolar units, without tidal volume modification. This phenomenon is called "pendelluft" and causes a local overstretch of alveoli, even during protective ventilation. Interest in "pendelluft" has increased recently, thanks to imaging (electrical impedance tomography [EIT], dynamic CT scan), as it has become possible to identify and describe when it occurs during the respiratory cycle [15]. Increasing the ventilatory support of a patient showing this alteration has been shown to reduce the degree of the phenomenon, which disappeared when fully controlled ventilation was initiated.
5. *Asynchronies*: In a mechanically ventilated patient, an appropriate interaction between the patient and the ventilator is fundamental during spontaneous breathing to prevent discomfort and prevent poor outcomes [16]. Discomfort and dyspnea, need for sedation, and prolonged mechanical ventilation are associated with an increase in intensive care unit (ICU) length of stay, muscle atrophy, and tracheostomy [17].

    It has been shown that in critically ill patients, patient–ventilator asynchronies occur frequently. Depending on the phase of the cycle, there are four different asynchrony patterns. We want to focus our attention on double triggering, which has the direct consequence of delivering a noncontrolled very high tidal volume. Double triggering occurs when prolonged diaphragm activation is detected during the ventilator expiratory phase as a new trigger, resulting in a tidal volume increase up to two times. A non-protective tidal volume is associated with an increased risk of VILI. It is essential to detect and quantify double-triggering asynchronies in any mechanically ventilated spontaneously breathing patient [16].

6.5 Monitoring and Respiratory Mechanics

Daily evaluation of a ventilated patient with spontaneous breathing should include assessment of the interaction between the respiratory drive, the condition of the lung, the amount of support with the ventilator, and the patient–ventilator interaction. Some parameters are commonly measured, such as tidal volume and minute ventilation. Others are only recently starting to be studied and used in clinical practice.

6.5.1 Plateau Pressure, Driving Pressure, and Respiratory System Compliance

In controlled mechanical ventilation, a daily evaluation of respiratory mechanics, to define the degree of respiratory system disease, is common practice, in particular, respiratory compliance as an indicator of the distensibility of the system and driving pressure as an indicator of burden of disease, also correlated with survival [18]. To measure compliance and driving pressure, an inspiratory hold is performed to obtain the plateau pressure, the airway pressure at zero flow, corresponding to the alveolar pressure.

The active participation of the patient's drive and effort during spontaneous breathing increases the level of complexity. During spontaneous breathing, the airway pressure (P_{aw}) trace shows only one part of the real pressure generated in the lung, i.e., the support of the ventilator; it is not possible to show the amount of pressure generated by the patient's respiratory muscles. Esophageal manometry is the gold standard technique to assess the negative pressure generate by the patient during inspiration and to calculate work of breathing [19]. Nonetheless, some recent data demonstrated that a plateau pressure obtained with an inspiratory hold in spontaneous breathing provide a good estimation of driving pressure and muscle pressure (P_{musc}) [20]. The difference between P_{aw} and plateau pressure (P_{plat}) is the Pressure Muscle Index (PMI), which is the pressure increase in the respiratory system due to patient relaxation, an index of patient elastic workload [21].

In a majority of cases, it is possible to obtain a good estimate of the P_{plat} and so calculate respiratory system compliance and driving pressure (Fig. 6.1). Measurement of P_{plat} is feasible in all the more common forms of ventilatory support, such as pressure support ventilation and neurally adjusted ventilatory assist (NAVA) [22]. A very recent retrospective study has shown that in patients with ARDS, P_{plat}, driving pressure, and respiratory system compliance are closely associated with outcome [23].

6.5.2 Pendelluft Phenomenon

Because it is a regional and dynamic phenomenon, the assessment of pendelluft requires an imaging monitoring technique, such as EIT. Moreover, description of this phenomenon is very recent and its clinical relevance is still to be defined.

6.5.3 Asynchronies

To recognize a non-physiologic interaction between the ventilator and the patient, it is necessary to combine physiologic knowledge of pulmonary physiology and ventilatory waveforms. Some asynchronies can be identified by analyzing airway pressure and flow traces on the ventilator. For example, a respiratory cycle that lacks an expiratory phase, because it is replaced by a new cycle, strongly indicates

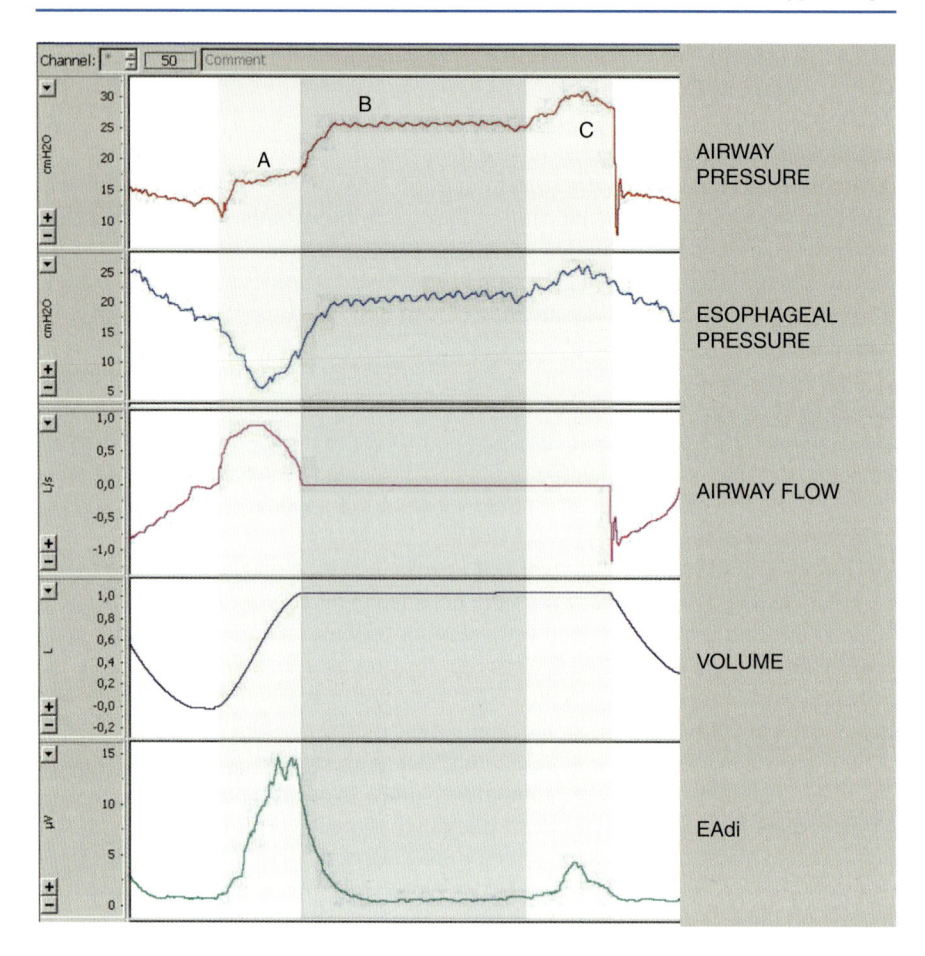

Fig. 6.1 Ventilatory traces of a patient in pressure support ventilation. After delivery of tidal volume (**A**), an inspiratory hold was performed, and a readable plateau pressure is shown (**B**). Esophageal pressure and electrical activity of the diaphragm (EA_{di}) traces confirm that in the flat part of the airway pressure, no muscular activity was observed. Interestingly at the end of the maneuver, muscular activation was detected (**C**) both by esophageal pressure and EA_{di} traces, corresponding to an increase in airway pressure

occurrence of double triggering. However, to better recognize the presence and degree of patient muscular activity, advanced monitoring, such as esophageal pressure and electrical activity of the diaphragm (EA_{di}) may be used [24, 25].

6.6 Conclusion

During spontaneous breathing and assisted ventilation, the risk of VILI is present. The additional mechanisms related to spontaneous breathing and the lack of monitoring of the additional pressure generated from the patient puts the patient at even greater risk in comparison with fully controlled ventilation. A careful evaluation of the patient is necessary to promote the weaning process without increasing the risk of VILI. Although esophageal pressure represents a standard, promising data also indicate the feasibility of plateau and driving pressure measurement during assisted ventilation.

References

1. Slutsky AS, Ranieri VM. Ventilator-induced lung injury. N Engl J Med. 2013;369:2126–36.
2. Dreyfuss D, Saumon G. Ventilator-induced lung injury: lessons from experimental studies. Am J Respir Crit Care Med. 1998;157:294–323.
3. Bellani G, Grasselli G, Teggia-Droghi M, et al. Do spontaneous and mechanical breathing have similar effects on average transpulmonary and alveolar pressure? A clinical crossover study. Crit Care. 2016;20:142.
4. Tremblay L, Valenza F, Ribeiro SP, Li J, Slutsky AS. Injurious ventilatory strategies increase cytokines and c-fos m-RNA expression in an isolated rat lung model. J Clin Invest. 1997;99:944–52.
5. Mascheroni D, Kolobow TH, Fumagalli R, Moretti MP, Chen V, Buckhold D. Acute respiratory failure following pharmacologically induced hyperventilation: an experimental animal study. Intensive Care Med. 1988;15:8–14.
6. Acute Respiratory Distress Syndrome Network, Brower RG, Matthay MA, et al. Ventilation with lower tidal volumes as compared with traditional tidal volumes for acute lung injury and the acute respiratory distress syndrome. N Engl J Med. 2000;342:1301–8.
7. Fan E, Del Sorbo L, Goligher EC, et al. An official American Thoracic Society/European Society of Intensive Care Medicine/Society of Critical Care Medicine clinical practice guideline: mechanical ventilation in adult patients with acute respiratory distress syndrome. Am J Respir Crit Care Med. 2017;195:1253–63.
8. Levine S, Nguyen T, Taylor N, et al. Rapid disuse atrophy of diaphragm fibers in mechanically ventilated humans. N Engl J Med. 2008;358:1327–35.
9. Brochard L, Slutsky A, Pesenti A. Mechanical ventilation to minimize progression of lung injury in acute respiratory failure. Am J Respir Crit Care Med. 2017;195:438–42.
10. Bellani G, Laffey JG, Pham T, et al. Noninvasive ventilation of patients with acute respiratory distress syndrome. Insights from the LUNG SAFE Study. Am J Respir Crit Care Med. 2017;195:67–77.
11. Carteaux G, Millán-Guilarte T, De Prost N, et al. Failure of noninvasive ventilation for de novo acute hypoxemic respiratory failure: role of tidal volume. Crit Care Med. 2016;44:282–90.
12. Mead J, Takishima TA, Leith DA. Stress distribution in lungs: a model of pulmonary elasticity. J Appl Physiol. 1970;28:596–608.
13. Bhattacharya M, Kallet RH, Ware LB, Matthay MA. Negative-pressure pulmonary edema. Chest. 2016;150:927–33.
14. Goldberg HS, Mitzner WA, Batra GO. Effect of transpulmonary and vascular pressures on rate of pulmonary edema formation. J Appl Physiol. 1977;43:14–9.
15. Yoshida T, Torsani V, Gomes S, et al. Spontaneous effort causes occult pendelluft during mechanical ventilation. Am J Respir Crit Care Med. 2013;188:1420–7.
16. de Haro C, Ochagavia A, López-Aguilar J, et al. Patient-ventilator asynchronies during mechanical ventilation: current knowledge and research priorities. Intensive Care Med Exp. 2019;7:43.
17. Thille AW, Rodriguez P, Cabello B, Lellouche F, Brochard L. Patient-ventilator asynchrony during assisted mechanical ventilation. Intensive Care Med. 2006;32:1515–22.
18. Amato MB, Meade MO, Slutsky AS, et al. Driving pressure and survival in the acute respiratory distress syndrome. N Engl J Med. 2015;372:747–55.

19. Akoumianaki E, Maggiore SM, Valenza F, et al. The application of esophageal pressure measurement in patients with respiratory failure. Am J Respir Crit Care Med. 2014;189:520–31.
20. Bellani G, Grassi A, Sosio S, Foti G. Plateau and driving pressure in the presence of spontaneous breathing. Intensive Care Med. 2019;45:97–8.
21. Foti G, Cereda M, Banfi G, Pelosi P, Fumagalli R, Pesenti A. End-inspiratory airway occlusion: a method to assess the pressure developed by inspiratory muscles in patients with acute lung injury undergoing pressure support. Am J Respir Crit Care Med. 1997;156:1210–6.
22. Grasselli G, Castagna L, Abbruzzese C, et al. Assessment of airway driving pressure and respiratory system mechanics during neurally adjusted ventilatory assist. Am J Respir Crit Care Med. 2019;200:785–8.
23. Pham T, Neto AS, Pelosi P, et al. Outcomes of patients presenting with mild acute respiratory distress syndrome: insights from the LUNG SAFE study. Anesthesiology. 2019;130:263–83.
24. Akoumianaki E, Lyazidi A, Rey N, et al. Mechanical ventilation-induced reverse-triggered breaths: a frequently unrecognized form of neuromechanical coupling. Chest. 2013;143:927–38.
25. Colombo D, Cammarota G, Alemani M, et al. Efficacy of ventilator waveforms observation in detecting patient-ventilator asynchrony. Crit Care Med. 2011;39:2452–7.

Part III
Biomarkers

The Future of ARDS Biomarkers: Where Are the Gaps in Implementation of Precision Medicine?

P. Yang, A. M. Esper, and G. S. Martin

7.1 Introduction

The acute respiratory distress syndrome (ARDS) is a severe form of acute inflammatory lung injury associated with high mortality rates ranging between 27 and 45% depending on severity [1]. Recent literature reported that ARDS is a common clinical syndrome in the intensive care unit (ICU), representing 10.4% of all ICU admissions and 23.4% of patients requiring mechanical ventilation [2]. However, only 51.3–78.5% of ARDS cases are recognized by clinicians, suggesting that clinicians often underdiagnose ARDS when treating patients [2]. As a result, only a fraction of the patients receive treatment interventions for ARDS, such as low tidal volume ventilation, high positive end-expiratory pressure (PEEP), neuromuscular blockade and prone positioning [2]. One of the main challenges in ARDS diagnosis and management is the lack of a simple diagnostic test, resulting in reliance on a consensus definition that tries to encompass a complex syndrome with marked clinical and pathophysiologic heterogeneity [3]. In order to address this problem,

P. Yang (✉)
Division of Pulmonary, Allergy, Critical Care and Sleep Medicine, Emory University, Atlanta, GA, USA
e-mail: pyang5@emory.edu

A. M. Esper
Division of Pulmonary, Allergy, Critical Care and Sleep Medicine, Emory University, Atlanta, GA, USA

Grady Health System, Atlanta, GA, USA

G. S. Martin
Division of Pulmonary, Allergy, Critical Care and Sleep Medicine, Emory University, Atlanta, GA, USA

Grady Health System, Atlanta, GA, USA

Emory Critical Care Center, Atlanta, GA, USA

numerous studies have focused on identifying biomarkers that can aid in the management of ARDS. Biomarkers can provide clues about the pathophysiologic mechanisms involved in ARDS and, when combined with other clinical data, can help in the diagnosis, risk stratification, and treatment of ARDS [4]. However, studies have tested a wide range of biomarkers using a variety of different methods, and are often retrospective studies with small sample sizes. As a result, the optimal way to utilize the biomarkers for clinical management of ARDS is still unclear. In this chapter, we review the current evidence for biomarkers in several aspects of ARDS management and to identify the gaps that need to be addressed before they are routinely applied in clinical medicine.

7.2 Current State of Biomarkers in ARDS

7.2.1 Biomarkers for Diagnosis of ARDS

A number of biomarkers have been studied to aid in the diagnosis of ARDS, with various levels of correlation with ARDS diagnosis. One of the biomarkers that has been shown to associate strongly with ARDS diagnosis is soluble receptor for advanced glycation end-products (sRAGE), which is the extracellular domain of a multiligand receptor expressed on alveolar type 1 cells and is a marker of lung epithelial injury [5]. In a study by Jabaudon et al., plasma sRAGE levels were found to be elevated in patients with acute lung injury or ARDS, and correlated with clinical and radiographic severity of disease [5]. Another study by Fremont et al. also found that plasma levels of sRAGE, along with several other biomarkers, were significantly elevated in trauma patients who developed acute lung injury/ARDS compared to controls [6]. A recent meta-analysis evaluating the strength of association of several biomarkers with ARDS diagnosis and mortality also found that sRAGE had a high odds ratio for ARDS diagnosis [4].

Another biomarker that has been studied in the diagnosis of ARDS is angiopoietin-2 (Ang-2), a molecule that leads to impairment of lung endothelial barrier function and serves as a marker of lung endothelial injury [7]. In one study, elevated plasma level of Ang-2 in critically ill patients receiving mechanical ventilation was shown to be predictive of acute lung injury/ARDS and to correlate with severity of disease [7]. Another study found that elevated Ang-2 levels were strongly associated with increased development of acute lung injury in critically ill patients [8]. The same study also found that the combination of elevated Ang-2 level and the Lung Injury Prediction Score (LIPS), a clinical prediction score for acute lung injury, had improved performance for identifying patients who developed acute lung injury compared to either component alone [8]. The aforementioned study by Fremont et al. in a trauma ICU population also found that Ang-2 levels were significantly elevated in acute lung injury/ARDS patients compared to controls [6].

Surfactant protein-D (SP-D) is another marker of lung epithelial injury that has been studied in ARDS diagnosis. SP-D is one of the surfactant-associated proteins that are mainly synthesized in alveolar type 2 cells and is thought to be a marker of lung epithelial injury and inflammation [9]. One study found that plasma levels of SP-D were higher in patients with ARDS compared to matched controls without ARDS [9]. Another study found that SP-D had the highest area under the receiver operating characteristic curve (AUC) among a panel of biomarkers tested for ARDS diagnosis [10].

A few other examples of biomarkers that have been shown to correlate with ARDS diagnosis in some studies include von Willebrand factor (vWF), tumor necrosis factor-α (TNF-α), interleukin (IL)-6, and IL-8 [4, 6, 8, 11] (Table 7.1).

Table 7.1 Selected biomarkers and their studied use in the acute respiratory distress syndrome (ARDS)

Biomarker	Mechanism	Studied uses	References
Soluble receptor for advanced glycation end-products (sRAGE)	Extracellular domain of multiligand receptor expressed on alveolar type 1 cells; involved in propagating inflammatory response; elevated plasma levels can indicate lung epithelial injury	Correlation with: – ARDS diagnosis – ARDS severity – ARDS mortality and outcomes	[4–6, 18, 19]
Angiopoietin-2 (Ang-2)	Binds Tie2 receptors on lung endothelial cells; impairs endothelial barrier function and increases adhesion of inflammatory cells; elevated plasma levels can indicate lung endothelial injury	Correlation with: – ARDS diagnosis – ARDS severity – ARDS mortality Distinguishing ARDS phenotype	[6–8, 19]
Surfactant protein-D (SP-D)	Synthesized in alveolar type 2 cells and non-ciliated bronchiolar epithelium; contributes to regulation of lung inflammation; elevated plasma levels can indicate lung epithelial injury	Correlation with: – ARDS diagnosis – ARDS mortality and outcomes Distinguishing ARDS phenotype	[9, 10, 15–17, 19]
von Willebrand factor (vWF)	Glycoprotein involved with hemostasis; released by endothelial cells into systemic circulation in endothelial activation or injury	Correlation with: – ARDS diagnosis – ARDS mortality Distinguishing ARDS phenotype	[4, 6, 8, 11, 19]
Interleukin-6 (IL-6)	Nonspecific pro-inflammatory cytokine	Correlation with: – ARDS diagnosis – ARDS mortality Distinguishing ARDS phenotype	[4, 6, 19]
Interleukin-8 (IL-8)	Nonspecific pro-inflammatory cytokine	Correlation with: – ARDS diagnosis – ARDS mortality Distinguishing ARDS phenotype	[4, 6, 8, 19]
Tumor necrosis factor-α (TNF-α)	Nonspecific pro-inflammatory cytokine	Correlation with: – ARDS diagnosis – ARDS mortality	[4, 6]
Fas, Fas ligand	TNF family of cytokine and receptor, expressed in many cell types including lung epithelial cells; high concentrations in BALF can indicate pro-apoptotic activity and lung epithelial injury	Correlation with: – ARDS diagnosis – Overall severity of illness in ARDS patients	[13]

BALF bronchoalveolar lavage fluid

Given the wide array of biomarkers that have shown promising results for ARDS diagnosis, some studies have examined the utility of combining several biomarkers into a panel for ARDS diagnosis. One study found that a panel of biomarkers consisting of sRAGE, procollagen peptide III, brain natriuretic peptide, Ang-2, IL-8, IL-10 and TNF-α had high diagnostic accuracy for ARDS diagnosis [6]. The same group of investigators also studied a different set of biomarkers consisting of SP-D, sRAGE, IL-6, IL-8 and club cell secretory protein, and found that the panel had higher AUC for ARDS diagnosis compared to any one of the biomarkers by itself [10]. However, partially due to the wide variability in the biomarkers that have been tested and included in the panels, there is currently no consensus about which biomarker or a panel of biomarkers is the best for ARDS diagnosis.

While the biomarkers discussed thus far are measured from plasma samples, bronchoalveolar lavage fluid (BALF) has been studied as another potential source for biomarkers. Since BALF is obtained from the distal airspaces that are close to the site of lung injury, it is thought to better reflect the local lung environment [12]. One study found that Fas and Fas ligand, which are signal molecules involved in the apoptosis pathway, were found in higher concentrations in the pulmonary edema fluid from patients with ARDS than in that from control patients with hydrostatic edema [13]. This study also found higher Fas and Fas ligand concentrations in the pulmonary edema fluid of the ARDS patients than in simultaneously collected plasma samples, supporting the potential utility of BALF as a source of biomarkers. The counterargument is that ARDS can be a patchy process occurring as a result of both pulmonary and extrapulmonary causes, and systemic compartment sampling such as serum or plasma may be more suitable for monitoring the processes related to ARDS [14]. Additional limitations in using BALF for measuring biomarkers is that sampling requires an invasive procedure and the variable dilution of BALF samples could make quantitative assessments of biomarkers more difficult [12].

7.2.2 Biomarkers for Prognostication in ARDS

The use of biomarkers has also been studied for prognostication or risk stratification to predict several outcome measures in patients with ARDS. One study showed a smaller increase in SP-D level in ARDS patients ventilated with lung-protective strategy compared to those ventilated with the conventional strategy, indicating that SP-D may serve as a marker of ventilator-induced lung injury (VILI) in ARDS [15]. The same study also found a correlation between higher SP-D levels in ARDS patients and mortality, number of days on the ventilator, and length of stay in the hospital, supporting its value in prognostication of ARDS. Eisner et al. found a similar association between higher SP-D levels in ARDS and greater risk of death, fewer ventilator-free days, and fewer organ failure-free days [16], and Jensen et al. reported that higher levels of SP-D at the time of ICU admission were not only predictive of ARDS but were also associated with low likelihood of successfully weaning from the ventilator at 28 days [17]. Similarly, Calfee et al. reported that higher sRAGE levels were associated with increased severity of acute lung injury, increased mortality, and fewer ventilator-free and organ failure-free days [18]. Several other biomarkers, including sRAGE, Ang-2, IL-6 and IL-8, were shown to be elevated in non-survivors from ARDS and associated with higher mortality [12, 19], and the meta-analysis discussed previously reported that IL-4, IL-2, Ang-2 and Krebs von den Lungen-6 had the highest odds ratios for ARDS mortality [4]. Although procalcitonin (PCT) has not been extensively studied in ARDS overall, a study by Tseng et al. found that higher levels of plasma PCT were associated with increased mortality from ARDS caused by severe community-acquired pneumonia [20].

Because of this potential utility in predicting ARDS outcomes, biomarkers have also been studied in conjunction with existing clinical prediction models to enhance their performance. As discussed previously, the combination of Ang-2 level and LIPS had higher AUC for acute lung injury development than either component alone [8], and similar results were found for combining Ang-2 and LIPS in another study in a Han Chinese patient population [21]. SP-D and IL-8 have also been used in combination with the Acute Physiology and Chronic Health Evaluation (APACHE)-III score to develop a mortality prediction model for ARDS, which was validated using the patients from several prior ARDS trials [22]. These results suggest that biomarkers may have utility in prognostication and risk stratification of ARDS patients, both alone and in combination with currently available clinical prediction models for ARDS.

7.2.3 Biomarkers for Distinguishing Phenotypes of ARDS

ARDS has been recognized as a clinically and biologically heterogeneous syndrome, with different underlying etiologies of ARDS resulting in different mechanisms of lung injury and various clinical phenotypes [3, 19]. A better mechanistic understanding of ARDS may enable further improvements in classification and management of this complex and heterogeneous syndrome, and there has been a growing interest in addressing ARDS heterogeneity using biomarkers [14]. For example, an early study reported that SP-D and SP-A levels were highest in patients with pneumonia as the ARDS risk factor and lowest in those with trauma as the ARDS risk factor [16]. The same study also found that higher SP-D levels had the strongest association with the risk of death in patients with sepsis and pneumonia, but higher SP-D levels were related to a lower risk of death in patients with trauma. Another study by Ware et al. found that the level of vWF, a marker of endothelial injury, was lower in patients with ARDS from trauma compared to other causes, and lower in patients with indirect lung injury compared to direct lung injury [11]. Calfee et al. subsequently compared the levels of several biomarkers between patients with ARDS from direct versus indirect lung injury [19]. They found that patients with ARDS from direct lung injury had higher levels of SP-D, a marker of epithelial injury, and lower levels of Ang-2, a marker of endothelial injury. In the same study, the investigators also performed a secondary analysis of a multicenter trial and found that patients with ARDS from direct lung injury had lower levels of vWF, IL-6, and IL-8 than those with indirect ARDS. Although the result regarding vWF in this study differs from that of the study by Ware et al. [11], these findings nonetheless suggest that different risk factors or phenotypes of ARDS result in different profiles of biomarkers. As such, biomarkers may be helpful for distinguishing different phenotypes of ARDS and potentially identifying various pathophysiologic mechanisms involved in ARDS that can be targeted for future therapies.

7.3 Gaps in Implementation of Biomarkers in ARDS

7.3.1 Barriers to the Clinical Application of Biomarkers in ARDS

While the above studies have demonstrated the potential utility of biomarkers in ARDS diagnosis, classification, and prognostication, currently there are significant limitations in their application and implementation in the clinical management of ARDS. Numerous biomarkers for ARDS have been studied in various contexts, but there is no single biomarker that reliably predicts ARDS diagnosis or an outcome of interest [12]. Many of the studies discussed in this review have wide variations in the patient populations recruited, biomarkers that were tested, timing and methods of biomarker measurement, and the endpoints or outcomes of interest. Many studies were also limited by the retrospective nature of the study and/or small sample sizes. These factors make it difficult to determine the optimal way to utilize biomarkers in the clinical management of ARDS.

There are also practical aspects of biomarker testing in ARDS that need to be addressed in future studies. An ideal biomarker should have high sensitivity and specificity, and be cost effective and easy to measure in a time-sensitive manner to be useful in the management of ARDS, given the acuity of this syndrome [3, 12]. Even if a biomarker or a panel of biomarkers is found to be predictive for the diagnosis or for an outcome measure of ARDS, it must be feasible to use in real time in clinical practice with the above characteristics. There is also some debate about which body compartment may be the best to sample for ARDS-related biomarkers. As discussed previously, BALF is thought to better reflect the local lung environment during lung injury and can capture biomarkers that may not be present in extrapulmonary sites, but requires an invasive procedure for sampling [14]. Plasma samples, on the other hand, are much easier to collect and may be better suited for analyzing systemic processes that are also involved in ARDS pathogenesis [14]. Exhaled breath and exhaled breath condensate have also been examined as a noninvasive source of volatile organic compounds that can serve as ARDS biomarkers [23, 24], but their utility in ARDS management and the methods for measuring these compounds need to be further assessed. All in all, more studies are needed to determine which biomarker (or panel of biomarkers) will have the best utility for predicting the diagnosis of or outcome from ARDS with reasonable accuracy, as well as the cost effectiveness and ease of measurement to be useful in a clinical setting.

7.3.2 Gaps in Identifying Additional Uses of Biomarkers in ARDS

Although prior studies have examined the use of biomarkers in various aspects of ARDS management, a majority of studies appears to focus on diagnosis and/or prognostication in ARDS. Studies examining the role of biomarkers in other aspects of ARDS management are relatively lacking, and more studies are needed to investigate additional applications of biomarkers. For example, the use of biomarkers to monitor progression of ARDS or response to treatment interventions needs more investigation. Some studies showed that ARDS patients who were ventilated with a lung-protective strategy with lower tidal volumes had a smaller increase in plasma SP-D levels over time [15, 16]. These findings suggest that measuring biomarkers over time may have a role in monitoring the severity of lung injury and the response to treatment interventions in ARDS.

Further studies are also needed for application of biomarkers in differentiating the phenotypes of ARDS and aiding in the development of future therapies for ARDS. The clinical and pathophysiologic heterogeneity in ARDS is thought to have contributed to many failures in developing therapies for ARDS, and elevation of specific biomarkers may help identify biologic or molecular pathways that can be targeted in future therapies [3]. For example, ARDS from direct lung injury appears to be characterized by lung epithelial injury, and studies evaluating therapies targeting the epithelium (e.g., keratinocyte growth factor) may preferentially enroll these patients [19]. Elevation of sRAGE level has also been implicated in identifying the subgroup of ARDS patients who have epithelial injury and may benefit from tailored therapy [5, 25], though the exact molecular target in this pathway for potential therapy still remains to be elucidated. On the other hand, ARDS from indirect lung injury appears to be characterized by endothelial injury, and these patients may benefit from future therapies targeting the endothelium and the pathways for protecting the endothelial barrier function (e.g., recombinant Ang-1) [7, 19]. Biomarkers can potentially help improve the mechanistic understanding of different ARDS phenotypes and develop a classification system, which may then help select patients who are most likely to benefit from new therapies targeting specific biologic or molecular pathways [3, 14]. Such advancements can be an important step in the application of precision medicine in ARDS management.

7.3.3 Additional Tools for ARDS Biomarker Discovery

In addition to the protein biomarkers, a relatively new scientific method that may be helpful in tackling these challenges of ARDS diagnosis and management is metabolomics. Metabolomics is an emerging field of "-omics" that simultaneously analyzes a large number of metabolites and biological compounds in an untargeted approach to identify clinically relevant biomarkers and potential therapeutic targets [26]. Because metabolites represent a level downstream of genomics and proteomics, it is thought to be closer to the phenotype of disease and more reflective of the biological perturbations in a disease process [14]. Metabolomics has been applied in defining the phenotypes of other heterogeneous pulmonary diseases, such as asthma and chronic obstructive pulmonary disease, and has started to be used in studies of ARDS as well [14]. A pilot study by Stringer et al. using nuclear magnetic resonance (NMR) spectroscopy of plasma samples found higher levels of total glutathione, adenosine, and phosphatidylserine, and lower levels of sphingomyelin in patients with sepsis-induced acute lung injury compared to healthy volunteers [26]. Another study by Viswan et al. used NMR spectroscopy of mini-BALF from ARDS patients and identified 29 metabolites [27]. Among these, six metabolites (proline, lysine, arginine, taurine, threonine, glutamate) were used to construct a predictive model for distinguishing mild versus moderate/severe ARDS. A handful of other studies have also applied metabolomic approaches to ARDS and identified biological profiles of deranged energy metabolism, increased fibrosis and inflammation, and disturbed cellular turnover in ARDS [14]. However, many of these studies have mainly focused on deriving a distinct metabolic signature of ARDS compared to control subjects, and also suffer from variability in the study populations and the methods by which the samples are measured and analyzed. Thus, more studies are needed to determine the utility of metabolomics in ARDS, with standardization of patient recruitment and sample collection, preparation, and analysis [14].

7.4 Conclusion

Numerous biomarkers have been studied for diagnosis, classification, and prognostication of ARDS. While several biomarkers have shown promising results in helping to better understand, diagnose, classify, and manage ARDS, their application to clinical settings is currently limited due to the large number of biomarkers being tested and the wide variability in the method and the timing of measurement. Further studies are needed in order to determine which biomarkers will be sufficiently accurate for predicting the diagnosis of or outcome from ARDS, and also be practical and cost effective to be useful in clinical settings. More studies are also needed in order to standardize the methods of measuring the biomarkers and to prospectively validate their utility in clinical management of ARDS. Through these steps, biomarkers can help better characterize and phenotype ARDS patients, identify potential biological and molecular targets for treatment, and allow for a more precise and tailored approach to treating this complex clinical syndrome.

References

1. ARDS Definition Task Force, Ranieri V, Rubenfeld G, et al. Acute respiratory distress syndrome: the Berlin definition. JAMA 2012;307:2526–2533.
2. Bellani G, Laffey J, Pham T, et al. Epidemiology, patterns of care, and mortality for patients with acute respiratory distress syndrome in intensive care units in 50 countries. JAMA. 2016;315:788–800.
3. Reilly JP, Calfee CS, Christie JD. Acute respiratory distress syndrome phenotypes. Semin Respir Crit Care Med. 2019;40:19–30.

4. Terpstra ML, Aman J, Van Nieuw Amerongen GP, Groeneveld ABJ. Plasma biomarkers for acute respiratory distress syndrome: a systematic review and meta-analysis. Crit Care Med. 2014;42:691–700.
5. Jabaudon M, Futier E, Roszyk L, et al. Soluble form of the receptor for advanced glycation end products is a marker of acute lung injury but not of severe sepsis in critically ill patients. Crit Care Med. 2011;39:480–8.
6. Fremont RD, Koyama T, Calfee CS, et al. Acute lung injury in patients with traumatic injuries: utility of a panel of biomarkers for diagnosis and pathogenesis. J Trauma. 2010;68:1121–7.
7. Van Der Heijden M, Van Nieuw Amerongen GP, Koolwijk P, Van Hinsbergh VWM, Groeneveld ABJ. Angiopoietin-2, permeability oedema, occurrence and severity of ALI/ARDS in septic and non-septic critically ill patients. Thorax. 2008;63:903–9.
8. Agrawal A, Matthay MA, Kangelaris KN, et al. Plasma angiopoietin-2 predicts the onset of acute lung injury in critically ill patients. Am J Respir Crit Care Med. 2013;187:736–42.
9. Park J, Pabon M, Choi AMK, et al. Plasma surfactant protein-D as a diagnostic biomarker for acute respiratory distress syndrome: validation in US and Korean cohorts. BMC Pulm Med. 2017;17:204.
10. Ware LB, Koyama T, Zhao Z, et al. Biomarkers of lung epithelial injury and inflammation distinguish severe sepsis patients with acute respiratory distress syndrome. Crit Care. 2013;17:R253.
11. Ware LB, Eisner MD, Thompson BT, Parsons PE, Matthay MA. Significance of Von Willebrand factor in septic and nonseptic patients with acute lung injury. Am J Respir Crit Care Med. 2004;170:766–72.
12. García-Laorden MI, Lorente JA, Flores C, Slutsky AS, Villar J. Biomarkers for the acute respiratory distress syndrome: how to make the diagnosis more precise. Ann Transl Med. 2017;5:283.
13. Albertine KH, Soulier MF, Wang Z, et al. Fas and fas ligand are up-regulated in pulmonary edema fluid and lung tissue of patients with acute lung injury and the acute respiratory distress syndrome. Am J Pathol. 2002;161:1783–96.
14. Metwaly S, Cote A, Donnelly SJ, Banoei MM, Mourad AI, Winston BW. Evolution of ARDS biomarkers: will metabolomics be the answer? Am J Physiol Lung Cell Mol Physiol. 2018;315:L526–34.
15. Determann R, Royakkers A, Haitsma J, et al. Plasma levels of surfactant protein D and KL-6 for evaluation of lung injury in critically ill mechanically ventilated patients. BMC Pulm Med. 2010;10:6.
16. Eisner M, Parsons P, Matthay M, Ware L, Greene K, Acute Respiratory Distress Syndrome Network. Plasma surfactant protein levels and clinical outcomes in patients with acute lung injury. Thorax. 2003;58:983–8.
17. Jensen JUS, Itenov TS, Thormar KM, et al. Prediction of non-recovery from ventilator-demanding acute respiratory failure, ARDS and death using lung damage biomarkers: data from a 1200-patient critical care randomized trial. Ann Intensive Care. 2016;6:114.
18. Calfee CS, Ware LB, Eisner MD, et al. Plasma receptor for advanced glycation end products and clinical outcomes in acute lung injury. Thorax. 2008;63:1083–9.
19. Calfee CS, Janz DR, Bernard GR, et al. Distinct molecular phenotypes of direct vs indirect ards in single-center and multicenter studies. Chest. 2015;147:1539–48.
20. Tseng JS, Chan MC, Hsu JY, Kuo BIT, Wu CL. Procalcitonin is a valuable prognostic marker in ARDS caused by community-acquired pneumonia. Respirology. 2008;13:505–9.
21. Xu Z, Wu GM, Li Q, et al. Predictive value of combined LIPS and ANG-2 level in critically ill patients with ARDS risk factors. Mediat Inflamm. 2018;2018:1739615.
22. Zhao Z, Wickersham N, Kangelaris KN, et al. External validation of a biomarker and clinical prediction model for hospital mortality in acute respiratory distress syndrome. Intensive Care Med. 2017;43:1123–31.
23. Bos LDJ, Weda H, Wang Y, et al. Exhaled breath metabolomics as a noninvasive diagnostic tool for acute respiratory distress syndrome. Eur Respir J. 2014;44:188–97.

24. Bos LDJ, Schultz MJ, Sterk PJ. Exhaled breath profiling for diagnosing acute respiratory distress syndrome. BMC Pulm Med. 2014;14:1–9.
25. Jabaudon M, Blondonnet R, Pereira B, et al. Plasma sRAGE is independently associated with increased mortality in ARDS: a meta-analysis of individual patient data. Intensive Care Med. 2018;44:1388–99.
26. Stringer KA, Serkova NJ, Karnovsky A, Guire K, Paine R, Standiford TJ. Metabolic consequences of sepsis-induced acute lung injury revealed by plasma 1H-nuclear magnetic resonance quantitative metabolomics and computational analysis. Am J Physiol Lung Cell Mol Physiol. 2011;300:L4–L11.
27. Viswan A, Singh C, Rai RK, Azim A, Sinha N, Baronia AK. Metabolomics based predictive biomarker model of ARDS: a systemic measure of clinical hypoxemia. PLoS One. 2017;12:e0187545.

8

Utility of Inflammatory Biomarkers for Predicting Organ Failure and Outcomes in Cardiac Arrest Patients

H. Vuopio, P. Pekkarinen, and M. B. Skrifvars

8.1 Introduction

Even with properly executed cardiopulmonary resuscitation (CPR), prognosis after cardiac arrest is poor, and less than half of those who are successfully resuscitated fully recover neurologically [1]. After the return of spontaneous circulation (ROSC), many patients develop a sepsis-like systemic inflammation reaction that leads to multiple organ failure (MOF) [2]. This reaction is thought to be triggered by the whole-body ischemia–reperfusion injury that occurs during cardiac arrest [2]. In some patients, this reaction results in non-cerebral organ failure and is independently associated with both long-term outcomes and elevated treatment costs [3]. The inflammatory response's magnitude upon admission and within the first 24 h is associated with both the severity of organ failure—especially circulatory failure—and the application of continuous vasopressor infusions to maintain adequate blood pressure [4]. In this chapter, we discuss the inflammatory response's role in cardiac arrest patients alongside the means for measuring this response with some old and some more novel inflammatory biomarkers: highly sensitive C-reactive protein (hsCRP), procalcitonin (PCT), soluble suppression of tumorigenicity 2 (sST2), interleukin-6 (IL-6), pentraxin-3 (PTX3), and presepsin.

H. Vuopio · M. B. Skrifvars (✉)
Department of Emergency Medicine and Services, Helsinki University Hospital, Helsinki, Finland

University of Helsinki, Helsinki, Finland
e-mail: markus.skrifvars@hus.fi

P. Pekkarinen
Division of Intensive Care Medicine, Department of Anesthesiology, Intensive Care and Pain Medicine, Helsinki University Hospital, Helsinki, Finland

University of Helsinki, Helsinki, Finland

8.2 Pathophysiology of the Inflammatory Response

During cardiac arrest, prolonged whole-body ischemia causes wide cellular and tissue damage. The respiratory chain in the mitochondria of tissue cells becomes perturbed during hypoxia [5], leading to the release of reactive oxygen species (ROS). These oxygen radicals play an important role in the initial ischemia–reperfusion injury during cardiac arrest. The release of ROS is continuous during the low-flow duration of CPR and peaks shortly after reperfusion [6], while electric shock delivered for defibrillation can directly generate ROS [7]. Ischemia, oxygen radicals, and mechanical shear stress associated with CPR [8] all damage the endothelial structures, which activates the endothelium and initiates a systemic inflammatory reaction. The activated endothelium then begins expressing adhesion molecules [9] that recruit neutrophils and other leukocytes into tissues.

The apoptotic and necrotic cells damaged by ischemia provide potent surfaces for complement activation. Full-blown complement activation has been previously reported during CPR [9] and is observed upon a patient's arrival at the ICU [10, 11]. Neutrophil activation occurs during CPR and continues increasing during reperfusion [9]. Activation of the endothelium, neutrophils, and complement all induce blood clotting, which causes further problems that may lead to disseminated intravascular coagulation (DIC) [12], thus predisposing the patient to MOF.

Monocytes and tissue macrophages can directly sense the damage-associated molecular patterns (DAMP) released upon tissue injury with their pattern recognition receptors (PRRs) [12], which then activate the nucleotide-binding oligomerization domain, leucine-rich repeat and pyrin domain containing 3 (NLRP3) inflammasome, and cause the rapid secretion of IL-1β [13]. The inflammatory mechanisms are densely interconnected, and after the initial triggering event, the inflammatory response is enhanced by several positive feedback loops. Complement fragments are versatile enhancers of inflammation that further activate the coagulation cascade, endothelial cells, neutrophils, and monocytes/macrophages. The oxidative stress that begins as a metabolic disturbance in early cardiac arrest [6] may be further aggravated by neutrophil and macrophage respiratory burst induced by the complement and DAMPs. This reaction generates oxygen radicals in the lysosomes of the phagocytes that aim to destroy an invading pathogen. In consort, these actions can create a circulus vitiosus of sterile inflammation. These rapid early events are followed by inflammatory cytokines requiring *de novo* synthesis, such as IL-6 produced by macrophages and endothelial cells [14, 10]. These molecules produced by inflammatory cells have been a target of intensive research that aims to identify markers with value for early risk stratification in cardiac arrest patients.

The inflammatory reaction is followed by immune suppression, which protects the body from excess tissue damage but predisposes the patient to infectious complications [15]. One manifestation of this immune suppression is the hyporesponsiveness of circulating leukocytes to endotoxin stimulation, which is observed in patients after cardiac arrest. Interestingly, in the absence of bacteremia, endotoxins have been reported to be present in the blood of resuscitated patients [16]. This claim suggests that endotoxins and other bacterial components that leak from the ischemic gastrointestinal tract may be additional drivers of the post-cardiac arrest inflammatory responses.

8.3 Inflammatory Biomarkers and Their Performance in Clinical Studies of OHCA

Biomarkers of inflammation are thought to be potential tools for recognizing and determining the severity of post-cardiac arrest syndrome. Many inflammatory biomarkers have been studied as possible prognostic factors because they may constitute an easily obtained and repeated method of assessing patient outcomes in the clinical setting. These studies have primarily been conducted in out-of-hospital cardiac arrest (OHCA) patients due to the confounding effect of pre-arrest infections in in-hospital cardiac arrest (IHCA) patients.

IL-6 is a pro-inflammatory cytokine produced early during the inflammatory response. It induces fever and the synthesis of acute phase proteins, such as CRP and fibrinogen in the liver, and can funnel activated helper T lymphocytes into Th17 lineage, which promotes neutrophil-mediated inflammation. Values of IL-6 measured upon ICU admission have some prognostic value for outcomes [14, 17] that lessen when measured at later timepoints [14].

PCT is perhaps the most frequently studied inflammatory biomarker for outcome prediction in OHCA [18]. PCT secretion is induced by monocyte adherence to the blood vessel's endothelial layer and is also secreted by parenchymal cells in response to ischemia. Inflammatory signaling, such as the presence of IL-6, induces PCT production [19]. PCT appears to have predictive value for poor outcomes [20], especially when measured at later timepoints [4]. Upon ICU admission, PCT may predict hemodynamic instability in cardiac arrest patients in the following 48 h [4].

Presepsin (sCD14-ST) is the soluble subtype of CD-14, a coreceptor of the PRR Toll-like receptor-4 (TLR4) that recognizes endotoxin. After an inflammatory stimulus, CD-14 is cleaved on the cell surface and released into circulation as presepsin [21]. In a study our group conducted, presepsin was associated with poor outcomes in OHCA patients but was not an independent predictor after adjusting for clinical variables [4]. Recently, another group reported presepsin's independent predictive value [22] although did not adjust for ROSC delay, which likely explains the differing results.

Other inflammatory markers studied in cardiac arrest patients include PTX3, sST2, and the classical acute phase protein CRP. PTX3 is produced by dendritic cells and macrophages in response to TLR ligand binding and by cytokine stimulation [23], whereas sST2 is a soluble decoy receptor associated with the attenuation of immune responses [24]. Admission values of PTX3 and sST2 are associated with organ dysfunction and death at the ICU but have failed to express predictive value for long-term outcomes [25]. Studies on CRP have produced conflicting results [25, 26].

Thus far, few studies have compared the utility of several inflammatory biomarkers in the same sample for predicting outcomes in cardiac arrest patients. In an analysis of 157 OHCA patients resuscitated from ventricular fibrillation, we report that no biomarker measured on admission possesses any accuracy about predicting long-term outcomes (Fig. 8.1). On the other hand, at 48 h post-cardiac arrest, PCT appears to be the most accurate biomarker for predicting outcomes albeit with moderate accuracy (Fig. 8.2). It need, however, be noted that patients resuscitated from a shockable initial rhythm receive a more favorable prognosis with less MOF compared to patients resuscitated from a non-shockable rhythm.

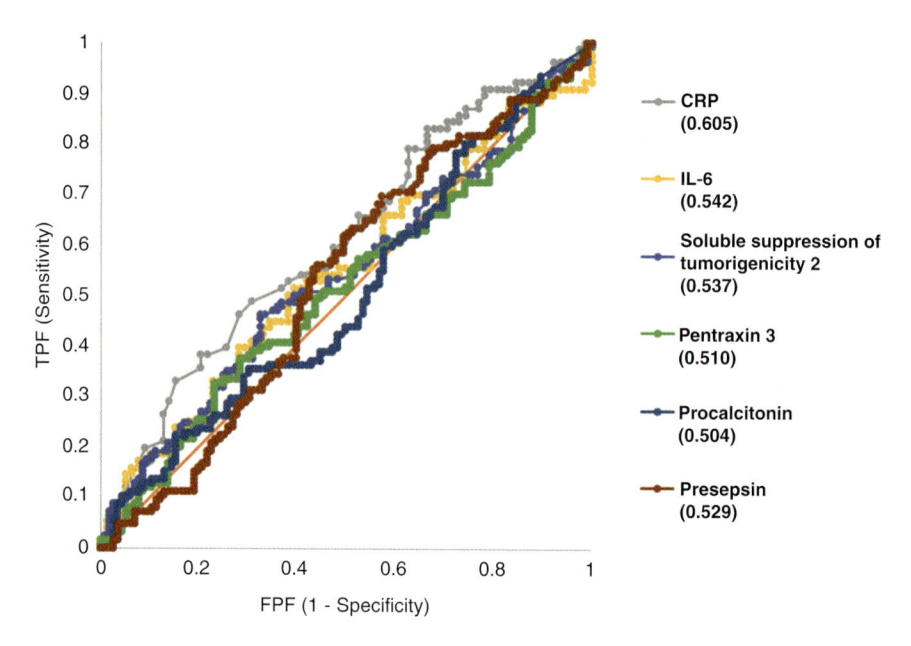

Fig. 8.1 The accuracy of inflammatory markers measured on hospital admission in post-cardiac arrest patients: the prediction of 1-year survival in 157 patients resuscitated from out-of-hospital ventricular fibrillation. The predictive accuracy is visualized with receiver operating characteristic curves. *TPF* true positive fraction; *FPF* false positive fraction

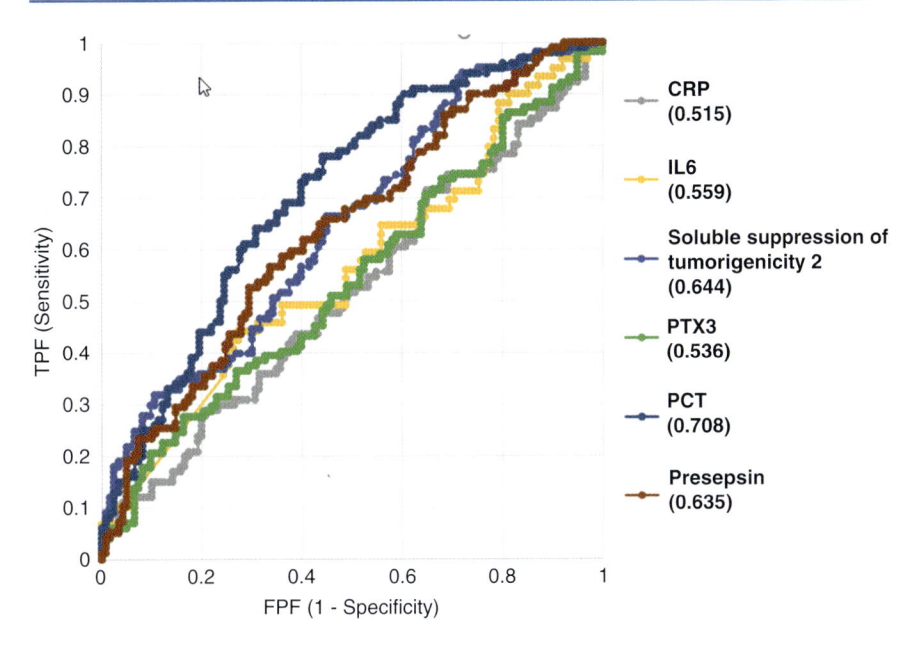

Fig. 8.2 The accuracy of inflammatory markers measured at 48 h post-cardiac arrest: the prediction of 1-year survival in 157 patients resuscitated from out-of-hospital ventricular fibrillation. The predictive accuracy is visualized with receiver operating characteristic curves. *TPF* true positive fraction; *FPF* false positive fraction

8.4 The Impact of Multiorgan Failure in Cardiac Arrest Patients

MOF following cardiac arrest is one of the main concerns in the ICU setting and is associated with high ICU morbidity and mortality [27]. Treatment for cardiac arrest patients is currently focused on neurological outcomes and treatment of the myocardium after ischemia. The dysfunction of other organs appears to affect the recovery of cardiac arrest patients although does not receive as much attention [3].

Organ failure scoring systems, such as the sequential organ failure assessment (SOFA), have been developed to assess the severity of organ dysfunction and provide predictive information for patient outcomes [28]. In an analysis of nearly 6000 cardiac arrest patients treated over a 10-year period, we demonstrate a significant association between SOFA scores (in tertiles) and long-term outcomes (Fig. 8.3). The SOFA scores do, however, include the level of consciousness measured by the Glasgow Coma Scale (GCS) score, which is likely to be paramount regarding these patients' outcomes; this fact has prompted the use of an extracranial SOFA or EC-SOFA (i.e., the SOFA score excluding the central nervous system). Two studies

Fig. 8.3 Association between organ dysfunction according to sequential organ failure assessment (SOFA) scores in tertiles during the first 24 h and outcome in 6000 cardiac arrest patients treated in Finland between 2003 and 2013

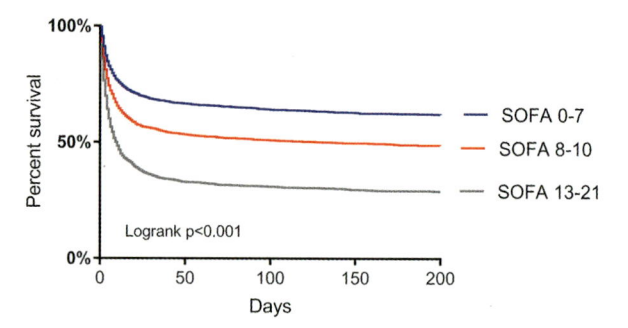

have reported an association between the EC-SOFA with in-hospital and 28-day mortality of cardiac arrest patients [29, 30]. By looking at the different subscores, a multicenter database study demonstrated that ICU OHCA and IHCA non-survivors achieved higher cardiovascular, respiratory and renal SOFA subscores, but only the renal subscore differences were statistically significant [31]. In a large multicenter database study our group conducted, EC-SOFA was an independent predictor of one-year mortality [3].

These recent studies indicate that the dysfunction of other organs apart from the central nervous and cardiovascular systems play an important role when predicting outcomes in cardiac arrest patients. These findings might also pave the way for novel therapeutic approaches in the ICU setting when treating these patients. The above-mentioned multicenter database study also determined that 16% of the cardiac arrest patients who eventually died had relatively preserved neurological function on their assessment in the ICU [31]. Many studies that address outcomes in cardiac arrest patients are currently focused on neurological recovery as an endpoint. Neurological recovery is often assessed long after ICU discharge, and non-survivors are thought to have poor neurological outcomes. Based on this multicenter study, additional repeated neurological assessments of cardiac arrest patients in the ICU might be important because their neurological recovery might be greater than a single long-term assessment may indicate [31].

8.5 The Role of Inflammation in Organ Failure and Outcomes After Cardiac Arrest

The ROS generated by ischemia–reperfusion injury lead to mitochondrial dysfunction and cause cytokines to be released throughout the body, which results in the activation of numerous macrophages, lymphocytes, and other cells in the immune system. This systemic inflammatory response created by the cytokines leads to multiple organ dysfunction and MOF [32], and the microcirculation and endothelial function are damaged due to the body's inflammatory response. The endothelium of blood vessels interacts with the circulating inflammation markers, such as IL-6 and tumor necrosis factor (TNF)-α. This interaction leads to the upregulation of cell adhesion molecules on the endothelium's surface, such as P- and E-selectin, which

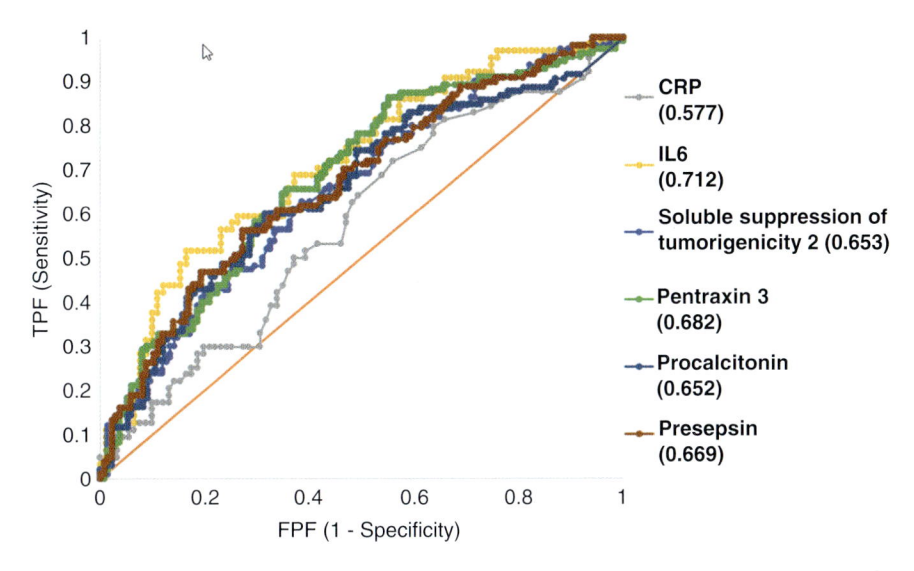

Fig. 8.4 The accuracy of different inflammatory markers measured upon hospital admission to predict organ failure (SOFA score >9) in 157 patients resuscitated from out-of-hospital ventricular fibrillation. *TPF* true positive fraction; *FPF* false positive fraction

in turn promotes the adhesion and transmigration of circulating leukocytes and leads to functional changes in the endothelium that include loss of vasomotor tone and increased permeability [33]. Increased vascular permeability leads to tissue edema due to protein-rich fluid leaking from the blood vessels. In the lungs, this increased permeability leads to interstitial and alveolar edema, both of which cause respiratory distress. The increased number of circulating phagocytic cells in the lung tissue causes further damage to the alveoli [34]. Several studies have reported associations between the magnitude of inflammatory markers (e.g., IL-6, PCT and PTX3) and organ dysfunction during the 24 h following cardiac arrest. In 157 patients resuscitated from OHCA with a shockable initial rhythm, we demonstrate that IL-6 measured upon hospital admission appears to be the most accurate inflammatory marker for predicting pending organ failure (Fig. 8.4).

8.6 Resuscitation Factors Associated with the Magnitude of the Inflammatory Response

Some studies have investigated the association between patient characteristics and factors at resuscitation as well as the magnitude of the inflammatory response. Patients who are unconscious after cardiac arrest have higher levels of IL-6 and hsCRP compared to those who remain conscious [35]. In one study, the sST2 and hsCRP levels were significantly higher in patients resuscitated from a non-shockable compared to a shockable rhythm [25]. Two studies have reported associations between increasing levels of PCT and PTX3 and the delay to ROSC [4, 25], and one of these also indicated an association between the use of epinephrine during CPR with increasing levels of PTX3, hsCRP and sST2 [25]. However, since the amount of time to ROSC and the use of epinephrine are markers of prolonged CPR, ascertaining the individual effect on the inflammatory response of any of the above is a difficult task. Overall, studies that investigate how these individual factors separately influence the developing inflammatory response in patients resuscitated from a shockable compared to a non-shockable rhythm are currently scarce.

8.7 Means of Treating Inflammation in Cardiac Arrest Patients

Several studies have attempted to alleviate the inflammatory response after cardiac arrest by aiming at both alleviating organ failure and improving patient outcomes. Thus far, the evidence is inconclusive, and no targeted management strategy yet exists. Targeted temperature management (TTM) is commonly employed in cardiac arrest patients, yet the optimal target temperature is currently unknown. In comparison to patients treated with no temperature control, TTM appeared in a small retrospective study to alleviate the inflammatory response [36], although this has not been conclusively confirmed in experimental studies of hypothermia post-cardiac arrest [37]. In a post hoc study from the TTM-Trial group, no difference was identified in IL-6 levels over time in cardiac arrest patients treated at a target of either 33 or 36 °C [38]. In a similar analysis performed by the same group that included a smaller subset of patients, the authors found no difference in IL-1β, IL-6, TNF-α, IL-4, IL-10, CRP or PCT based on whether a target temperature of 33 or 36 °C was applied [39].

A small, elegant, pilot randomized controlled trial investigated the use of steroids in OHCA patients and determined that the use of hydrocortisone as a bolus injection decreased levels of IL-6 but did not affect shock reversal or clinical outcomes, which might suggest that IL-6 plays a fairly limited role in the ongoing inflammatory response and circulatory shock in cardiac arrest patients. Another possible intervention may be the extracorporeal removal of cytokines with high cutoff venovenous hemodialysis (HC-CVVH), which was elegantly studied in the recent HYPERDIA trial [40]. In that French study, 35 patients with post-cardiac arrest shock were randomized to receive HC-CVVH or control care for 48 h. Interestingly, the study did not report a decrease in any of the multiple inflammatory markers that were studied; it is possible that the levels of most cytokines are too low to be removed by the treatment itself or that the intervention is pro-inflammatory in itself.

Several other aspects of post-cardiac arrest care may theoretically influence the inflammatory response. Extreme hyperoxia, which is reported to have harmful effects in cardiac arrest patients, has been linked with an inflammatory response in experimental studies [41]. Clinical studies, on the other hand, are scarce; one small study conducted in traumatic brain injury patients reported no difference in IL-6 levels of patients mechanically ventilated with 70% FiO_2 compared to those ventilated with 40% FiO_2 [42]. Another option is hemodynamic optimization using vasopressors and inotropes; in sepsis patients, the original early goal-directed therapy study by Rivers and colleagues indicated changes in inflammation with circulation optimization [43]. While some studies that include circulation optimization after cardiac arrest have been conducted, the results of any effect on inflammation markers have thus far not been reported [44, 45].

8.8 Incorporating Inflammatory Biomarkers into Prognostication Algorithms

Biomarkers play a role in the prognostication algorithms that are recommended and are currently in use. Most of these algorithms focus on the severity of the neurological injury; for example, neuron-specific enolase (NSE) seems to correlate fairly well with the severity of ischemic brain damage. In addition, the S100-B protein has been reported to have prognostic value in the first 24 h after cardiac arrest [46]. Most studies that analyze biomarkers as outcome predictors focus on independent examinations of specific biomarkers after cardiac arrest. As some inflammatory markers appear to be independently prognostically accurate, an appealing approach would involve incorporating some inflammatory markers into the armament of the biomarkers used. In a study conducted by Park and colleagues, various biomarkers were analyzed to determine whether or not multiple biomarkers provided a more accurate prediction for neurological outcomes of OHCA patients [47]. In that study, NSE combined with PCT seemed to express greater predictive value than either marker alone, although the difference between only measuring NSE was not statistically significant. Conversely, a study conducted by Annborn and colleagues evaluated the addition of several biomarkers into prognostication with NSE alone and did not identify any clear improvement after the addition of PCT to NSE [20].

8.9 Conclusion

Numerous studies seem to support the concept that post-cardiac arrest disease exhibits features similar to sepsis. Multiple biomarkers have been studied, most of which express a small although significant independent association with the severity of organ failure, shock, and outcomes. Of the studied biomarkers, IL-6 shows promise and appear to be a very early marker of pending organ failure. An inflammatory biomarker may play a role in identifying those cardiac arrest patients who are at special risk of severe circulatory shock. No inflammatory biomarker measured on ICU admission in patients resuscitated from a shockable initial rhythm appears to predict long-term outcomes when used in isolation; when measured at 48 h, however, PCT shows promise. Future studies must focus on whether or not there may be value in incorporating an inflammatory biomarker into the employed prognostication algorithms. Finally, despite their efforts, no studies have been able to conclusively identify any specific means that would modify the inflammatory response in cardiac arrest patients.

References

1. Dragancea I, Horn J, Kuiper M, et al. Neurological prognostication after cardiac arrest and targeted temperature management 33 °C versus 36 °C: results from a randomised controlled clinical trial. Resuscitation. 2015;93:164–70.
2. Neumar RW, Nolan JP, Adrie C, et al. Post-cardiac arrest syndrome: epidemiology, pathophysiology, treatment, and prognostication. A consensus statement from the International Liaison Committee on Resuscitation (American Heart Association, Australian and New Zealand Council on Resuscitation, European Resuscitation Council, Heart and Stroke Foundation of Canada, InterAmerican Heart Foundation, Resuscitation Council of Asia, and the Resuscitation Council of Southern Africa); the American Heart Association Emergency Cardiovascular Care Committee; the Council on Cardiovascular Surgery and Anesthesia; the Council on Cardiopulmonary, Perioperative, and Critical Care; the Council on Clinical Cardiology; and the Stroke Council. Circulation. 2008;118:2452–83.
3. Pekkarinen PT, Bäcklund M, Efendijev I, et al. Association of extracerebral organ failure with 1-year survival and healthcare-associated costs after cardiac arrest: an observational database study. Crit Care. 2019;23:67.
4. Pekkarinen P, Ristagno G, Wilkman E, et al. Procalcitonin and presepsin as prognostic markers after out-of-hospital cardiac arrest. Shock. 2018;50:395–400.
5. Vanden Hoek TL, Shao Z, Li C, Schumacker PT, Becker LB. Mitochondrial electron transport can become a significant source of oxidative injury in cardiomyocytes. J Mol Cell Cardiol. 1997;29:2441–50.
6. Idris A, Roberts L, Caruso L, et al. Oxidant injury occurs rapidly after cardiac arrest, cardiopulmonary resuscitation, and reperfusion. Crit Care Med. 2005;33:2043–8.
7. Caterine MR, Spencer KT, Pagan-Carlo LA, Smith RS, Buettner GR, Kerber RE. Direct current shocks to the heart generate free radicals: an electron paramagnetic resonance study. J Am Coll Cardiol. 1996;28:1598–609.
8. Fink K, Schwarz M, Feldbrügge L, et al. Severe endothelial injury and subsequent repair in patients after successful cardiopulmonary resuscitation. Crit Care. 2010;14:R104.
9. Böttiger B, Motsch J, Braun V, Martin E, Kirschfink M. Marked activation of complement and leukocytes and an increase in the concentrations of soluble endothelial adhesion molecules during cardiopulmonary resuscitation and early reperfusion after cardiac arrest in humans. Crit Care Med. 2002;30:2473–80.
10. Bisschops LLA, Hoedemaekers CWE, Mollnes TE, van der Hoeven JG. Rewarming after hypothermia after cardiac arrest shifts the inflammatory balance. Crit Care Med. 2012;40:1136–42.
11. Jenei ZM, Zima E, Csuka D, et al. Complement activation and its prognostic role in post-cardiac arrest patients. Scand J Immunol. 2014;79:404–9.
12. Ito T. PAMPs and DAMPs as triggers for DIC. J Intensive Care. 2014;2:67.
13. Asmussen A, Fink K, Busch HJ, et al. Inflammasome and toll-like receptor signaling in human monocytes after successful cardiopulmonary resuscitation. Crit Care. 2016;20:170.
14. Vaahersalo J, Skrifvars MB, Pulkki K, et al. Admission interleukin-6 is associated with post resuscitation organ dysfunction and predicts long-term neurological outcome after out-of-hospital ventricular fibrillation. Resuscitation. 2014;85:1573–9.
15. Beurskens CJ, Horn J, de Boer AMT, et al. Cardiac arrest patients have an impaired immune response, which is not influenced by induced hypothermia. Crit Care. 2014;18:R162.
16. Adrie C, Adib-Conquy M, Laurent I, et al. Successful cardiopulmonary resuscitation after cardiac arrest as a "sepsis-like" syndrome. Circulation. 2002;106:562–8.
17. Peberdy MA, Andersen LW, Abbate A, et al. Inflammatory markers following resuscitation from out-of-hospital cardiac arrest—a prospective multicenter observational study. Resuscitation. 2016;103:117–24.
18. Shin H, Kim JG, Kim W, et al. Procalcitonin as a prognostic marker for outcomes in post-cardiac arrest patients: a systematic review and meta-analysis. Resuscitation. 2019;138:160–7.
19. Davies J. Procalcitonin. J Clin Pathol. 2015;68:675–9.

20. Annborn M, Dankiewicz J, Erlinge D, et al. Procalcitonin after cardiac arrest—an indicator of severity of illness, ischemia-reperfusion injury and outcome. Resuscitation. 2013;84:782–7.
21. Chenevier-Gobeaux C, Borderie D, Weiss N, Mallet-Coste T, Claessens YE. Presepsin (sCD14-ST), an innate immune response marker in sepsis. Clin Chim Acta. 2015;450:97–103.
22. Qi Z, Zhang Q, Liu B, Shao F, Li C. Presepsin as a biomarker for evaluating prognosis and early innate immune response of out-of-hospital cardiac arrest patients after return of spontaneous circulation. Crit Care Med. 2019;47:e538–46.
23. Garlanda C, Bottazzi B, Bastone A, Mantovani A. Pentraxins at the crossroads between innate immunity, inflammation, matrix deposition, and female fertility. Annu Rev Immunol. 2005;23:337–66.
24. Kakkar R, Lee RT. The IL-33/ST2 pathway: therapeutic target and novel biomarker. Nat Rev Drug Discov. 2008;7:827–40.
25. Ristagno G, Varpula T, Masson S, et al. Elevations of inflammatory markers PTX3 and sST2 after resuscitation from cardiac arrest are associated with multiple organ dysfunction syndrome and early death. Clin Chem Lab Med. 2015;53:1847–57.
26. Dell'anna AM, Bini Viotti J, Beumier M, et al. C-reactive protein levels after cardiac arrest in patients treated with therapeutic hypothermia. Resuscitation. 2014;85:932–8.
27. Ferreira FL, Bota DP, Bross A, Mélot C, Vincent JL. Serial evaluation of the SOFA score to predict outcome in critically ill patients. JAMA. 2001;286:1754–8.
28. Vincent JL, Moreno R, Takala J, et al. The SOFA (sepsis-related organ failure assessment) score to describe organ dysfunction/failure. Intensive Care Med. 1996;22(7):707–10.
29. Cour M, Bresson D, Hernu R, Argaud L. SOFA score to assess the severity of the post-cardiac arrest syndrome. Resuscitation. 2016;102:110–5.
30. Roberts B, Kilgannon J, Chansky M, et al. Multiple organ dysfunction after return of spontaneous circulation in postcardiac arrest syndrome. Crit Care Med. 2013;41:1492–501.
31. Nobile L, Taccone FS, Szakmany T, et al. The impact of extracerebral organ failure on outcome of patients after cardiac arrest: an observational study from the ICON database. Crit Care. 2016;20:368.
32. Duran-Bedolla J, Montes de Oca-Sandoval MA, Saldaña-Navor V, Villalobos-Silva JA, Rodriguez MC, Rivas-Arancibia S. Sepsis, mitochondrial failure and multiple organ dysfunction. Clin Invest Med. 2014;37:E58–69.
33. Aird WC. The role of the endothelium in severe sepsis and multiple organ dysfunction syndrome. Blood. 2003;101:3765–77.
34. Malik AB, Stevens T, Bhattacharya J, Garcia JGN, Shasby MD. Mechanisms regulating endothelial cell barrier function. Am J Physiol Lung Cell Mol Physiol. 2000;279:L419.
35. Samborska-Sablik A, Sablik Z, Gaszynski W. The role of the immuno-inflammatory response in patients after cardiac arrest. Arch Med Sci. 2011;7:619–26.
36. Fries M, Stoppe C, Brücken D, Roissant R, Kuhlen R. Influence of mild therapeutic hypothermia on the inflammatory response after successful resuscitation from cardiac arrest. J Crit Care. 2009;24:453–7.
37. Callaway C, Rittenberger J, Logue E, McMichael M. Hypothermia after cardiac arrest does not alter serum inflammatory markers. Crit Care Med. 2008;36:2607–12.
38. Bro-Jeppesen J, Kjaergaard J, Stammet P, et al. Predictive value of interleukin-6 in post-cardiac arrest patients treated with targeted temperature management at 33 °C or 36 °C. Resuscitation. 2016;98:1–8.
39. Bro-Jeppesen J, Kjaergaard J, Wanscher M, et al. The inflammatory response after out-of-hospital cardiac arrest is not modified by targeted temperature management at 33 °C or 36 °C. Resuscitation. 2014;85:1480–7.
40. Geri G, Grimaldi D, Seguin T, et al. Hemodynamic efficiency of hemodialysis treatment with high cut-off membrane during the early period of post-resuscitation shock: the HYPERDIA trial. Resuscitation. 2019;140:170–7.
41. Llitjos JF, Mira JP, Duranteau J, Cariou A. Hyperoxia toxicity after cardiac arrest: what is the evidence? Ann Intensive Care. 2016;6:1–9.

42. Lång M, Skrifvars MB, Siironen J, et al. A pilot study of hyperoxemia on neurological injury, inflammation and oxidative stress. Acta Anaesthesiol Scand. 2018;62:801–10.
43. Rivers E, Kruse J, Jacobsen G, et al. The influence of early hemodynamic optimization on biomarker patterns of severe sepsis and septic shock. Crit Care Med. 2007;35:2016–24.
44. Ameloot K, De Deyne C, Eertmans W, et al. Early goal-directed haemodynamic optimization of cerebral oxygenation in comatose survivors after cardiac arrest: the Neuroprotect post-cardiac arrest trial. Eur Heart J. 2019;40:1804–14.
45. Jakkula P, Pettilä V, Skrifvars MB, et al. Targeting low-normal or high-normal mean arterial pressure after cardiac arrest and resuscitation: a randomised pilot trial. Intensive Care Med. 2018;44:2091–101.
46. Shinozaki K, Oda S, Sadahiro T, et al. Serum S-100B is superior to neuron-specific enolase as an early prognostic biomarker for neurological outcome following cardiopulmonary resuscitation. Resuscitation. 2009;80:870–547.
47. Park JH, Wee JH, Choi SP, Oh JH, Cheol S. Assessment of serum biomarkers and coagulation/fibrinolysis markers for prediction of neurological outcomes of out of cardiac arrest patients treated with therapeutic hypothermia. Clin Exp Emerg Med. 2019;6:9–18.

Troponin Elevations after Cardiac Surgery: Just "Troponitis"?

D. E. C. van Beek, I. C. C. van der Horst, and T. W. L. Scheeren

9.1 Introduction

Cardiac troponins (cTn) are a crucial part of the contractile apparatus within cardiac myocytes. There are different types of cTn: troponin C (cTn-C), troponin I (cTn-I), and troponin T (cTn-T). Contraction of the cardiac myocytes starts with binding of calcium to cTn-C. This binding results in a conformational change in tropomyosin, cTn-I, and cTn-T. This conformational change allows the myosin head to attach to actin, facilitating the acto-myosin cross-bridge to cycle, resulting in a power stroke. The subtypes cTn-I and cTn-T have been well established as biomarkers for myocardial injury with high sensitivity and specificity, since they are only detectable in human plasma when cardiac myocytes are damaged [1]. In 2009, highly sensitive cTn assays were introduced that enable detection of even very low levels of cTn, thus enabling identification of very limited myocardial injury [2], but may also lead to overdiagnosis of clinically irrelevant myocardial injury by detection of minor increases in cTn, a phenomenon referred to as "troponitis."

After cardiac surgery, there will inevitably be a substantial elevation in cTn levels [3, 4]. The cTn levels found after cardiac surgery are directly related to myocardial apoptosis and myocardial injury. However, this does not say anything about the cause of the myocardial injury. For example, use of cardiopulmonary bypass (CPB) or even simple direct manipulation of the heart can both result in myocardial

---

D. E. C. van Beek · T. W. L. Scheeren (✉)
Department of Anesthesiology, University of Groningen, University Medical Center Groningen, Groningen, The Netherlands
e-mail: t.w.l.scheeren@umcg.nl

I. C. C. van der Horst
Department of Intensive Care, Maastricht University, Maastricht University Medical Center+, Maastricht, The Netherlands

damage [5]. Because of this, clinical interpretation of elevated cTn post-cardiac surgery may be that it is simply "troponitis"; an inevitable and irrelevant consequence of cardiac surgery.

Nevertheless, cTn is key to diagnosing a postoperative myocardial infarction (MI). It has been shown that cTn is superior in detecting MI after cardiac surgery compared to electrocardiogram (EKG) changes and other biomarkers [6]. However, how cTn should be used most optimally for this diagnosis is not yet clear.

A secondary interest is in the use of cTn as a prognostic marker after cardiac surgery. The biomarker has already proved to be a useful marker for cardiovascular mortality in the general population [7]. In addition, cTn elevations after noncardiac surgery are related to mortality [8].

In this chapter, we will discuss the use of cTn for both diagnostic and prognostic purposes after cardiac surgery and the corresponding challenges. We particularly try to answer the question of whether cTn elevation after cardiac surgery is merely "troponitis" or if it should be considered an (important) factor for clinical decision-making?

9.2 Troponin and the Diagnosis of Postoperative Myocardial Infarction After Cardiac Surgery

After coronary artery bypass grafting (CABG), there is a concern of early graft failure, which can result in a postoperative MI. The incidence of early graft failure is approximately 12%, depending on the definition used [9]. Immediately after CABG, myocardial injury often occurs, but myocardial injury is not equal to MI. For a diagnosis of postoperative MI, it is essential that the presence of myocardial injury is combined with additional criteria (for details see below) [1].

Early graft failure results not merely from thrombotic occlusion, it can also be related to dissection of the graft, spasm of the graft, incomplete revascularization, and incorrect graft anastomosis [10]. When graft failure after CABG leads to a postoperative MI, the patient is at increased risk of major adverse cardiac events and mortality [11]. Immediate coronary angiography is recommended if a postoperative MI is suspected, as the angiography can direct intervention [11], and delayed angiography is associated with increased mortality [9, 12]. Adequate therapy in the case of early graft failure is associated with improved patient outcome [10]. This warrants prompt identification of patients with early graft failure after CABG. A key factor is determination of cTn after CABG to detect early graft failure, but the timing of sampling and the interval between samples need to be optimized.

As mentioned above, a diagnosis of postoperative MI is based on the presence of elevated cTn in combination with at least one additional criterion [1]. CTn levels are considered elevated according to the following criteria [1]: (1) If baseline cTn values were normal preoperatively → cTn values >10 times the 99th percentile are considered elevated and (2) if baseline cTn values were elevated (but stable or falling) preoperatively → cTn values that increase >20% *and* are >10 times the 99th percentile are considered elevated. Additional criteria are [1]: (1) new pathological Q waves on an EKG; (2) angiographic documented new graft or native coronary artery occlusion; and (3) evidence of new loss of viable myocardium or new regional wall motion abnormalities on echocardiogram.

Despite these criteria, a meta-analysis showed that early graft failure was proved in only 62% of patients undergoing angiography after CABG for the clinical suspicion of postoperative MI [13]. Currently, identifying the group of patients who could benefit from early therapeutic interventions is therefore suboptimal. The complex relationships at play in postoperative MI are largely explanatory of this situation (Fig. 9.1). Let us imagine a patient with or without certain risk factors for myocardial injury after cardiac surgery. This patient is admitted to the intensive care unit (ICU) after cardiac surgery. During surgery, the patient was exposed to potential surgery-related risk factors for myocardial injury. In the subsequent hours, cTn increases and we have to consider the patient- and surgery-related factors that resulted in myocardial injury (and thus the increased cTn levels). At the second sampling, the cTn has further increased, so we have to consider that excessive amounts of myocardial injury will put the patient at risk of adverse outcomes. Simultaneously, the patient is also at risk for early graft failure, which can occur postoperatively independent of the direct myocardial injury. Once graft failure occurs, the patient is at risk of postoperative MI with subsequent myocardial injury, which again puts the patient at risk of adverse outcomes. The complex interactions thus all drive toward cTn elevation. Figure 9.1 helps to understand the difficulty of using a biomarker for myocardial injury in the diagnosis of MI after cardiac surgery. Ideally, we should separate one particular cause of myocardial injury from other causes, using a single biomarker of myocardial injury. To do that, it is essential to first determine how the myocardial injury, and thus cTn levels, can differentiate between patients with and without postoperative MI.

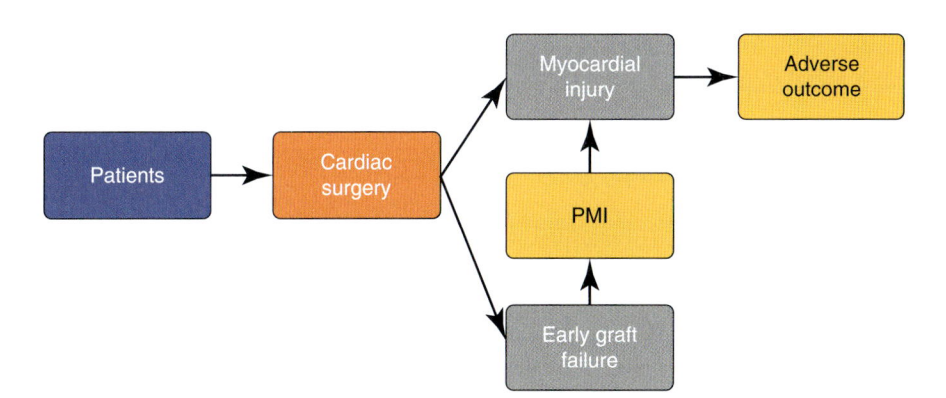

Fig. 9.1 The relationships between patient-related factors, surgery-related factors, myocardial injury, early graft failure, and poor outcome. *PMI* postoperative myocardial infarction

9.2.1 Cutoff Level of Troponin

When comparing the cTn levels of patients with and without postoperative MI, cTn levels are 1.5–5 times higher in patients with MI (depending on the assay used, the timing of the measurement and the diagnostic criteria for MI) [4, 14–16]. Considering these large differences, it should provide opportunities to find discriminating cutoff levels.

When the recommended ">10 times the 99th percentile cutoff" for cTn is combined with either EKG or echocardiographic evidence of postoperative MI, this composite is significantly associated with 30-day mortality [3]. However, as many as 93% of the patients in this study ($n = 522$) had a cTn >10 times the 99th percentile after cardiac surgery [3]. In a different study ($n = 826$), as many as 98% had a cTn > 10 times the 99th percentile [4]. If almost all patients have cTn levels above the recommended cutoff level, we question whether it can still be a useful cutoff level for the differentiation between patients with and without postoperative MI?

The "normal" cTn release after cardiac surgery in patients without MI was identified as 18 times the 99th percentile [17]. Studies evaluating potential cTn cutoff levels for the diagnosis of postoperative MI thus recommend cutoff levels between 19 and 170 times the 99th percentile [6, 18–21]. These recommendations clearly indicate that the suggested level of >10 times the 99th percentile is not the most optimal discriminative cutoff level to diagnose postoperative MI.

9.2.2 Timing of Troponin Measurements

The recommended timepoint of cTn measurements for separating patients with and without postoperative MI ranges from 8 h after aortic unclamping [20] to 48 h postoperatively [19], with most studies finding significant differences 12 h after surgery/aortic unclamping [6, 18, 20, 21]. Conversely, in one study, the cTn values did not differ significantly in patients with and without postoperative MI until 24–72 h after surgery [22]. Ideally, graft failure is diagnosed as soon as possible to prevent further myocardial injury.

9.2.3 Delta Troponin

A relatively new method of interpreting cTn levels is to look at the difference (delta) between two successive cTn measurements. When all patients ($n = 29$, 2% of the included patients) in whom the cTn-I 12 h postoperatively was higher than at 6 h postoperatively received a coronary angiogram, lesions were found in 16 patients (55%) [23]. The authors calculated the delta troponin as the ratio between cTn measurements taken at 12 h and those taken at 6 h postoperatively. The cTn ratio was 2.1 ± 1.4 in patients with lesions and 1.4 ± 0.3 in patients without lesions, and a cutoff ratio of 1.3 had a sensitivity of 88% and a specificity of 62% to detect postoperative MI [23].

9.2.4 Timing of the Peak cTn Level

Interestingly, in one study the cTn-I peaked after 24 h regardless of the presence or not of postoperative MI, whereas cTn-T peaked after 48 h in patients without postoperative MI and after 120 h in those with postoperative MI [24]. CTn levels that do not decrease 24 h after surgery were associated with increased mortality (20% versus 2.1%) in a different study [25]. Patients with a composite adverse outcome (ventricular or supraventricular arrhythmia, need for intra-aortic balloon pump for >12 h, postoperative MI) had their peak cTn level about 36 h after surgery, whereas the peak level in the group without this outcome was already seen after 24 h [26].

9.2.5 Postoperative MI and Valve Surgery

Patients undergoing isolated valve surgery cannot have early graft failure; they are, however, still at risk of postoperative MI. The incidence of postoperative MI in valve surgery is also around 11% [27]. The optimal cutoff level for cTn varied between 52 times the 99th percentile at ICU admission and 76 times the 99th percentile 16 h after surgery [27]. The cTn levels after valve surgery are generally higher than those after CABG surgery [28], which is probably a consequence of the cardiotomy required for valve surgery. To establish the diagnosis of postoperative MI in valve surgery, a higher cutoff level for cTn should be accepted, to prevent a false positive diagnosis. The occurrence of postoperative MI is associated with adverse outcome after valve surgery as well, with a higher incidence of complications and mortality [27].

Unfortunately, most studies focus on evaluating one particular method of cTn evaluation (either peak levels or delta or timing), furthermore they use different timepoints of measuring cTn and different criteria for the diagnosis of postoperative MI, making it impossible to determine which method works best. We conclude that very high postoperative levels of cTn and late timing of the peak level of cTn can be indications of ongoing myocardial injury, requiring further evaluation.

9.3 Troponin and Prognosis After Cardiac Surgery

Elevated cTn levels after cardiac surgery have been directly linked to many adverse outcomes, including ICU length of stay [29], ventilator hours [4], new-onset atrial fibrillation postoperatively [30], hospital length of stay [4, 31], in-hospital mortality [32], 30-day mortality [33] and even 5-year mortality [31].

9.3.1 Preoperative Troponin and Increased Perioperative Risk in Cardiac Surgery

An elevated *pre*operative cTn (i.e., a value above the upper reference limit) can be used to identify patients with an increased perioperative risk. Increased preoperative cTn levels have been widely associated with adverse outcomes after CABG (e.g., postoperative MI [34], low cardiac output syndrome [34], cardiac arrest [35], in-hospital mortality [34] and 6-month mortality [36]).

9.3.2 What We Can Learn from Myocardial Injury After Noncardiac Surgery

Detection of myocardial injury after noncardiac surgery using high-sensitive cTn has been increasingly studied in recent years, as it is associated with 30-day mortality (HR 3.20) [8]. Of note, 93% of these patients with myocardial injury after noncardiac surgery did not experience ischemic symptoms [8], indicating that at least in noncardiac surgery cTn elevations are highly prognostically relevant, regardless of concomitant ischemic symptoms. In myocardial injury after noncardiac surgery, the relevance of these elevations has also been demonstrated by the improvement in outcome with early interventions. Early consultation of a cardiologist and subsequent modification of the risk factor(s) resulted in similar survival rates for patients with and without myocardial injury after noncardiac surgery [37]. Whether interventions can also improve outcome when cTn is elevated after cardiac surgery remains uncertain at this point.

9.4 Important Considerations When Interpreting Troponin After Cardiac Surgery

Many patient- and surgery-related factors that affect postoperative cTn have been identified (Box 9.1). These factors do not only affect cTn level by itself, they also affect the risk for adverse outcomes (Fig. 9.2), which is a classic example of confounding. Confounding is a major concern in etiologic research; however, for

---

Box 9.1 Patient- and Surgery-Related Factors Related to Increased or Decreased Cardiac Troponin (cTn) Levels After Cardiac Surgery

Patient-related factors	Surgery-related factors
Increased troponin	
• Male [39]	• Aortic cross clamp time [32, 45]
• Higher preoperative creatinine [14]	• Cardiopulmonary bypass time [4, 14, 32, 45]
• NYHA IV [14]	• Number of perioperative defibrillations [4, 46]
• Reduced LVEF [14]	• Number of distal anastomoses [4]
• Higher CRP [14]	• Use of the intra-aortic balloon pump [4]
• Higher preoperative cTn [32]	
Decreased troponin	
• Higher BSA [14]	• Warm cardioplegia [4]
	• Off-pump CABG compared to on-pump CABG [4, 47]

NYHA New York Heart Association classification, *LVEF* left ventricular ejection fraction, *CRP* C-reactive protein, *BSA* body surface area, *CABG* coronary artery bypass grafting

Fig. 9.2 The relationships between troponin, patient-related factors, surgery-related factors, and adverse outcomes after cardiac surgery

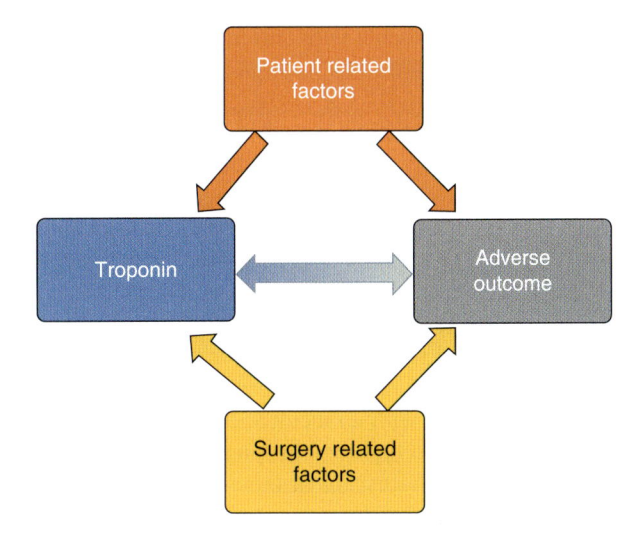

prognostic purposes it does not have to be a limitation. It is, however, important to interpret troponin levels in clinical practice in the light of the presence of these confounders. We will discuss a few of the most important factors.

9.4.1 Gender

For some highly sensitive cTn analyzers, it is recommended that a sex-specific cut-off value be used because it improves diagnostic and prognostic information [1]. The underlying cause is that cTn levels correlate with left ventricular mass, and women have on average less left ventricular mass [38].

Considering the physiological nature of the sex differences in cTn levels, it is likely that these differences also play a role after cardiac surgery. Sex has been identified as a factor with significant influence on postoperative cTn levels after uncomplicated cardiac surgery [39]. The cTn levels in males after cardiac surgery were consistently 13–37% higher at all seven timepoints (timing ranging from 6 h to 120 h after surgery) than in females [39], with the differences most pronounced immediately after surgery (timepoint 6 h) and very late after surgery (timepoints 96 h and 120 h) [39]. The exact differences in cTn between males and females in patients with a complicated postoperative course are not yet clear.

9.4.2 Kidney Function

There are two types of decreased kidney function that can occur in patients undergoing cardiac surgery. There are patients who already had impaired kidney function before surgery due to chronic kidney disease, and all patients are also at risk of developing acute kidney injury (AKI) after cardiac surgery.

In 7–71% of patients with chronic kidney disease (depending on the cTn analyzer used), cTn elevations were present without an acute MI [40]. These elevated levels are not believed to be caused by a decreased clearance of cTn, and there are many different hypotheses on what causes them (e.g., micro-infarctions, left ventricular hypertrophy, and heart failure) [40]. In general, if a patient already has an elevated cTn level before cardiac surgery, it is recommended to use a delta cTn >20% as a cutoff point postoperatively [1]. It is not known whether this also specifically applies for patients with a cTn elevation related to chronic kidney disease; however, we believe that the rationale of using a delta instead of an absolute level of cTn makes sense for all causes of cTn elevation.

As mentioned earlier, some cardiac surgery patients will already have impaired kidney function before surgery, but all cardiac surgery patients are at risk of postoperative AKI. AKI, with an incidence of about 30% after cardiac surgery, is associated with a fivefold higher in-hospital mortality rate [41]. When the AKI results in the need for renal replacement therapy (RRT; incidence 2–5%), the mortality rate increases to 50% [41]. In patients with AKI after CABG, there are indications that there is probably delayed clearance of cTn [42], this in contrast to chronic kidney disease where delayed clearance likely does not play a role [40].

In a small study ($n = 28$) in patients undergoing CABG surgery, impaired kidney function resulted in higher cTn levels postoperatively and a longer half-life of cTn [43]. A larger study ($n = 847$) showed an inverse linear relationship between glomerular filtration rate and cTn levels postoperatively [4]. In one study ($n = 805$), the optimal threshold for the diagnosis of postoperative MI after valve surgery was 19% higher in patients with impaired postoperative renal function [44]. All these findings indicate that kidney function needs to be taken into account when interpreting cTn levels post-cardiac surgery.

9.4.3 Duration of the Cardiopulmonary Bypass

The duration of CPB is directly associated with increased cTn levels [4, 14]. Therefore, it is not surprising that the fact of avoiding CPB in off-pump CABG results in lower postoperative cTn levels than on-pump CABG [4]. It is thus useful to know the presence and duration of the CBP when interpreting postoperative cTn levels.

9.5 Conclusion

Despite the many studies that have focused on this topic, the question on how to optimally use cTn measurements after cardiac surgery is still not answered. Interpreting cTn levels after cardiac surgery remains complicated because of the complex interactions, making it tempting to disregard elevations as "troponitis." However, because cTn is a reliable marker of myocardial injury and has a direct and strong relation to adverse outcomes, postoperative cTn elevations cannot be

> **Box 9.2 Summary Considerations for Clinical Practice When Using Cardiac Troponin (cTn)**
>
> *Regarding use of cTn for diagnosis of postoperative myocardial infarction (MI)*
> - Postoperative MI is common in both coronary and valve surgery
> - The diagnosis of postoperative MI is not made merely on cTn levels, which are inevitably elevated after cardiac surgery
> - A cutoff of cTn >10 times the 99th percentile is likely not specific enough to discriminate between patients with and without postoperative MI. A cTn level of at least 19 times the 99th percentile seems more appropriate
> - Cutoff levels are different in different types of cardiac surgery
> - There are indications that the best timepoint for a cTn measurement to discriminate between patients with and without postoperative MI is 12 h after cardiac surgery
> - A cTn peak level later than 24 h after cardiac surgery could potentially indicate ongoing myocardial damage, requiring further evaluation
> - Once there is a suspicion of postoperative MI, immediate coronary angiography is recommended
>
> *Regarding using cTn for prognostic purposes*
> - Preoperative cTn levels above the upper reference limit and elevated cTn levels after cardiac surgery are prognostic for important adverse outcomes after cardiac surgery
>
> *Regarding factors affecting cTn levels after cardiac surgery*
> - Women have lower cTn levels than men (>10% lower), therefore consider using gender-specific cutoff levels for cTn
> - In chronic kidney disease, there is potentially already an elevated preoperative cTn; consider using a delta cTn instead of a cTn threshold postoperatively
> - In acute kidney injury (AKI) there is possibly a decreased clearance of cTn, making interpretation of the levels very challenging. Consider using a threshold for cTn that is 19% higher for patients with AKI
> - There is a relationship between the presence and duration of cardiopulmonary bypass (CPB) and cTn levels, therefore take the CBP time under consideration when interpreting cTn levels after cardiac surgery

considered irrelevant. Moreover, cTn levels may be more than a diagnostic tool or a predictor; perhaps they can be even considered as an outcome on their own. To guide diagnostics and interventions in patients after cardiac surgery, optimal cutoff levels should take into account factors such as sex, kidney function, timing and type of surgery (Box 9.2).

References

1. Thygesen K, Alpert JS, Jaffe AS, et al. Fourth universal definition of myocardial infarction (2018). Glob Heart. 2018;13:305–38.
2. Keller T, Zeller T, Peetz D, et al. Sensitive troponin I assay in early diagnosis of acute myocardial infarction. N Engl J Med. 2009;361:868–77.
3. Wang TK, Stewart RA, Ramanathan T, Kang N, Gamble G, White HD. Diagnosis of MI after CABG with high-sensitivity troponin T and new ECG or echocardiogram changes: relationship with mortality and validation of the universal definition of MI. Eur Heart J Acute Cardiovasc Care. 2013;2:323–33.

4. Mohammed AA, Agnihotri AK, van Kimmenade RRJ, et al. Prospective, comprehensive assessment of cardiac troponin T testing after coronary artery bypass graft surgery. Circulation. 2009;120:843–50.
5. Chowdhury UK, Sheil A, Kapoor PM, et al. Short-term prognostic value of perioperative coronary sinus-derived-serum cardiac troponin-I, creatine kinase-MB, lactate, pyruvate, and lactate-pyruvate ratio in adult patients undergoing open heart surgery. Ann Card Anaesth. 2016;19:439–53.
6. Thielmann M, Massoudy P, Marggraf G, et al. Role of troponin I, myoglobin, and creatine kinase for the detection of early graft failure following coronary artery bypass grafting. Eur J Cardiothorac Surg. 2004;26:102–9.
7. Blankenberg S, Salomaa V, Makarova N, et al. Troponin I and cardiovascular risk prediction in the general population: the BiomarCaRE consortium. Eur Heart J. 2016;37:2428–37.
8. Devereaux PJ, Biccard BM, Sigamani A, et al. Association of postoperative high-sensitivity troponin levels with myocardial injury and 30-day mortality among patients undergoing non-cardiac surgery. JAMA. 2017;317:1642.
9. Preußer MJ, Landwehrt J, Mastrobuoni S, et al. Survival results of postoperative coronary angiogram for treatment of perioperative myocardial ischaemia following coronary artery bypass grafting: a single-centre experience. Interact Cardiovasc Thorac Surg. 2018;26:237–42.
10. Sef D, Szavits-Nossan J, Predrijevac M, et al. Management of perioperative myocardial ischaemia after isolated coronary artery bypass graft surgery. Open Heart. 2019;6:e001027.
11. Windecker S, Kolh P, Alfonso F, et al. 2014 ESC/EACTS guidelines on myocardial revascularization. Eur Heart J. 2014;35:2541–619.
12. Davierwala PM, Verevkin A, Leontyev S, Misfeld M, Borger MA, Mohr FW. Impact of expeditious management of perioperative myocardial ischemia in patients undergoing isolated coronary artery bypass surgery. Circulation. 2013;128(Suppl. 1):S226–34.
13. Biancari F, Anttila V, Dell'Aquila AM, Airaksinen JKE, Brascia D. Control angiography for perioperative myocardial ischemia after coronary surgery: meta-analysis. J Cardiothorac Surg. 2018;13:24.
14. Koppen E, Madsen E, Greiff G, et al. Perioperative factors associated with changes in troponin T during coronary artery bypass grafting. J Cardiothorac Vasc Anesth. 2019;33:3309–19.
15. Noora J, Ricci C, Hastings D, Hill S, Cybulsky I. Determination of troponin I release after CABG surgery. J Card Surg. 2005;20:129–35.
16. Jacquet L, Noirhomme P, El Khoury G, et al. Cardiac troponin I as an early marker of myocardial damage after coronary bypass surgery. Eur J Cardiothorac Surg. 1998;13:378–84.
17. Banning A, Musumeci F, Penny W, Tovey JA. Reference intervals for cardiac troponin T, creatine kinase and creatine kinase-MB isoenzyme following coronary bypass graft surgery. Ann Clin Biochem. 1996;33:561–2.
18. Thielmann M, Massoudy P, Schmermund A, et al. Diagnostic discrimination between graft-related and non-graft-related perioperative myocardial infarction with cardiac troponin I after coronary artery bypass surgery. Eur Heart J. 2005;26:2440–7.
19. Carrier M, Pellerin M, Perrault LP, Solymoss BC, Pelletier LC. Troponin levels in patients with myocardial infarction after coronary artery bypass grafting. Ann Thorac Surg. 2000;69:435–40.
20. Sadony V, Körber M, Albes G, et al. Cardiac troponin I plasma levels for diagnosis and quantitation of perioperative myocardial damage in patients undergoing coronary artery bypass surgery. Eur J Cardiothorac Surg. 1998;13:57–65.
21. Mair J, Larue C, Mair P, Balogh D, Calzolari C, Puschendorf B. Use of cardiac troponin I to diagnose perioperative myocardial infarction in coronary artery bypass grafting. Clin Chem. 1994;40:2066–70.
22. Cattozzo G, Finazzi S, Ferrarese S, Sala A, D'Eril GVM. Serum cardiac troponin I after conventional and minimal invasive coronary artery bypass surgery. Clin Chem Lab Med. 2001;39:392–5.
23. Perrotti A, Luporsi P, Durst C, Vernerey D, Chocron S. Early detection of asymptomatic bypass graft abnormalities using a cardiac troponin I ratio following coronary artery bypass surgery. J Card Surg. 2015;30:319–23.

24. Peivandi AA, Dahm M, Opfermann UT, et al. Comparison of cardiac troponin I versus T and creatine kinase MB after coronary artery bypass grafting in patients with and without perioperative myocardial infarction. Herz. 2004;29:658–64.
25. Moon MH, Song H, Wang YP, Jo KH, Kim CK, Cho KD. Changes of cardiac troponin I and operative mortality of coronary artery bypass. Asian Cardiovasc Thorac Ann. 2014;22:40–5.
26. Tzimas PG, Milionis HJ, Arnaoutoglou HM, et al. Cardiac troponin I versus creatine kinase-MB in the detection of postoperative cardiac events after coronary artery bypass grafting surgery. J Cardiovasc Surg. 2008;49:95–101.
27. Cubero-Gallego H, Lorenzo M, Heredia M, Gómez I, Tamayo E. Diagnosis of perioperative myocardial infarction after heart valve surgery with new cut-off point of high-sensitivity troponin T and new electrocardiogram or echocardiogram changes. J Thorac Cardiovasc Surg. 2017;154:895–903.
28. Mastro F, Guida P, Scrascia G, et al. Cardiac troponin I and creatine kinase-MB release after different cardiac surgeries. J Cardiovasc Med. 2015;16:456–64.
29. Salamonsen RF, Schneider H-G, Bailey M, Taylor AJ. Cardiac troponin I concentrations, but not electrocardiographic results, predict an extended hospital stay after coronary artery bypass graft surgery. Clin Chem. 2004;51:40–6.
30. Leal JC, Petrucci O, Godoy MF, Braile DM. Perioperative serum troponin I levels are associated with higher risk for atrial fibrillation in patients undergoing coronary artery bypass graft surgery. Interact Cardiovasc Thorac Surg. 2012;14:22–5.
31. Muehlschlegel JD, Perry TE, Liu KY, et al. Troponin is superior to electrocardiogram and creatinine kinase MB for predicting clinically significant myocardial injury after coronary artery bypass grafting. Eur Heart J. 2009;30:1574–83.
32. Paparella D, Cappabianca G, Visicchio G, et al. Cardiac troponin I release after coronary artery bypass grafting operation: effects on operative and midterm survival. Ann Thorac Surg. 2005;80:1758–64.
33. Machado M, Rodrigues F, Grigolo I, et al. Early prognostic value of high-sensitivity troponin T after coronary artery bypass grafting. Thorac Cardiovasc Surg. 2019;67:467–74.
34. Thielmann M, Massoudy P, Neuhäuser M, et al. Prognostic value of preoperative cardiac troponin I in patients with non-ST-segment elevation acute coronary syndromes undergoing coronary artery bypass surgery. Chest. 2005;128:3526–36.
35. Buratto E, Conaglen P, Dimitriou J, et al. Predicting adverse outcomes in elective coronary artery bypass graft surgery using pre-operative troponin I levels. Heart Lung Circ. 2014;23:711–6.
36. Paparella D, Scrascia G, Paramythiotis A, et al. Preoperative cardiac troponin I to assess midterm risks of coronary bypass grafting operations in patients with recent myocardial infarction. Ann Thorac Surg. 2010;89:696–702.
37. Hua A, Pattenden H, Leung M, et al. Early cardiology assessment and intervention reduces mortality following myocardial injury after non-cardiac surgery (MINS). J Thorac Dis. 2016;8:920–4.
38. Shah ASV, Griffiths M, Lee KK, et al. High sensitivity cardiac troponin and the under-diagnosis of myocardial infarction in women: prospective cohort study. BMJ. 2015;350:g7873.
39. Ge W, Gu C, Chen C, et al. High-sensitivity troponin T release profile in off-pump coronary artery bypass grafting patients with normal postoperative course. BMC Cardiovasc Disord. 2018;18:157.
40. Freda BJ, Tang WHW, Van Lente F, Peacock WF, Francis GS. Cardiac troponins in renal insufficiency: review and clinical implications. J Am Coll Cardiol. 2002;40:2065–71.
41. O'Neal JB, Shaw AD, Billings FT IV. Acute kidney injury following cardiac surgery: current understanding and future directions. Crit Care. 2016;20:187.
42. Omar AS, Mahmoud K, Hanoura S, et al. Acute kidney injury induces high-sensitivity troponin measurement changes after cardiac surgery. BMC Anesthesiol. 2017;17:15.
43. Wiessner R, Hannemann-Pohl K, Ziebig R, et al. Impact of kidney function on plasma troponin concentrations after coronary artery bypass grafting. Nephrol Dial Transplant. 2007;23:231–8.
44. Cubero-Gallego H, Heredia-Rodriguez M, Tamayo E. Influence of impairment in renal function on the accuracy of high-sensitivity cardiac troponin T for the diagnosis of

perioperative myocardial infarction after heart valve surgery. Interact Cardiovasc Thorac Surg. 2018;27:234–7.
45. Cosgrave J, Foley B, Ho E, et al. Troponin T elevation after coronary bypass surgery: clinical relevance and correlation with perioperative variables. J Cardiovasc Med. 2006;7:669–74.
46. Rodriguez-Castro D, Farrero E, Javierre C, et al. Troponin repercussion of defibrillation at the end of cardiopulmonary bypass. J Card Surg. 2007;22:192–4.
47. Brown J, Hernandez F, Klemperer J, et al. Cardiac troponin T levels in on- and off-pump coronary artery bypass surgery. Heart Surg Forum. 2007;10:E42–6.

Biomarkers of Sepsis During Continuous Renal Replacement Therapy: Have We Found the Appropriate Biomarker to Use Under This Condition?

P. M. Honore, S. Redant, and D. De Bels

10.1 Introduction

Numerous biomarkers exist to detect and quantify sepsis and infection [1].Those markers are also extremely useful to monitor the resolution of infection and to indicate when we can stop antimicrobials. Today almost 180 biomarkers have been identified [1]. One of the major caveats of these biomarkers is the fact that because of their removal during continuous renal replacement therapy (CRRT), they are no longer reliable in accurately reflecting the severity of infection [2]. So far the search continues for a novel biomarker that is not removed at all by CRRT, unfortunately without any success and so the odyssey continues. The aim of this structured review is to look at some potential biomarkers of sepsis and see if they are suitable for monitoring without any interference during CRRT allowing them to accurately depict the level of infection. For the three most used biomarkers, we provide a broad description including structure and function on top of CRRT removal whereas for the seven others, we will only focus on potential CRRT removal by convection or by hemoadsorption (Fig. 10.1).

10.2 Description of the Putative Candidates

10.2.1 The Most Frequently Used Clinical Biomarkers

10.2.1.1 C-reactive Protein

C-reactive protein (CRP) is a member of the pentraxin superfamily and was first discovered in 1930 by Tillett and Francis [3]. Indeed, the first characterization of this protein was based on the initial observation that a distinct third fraction

---

P. M. Honore (✉) · S. Redant · D. De Bels
ICU Department, Centre Hospitalier Universitaire Brugmann, Brussels, Belgium
e-mail: Patrick.Honore@CHU-Brugmann.be

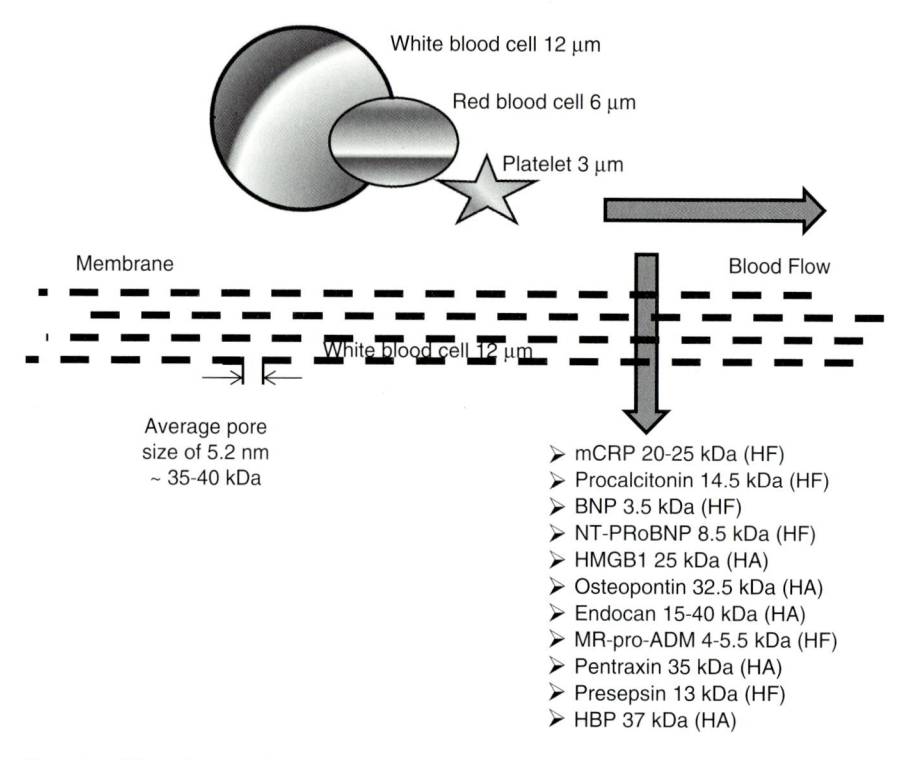

Fig. 10.1 Biomarkers: molecular weight and removal by continuous renal replacement therapy (CRRT) membranes. *HF* hemofiltration, *HA* hemoadsorption, *mCRP* monomeric C-reactive protein, *BNP* brain natriuretic peptide, *NT-ProBNP* N-terminal prohormone of BNP, *HMGB-1* high mobility group 1 protein, *HBP* heparin binding protein

identified from the sera of patients with pneumococcus infection could precipitate the "C" polysaccharide derived from the pneumococcus cell wall. Subsequently, Avery and McCarty described CRP as an acute phase reactant after demonstrating that CRP levels were elevated in patients with a range of inflammatory conditions [4]. Some 40 years after the original description of CRP, phosphocholine was shown to be the specific ligand for CRP binding within the pneumococcal cell wall [2]. Today, CRP is widely used at the bedside as a marker of inflammation and infection [4]. However, importantly, there is now a large body of evidence from prospective clinical trials that CRP levels may serve as a predictor of cardiovascular events, thus bringing the biological role of CRP into focus [4]. New insight into the different structural isoforms of CRP has led to a greater appreciation of its pro-inflammatory and prothrombotic role, which is relevant to a broad range of disease states [4].

CRP Structure and Function

CRP is predominantly synthesized by the liver as a pentamer composed of five identical, non-covalently linked 23 kDa protomers [4]. Each protomer has a binding face with a phosphocholine-binding site, which binds apoptotic cell membranes and bacterial cell walls [4]. The opposite face of the binding face, known as the effector face, binds the globular domain of the complement factor 1q (C1q) and Fc gamma receptors, thus providing a mechanism to activate the innate immune system [4]. However, the location of these binding sites on the pentameric form of CRP (pCRP) appears to be cryptic, thus supporting the concept that pCRP does not possess intrinsic pro-inflammatory properties [4].

Potential Elimination by CRRT

CRP is predominantly present as a monomer (mCRP) in the blood of septic patients [5] and is removed by all forms of CRRT because of its relatively small molecular weight (22–25 kDa), which lies below the cutoff permeability limits of all classic dialysis membranes [4]. However, although mCRP is adequately filtered, substantial amounts are also adsorbed on the dialysis membrane [2, 6]. Therein lies a clinically relevant but poorly recognized problem! In fact, highly adsorptive dialysis membranes are increasingly applied to CRRT in many intensive care units (ICUs) worldwide. The use of such membranes will inherently accentuate mCRP removal. As a result, plasma levels of these biomarkers may be falsely low during CRRT, thereby losing all potential to help clinicians diagnose or evaluate infection. One of the best recent studies looking at mCRP elimination during CRRT was by Matsui et al. [7].

10.2.1.2 Procalcitonin

Procalcitonin (PCT) is the peptide precursor of the hormone calcitonin. It is well known to be produced by the parafollicular cells of the thyroid, but it is also secreted from lung and intestinal neuroendocrine cells. The latter two sources of PCT provide its true clinical utility, as they increase its production in response to a pro-inflammatory stimulus, particularly when the stimulus is of bacterial origin. Baseline levels in most adults are <10 pg/ml, but can rapidly increase to more than 400 times baseline (>4000 pg/ml), for example when endotoxin enters the bloodstream [8]. Unlike CRP, PCT is not an acute phase reactant although this is still under debate [8].

Structure and Function

PCT is a member of the calcitonin peptide superfamily. It is a 116 amino acid peptide with an approximate molecular weight of 14.5 kDa, and its structure can be divided into three sections [9]. During inflammation induced by endotoxin shedding or microbial toxin and/or inflammatory mediators, such as interleukin (IL)-6 or circulating tumor necrosis factor (TNF)-α, there is induction together with gene activation in adipoctyes. Consequently, increased levels of PCT under these conditions never get cleaved to produce calcitonin. In a healthy individual, PCT in endocrine cells is produced by gene activation due for example to elevated calcium levels, glucocorticoids, glucagon or gastrin and is cleaved to form calcitonin, which is released into the blood [9].

Potential Elimination by CRRT

In septic patients undergoing continuous veno-venous hemofiltration (CVVH), PCT was detectable in the ultrafiltrate of all subjects [10]. Most of the PCT mass is eliminated by convective flow, but adsorption also contributes to elimination during the first hours of treatment [10]. Another important issue is the emergence of highly adsorptive dialysis membranes [6] in many ICUs worldwide, which may accentuate CRP and PCT removal even more [6, 11].

10.2.1.3 Brain Natriuretic Factors

The increased levels of B-type natriuretic peptide (BNP) and N-terminal prohormone of brain natriuretic peptide (NT-proBNP) are related to dysfunction of the cardiovascular system and systemic inflammation. In recent years, BNP and NT-proBNP have been the focus of studies evaluating their suitability for accurately reflecting severity and prognosis of sepsis and infection [12].

Structure

BNP and NT-proBNP have molecular weights of 3.5 kDa and 8.5 kDa, respectively [13].

Potential Elimination by CRRT

Whether the recently introduced biomarkers of sepsis, BNP and NT-proBNP, may perform better under CRRT conditions than other biomarkers is highly arguable. Indeed, as might be expected from their low molecular size [13], both markers will be effectively cleared by high- and low-flux membranes [14] very easily.

10.2.2 Cytokine/Chemokine Biomarkers of Sepsis

10.2.2.1 High Mobility Group 1 Protein (HMGB-1)

Although its relatively small molecular weight does not prohibit removal by routine convective hemofiltration (molecular weight of 25 kDa), HMGB-1 is effectively cleared by highly adsorptive dialysis membranes only through adsorption [15]. Highly adsorptive dialysis membranes, in particular the surface-treated acrylonitrile 69 filter (AN69-ST), are increasingly used for CRRT in ICU patients [15].

10.2.2.2 Osteopontin

Osteopontin is a highly negatively charged protein. Its nascent molecular weight approximates 32 kDa with slight variations due to post-translational modification or proteolytic cleavage. Osteopontin is not eliminated by slow extended dialysis. This is not surprising because the 5-kDa membrane cutoff point for molecular diffusion with this technique lies largely below the molecular weight of osteopontin. Theoretically, continuous hemofiltration may remove osteopontin from the circulation but evidence is lacking [16]. Moreover, CRRT is increasingly performed with novel membranes, such as the AN69-ST membrane [6]. Surface treatment implies coating with a polyethylene imine biopolymer resulting in a more neutral membrane surface composed of areas with a high density of positive charges. In addition to being highly biocompatible and permeable, this membrane displays potent adsorptive capacity.

10.2.3 Biomarkers of Sepsis Related to Vascular Endothelial Damage

10.2.3.1 Endocan

Endocan as a novel endothelium-derived soluble dermatan sulfate proteoglycan, has a molecular mass of around 15–40 kDa [17, 18]. Contemporary CRRT membranes are able to remove molecules as large as 35 kDa. Hence, endocan could be removed by CRRT [6]. When new highly adsorptive membranes are used, the ability of CRRT to eliminate endocan may even be enhanced [6]. Therefore, the reliability of endocan during CRRT could be altered. De Freitas Caires et al. showed that endocan appears as a consistently good biomarker as good as PCT and could potentially be used as a tool for antimicrobial de-escalation therapy in the future (obviously requiring new studies) as is the case now for PCT [19]. Accordingly (if endocan is used for de-escalation in the future), falsely low endocan levels in CRRT patients could lead to earlier de-escalation of antibiotics and reduced level of care for septic patients especially when using highly adsorptive membrane filters. In Europe, 80% of ICUs use highly adsorptive membrane filters, such as AN69-ST [2]. There has been no investigation on the performance of endocan in patients who receive CRRT. Such studies are urgently needed.

10.2.4 Biomarkers of Sepsis Related to Vasodilation

10.2.4.1 Proadrenomedullin (MR-proADM)

The molecular weight of MR-proADM is between 4 and 5.5 kDa, and, therefore, it may also be removed by CRRT. Indeed, Mueller et al. showed a significant decrease in MR-proADM (45–65%) if a high-flux membrane was used [20] (especially with a cutoff of 35,000 Da as used in contemporary CRRT membranes) [6]. In a study by Elke et al., 20.5% of the survivors and 58.1% of the non-survivors received CRRT, and the values of MR-proADM were, respectively, 4.0 and 8.2 nmol/l in survivors and non-survivors ($p < .001$) [21]. As the average MR-proADM levels in each group could have been impacted by differences in the CRRT prevalence [22], lower values in the non-survivor group may have given the clinician the false impression that the patient was getting better and could lead to de-escalation of therapy including antimicrobials. Again, studies are urgently needed to confirm or not this elimination by convection during CRRT.

10.2.5 Other Acute Phase Reactant Protein Biomarkers

10.2.5.1 Pentraxin

Necrotizing soft tissue infection is a devastating condition with high morbidity and a dismal prognosis [23]. Timely and adequate surgery and early aggressive treatment of associated sepsis are imperative to improve survival. Pentraxin-3 (PTX3) is a glycoprotein released by endothelial and inflammatory cells upon stimulation by cytokines and endotoxins. In contrast with CRP, which is produced in the liver in response to systemic inflammation, PTX3 is thought to better reflect local vascular inflammation and bacterial load [23]. PTX3 might thus be a more appropriate marker of severity and prognosis of necrotizing soft tissue infection. This suggestion is corroborated by Hansen et al. [23], who reported a significant association between high baseline PTX3 levels and occurrence of septic shock, amputation, dialysis need, and risk of death in a large cohort of patients with necrotizing soft tissue infection [23]. PTX3 also performed better than the "classical" inflammatory markers, CRP and PCT. Although PTX3 is a monomer, it can form a plasma octamerin composed of two covalently linked tetramers with a molecular weight >400 kDa [23]. Nevertheless, most of the PTX3 in the plasma is in monomeric form [23]. Finally, many patients with necrotizing soft tissue infection develop acute kidney injury (AKI), necessitating CRRT (25% of the patients studied by Hansen et al.). PTX3 has a molecular weight of approximately 35 kDa [23] and thus in theory can be removed by CRRT. Recently, Schilder et al. [24] demonstrated some adsorption but no elimination of PTX3 by convection across the system of CVVH, resulting in unaltered plasma levels. Whether this is also relevant when CVVH is performed at higher convection flux or with different types of dialysis membranes (especially highly adsorptive) remains to be determined. It stands to reason that the highly adsorptive membrane filters used nowadays will probably remove even more PTX3 compared to the study by Schilder et al. [24, 25].

10.2.6 Cell Marker Biomarkers of Sepsis

10.2.6.1 Presepsin

Recently, soluble cluster of differentiation 14 subtype (sCD14-ST), also known as presepsin, has been identified as a potential biomarker of sepsis [26]. Presepsin is fragmented from a larger glycoprotein and has a molecular weight of approximately 13 kDa. This is of particular concern because it theoretically exposes presepsin to significant convective elimination. Presepsin clearance may be even higher than expected because the molecule may "stick" to the highly adsorptive membranes incorporated in modern CRRT devices [6]. Thus, presepsin cannot be proposed as an accurate and clinically relevant sepsis biomarker until its behavior during CRRT is better specified [27].

10.2.7 Coagulation Biomarkers of Sepsis

10.2.7.1 Heparin Binding Protein (HBP)

HBP, also called cationic antimicrobial protein, has a molecular weight of 37 kDa [28] and thus could be removed by CRRT through convection [6] as the molecular weight of HBP falls just below the 40 kDa cutoff of classical membranes. The increased use of highly adsorptive membranes could in turn enhance the ability of CRRT to eliminate HBP through adsorption [6]. Therefore, the reliability of HBP during CRRT could be altered. Accordingly, a falsely low HBP in CRRT patients could, in turn, lead to an impression that the patient is improving and could lead perhaps to a too early reduction in the level of care for such patients [29].

10.3 Discussion

As we can see, out of the three main biomarkers used almost every day in the ICU, none is able to accurately predict the severity of sepsis and infection during CRRT [2, 30]. Regarding the other biomarkers, it has not yet been proved that any of the seven described here are not removed by CRRT especially with highly adsorptive membrane filters [6]. This is why it is really urgent to address CRRT elimination issues by appropriate studies to see if some new biomarkers are not removed by CRRT. This could offer the clinician a great tool to be able to correctly monitor infection during CRRT. The situation is becoming even more complex as more and more sorbents are used in refractory septic shock in series with CRRT [31]. These sorbents, like CytoSorb®, have a greater cutoff up to 65 kDa and may induce an even greater problem to find a new sepsis biomarker that is not eliminated by sorbents in series with CRRT [32]. Table 10.1 summarizes all the biomarkers described in this review with their molecular weights, ability to be removed by convection or/and adsorption and whether a study has already been done or not.

Table 10.1 Biomarkers: molecular weights and potential for removal by hemofiltration or hemoadsorption with summary of presence of available studies and studies that need to be realized

Biomarker	Molecular weight (kDa)	Hemofiltration	Hemoadsorption	Studies existing	Studies needed
pCRP	120	−	+?	−	+
mCRP	20–25	+	+	+	+
Procalcitonin	14.5	+	+	+	+
BNP	3.5	+	−	+	+
NT-ProBNP	8.5	+	−	+	+
HMGB-1	25	−	+	+	−
Ostepontin	32.5	−	+?	−	+
Endocan	15–40	−	+?	−	+
Proadrenomedullin (MR-pro-ADM)	4–5.5	+	−	−	+
Pentraxin	35	−	+	+	+
Presepsin	13	+	−	+	+
Heparin-binding protein	37	−	+?	−	+

pCRP pentamer C-reactive protein, *mCRP* monomeric C-reactive protein, *BNP* brain natriuretic peptide, *NT-ProBNP* N-terminal prohormone of BNP, *HMGB-1* high mobility group 1 protein

10.4 Conclusion

So far, every putative biomarker candidate can potentially be removed by CRRT, especially with the new adsorptive membranes, so we are still without any accurate biomarker of infection in CRRT-treated patients. We need to perform studies to assess whether new biomarker candidates are eliminated or not by CRRT. This would enable us to have a reliable marker of infection during CRRT. The task is becoming even more complex as sorbents have increased the cutoff up to 65 kDa making it even more complicated to find the suitable candidate to accurately monitoring infection when a sorbent is in series with a CRRT device.

References

1. Pierrakos C, Vincent JL. Sepsis biomarkers: a review. Crit Care. 2010;14:R15.
2. Honore PM, Jacobs R, De Waele E, Van Gorp V, Spapen HD. Biomarkers of inflammation during continuous renal replacement therapy: sensors, players, or targets? Blood Purif. 2014;38:102–3.
3. Tillett WS, Francis T. Serological reactions in pneumonia with a non-protein somatic fraction of pneumococcus. J Exp Med. 1930;52:561–71.
4. McFadyen JD, Kiefer J, Braig D, et al. Dissociation of C-reactive protein localizes and amplifies inflammation: evidence for a direct biological role of C-reactive protein and its conformational changes. Front Immunol. 2018;9:1351.
5. Taylor KE, van den Berg CW. Structural and functional comparison of native pentameric, denatured monomeric and biotinylated C-reactive protein. Immunology. 2007;120:404–11.
6. Dahaba AA, Elawady GA, Rehak PH, List WF. Procalcitonin and proinflammatory cytokine clearance during continuous venovenous haemofiltration in septic patients. Anaesth Intensive Care. 2002;30:269–74.
7. Matsui T, Nakagawa T, Kikuchi H, Horio H, Hashimura K. The effect of continuous renal replacement therapy with the AN69ST membrane on inflammatory markers and the level of consciousness of hemodialysis patients with stroke: comparison with hemodialysis with low blood flow rate. Pril (Makedon Akad Nauk Umet Odd Med Nauki). 2018;39:29–35.
8. Taylor R, Jones A, Kelly S, et al. A review of the value of procalcitonin as a marker of infection. Cureus. 2017;9:e1148.
9. Vijayan AL, Ravindran S, Saikant R, Lakshmi S, Kartik R. Procalcitonin: a promising diagnostic marker for sepsis and antibiotic therapy. J Intensive Care. 2017;5:51.
10. Level C, Chauveau P, Guisset O, et al. Mass transfer, clearance and plasma concentration of procalcitonin during continuous veno-venous hemofiltration in patients with septic shock and acute oliguric renal failure. Crit Care. 2003;6:R160–6.
11. Honore PM, Jacobs R, Joannes-Boyau O, et al. Newly designed CRRT membranes for sepsis and SIRS—a pragmatic approach for bedside intensivists summarizing the more recent advances: a systematic structured review. ASAIO J. 2013;59:99–106.
12. N L, Zhang Y, Fan S, Xing J, Liu H. BNP and NT-proBNP levels in patients with sepsis. Front Biosci (Landmark Ed). 2013;18:1237–43.
13. Pirracchio R, Salem R, Mebazaa A. Use of B natriuretic peptide in critically ill patients. Biomark Med. 2009;3:541–7.
14. Wahl HG, Graf S, Renz H, Fassbinder W. Elimination of the cardiac natriuretic peptides B-type natriuretic peptide (BNP) and N-terminal proBNP by hemodialysis. Clin Chem. 2004;50:1071–4.
15. Yumoto M, Nishida O, Moriyama K, et al. In vitro evaluation of high mobility group box 1 protein removal witvarious membranes for continuous hemofiltration. Ther Apher Dial. 2011;15:385–93.

16. Honore PM, Jacobs R, Hendrickx I, De Waele E, Van Gorp V, Spapen HD. To counteract or to clear high-mobility group box-1 protein in influenza A (H1N1) infection? That may become the question. Crit Care. 2015;19:401.
17. Honore PM, De Bels D, Attou R, Redant S, Gallerani A, Kashani K. Endocan removal during continuous renal replacement therapy: does it affect the reliability of this biomarker? Crit Care. 2019;23:184.
18. Hureau M, Gaudet A, De Freitas Caires N, et al. Endocan is a reliable biomarker during continuous renal replacement therapy. Crit Care. 2019;23:296.
19. De Freitas Caires N, Gaudet A, Portier L, Tsicopoulos A, Mathieu D, Lassalle P. Endocan, sepsis, pneumonia, and acute respiratory distress syndrome. Crit Care. 2018;22:280.
20. Mueller T, Gegenhuber A, Kronabethleitner G, Leitner I, Haltmayer M, Dieplinger B. Plasma concentrations of novel cardiac biomarkers before and after hemodialysis session. Clin Biochem. 2015;48:1163–6.
21. Elke G, Bloos F, Wilson DC, et al. The use of mid-regional proadrenomedullin to identify disease severity and treatment response to sepsis—a secondary analysis of a large randomised controlled trial. Crit Care. 2018;22:79.
22. Honore PM, De Bels D, Attou R, Redant S, Kashani K. The challenge of removal of sepsis markers by continuous hemofiltration. Crit Care. 2019;23:173.
23. Hansen MB, Rasmussen LS, Garred P, Bidstrup D, Madsen MB, Hyldegaard O. Pentraxin-3 as a marker of disease severity and risk of death in patients with necrotizing soft tissue infections: a nationwide, prospective, observational study. Crit Care. 2016;20:40.
24. Schilder L, Nurmohamed SA, ter Wee PM, et al. Putative novel mediators of acute kidney injury in critically ill patients: handling by continuous venovenous hemofiltration and effect of anticoagulation modalities. BMC Nephrol. 2015;16:178.
25. Honore PM, Spapen HD. Pentraxin-3 to better delineate necrotizing soft tissue infection: not really! Crit Care. 2016;20:173.
26. Zhang X, Liu D, Liu YN, Wang R, Xie LX. The accuracy of presepsin (sCD14-ST) for the diagnosis of sepsis in adults: a meta-analysis. Crit Care. 2015;19:323.
27. Honore PM, Jacobs R, Hendrickx I, De Waele E, Van Gorp V, Spapen HD. Presepsin and sepsis-induced acute kidney injury treated with continuous renal replacement therapy: will another promising biomarker bite the dust? Crit Care. 2015;19:428.
28. Honore PM, De Bels D, Barreto Gutierrez L, Redant S, Spapen HD. Heparin-binding protein in sepsis: player! predictor! positioning? Ann Intensive Care. 2019;9:71.
29. Tverring J, Vaara ST, Fisher J, Poukkanen M, Pettilä V, Linder A, FINNAKI Study Group. Heparin-binding protein (HBP) improves prediction of sepsis-related acute kidney injury. Ann Intensive Care. 2017;7:105.
30. Honore PM, Jacobs R, Hendrickx I, De Waele E, Van Gorp V, Spapen HD. 'Biomarking' infection during continuous renal replacement therapy: still relevant? Crit Care. 2015;19:232.
31. Schadler D, Pausch C, Heise D, et al. The effect of a novel extracorporeal cytokine hemoadsorption device on IL-6 elimination in septic patients: a randomized controlled trial. PLoS One. 2017;12:e0187015.
32. Honore PM, Hoste E, Molnár Z, et al. Cytokine removal in human septic shock: where are we and where are we going? Ann Intensive Care. 2019;9:56.

Part IV
Fluids

Do Intensivists Need to Care About the Revised Starling Principle?

R. G. Hahn

11.1 Introduction: Concerns Among Clinicians

Microcirculatory researchers have recently re-evaluated the principles of transvascular fluid exchange. The new aspects were summarized for anesthetists and intensivists in an influential and widely cited review article by Woodcock and Woodcock in 2012 [1]. The new evaluations have been transmitted via numerous lectures and articles worldwide and have even been the leading topic of a book [2]. Those who are popularizing the new concepts provide explanations for how fluid therapy works in humans and even give recommendations, despite the fact that the revised physiology rests primarily on experiments on mesenteric capillaries of primitive animals, such as frogs.

A multitude of "pro" articles claim a clinical importance for the revised Starling and glycocalyx principles. The present "con" article points out that the new concepts are sometimes difficult to reconcile with actual studies in humans.

11.2 Glycocalyx Degradation

The luminal side of the endothelium is covered with a layer of loose tissue containing glycoproteins and glycosaminoglycans called the glycocalyx layer. Beyond any doubt, this layer is relevant to many functions in the vascular system [3], but the key issue for anesthetists and intensivists is how easily injury or fragmentation (shedding) of the glycocalyx occurs, and to what degree this type of injury impairs the intravascular persistence of infusion fluids.

R. G. Hahn (✉)
Research Unit, Södertälje Hospital, Södertälje, Sweden

Karolinska Institutet at Danderyds Hospital (KIDS), Stockholm, Sweden
e-mail: robert.hahn@sll.se

Glycocalyx shedding is suggested to result from hypervolemia, surgery, ischemia, and severe infection [1]. Several hundred published clinical studies have reported acute elevations of the plasma concentration of glycocalyx layer constituents, implying damage to the endothelium. However, the observed three- to fourfold elevations of syndecan-1 and heparan sulfate can also be explained by changes in kidney function [4], which is often affected after surgery, trauma and intensive care.

Acute shedding probably needs to be associated with at least a tenfold elevation of the plasma concentrations of glycocalyx components to exclude the kidney as a confounder, but it most certainly occurs in cardiac surgery and in severely ill patients. Importantly, several key scenarios have been studied that show only minimal, if any, signs of glycocalyx shedding. These include cholecystitis, appendectomy [5], hysterectomy [6], hypervolemia [5, 6] and lengthy (6 h) abdominal surgery [7, 8]. However, the occurrence of acute shedding seems unlikely in most situations encountered in routine hospital work.

Correction of the plasma concentration of degradation products for plasma albumin has occasionally been applied, but its validity is unproven due to a lack of pharmacokinetic characteristics for these substances [9].

11.3 Increased Capillary Leakage?

A fourfold increased rate in the capillary leakage of albumin has been found in septic patients [10]. However, we do not know whether the increased loss was replaced by albumin from an increased lymphatic flow, or if the intravascular persistence of infusion fluid was affected. Severe disease is always associated with hypoalbuminemia, but it does not seem to be coupled with impaired intravascular persistence of infusion fluid or albumin [8].

Capillary leakage resulting from glycocalyx fragmentation has been difficult to demonstrate in complex biological systems. Rehm et al. [11] pointed out this possibility by using indocyanine green to demonstrate massive capillary leakage immediately after induction of general anesthesia for abdominal hysterectomy, where hypervolemia was induced with colloid fluid. Only 40% of the infused volume remained after a short equilibration time [12, 13].

Inspired by this finding, Nemme et al. induced hypervolemia with a rapid infusion of Ringer's in the same setting, but found no increase in glycocalyx shedding products in the bloodstream at all [6]. At the same time, the possibility was raised that Rehm's widely cited finding was due to overlooking the transit time of the indocyanine green tracer between the site of injection and the site of elimination (the liver) [14].

Rehm's group used an isolated heart model to convincingly demonstrate increased leakage of fluid upon administration of natriuretic peptides, which cause glycocalyx shedding, but the glycocalyx layer was unlikely to have remained intact after such a complex manual preparation [15].

Later, the occurrence of increased capillary leakage of albumin or fluid due to glycocalyx shedding was refuted in cholecystitis, appendectomy [5] and abdominal surgery [7, 8]. In the rat, Can Ince's group could not find any evidence that the glycocalyx serves as a barrier to fluid distribution [16].

11.4 "Non-absorption Rule"

Another claim is that an increased intravascular oncotic pressure cannot reverse fluid filtration in the capillaries because of the existence of a presumed colloid-free spatium below the glycocalyx layer (the "non-absorption rule"). This is said to explain why one cannot successfully treat edema by infusing colloid fluids. Naturally, the clinician then begins to question whether infusing 20% albumin is meaningful for that purpose.

A recent study by my group shows that infusion of 20% albumin results in allocation of three times as much fluid to the circulating plasma than the infused volume [17], which degree is expected because recruitment of fluid also concentrates the albumin concentration of the interstitium. Moreover, the same recruitment was shown in volunteers and in postoperative patients who had undergone surgery with a mean operating time of 6 h, and who had a much lower plasma albumin concentration at baseline [8].

These findings do not support the "non-absorption rule," although the possibility remains that the recruited fluid stems from the lymph rather than from the interstitial fluid. Recruitment of fluid from the glycocalyx layer has been claimed to occur, but is unproven [1] and further would be expected to cause some disintegration of this structure (shedding), which does not occur as a result of fluid recruitment with 20% albumin [17].

11.5 Capillary Filtration

A finding in primitive animals related to the "non-absorption rule" is that fluid is filtered throughout the length of most capillaries. No absorption occurs at the distal end, except transiently in hypovolemic states. This claim creates difficulties in understanding how hypertonic (7.5%) saline can greatly increase the plasma volume when given to normovolemic volunteers [18]. Infusion of 7.5% saline in 6% dextran 70 increases the plasma volume even more, by twice as much as 7.5% saline alone, which is consistent with the idea that osmotically withdrawn intracellular fluid is further transported to the plasma by a transendothelial absorption process [18] (Fig. 11.1). The reversal of the arteriovenous difference in plasma dilution in the hand only 2 min after the end of an infusion of crystalloid fluid is also difficult to reconcile [19]. This latter finding suggests that filtered fluids in the hand muscles become absorbed locally, despite the fact that the filtration pressure must be markedly raised.

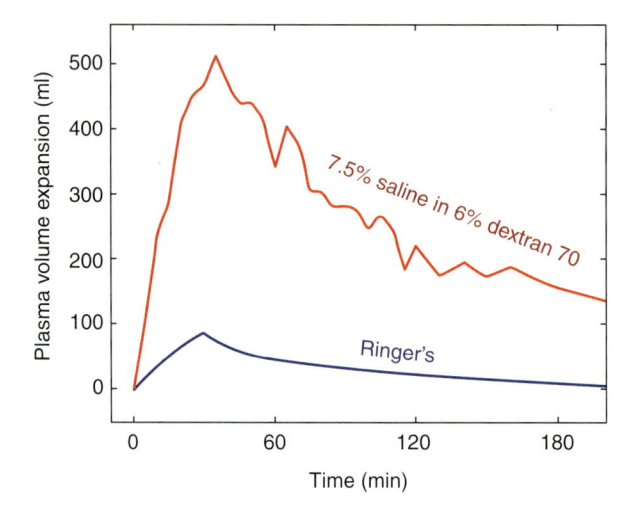

Fig. 11.1 Plasma volume expansion based on hemoglobin dilution. Red curve: in a representative male volunteer receiving 250 ml of 7.5% saline in 6% dextran 70 over 30 min. Blue curve: the same amount of Ringer's solution in a group of 10 volunteers simulated by volume kinetics (data from [18])

The revision of the traditional models for transvascular fluid exchange emphasizes filtration while downplaying, in particular, the impact of the interstitial colloid pressure, since the colloid gradient is claimed to exist between the plasma and an almost protein-free "protected region" of the subglycocalyx space [1]. This model scarcely agrees with our results from cardiopulmonary bypass (CPB), where the priming solution (Ringer's) had a normal distribution half-life of 8 min [20]. Connecting the patient to the circuit would then imply that the hydrostatic pressure is kept constant while the intravascular colloid pressure is dramatically reduced by dilution with the crystalloid fluid in the circuit. In this setting, no distribution at all would have occurred if the subglycocalyx region had been protein free.

11.6 Are Colloids and Crystalloids Equal?

Microcirculatory researchers claim that the traditional Starling principle predicts that crystalloid fluid has only a transient effect on the blood volume in hypovolemic humans [21]. This is actually the case, and rebound hypovolemia is therefore an expected but widely overlooked problem [22]. However, these researchers now propose an alternative interpretation, the revised Starling principle, which predicts that crystalloids are retained to a greater extent in the hypovolemic setting. This is said to explain why crystalloids are far more effective in the operating room and in trauma than in volunteers [21].

In clinical patients, an excess intravascular accumulation of crystalloid fluid has been known for almost 30 years to require the development of arterial hypotension, i.e., relative or absolute hypovolemia is not sufficient [23, 24]. In humans, a reduction in the mean arterial pressure (MAP) to a steady state 20% below baseline temporarily arrests the distribution of crystalloid fluid to the interstitium, making it an effective plasma volume expander [25]. This effect is easy to explain by the traditional Starling equation, since a reduction in the intravascular pressure should create difficulties for infused fluid to distribute against an interstitial fluid at a normal pressure. However, the effective plasma volume expansion is likely to last only until the infusion has built up a new Starling equilibrium. Thereafter, the distribution function is the same as that observed in conscious volunteers [26].

Kinetic analyses in humans do not support a more than transient slowdown of the rate of distribution of fluid in extrarenal capillaries in this setting. The increased effectiveness of crystalloid fluid in lengthy surgery or intensive care is not due to a slow distribution but due to renal fluid retention, which is proportional to the patient's age and inversely to the MAP [27]. Therefore, the rate of elimination is the main factor that determines plasma volume expansion during long observation times, and this fact has cast doubts over the relative potency of these fluids in several intensive care studies [28].

11.7 Hemodilution and the Glycocalyx

Objections to the use of hemoglobin (Hb) concentration to estimate the distribution of infused fluid are usually based on microcirculatory considerations. Hb concentration is claimed to be a misleading index of plasma volume change because red blood cells (RBCs) do not pass into the glycocalyx layer; therefore, Hb only indicates the circulating blood volume [13, 29].

This consideration is not valid because the Hb concentration is only the inverse of the blood water concentration and has nothing to do with the blood volume. The glycocalyx will be indicated by the Hb concentration as long as infused water passes into the glycocalyx. This can be understood from the following example:

Assume that we infuse two fluids on separate occasions that distribute into different body fluid compartments (let us say the plasma and the total body water). Naturally, the hemodilution will be greater for the first and smaller for the second infusion. Nevertheless, a correct volume of distribution for the infused fluid will be obtained in both cases by dividing the infused volume with the Hb dilution. The fact that RBCs cannot distribute into the total body water is not relevant as long as the infused water volume does distribute there. Hence, the hemodilution reflects how the infused water is distributed, and whether this is occurring inside or outside the circulating blood does not matter.

Microcirculatory researchers also discredit the use of Hb because RBCs circulate at a different rate than the plasma [21]. This objection might be valid for radioactive tracers but not for hemodilution, which will be the same even if the RBCs are transported at a rate of zero. The blood Hb concentration mirrors the blood-water concentration and nothing else.

11.8 Volume Kinetics

The most sophisticated use of Hb dilution is to apply volume kinetics to serial measurements and calculate the distribution and elimination of an infusion fluid [27]. This analysis detects a "wall" between a central compartment (the plasma) and a peripheral compartment (probably the interstitium) and indicates where the infused fluid is located, regardless of the degree of hemodilution. Hence, if hemodilution is doubled, the plotted fluid distribution will be the same, although a scaling factor between the hemodilution and the volume change (i.e., V_c, the plasma volume) will be cut in half.

The example shown in Fig. 11.2 compares the modeled plasma volume expansion and the plasma dilution as derived by population volume kinetics, based on four published studies where blood Hb and plasma albumin were measured at precisely timed intervals during and after infusion of a crystalloid fluid [6, 26, 30, 31]. Both albumin and Hb show practically identical intravascular fluid volumes (Fig. 11.2, upper). The scaling factor between the volume change and dilution was

Fig. 11.2 Plasma volume expansion (upper) and the corresponding plasma dilution (lower) when 1.5 l of crystalloid fluid is infused over 30 min. Computer simulations based on population kinetic data from 128 infusion experiments (2009 data points), where blood hemoglobin (Hb) concentration and plasma albumin had been measured at precisely timed intervals. Compilation of measurements from four studies [6, 26, 30, 31] using methods described in [27]

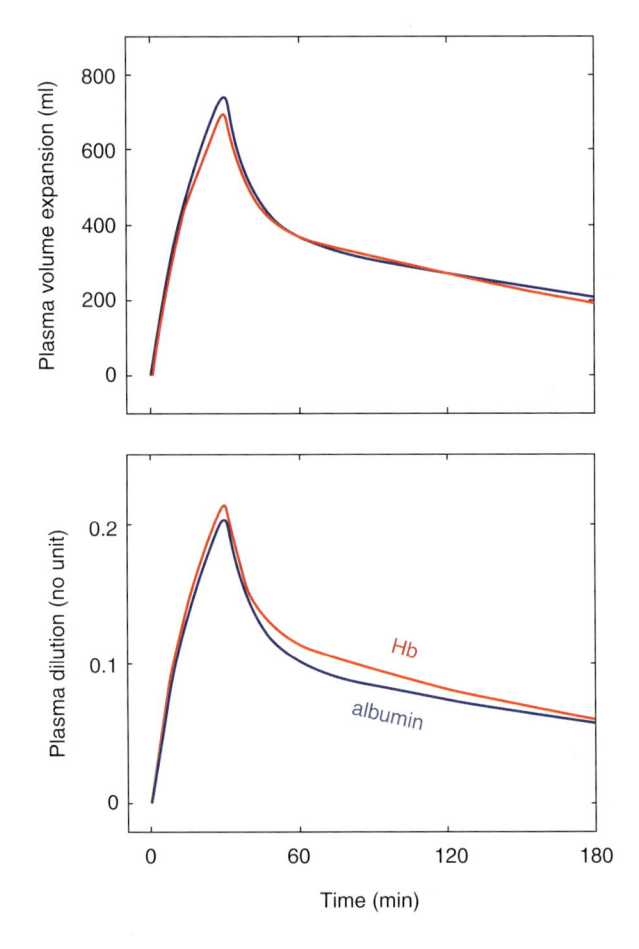

3.25 l for Hb and 3.63 l for albumin, and this is the closest we can get to an estimate of the plasma volume using dilution kinetics. Figure 11.2 (lower panel) indicates a somewhat smaller plasma dilution for plasma albumin than for Hb, which agrees well with the "f-cell ratio", or "hematocrit factor", (usually 0.88–0.92; here, it is 3.25/3.63 = 0.895), which is reported when the blood volume is measured using radioactive tracers.

11.9 Conclusion

The relevance of the revised Starling principle and the glycocalyx model to clinical work is not yet proven, and their use can even create difficulties in explaining the results of some studies in humans. Acute degradation of the glycocalyx apparently requires the occurrence of a more severe physiological insult than was previously believed. Misinterpretation of elevated plasma concentrations of glycocalyx degradation products due to changes in kidney function can be suspected. Shortened intravascular persistence of infusion fluids after shedding of the glycocalyx layer has not yet been demonstrated in humans. Lastly, the author argues against objections raised by microcirculatory researchers regarding the use of hemodilution to study fluid distribution.

References

1. Woodcock TE, Woodcock TM. Revised Starling equation and the glycocalyx model of transvascular fluid exchange: an improved paradigm for prescribing intravenous fluid therapy. Br J Anaesth. 2012;108:384–94.
2. Farag E, Kurz A. Perioperative fluid management. Cham: Springer; 2016.
3. Kolsen-Petersen JA. The endothelial glycocalyx: the great luminal barrier. Acta Anaesthesiol Scand. 2015;59:137–9.
4. Hahn RG, Hasselgren E, Björne H, Zdolsek M, Zdolsek J. Biomarkers of endothelial injury in plasma are dependent on kidney function. Clin Hemorheol Microcirc. 2019;72:161–8.
5. Li Y, Yi S, Zhu Y, Hahn RG. Volume kinetics of Ringer's lactate in acute inflammatory disease. Br J Anaesth. 2018;121:574–80.
6. Nemme J, Hahn RG, Krizhanovskii C, Ntika S, Sabelnikovs O, Vanags I. Minimal shedding of the glycocalyx layer during abdominal hysterectomy. BMC Anesthesiol. 2017;17:107.
7. Statkevicus S, Bonnevier J, Fisher J, et al. Albumin infusion rate and plasma volume expansion: a randomized clinical trial in postoperative patients after major surgery. Crit Care. 2019;23:191.
8. Hasselgren E, Zdolsek M, Zdolsek JH, et al. Long intravascular persistence of albumin 20% in postoperative patients. Anesth Analg. 2019;129:1232–9.
9. Chappell D, Bruegger D, Potzel J, et al. Hypervolemia increases release of atrial natriuretic peptide and shedding of the endothelial glycocalyx. Crit Care. 2014;18:538.
10. Fleck A, Raines G, Hawker F, et al. Increased vascular permeability: a major cause of hypoalbuminaemia in disease and injury. Lancet. 1985;325:781–4.
11. Rehm M, Haller M, Orth V, et al. Changes in blood volume and hematocrit during acute perioperative volume loading with 5% albumin or 6% hetastarch solutions in patients before radical hysterectomy. Anesthesiology. 2001;95:849–56.

12. Jacob M, Chappell D, Rehm M. Clinical update: perioperative fluid management. Lancet. 2007;369:1984–6.
13. Chappell D, Jacob M, Hofmann-Kiefer K, Conzen P, Rehm M. A rational approach to perioperative fluid management. Anesthesiology. 2008;109:723–40.
14. Hahn RG. Must hypervolaemia be avoided? A critique of the evidence. Anaesthesiol Intensive Ther. 2015;47:94–101.
15. Jacob M, Saller T, Chappell D, Rehm M, Welsch U, Becker BF. Physiological levels of A-, B- and C-type natriuretic peptide shed the endothelial glycocalyx and enhance vascular permeability. Basic Res Cardiol. 2013;108:347.
16. Guerci P, Ergin B, Uz Z, et al. Glycocalyx degradation is independent of vascular barrier permeability increase in nontraumatic hemorrhagic shock in rats. Anesth Analg. 2019;129:598–607.
17. Zdolsek M, Hahn RG, Zdolsek JH. Recruitment of extravascular fluid by hyperoncotic albumin. Acta Anaesthesiol Scand. 2018;62:1255–60.
18. Drobin D, Hahn RG. Kinetics of isotonic and hypertonic plasma volume expanders. Anesthesiology. 2002;96:1371–80.
19. Svensén CH, Rodhe PM, Olsson J, Borsheim E, Aarsland A, Hahn RG. Arteriovenous differences in plasma dilution and the distribution kinetics of lactated Ringer's solution. Anesth Analg. 2009;108:128–33.
20. Törnudd M, Hahn RG, Zdolsek JH. Fluid distribution kinetics during cardiopulmonary bypass. Clinics. 2014;69:535–41.
21. Michel CC, Arkill KP, Curry FE. The revised Starling principle and its relevance to perioperative fluid therapy. In: Farag E, Kurz A, editors. Perioperative fluid management. Cham: Springer; 2016. p. 31–74.
22. Hahn RG, Drobin D, Li Y, Zdolsek J. Kinetics of Ringer's solution in extracellular dehydration and hemorrhage. Shock. 2019. https://doi.org/10.1097/SHK.0000000000001422. [Epub ahead of print]
23. Hahn RG. Haemoglobin dilution from epidural-induced hypotension with and without fluid loading. Acta Anaesthesiol Scand. 1992;36:241–4.
24. Drobin D, Hahn RG. Time course of increased haemodilution in hypotension induced by extradural anaesthesia. Br J Anaesth. 1996;77:223–6.
25. Hahn RG, Lyons G. The half-life of infusion fluids: an educational review. Eur J Anaesthesiol. 2016;33:475–82.
26. Ewaldsson C-A, Hahn RG. Kinetics and extravascular retention of acetated Ringer's solution during isoflurane and propofol anesthesia for thyroid surgery. Anesthesiology. 2005;103:460–9.
27. Hahn RG. Arterial pressure and the rates of elimination of crystalloid fluid. Anesth Analg. 2017;124:1824–33.
28. Hahn RG. Why are crystalloid and colloid fluid requirements similar during surgery and intensive care? Eur J Anaesthesiol. 2013;30:515–8.
29. Chappell D, Jacob M. A rational approach to fluid and volume management. In: Cannessson M, Pearse R, editors. Perioperative hemodynamic monitoring and goal directed therapy. From theory to practice. Cambridge: Cambridge University Press; 2014. p. 74–84.
30. Nilsson A, Randmaa I, Hahn RG. Haemodynamic effects of irrigating fluids studied by Doppler ultrasonography in volunteers. Br J Urol. 1996;77:541–6.
31. Hahn RG, Stalberg HP, Ekengren J, Rundgren M. Effects of 1.5% glycine solution with and without ethanol on the fluid balance in elderly men. Acta Anaesthesiol Scand. 1991;35:725–30.

Right Ventricular Dysfunction and Fluid Administration in Critically Ill Patients

F. Gavelli, X. Monnet, and J.-L. Teboul

12.1 Introduction

In critically ill patients, right ventricular (RV) function is often acutely impaired [1, 2]. This may be due to either an acute decrease in contractility related to sepsis-induced myocardial depression or an acute increase in pulmonary vascular resistance (PVR) [2, 3]. The latter can be secondary to acute pathological conditions, such as severe pulmonary embolism or acute respiratory distress syndrome (ARDS). An increase in PVR may also occur as a result of the effects of mechanical ventilation on the pulmonary vasculature [4], which we will classify hereafter as a "functional cause" of RV dysfunction. Whatever the mechanism, the RV dysfunction is often associated with RV enlargement, which can be easily detected by echocardiography [5, 6]. An increase in the RV end-diastolic area (RVEDA)/left ventricular end-diastolic area (LVEDA) is one of the major elements for the definition of RV dysfunction.

It is generally thought that the presence of RV enlargement or RV dysfunction is a contraindication for fluid administration in shock states. However, this idea must be debated and the objective of this chapter is to emphasize the distinction between situations where fluid administration is always deleterious (structural causes of RV dysfunction) and situations where fluid administration can be useful (functional cause of RV dysfunction).

12.2 Fluid Administration in Cases of Structural Causes of Acute RV Dysfunction

As mentioned earlier, acute decreases in RV contractility may occur in cases of sepsis or septic shock. This is generally associated with left ventricular (LV) dysfunction. In general, but not always, the right ventricle is moderately to severely dilated [3]. Another major category of acute RV dysfunction encountered in critically ill patients is referred to as the acute increase in RV afterload due to structural abnormalities of the pulmonary vascular tree. The main causes are severe acute pulmonary embolism (involving the proximal arteries) and ARDS (involving the small vessels). In ARDS, the alteration of the small pulmonary vasculature is multifactorial: pulmonary vasoconstriction related either to hypoxemia or to release of inflammatory mediators, formation of microthrombi, and microvascular remodeling [7, 8]. In the case of an acute increase in RV afterload, the right ventricle has no adaptive mechanism other than its dilatation [9]. Due to the biventricular interdependence mechanism, RV dilatation may impede LV filling and thus decrease the LV stroke volume. The most severe form of RV failure—also called acute *cor pulmonale*—during pulmonary embolism or ARDS is associated with RV dilatation and leftward shift of the interventricular septum, both signs easily visualized by echocardiography [2].

Fluid resuscitation is the cornerstone of the management of circulatory shock. However, administration of fluid in patients with shock associated with or due to RV dysfunction secondary to structural causes such as pulmonary embolism, septic myocardial depression or ARDS may be harmful for the following reasons. First, according to the Frank-Starling mechanism, a dilated right ventricle should operate on the flat part of its systolic function curve. Therefore, a further increase in RV preload with fluid administration cannot increase the RV stroke volume (preload unresponsiveness state). This was clearly demonstrated in shocked patients with acute pulmonary embolism, in whom an increase in cardiac output after fluid administration was observed only when the right ventricle was not dilated [10]. Second, the two ventricles are surrounded by the pericardium, which is a poorly expandable membrane. Therefore, according to the biventricular interdependence mechanism, the fluid-induced increase in the pressure and volume of a previously dilated right ventricle will result in a further leftward septal displacement, which further limits the filling of the left heart and results in decreases in LV stroke volume and cardiac output [11].

Third, considering the hyperbolic end-diastolic RV pressure-volume relationship, a further increase in preload of a previously dilated right ventricle should increase the RV end-diastolic pressure much more than it would do in the case of a non-dilated right ventricle. This will increase all the right-side pressures and, hence, the downstream pressure of the perfusion of some important organs. This could thus negatively affect the function of organs such as the kidney [12, 13].

In summary, in the case of a dilated right ventricle due to structural causes, such as septic myocardial depression or structural abnormalities of the pulmonary vasculature, fluid administration does not increase cardiac output or may even decrease it. In addition, the increase in pressure upstream of the right heart may have deleterious consequences on the perfusion and hence on the function of important organs.

12.3 Fluid Administration in Cases of Acute RV Dysfunction Related to Mechanical Ventilation (Functional Causes of RV Dysfunction)

12.3.1 Pulmonary Vascular Resistance and Lung Volume

The relationship between PVR and lung volume is complex and determined by the presence of two types of pulmonary microvessels, the extra-alveolar and intra-alveolar microvessels, and by the hydrostatic distribution of the pulmonary vascular pressures [14].

The extra-alveolar microvessels are located outside the alveolar space, are subjected to the intrathoracic pressure (or pleural pressure [P_{pl}]), and are stretched by the increase in lung volume. This results in a decrease in the resistance of the extra-alveolar vessels [15] that is exponential from the residual volume to the total lung capacity (TLC), being maximal for low lung volumes and becoming lower as alveoli are stretched further. Above the functional respiratory capacity (FRC), the decrease in the resistance of the extra-alveolar vessels with lung volume is only minimal (Fig. 12.1).

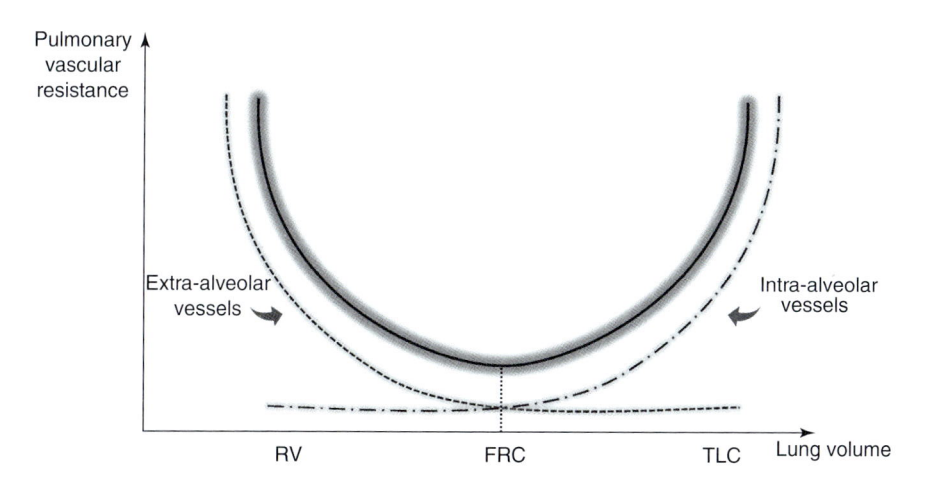

Fig. 12.1 Relationship between lung volume and pulmonary vascular resistance. *FRC* functional residual capacity, *RV* residual volume, *TLC* total lung capacity

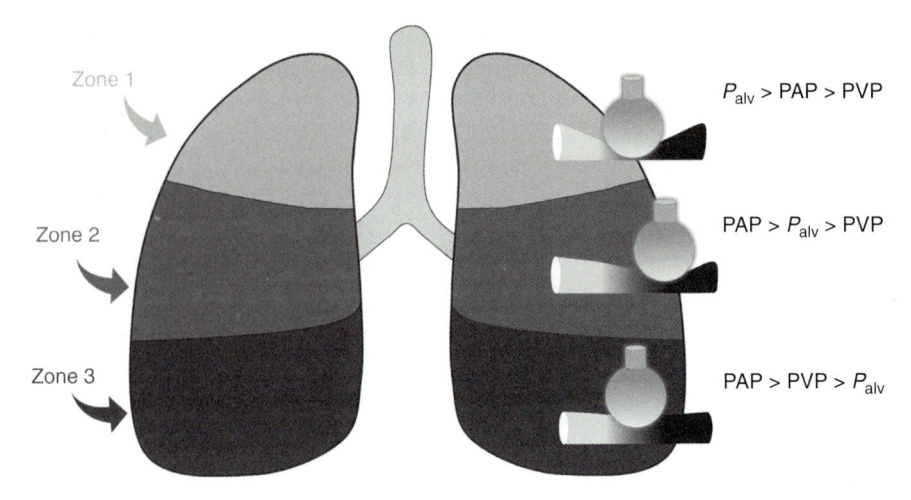

Fig. 12.2 West zones according to the ventilation/perfusion ratio. P_{alv} alveolar pressure, *PAP* pulmonary arterial pressure, *PVP* pulmonary venous pressure

The intra-alveolar vessels are in the proximity of the alveoli and are exposed to the transpulmonary pressure (P_L), which is the difference between the alveolar pressure (P_{alv}) and the P_{pl}. The increase in lung volume from the FRC to the TLC is associated with an increase in the P_L, which is more pronounced in cases of low compliance of the respiratory system, such as in ARDS [16]. Due to the vertical hydrostatic pressure gradient, the local pulmonary vascular pressures (local pulmonary artery and venous pressures) are higher in the dependent regions of the lung compared to the nondependent regions. This is not the case for the P_{alv} and the P_L, which are more homogeneously distributed from the base to the top of the lungs. Therefore, the intra-alveolar vessels in the dependent regions are more likely to be totally open since the pressure at their entry (local pulmonary arterial pressure) as well as the pressure at their exit (local pulmonary venous pressure) are higher than the P_L (Fig. 12.2). The pulmonary blood flow in these regions (West zone 3) is maximal and the resistance of the intra-alveolar vessels is minimal [17]. In the nondependent lung regions, the P_L can be higher than both the local pulmonary arterial and venous pressures, so that the intra-alveolar vessels are squeezed and the perfusion is absent (West zone 1) (Fig. 12.2) [17]. In the intermediate lung regions, the P_L can be lower than the local pulmonary arterial pressure but higher than the local pulmonary venous pressure, so that the intra-alveolar vessel can be compressed at its venous side (West zone 2) (Fig. 12.2) [17]. This results in a slower blood flow (waterfall effect) and an increased resistance of the intra-alveolar vessels. Therefore, for given pulmonary artery and venous pressures, the increase in the resistance of the intra-alveolar vessels is exponential from the FRC to the TLC due to the progressive increase in P_L and, thus, the progressive extent of the West zones 1 and 2. In cases of high pulmonary venous pressures (for example due to congestive heart failure), the extent of West zone 2 is inherently reduced resulting in a lower slope of the exponential increase in the resistance of the intra-alveolar vessels with lung

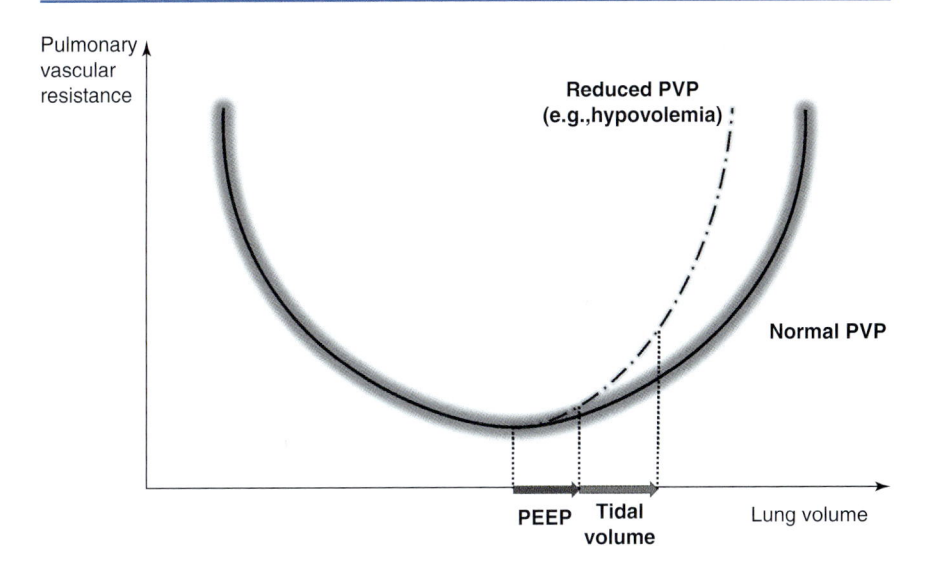

Fig. 12.3 Effects of positive end-expiratory pressure (PEEP) and tidal volume on pulmonary vascular resistance, in cases of normal and low pulmonary venous pressure (PVP)

volume. Conversely, if pulmonary venous pressure is low due to a decreased central blood volume, the extent of West zone 2 will be increased and the slope of the exponential increase in the resistance of the intra-alveolar vessels with lung volume will be higher (Fig. 12.3).

The combined effects of lung volume on the resistance of the two types of pulmonary microvessels can be represented by plotting both curves on the same graph: the resulting U-shaped curve (Fig. 12.1) has the lowest inflection at the point corresponding to the FRC, meaning that the global PVR is at its minimum when the respiratory system is at rest [15, 18].

12.3.2 Mechanical Ventilation and RV Afterload

During mechanical ventilation, the active insufflation produces an increase in P_{alv}, and thus tends to enhance the West zone 2 conditions, as the pulmonary venous pressure cannot increase to the same extent as the P_{alv}. Indeed, the P_{pl} (which influences the pulmonary vascular pressures) increases less than the P_{alv} during mechanical insufflation. Obviously, this cyclic increase in PVR should be more pronounced when the tidal volume is high [19]. Lowering tidal volume, as is currently recommended in patients with ARDS, must thus lower the increase in PVR and its negative impact on the RV function during mechanical insufflation.

In addition to the cyclic effects of mechanical ventilation on the RV afterload, the effects of a positive end-expiratory pressure (PEEP) must also be discussed since it is also recommended in ARDS patients [20].

By recruiting the collapsed alveoli, PEEP may relieve the hypoxic vasoconstriction, reducing the vascular resistance to pulmonary blood flow. In addition, if PEEP recruits lung units, the initially low end-expiratory lung volume increases towards the FRC resulting in a decrease in the resistance of the extra-alveolar vessels. Application of a low tidal volume should then result in an only small increase in PVR during insufflation. If PEEP over-distends more than it recruits lung units, the PVR should increase at end-expiration. Application of a tidal volume should then further increase the PVR during insufflation. These mechanisms explain why in patients with ARDS some investigators found an increased incidence of acute *cor pulmonale* with increased plateau pressure, which combines the total PEEP and the alveolar pressure related to tidal volume application [21].

As already mentioned, in the presence of a low pulmonary venous pressure (e.g., due to low central blood volume), the West zone 2 conditions are enhanced, so that the increase in the resistance of the intra-alveolar vessels and, hence, PVR would be amplified. Consequently, in cases of low central blood volume, the increase in RV afterload due to PEEP ventilation should be amplified (Fig. 12.3). Obviously, this effect would be more pronounced when tidal volume is high, when PEEP is high, when PEEP over-distends more than it recruits lung units, and in ARDS where the end-expiratory P_L is high due to the lung stiffness [22].

One option to decrease the negative impact of PEEP on RV function is to decrease its level. However, such a PEEP level should sometimes be maintained to avoid profound hypoxemia. Another option to reduce the PEEP-induced increase in RV afterload is to increase the pulmonary venous pressure in order to transform West zone 2 to zone 3 conditions. This has been illustrated in a study including patients with ARDS ventilated with a tidal volume of 6 ml/kg [23]. The level of PEEP was increased from 5 cmH_2O to the maximal value compatible with a plateau pressure of 30 cmH_2O (on average 13 ± 4 cmH_2O). The increase in PEEP resulted in an improved PaO_2/FiO_2 from 108 ± 40 to 135 ± 30 mmHg. The hemodynamic effects of PEEP were evaluated with echocardiography and pulmonary artery catheter. The increase in PEEP was associated with a significant decrease in cardiac output and significant increases in the difference between mean pulmonary artery pressure (mPAP) and pulmonary artery occlusion pressure (PAOP), in the PVR and in the RVEDA/LVEDA ratio (from 0.66 ± 0.20 to 0.72 ± 0.20), all findings consistent with an increase in RV afterload. Importantly, performance of passive leg raising (PLR) (simulating a fluid challenge) at the high level of PEEP resulted in the return of cardiac output, mPAP-PAOP, PVR and RVEDA/LVEDA to their baseline values. In other words, increasing central blood volume with PLR decreased the RV afterload suggesting that West zone 2 conditions were transformed into zone 3 conditions.

Thus, as a reduced central blood volume may amplify the deleterious impact of mechanical ventilation and PEEP application on RV function, increase in the central blood volume could be a good option to reduce RV dysfunction without affecting the beneficial respiratory effects of PEEP.

However, it should be remembered that administering fluids in the presence of a dilated right ventricle may be beneficial only in the case of functional RV impairment due to mechanical ventilation. Moreover, as the pathophysiologic hallmark of

ARDS is an increase in pulmonary vascular permeability, the benefit/risk balance of infusing fluids should be carefully assessed. In case of any doubt, especially in ARDS where both structural and functional causes of RV dysfunction may coexist, performing a PLR test may be helpful to investigate to what extent increasing the central blood volume could improve RV function. Measuring the changes in the RV function echocardiographic indices during PLR is of great interest in this context.

12.4 Conclusion

In critically ill patients, acute RV dysfunction can be secondary to structural or functional causes. The decision whether to administer fluids to these patients depends on the mechanism of the RV dysfunction. In cases of structural causes of RV dysfunction, administration of fluids is potentially harmful as it results in unchanged or even decreased cardiac output and increased right-side pressures with potential subsequent organ dysfunction. In the case of acute RV dysfunction due to mechanical ventilation, administration of fluids may be beneficial, by reopening lung microvessels and hence reducing PVR and eventually increasing cardiac output. Performance of a PLR test before making the decision to administer fluids can be helpful in cases of doubt.

References

1. Osman D, Monnet X, Castelain V, et al. Incidence and prognostic value of right ventricular failure in acute respiratory distress syndrome. Intensive Care Med. 2009;35:69–76.
2. Vieillard-Baron A, Naeije R, Haddad F, et al. Diagnostic workup, etiologies and management of acute right ventricle failure: a state-of-the-art paper. Intensive Care Med. 2018;44:774–90.
3. Ehrman RR, Sullivan AN, Favot MJ, et al. Pathophysiology, echocardiographic evaluation, biomarker findings, and prognostic implications of septic cardiomyopathy: a review of the literature. Crit Care. 2018;22:112.
4. Mahmood SS, Pinsky MR. Heart-lung interactions during mechanical ventilation: the basics. Ann Transl Med. 2018;6:349.
5. Orde S, Slama M, Yastrebov K, Mclean A, Huang S. Subjective right ventricle assessment by echo qualified intensive care specialists: assessing agreement with objective measures. Crit Care. 2019;23:1–9.
6. Vignon P. What is new in critical care echocardiography? Crit Care. 2018;22:40.
7. Tomashefski JF, Davies P, Boggis C, Greene R, Zapol WM, Reid LM. The pulmonary vascular lesions of the adult respiratory distress syndrome. Am J Pathol. 1983;112:112–26.
8. Koyama K, Katayama S, Tonai K, Shima J, Koinuma T, Nunomiya S. Biomarker profiles of coagulopathy and alveolar epithelial injury in acute respiratory distress syndrome with idiopathic/immune-related disease or common direct risk factors. Crit Care. 2019;23:283.
9. Repessé X, Vieillard-Baron A. Right heart function during acute respiratory distress syndrome. Ann Transl Med. 2017;5:29.
10. Mercat A, Diehl JL, Meyer G, Teboul JL, Sors H. Hemodynamic effects of fluid loading in acute massive pulmonary embolism. Crit Care Med. 1999;27:540–4.
11. Pinsky MR. The right ventricle: interaction with the pulmonary circulation. Crit Care. 2016;20:266.

12. Legrand M, Dupuis C, Simon C, et al. Association between systemic hemodynamics and septic acute kidney injury in critically ill patients: a retrospective observational study. Crit Care. 2013;17:R278.
13. Chen X, Wang X, Honore PM, Spapen HD, Liu D. Renal failure in critically ill patients, beware of applying (central venous) pressure on the kidney. Ann Intensive Care. 2018;8:91.
14. Roos A, Thomas LJ, Nagel EL, Prommas DC. Pulmonary vascular resistance as determined by lung inflation and vascular pressures. J Appl Physiol. 1961;16:77–84.
15. Whittenberger JL, McGregor M, Berglund E, Borst HG. Influence of state of inflation of the lung on pulmonary vascular resistance. J Appl Physiol. 1960;15:878–82.
16. Pelosi P, Rocco PRM, Gama de Abreu M. Close down the lungs and keep them resting to minimize ventilator-induced lung injury. Crit Care. 2018;22:72.
17. West JB, Dollery CT, Naimark A. Distribution of blood flow in isolated lung; relation to vascular and alveolar pressures. J Appl Physiol. 1964;19:713–24.
18. Shekerdemian L, Bohn D. Cardiovascular effects of mechanical ventilation. Arch Dis Child. 1999;80:475–80.
19. Howell JB, Permutt S, Proctor DF, Riley RL. Effect of inflation of the lung on different parts of pulmonary vascular bed. J Appl Physiol. 1961;16:71–6.
20. Fan E, Brodie D, Slutsky AS. Acute respiratory distress syndrome: advances in diagnosis and treatment. JAMA. 2018;319:698–710.
21. Jardin F, Vieillard-Baron A. Is there a safe plateau pressure in ARDS? The right heart only knows. Intensive Care Med. 2007;33:444–7.
22. Teboul JL, Pinsky MR, Mercat A, et al. Estimating cardiac filling pressure in mechanically ventilated patients with hyperinflation. Crit Care Med. 2000;28:3631–6.
23. Fougères E, Teboul J-L, Richard C, Osman D, Chemla D, Monnet X. Hemodynamic impact of a positive end-expiratory pressure setting in acute respiratory distress syndrome: importance of the volume status. Crit Care Med. 2010;38:802–7.

Intravenous Fluids: Do Not Drown in Confusion!

J. N. Wilkinson, F. M. P. van Haren, and M. L. N. G. Malbrain

13.1 Introduction

Intravenous fluids are some of the most commonly prescribed therapeutics on a daily basis. They should however be considered as any other drug with their indications, contraindications, benefits, risks, adverse effects and complications. Often, the task of prescribing intravenous fluids is delegated to the most junior members of the team. Or, in many circumstances, there is no intravenous fluid prescription available and the decision to start and choose the right fluid is left to the attending nurse. Evidence suggests that when available, fluid prescriptions are rarely documented correctly despite the presence of clear guidelines [1]. This is thought to be due to lack of knowledge and experience, which often leads to confusion. Consequently, this puts many patients at increased risk of serious harm and may incur unnecessary costs to healthcare insurance companies. It is therefore imperative to carefully assess the individual patients, their requirements, and the clinical picture to tailor intravenous fluid plans safely [2].

Ideally, fluids should be prescribed during rounds by the team that knows the patient and their history. Nonparent team prescriptions, particularly out of hours, require extra care and should not be done as a duplication of the last prescription to save time. Clearly, there are emergency situations in which fluids may need to be prescribed outside of this policy.

J. N. Wilkinson
Department of Intensive Care and Anesthesia, Northampton General Hospital, Northampton, UK

F. M. P. van Haren
Intensive Care Unit, The Canberra Hospital, Woden, ACT, Australia

Australian National University Medical School, Canberra, Australia

M. L. N. G. Malbrain (✉)
Intensive Care Unit, University Hospital Brussels (UZB), Jette, Belgium

Faculty of Medicine and Pharmacy, Vrije Universiteit Brussel (VUB), Campus Jette, Jette, Belgium

There are many controversial areas in the field of fluid administration. For example, in patients with septic shock, administration of fluids for resuscitation during initial hemodynamic stabilization may be associated with harm and we are faced with many unresolved questions regarding the type, dose, and timing of fluid administration. In addition, fluids may be used for maintenance of the intravascular fluid status, for replacement of fluid losses, and for nutrition to cover the daily calorie needs [3–5].

In this chapter, we provide definitions of terms important in the context of fluid therapy in hospitalized patients, amongst the sickest of whom are those with septic shock. We discuss different fluid management strategies including early adequate goal-directed fluid management, late conservative fluid management, and late goal-directed fluid removal. Also, we expand on the concept of the "four Ds" of fluid therapy, namely drug, dosing, duration, and de-escalation [5].

13.2 The Goals of Fluid Stewardship

Fluid stewardship is defined as a series of coordinated interventions, introduced to select the optimal type of fluid, dose, and duration of therapy that results in the best clinical outcome, prevention of adverse events, and cost reduction [6].

The primary goal of fluid stewardship is to optimize clinical outcomes while minimizing unintended consequences of intravenous fluid administration by taking into account indications, contraindications, toxicity, adverse events, fluid dynamics and kinetics. The appropriate use of intravenous fluids is an essential part of patient safety and deserves careful oversight and guidance and it is, therefore, necessary for the bedside clinician to understand fluid physiology. Given the association between fluid (mis)use and deleterious effects on patient morbidity and mortality, the frequency of inappropriate fluid prescription could be used in the future as a surrogate marker for the avoidable impact on iatrogenic fluid overload and subsequent end-organ dysfunction and failure [6]. A secondary goal of fluid stewardship is to reduce healthcare costs without adversely impacting on the quality of care.

The combination of effective fluid stewardship (with doctors and nurse ambassadors) with a comprehensive fluid bundle and organ function monitoring program may limit the deleterious effects of inappropriate fluid prescription and fluid overload and reduce costs [6, 7].

13.3 Framework for Intravenous Fluid Prescription

The process of intravenous fluid treatment is divided into four stages, based on an audit framework developed by the National Institute for Health and Care Excellence (NICE) [6, 8, 9].

1. Assessment of intravenous fluid need: Only the three major indications need to be examined thoroughly for the purpose of a clinical audit: resuscitation; maintenance; and replacement or redistribution.

2. Clear prescription: Every intravenous fluid prescription has to be detailed to ensure correct administration and that a fluid management plan is available to warrant the continuity of care.
3. Quality standards: The information in the hospital's fluid guideline or bundle is used to create different quality standards.
4. Appropriateness: These standards represent the necessary elements to do a full and qualitative check of appropriateness.

If all standards are met, the therapy will be classified as appropriate for that patient.

13.4 The Four Ds of Fluid Therapy: A Guide to Key Performance Indicators

13.4.1 Drug

Fluids, in analogy to antibiotics, should be treated as drugs and inappropriate fluid therapy should be avoided. All resuscitation, replacement, and even maintenance fluids can contribute to the formation of interstitial edema, particularly in patients with systemic inflammation associated with altered endothelial function [10]. As such the best fluid may be the one that has not been given (unnecessary). Critical care physicians should consider fluids as drugs that have contraindications and potential side effects, and pay particular attention to the different compounds and their specificities (crystalloids vs. colloids, synthetic vs. blood-derived, balanced vs. unbalanced, intravenous vs. oral). For each type of fluid, there are distinct indications and specific adverse effects. The osmolality, tonicity, pH, levels of chloride, sodium, potassium, and other metabolizable compounds (lactate, acetate, malate), as well as clinical factors (underlying conditions, kidney or liver failure, presence of capillary leak, albumin levels, fluid balance), must all be considered when choosing the type of fluid for a given patient at a given time [5].

13.4.2 Dose

"*Sola dosis facit venenum*" or "the dose makes the poison." This is true for drugs but also for intravenous fluids. There are various important considerations for fluid prescription:

- Pharmacokinetics: Most intravenous fluids administered, whatever their morphology, tend to remain within the intravascular compartment for 1 h or less. However, their half-life will alter according to co-pathology (infection, inflammation, surgery, and anesthesia).
- Volume kinetics: Crystalloids or colloids, when infused, will exert a similar volume expansion effect and their distribution may be slowed down. Their

isotonic or hypotonic maintenance solutions should be used. Data in children showed that hypotonic solutions carry the risk of hyponatremia and neurologic complications. Studies in adults are scarce and indicate that administration of isotonic solutions will result in a more positive fluid balance as compared to hypotonic solutions. This was confirmed in a recent pilot study in healthy volunteers showing that isotonic solutions caused lower urine output, characterized by decreased aldosterone concentrations indicating (unintentional) volume expansion, than hypotonic solutions and were associated with hyperchloremia. Despite their lower sodium and potassium content, hypotonic fluids were not associated with hyponatremia or hypokalemia [11].

There are several important points to consider in terms of maintenance fluids. First, many drugs are administered in large volumes of fluid. These are often forgotten and may result in fluid creep. Second, hypervolemic patients may require fluid restriction or even active fluid removal with diuretics. Third, occult losses, such as febrile states, leading to excessive evaporative losses in sweat should not be forgotten. Fourth, urine output does not need to be replaced unless excessive in volume (e.g., in diabetes insipidus or the diuretic phase of resolving renal failure). Finally, postoperative patients may be polyuric. This may be due to excessive intraoperative fluid provision, or secondary to the surgical stress response itself. Here, increased antidiuretic hormone release leads to retention of sodium and water but diuresis of potassium-containing urine.

13.6.3 Replacement

Replacement fluids are slightly different to maintenance solutions in that they are designed to replace more specific, known losses: for example, the output from drains or stomata, fistulas, fever, open wounds (evaporation during surgery, severe burn injury), polyuria (salt-wasting nephropathy or diabetes insipidus), and others. Several recent guidelines advise matching the amount of fluid and electrolytes as closely as possible to the fluid that is being or has been lost. An overview of the composition of the different body fluids can be found in the NICE guidelines [9]. Replacement fluids are usually isotonic balanced solutions. One example where one may choose 0.9% saline would be in patients where the fluid deficit is due to a loss of chloride-rich gastric fluid. Some commonly used solutions are shown in Table 13.1.

Table 13.1 Electrolyte constitution of the most popular intravenous fluids

Fluid	Na	K	Cl	Mg	Ca	Other	Osmolality
0.9% NaCl	154	0	154	0	0	0	308
0.18% NaCl/4% dextrose	30	0	30	0	0	Glu 40 g/l	284
0.45% NaCl/5% dextrose	77	0	77	0	0	Glu 50 g/l	406
Hartmann's	131	5	111	0	2	Lactate 29	274
Plasmalyte 148	140	5	98	1.5	0	Acetate 27/gluconate 23	297
5% Dextrose	0	0	0	0	0	Glu 50 g/l	278

13.6.4 Nutrition

Often overlooked, it is important to consider parenteral nutrition as another source of intravenous fluid that may contribute to fluid overload. Likewise, nutritional therapy in the critically ill should be seen as "medication," helping the healing process. As such we should consider the four Ds of nutritional therapy in analogy to how we deal with antibiotics and fluids: drug (type of feeding), dose (caloric and protein load), duration (when and how long) and de-escalation (stop enteral nutrition and/or parenteral nutrition when oral intake improves) [12].

13.7 The Four Questions of Fluid Therapy

1. When to Start Intravenous Fluid?
   This refers to the benefits of fluid administration guided by macro-hemodynamics (volumetric monitoring, fluid responsiveness, point-of-care ultrasound [POCUS]).
2. When to Stop Intravenous Fluid?
   This refers to the potential risks of ongoing fluid administration. The decision to stop intravenous fluids could be supported by the absence of fluid responsiveness or by transpulmonary thermodilution measurements if available. POCUS may also have a role here.
3. When to Start Fluid Removal?
   This is becoming a key area within more advanced fluid management. Fluid can be actively removed by the use of diuretics or ultrafiltration. Much of this may relate to the mobilization of edema in critically ill patients, very well described by Morris and Plumb [13] (Table 13.2).
4. When to Stop Fluid Removal?
   This refers to the risks of too much fluid removal, with resultant intravascular volume depletion or dehydration.

Table 13.2 The diuretic regime used to achieve a negative fluid balance in acute respiratory distress syndrome (ARDS)

Agent	Dose	Rationale	Comments
Furosemide	Variable infusion 10–50 mg/h	Loop diuretic; establishes polyuria through antagonizing the medullary concentrating gradient. May act as a pulmonary vasodilator	Target 400 ml/h maximum urine output. Plasma electrolytes measured every 6 h
Aminophylline	Fixed infusion 10 mg/h	At this low dose aminophylline is associated with natriuresis, possibly via antagonism of adenosine	Combined furosemide and aminophylline is common in Australasian and European practice with relatively few published data

(continued)

Table 13.2 (continued)

Agent	Dose	Rationale	Comments
Acetazolamide	Bolus 500 mg 12 hourly if pH >7	A carbonic anhydrase inhibitor acting principally at the proximal convoluted tubule 45 promoting natriuresis in association with bicarbonaturia, antagonizing the development of alkalosis	Acetazolamide is unlikely to have an effect if the urine is already maximally alkalinized (pH 8.0–8.5)
Spironolactone	100 mg NG 12 hourly	A prodrug yielding canrenoic acid as a metabolite acts as an aldosterone antagonist. Acting via the distal convoluted tubule to ensure potassium retention, bicarbonaturia, and associated natriuresis	Canrenoic acid may be administered parenterally but is not licensed or manufactured in the UK. The pyrazine derivative amiloride may also be a suitable alternative

Adapted from [13] with permission

13.8 The Four Phases of Fluid Therapy: The ROSE Concept

The ROSE concept of fluid therapy consists of a resuscitation phase, to save lives with a focus on patient rescue; an optimization phase, to avoid fluid overload and focus on organ rescue (maintenance); a stabilization phase, conservative fluid management and focus on organ support (homeostasis); and an evacuation phase with a focus on organ recovery and resolution of fluid overload. Figure 13.1 summarizes the different phases during fluid management [14].

13.9 The Four Hits of Shock

1. First hit—in the initial insult, which can be sepsis (but also burns, pancreatitis, or trauma), the patient will enter the "ebb" phase of shock.
2. The second hit—occurs within hours and refers to ischemia and reperfusion. Fluid accumulation reflects the severity of illness (and might be considered a "biomarker" for it). The greater the fluid requirement, the sicker the patient and the more likely the organ failure (e.g., acute kidney injury [AKI]) may occur.
3. Third hit—global increased permeability syndrome, a state of ongoing positive cumulative fluid balance and new-onset organ failure. After the second hit, the patient can either recover, entering the "flow" phase with spontaneous evacuation of the excess fluids that have been administered previously, or, as is the case in many ICU patients, remain in a "no-flow" state followed by a third hit usually resulting from global increased permeability syndrome with ongoing fluid accumulation due to capillary leak [14].
4. The fourth hit—usually occurs secondary to overaggressive fluid removal. This induces hypovolemia, which may trigger hemodynamic deterioration and hypoperfusion. On the other hand, fluid overload can account for this, causing organ failure, deterioration, and death at the extreme.

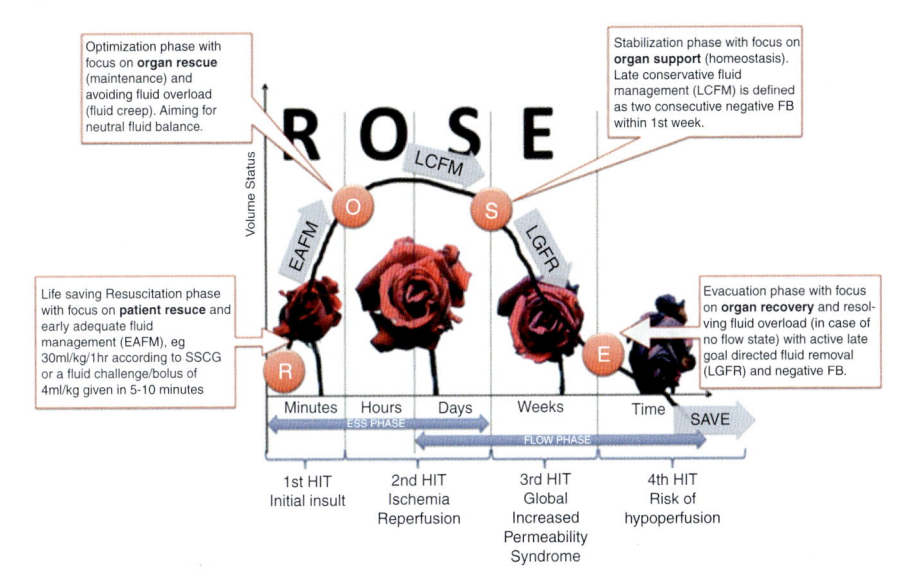

Fig. 13.1 The four hits of shock. Graph showing the four-hit model of shock with evolution of patients' cumulative fluid volume status over time during the five distinct phases of resuscitation: resuscitation (R), optimization (O), stabilization (S), and evacuation (E) (ROSE), followed by a possible risk of hypoperfusion in case of too aggressive de-resuscitation. On admission patients are hypovolemic, followed by normovolemia after fluid resuscitation (EAFM, early adequate fluid management), and possible fluid overload, again followed by a phase going to normovolemia with late conservative fluid management (LCFM) and late goal-directed fluid removal (LGFR) or de-resuscitation. In case of hypovolemia, O_2 cannot get into the tissue because of convective problems; in case of hypervolemia, O_2 cannot get into the tissue because of diffusion problems related to interstitial and pulmonary edema and gut edema (ileus and abdominal hypertension) (adapted from [14, 20] under the terms of the Open Access CC by License 4.0)

13.10 Important Definitions

13.10.1 Fluid Balance

This is the input versus output with a resultant overall state within a 24-h period, classically described as negative, neutral, or positive. Daily fluid balance does not usually include insensible losses unless the patient is being cared for in an ICU bed that can weigh the patient.

13.10.2 Cumulative Fluid Balance

This is the sum of fluid accumulated over a set period of time, assessed by calculating the sum of daily fluid balances over that period. The cumulative fluid balance during the first week of the ICU stay is considered to be a prognostic marker [15].

13.10.3 Fluid Loss and Gain

Fluid loss is defined as a negative fluid balance, regardless of intravascular status, and fluid gain is the opposite.

13.10.4 Dehydration (Fluid Underload)

This is excessive loss of body water and has a wide range of etiologies, including gastrointestinal loss of fluid (vomiting or diarrhea), heat exposure, prolonged vigorous exercise, kidney disease, and medication (e.g., diuretics). Dehydration is classified as mild (5–7.5%), moderate (7.5–10%), or severe (>10%). Percentage fluid loss = cumulative balance (l) divided by baseline body weight × 100.

13.10.5 Overhydration (Fluid Overload or Fluid Accumulation)

Percentage fluid accumulation = cumulative fluid balance (l) divided by baseline body weight × 100. Overhydration or fluid overload at any stage is the opposite of dehydration and is defined by a cutoff value of 10% of fluid accumulation. Fluid overload is universally associated with worse ICU outcomes. Fluid administration potentially induces a vicious cycle, where interstitial edema induces organ dysfunction that contributes to fluid accumulation (Fig. 13.2).

13.10.6 Hypovolemia

Hypovolemia is the term used to describe a patient with insufficient intravascular volume (Table 13.3). It does not refer to total body fluid, but rather to the intravascular compartment. Total body fluid comprises approximately 60% of the body

Fig. 13.2 The vicious cycle of septic shock resuscitation. *IAH* intra-abdominal hypertension (adapted from [21] with permission)

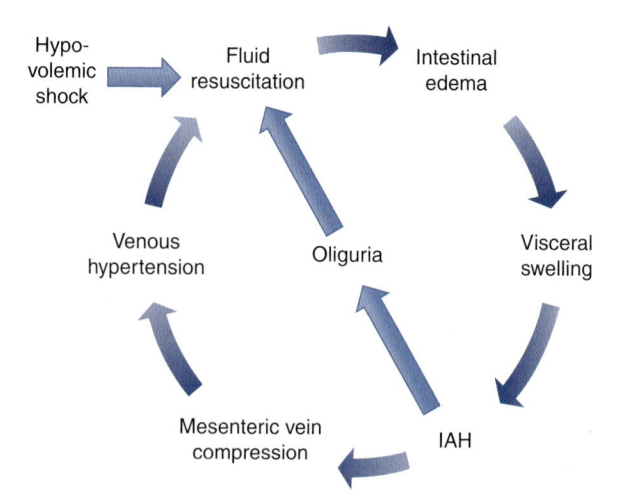

Table 13.3 Clinical, laboratory, imaging and hemodynamic signs of hypovolemia

Clinical signs	Laboratory signs	Imaging signs	Hemodynamic signs
Body weight ↓	Lactate ↑ S(c)vO₂ ↓	Normal chest X-ray, absence of Kerley-B lines, no pleural effusion	MAP (<55 mmHg) ↓, HR ↑ = ↓
Fluid balance ↓	Albumin leak index ↑ (ratio urine albumin/urine creatinine)	Abdominal US: no ascites	CVP ↓, PAOP ↓
Cumulative fluid balance ↓	Hemoconcentration: hemoglobin ↑	TTE: low E/e', LVOT VTI variations ↑	GEF/GEDVI (<680) ↓
Absence of pitting edema	Total protein ↑ and albumin ↑	IVCCI ↑ >50% (IVC ↑ <1.5 cm)	RVEF/RVEDVI (<80) ↓
Decreased skin turgor	Serum Na ↑	Left atrium volume ↓	Presence of FR (CI increase >15%)
Absence of second and third space fluid accumulation	CLI ↑ = ↓ (ratio serum CRP/serum albumin)	Normal lung US: no B-lines	PPV ↑, SVV ↑, SPV ↑, Δdown ↑ (>12–15%)
JVP normal and HJR absent	Serum osmolality ↑, COP ↑		Positive PLR (CI increase >10%)
Capillary refill time (>2 s) ↑	BNP and NT-pro-BNP ↓ (In)activation RAAS		Positive EOT (CI increase >5%)
No orthopnea or platydeoxia	Urine electrolytes: Na ↓ osm ↑		
Dry mucosa, thirst			
Mottled skin (livedo), peripheral cyanosis			
Central to peripheral temperature difference ↑			
Drop in urine output ↓ <0.5 ml/kg/h			

Adapted from [23] with permission

HJR hepatojugular reflex, *JVP* jugular venous pressure, *BNP* brain natriuretic peptide, *CLI* capillary leak index, *COP* colloid oncotic pressure, *CRP* C-reactive protein, *Na* sodium, *RAAS* renin-angiotensin-aldosterone system, *ScvO₂* mixed central venous oxygen saturation, *CI* cardiac index, *CVP* central venous pressure, *EOT* end-expiratory occlusion, *FR* fluid responsiveness, *GEF* global ejection fraction, *GEDVI* global end-diastolic volume index, *HR* heart rate, *MAP* mean arterial blood pressure, *PAOP* pulmonary artery occlusion pressure, *PLR* passive leg raising, *PPV* pulse pressure variation, *RVEF* right ventricular ejection fraction, *RVEDVI* right ventricular end-diastolic volume index, *SPV* systolic pressure variation, *SVV* stroke volume variation, *TTE* transthoracic echocardiography, *E/e'* noninvasive tissue Doppler estimate of left atrial filling pressure, *LVOT* left ventricular outflow tract, *VTI* velocity time integral, *IVCCI* inferior vena cava collapsibility index weight for men and 50% for women. Blood volume can be estimated according to Gilcher's rule of fives at 70 ml/kg for men and 65 ml/kg for women. Blood loss is frequently followed by recruitment of interstitial fluid from compartments distant to the central compartment. Vasoconstriction of the splanchnic mesenteric vasculature is one of the first physiologic responses.

Sodium and water retention results from activation of the renin-angiotensin-aldosterone system (RAAS), which replenishes the interstitial reserves and maintains transcapillary perfusion. As a result, the body may lose up to 30% of blood volume before hypovolemia becomes clinically apparent. Therefore, undiagnosed hypovolemia may be present long before clinical signs and symptoms occur. Hypovolemia can also occur in edematous patients, where total body water is increased but intravascular volume is reduced (e.g., patients with eclampsia).

Finally, some patients are fluid responsive, but not necessarily hypovolemic. Even the most basic of paradigms, such as the description of early sepsis and distributive shock as a hypovolemic state needing aggressive fluid resuscitation, have recently been called into question, with data suggesting improved outcomes with less or even no administered intravenous fluid. There has been a greater focus on the health and function of the microcirculation and the endothelial glycocalyx, with potential new treatment paradigms calling for less fluid, and earlier vasopressor use has become the focus. These elements make an accurate assessment of fluid status in the critically ill a challenging task.

13.10.7 Hypervolemia

Hypervolemia is the opposite of hypovolemia and is defined by intravascular overfilling.

This can be monitored in different ways: the absence of fluid responsiveness, increased barometric or volumetric preload indicators, and ultrasound findings.

13.10.8 Fluid Bolus

A fluid bolus is the rapid infusion of fluid over a short period of time. In clinical practice, a fluid bolus is usually given to correct hypovolemia, hypotension, inadequate blood flow or impaired microcirculatory perfusion. A fluid bolus typically includes the infusion of 4–6 ml/kg given over a maximum of 20 min.

13.10.9 Fluid Challenge

A fluid challenge is a dynamic functional test to assess a patient's fluid responsiveness by giving a fluid bolus of at least 4 ml/kg over 5–10 min and simultaneously monitoring the hemodynamic status to be able to identify fluid responsive patients. Recently, it has been shown that in clinical practice there is marked variability in how fluid challenge tests are performed and what clinicians' beliefs are regarding the predicted physiologic effects of administering a fluid bolus.

13.10.10 Fluid Responsiveness

Fluid responsiveness indicates a condition in which a patient will respond to fluid administration by a significant increase in stroke volume and/or cardiac output or their surrogates. A threshold of 15% is most often used for this definition. Physiologically, fluid responsiveness means that cardiac output depends on cardiac preload; that is, the slope of the Frank-Starling relationship is steep.

Many studies have shown that fluid responsiveness, which is a normal physiologic condition, exists in only half of ICU patients receiving a fluid challenge. Fluid responsiveness does not mean that the patient needs fluids.

13.10.11 Prediction of Fluid Responsiveness

This is a process that consists of predicting—before fluid administration—whether or not fluid administration will increase cardiac output. It avoids unnecessary fluid administration and contributes to reducing the cumulative fluid balance. It may also guide fluid removal, making sure that it will not result in hemodynamic impairment.

Prediction of fluid responsiveness cannot be achieved with static markers of cardiac preload, such as the CVP, the pulmonary artery occlusion pressure (PAOP) and its echocardiographic estimates, or the left ventricular end-diastolic dimensions. It is based on a dynamic assessment of the cardiac output/preload relationship. The classic fluid challenge shows whether a patient is fluid responsive, but is inherently associated with fluid boluses administered to patients that are not fluid responsive.

Respiratory variations in stroke volume and its surrogates (arterial pulse pressure, aortic blood flow, maximal velocity in the left ventricular outflow tract, amplitude of the plethysmographic signal) in patients under mechanical ventilation are more reliable predictors of fluid responsiveness but are not reliable in some conditions, including the presence of spontaneous breathing activity, cardiac arrhythmias, ventilation at low tidal volume, and low lung compliance.

Respiratory variation in the diameter of the inferior and superior vena cavae shares the same limitations, except for cardiac arrhythmias. Passive leg raising (see below) and the end-expiratory occlusion test are reliable in these circumstances.

The threshold to define fluid responsiveness depends on the change in cardiac preload induced by the test (e.g., 15% for the fluid challenge, 10% for the passive leg raising test, 5% for the end-expiratory occlusion test).

13.11 Noninvasive Tests of Fluid Responsiveness

13.11.1 Passive Leg Raising Test

The passive leg raising test is aimed at evidencing fluid responsiveness (Fig. 13.3).

It consists of moving a patient from the semi-recumbent position to a position where the legs are lifted at 45° and the trunk is horizontal. The transfer of venous

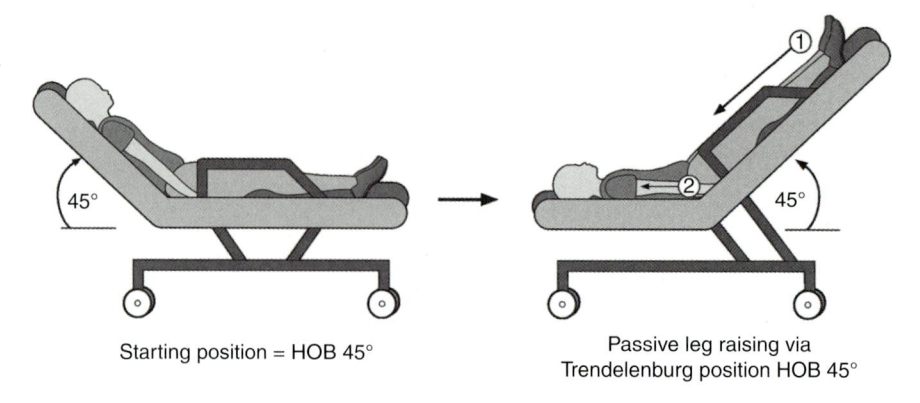

Fig. 13.3 Trolley-assisted passive leg raise test. In order to perform a correct passive leg raise test, one should not touch the patient in order to avoid sympathetic activation. The passive leg raise is performed by turning the bed from the starting position (head of bed [HOB] elevation 30–45°) to the Trendelenburg position. The passive leg raise test results in an autotransfusion effect via the increased venous return from the legs (1) and the splanchnic mesenteric pool (2). Monitoring of stroke volume is required as a positive passive leg raise test is defined by an increase in stroke volume of at least 10% (adapted from [22] with permission)

blood from the inferior limbs and the splanchnic compartment toward the cardiac cavities mimics the increase in cardiac preload induced by fluid infusion. In general, the threshold to define fluid responsiveness with the passive leg raising test is a 10% increase in stroke volume and/or cardiac output [16].

13.11.2 End-Expiratory Occlusion Test

This is a test of fluid responsiveness that consists of stopping mechanical ventilation at end expiration for 15 s and measuring the resultant change in cardiac output. The test increases cardiac preload by stopping the cyclic impediment of venous return that occurs at each insufflation of the ventilator.

An increase in the cardiac output above the threshold of 5% indicates preload/fluid responsiveness. When the test is performed with echocardiography, it is better to add the effects of an end-inspiratory occlusion, because the diagnostic threshold of changes in stroke volume is more compatible with the precision of echocardiography.

13.12 Classification of Fluid Dynamics

13.12.1 Ebb Phase

This refers to the initial phase of (septic) shock when the patient shows hyperdynamic circulatory shock with decreased systemic vascular resistance due to vasodilation, increased capillary permeability, and severe absolute or relative intravascular hypovolemia. Fluid management can be extremely challenging during the ebb phase and if done poorly can result in excessive morbidity for the patient [14].

13.12.2 Flow Phase

This refers to the phase of septic shock after initial stabilization where the patient will mobilize excess fluid spontaneously. A classic example is when a patient enters a polyuric phase when recovering from sepsis-induced AKI. In contrast to the "ebb" phase, the "flow" phase refers to the time period after the acute circulatory shock has been resolved. In this post-shock phase, metabolic turnover is increased, the innate immune system is activated, and a hepatic acute-phase response is induced. This hypercatabolic metabolic state is characterized by an increase in oxygen consumption and energy expenditure [14].

13.13 Ongoing Fluid Management

13.13.1 Late Conservative Fluid Management

This is the phase geared to avoid fluid overload. Recent studies show that two consecutive days of negative fluid balance within the first week of the ICU stay is a strong and independent predictor of survival. Late conservative fluid management must be adapted according to the variable clinical course of septic shock during the first days of ICU treatment; for example, patients with persistent systemic inflammation maintain transcapillary albumin leakage and do not reach the flow phase (see further) mounting up positive fluid balances [14].

13.13.2 Late Goal-Directed Fluid Removal

Late goal-directed fluid removal describes situations where more aggressive and active fluid removal employing diuretics or renal replacement therapy (RRT) with net ultrafiltration is needed, with or without combination with hypertonic solutions, to mobilize the excess interstitial edema [14]. This is also referred to as de-resuscitation, a term that was coined for the first time in 2014 [5].

13.14 Fluid Overload

13.14.1 Intra-abdominal Hypertension

Peripheral and generalized edema is not only of cosmetic concern, as believed by some, but harmful to the patient as a whole because it can cause organ edema and dysfunction. One potential detrimental effect is abdominal hypertension (defined as a sustained increase in intra-abdominal pressure > 12 mmHg). Figure 13.4 details all the potential harmful consequences of fluid overload on different end-organ systems, with consequential effects on patient morbidity and mortality.

Respiratory
Pulmonary edema↑
Pleural effusion↑
Altered pulmonary and
chest wall elastance (cfr IAP↑)
PaO2↓ PaCO2↑ PaO2/FiO2↓
Extravascular lung water↗
Lung volumes↓ (cfr IAP↑)
Prolonged ventilation↑
Difficult weaning↑
Work of breathing↑

Central nervous system
Cerebral edema, impaired
cognition, delirium
ICP↑ CPP↓ IOP↑
ICH, ICS, OCS

Cardiovascular
Myocardial edema↑
Conduction disturbance
Impaired contractility
Diastolic dysfunction
CVP↑ and PAOP↑
Venous return↓
SV↓ and CO↓
Myocardial depression
Pericardial effusion↑
GEF↓ GEDVI↑ CARS↑

Hepatic
Hepatic congestion↑
Impaired synthetic function
Cholestatis↑
Cytochrome P450 activity↓
Hepatic compartment syndrome

Gastrointestinal/visceral
Ascites formation↑ Gut edema↑
Malabsorption↑ Ileus↑
Bowel contractility↓
IAP↑ and APP (=MAP-IAP)↓
Success enteral feeding↓
Intestinal permeability↑
Bacterial translocation↑
Splanchnic microcirculatory flow↓
ICG-PDR↓, pHi↓

Abdominal Wall
Tissue edema↑
Poor wound
healing↑
Wound infection↑
Pressure ulcers↑
Abdominal
compliance↓

Renal
Renal interstitial edema
Renal venous pressure↑
Renal blood flow↓
Interstitial pressure↑
Salt + water retention↑
Uremia↑ GFR↓ RVR↑
Renal CS

Fluid Overload

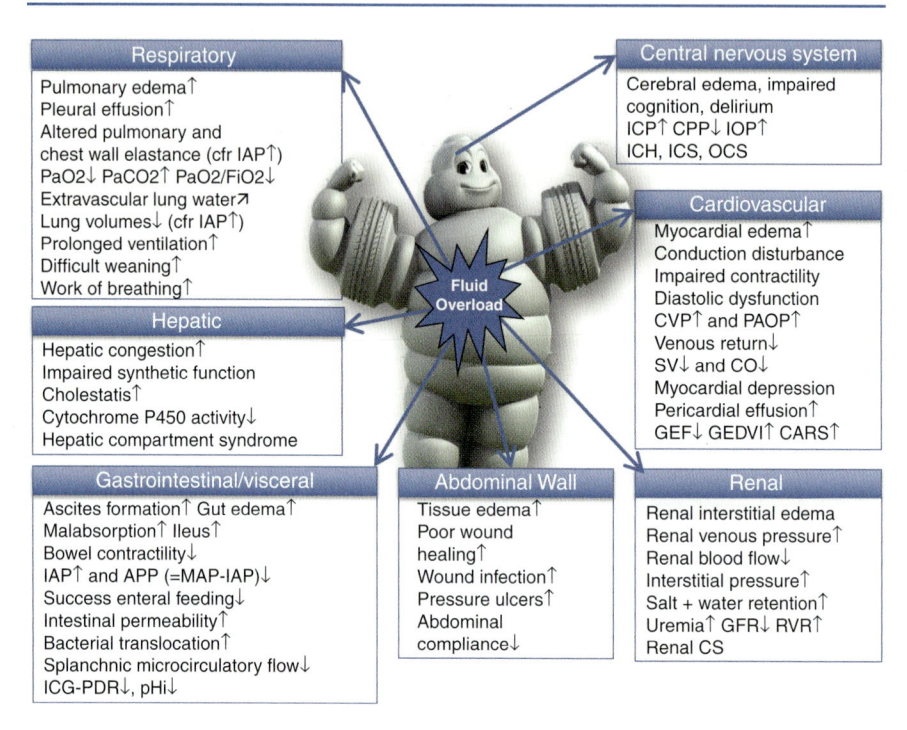

Fig. 13.4 Potential adverse consequences of fluid overload on end-organ function. *APP* abdominal perfusion pressure, *IAP* intra-abdominal pressure, *IAH* intra-abdominal hypertension, *ACS* abdominal compartment syndrome, *CARS* cardio-abdominal-renal syndrome, *CO* cardiac output, *CPP* cerebral perfusion pressure, *CS* compartment syndrome, *CVP* central venous pressure, *GEDVI* global end-diastolic volume index, *GEF* global ejection fraction, *GFR* glomerular filtration rate, *ICG-PDR* indocyanine green plasma disappearance rate, *ICH* intracranial hypertension, *ICP* intracranial pressure, *ICS* intracranial compartment syndrome, *IOP* intraocular pressure, *MAP* mean arterial pressure, *OCS* ocular compartment syndrome, *PAOP* pulmonary artery occlusion pressure, *pHi* gastric tonometry, *RVR* renal vascular resistance, *SV* stroke volume (adapted from [14, 17] with permission)

13.14.2 Global Increased Permeability Syndrome

Some patients will not transgress to the "flow" phase spontaneously and will remain in a persistent state of global increased permeability syndrome and ongoing fluid accumulation. This is also referred to as "the third hit of shock."

13.15 Intravenous Fluid Bundles: The Northampton Example

Previous retrospective reviews of prescriptions within one of the author's hospitals identified poor control of the process. There were elements of intravenous fluid prescribing practice that were placing patients at risk. For example, only 16% had the correct volumes prescribed for maintenance fluids, many were receiving excessive amounts of sodium within their intravenous fluid prescriptions yet minimal potassium, and only 25% contained the correct amount of glucose.

As a result, a new intravenous fluid bundle and guideline were produced [17]. This led to significant improvements in the measured outcomes and balancing measures. After the bundle introduction, all patients had a documented review of both fluid status and balance. The incidence of deranged electrolyte values decreased from 48% to 35%; the incidence of AKI decreased from 14% to 10%; and the average number of days between the last electrolyte measurements and a fluid prescription decreased from 2.2 days to 1.0 day.

13.15.1 Education Is Key

Continuous education programs, targeting key users in hospitals, are paramount to ensure that safe intravenous fluid prescription is propagated within day-to-day practice. Intended changes must be simple, sustainable, and understandable so that the inertia of good care does not grind to a halt. This can involve identification of an overall lead clinician, supported by a senior nurse, who will oversee proceedings and be available for advice/troubleshooting.

13.16 Busting the Myths!

13.16.1 Chasing the Wrong Target: Optimal Perfusion Does Not Require Excessive Volume

A common misconception is that providing more intravascular volume via the provision of intravenous fluids is relatively harmless. Organ perfusion (blood flow) is dependent on the pressure gradient from the arterial to the venous side of the organ. Arterial flow is constant over a wide range of blood pressures due to autoregulation. Therefore, organ blood flow is dependent on venous pressures. Hypervolemia increases venous pressures and reduces organ blood flow, as it increases downstream pressure, effectively clogging up the system. It has been well demonstrated that AKI is often a direct result of fluid overload.

13.16.2 Urine Output: Not the Golden Bullet!

Another misconception is that "what goes out must be chased." We often look at urine output as a marker of fluid requirement; however, unwell patients, who have suffered trauma or have undergone surgery, often have a reduced urine output due to increased sodium retention (and thus water) by the kidneys. Over time, patients can be seen to develop edema, hypokalemia and hypernatremia. If normal saline has been given as a resuscitation fluid or maintenance fluid, the potential situation of hyperchloremic acidosis can ensue, on top of these other electrolyte imbalances.

Surprisingly, normal saline containing no potassium will result in a higher increase in potassium levels in patients with renal impairment compared to a balanced solution (lactated Ringer's) containing 5 mmol/l of potassium. This is due to concomitant metabolic acidosis due to a decreased strong ion difference (SID) [18].

13.16.3 Sepsis and Septic Shock

Less than 50% of hemodynamically unstable patients are "fluid responders," and it is unproven in humans that fluid boluses in septic shock improve cardiac output, organ perfusion, or relevant patient outcomes. Eighty-five percent of an infused bolus of crystalloid goes to the interstitial space after 4 h in health and 95% of an infused bolus of crystalloid goes to the interstitial space in sepsis in under 90 min.

Evidence is mounting against excessive fluid resuscitation in this group. Patients are in a state of distributive shock whereby excessive intravenous fluid simply pools within an ineffective body compartment (certainly not the intravascular compartment). The key here is to provide earlier vasopressor support within a critical care environment. This is the paradigm of the "less is more" approach. Hence, the safety mechanism provides advice of cessation of giving any resuscitation volume over and above 2000 ml in ward-based areas.

We also consider the recommended Surviving Sepsis Campaign dosage of 30 ml/kg resuscitation fluid to be excessive. The predominant expert opinion is that it may apply to those who are profoundly shocked with sepsis/systemic inflammatory response syndrome (SIRS) but should always be paralleled with sensible invasive or more advanced monitoring within a critical care environment [19].

13.17 Conclusion

Intravenous fluids are one of the most commonly prescribed drugs worldwide and should be considered with the same level of respect within prescription safety. Good education, regular audit, and a solid leadership within fluid stewardships will help to minimize any morbidity and mortality related to malprescription of these drugs.

Acknowledgements This chapter is endorsed by the International Fluid Academy (IFA). The mission statement of the IFA is to foster education, promote research on fluid management and hemodynamic monitoring, and thereby improve survival of critically ill by bringing together physicians, nurses, and others from throughout the world and from a variety of clinical disciplines. The IFA is integrated within the not-for-profit charitable organization iMERiT, International Medical Education and Research Initiative, under Belgian law. The IFA website (http://www.fluidacademy.org) is now an official SMACC-affiliated site (Social Media and Critical Care) and its content is based on the philosophy of FOAM (Free Open Access Medical education—#FOAMed). The site recently received the HONcode quality label for medical education (https://www.healthonnet.org/HONcode/Conduct.html?HONConduct519739).

Parts of this manuscript were previously presented at the IFAD meetings under the Open Access CC BY License 4.0 [5, 7, 14, 17].

References

1. Intravenous fluid therapy in adults in hospital. Available at: https://www.nice.org.uk/guidance/cg174. Accessed 2/8/19.
2. van Haren F. Personalised fluid resuscitation in the ICU: still a fluid concept? Crit Care. 2017;21:313.
3. Byrne L, Obonyo NG, Diab SD, et al. Unintended consequences; fluid resuscitation worsens shock in an ovine model of endotoxemia. Am J Respir Crit Care Med. 2018;198:1043–54.
4. Byrne L, Van Haren F. Fluid resuscitation in human sepsis: time to rewrite history? Ann Intensive Care. 2017;7:4.
5. Malbrain ML, Marik PE, Witters I, et al. Fluid overload, de-resuscitation, and outcomes in critically ill or injured patients: a systematic review with suggestions for clinical practice. Anaesthesiol Intensive Ther. 2014;46:361–80.
6. Malbrain ML, Rice T, Mythen M, Wuyts S. It is time for improved fluid stewardship. ICU Manag Pract. 2018;18(3):158–62.
7. Malbrain ML, Van Regenmortel N, Owczuk R. It is time to consider the four D's of fluid management. Anaesthesiol Intensive Ther. 2015;47:1–5.
8. Sansom LT, Duggleby L. Intravenous fluid prescribing: improving prescribing practices and documentation in line with NICE CG174 guidance. BMJ Qual Improv Rep. 2014;3:u205899.w2409.
9. Padhi S, Bullock I, Li L, Stroud M, et al. Intravenous fluid therapy for adults in hospital: summary of NICE guidance. BMJ. 2013;347:f7073.
10. Van Regenmortel N, Verbrugghe W, Roelant E, Van den Wyngaert T, Jorens PG. Maintenance fluid therapy and fluid creep impose more significant fluid, sodium, and chloride burdens than resuscitation fluids in critically ill patients: a retrospective study in a tertiary mixed ICU population. Intensive Care Med. 2018;44:409–17.
11. Van Regenmortel N, De Weerdt T, Van Craenenbroeck AH, et al. Effect of isotonic versus hypotonic maintenance fluid therapy on urine output, fluid balance, and electrolyte homeostasis: a crossover study in fasting adult volunteers. Br J Anaesth. 2017;118:892–900.
12. De Waele E, Honore PM, Malbrain M. Does the use of indirect calorimetry change outcome in the ICU? Yes it does. Curr Opin Clin Nutr Metab Care. 2018;21:126–9.
13. Morris C, Plumb J. Mobilising oedema in the oedematous critically ill patient with ARDS: do we seek natriuresis not diuresis? J Intensive Care Soc. 2010;12:92–7.
14. Malbrain MLNG, Van Regenmortel N, Saugel B, et al. Principles of fluid management and stewardship in septic shock: it is time to consider the four D's and the four phases of fluid therapy. Ann Intensive Care. 2018;8:66.
15. Cordemans C, De Laet I, Van Regenmortel N, et al. Fluid management in critically ill patients: the role of extravascular lung water, abdominal hypertension, capillary leak, and fluid balance. Ann Intensive Care. 2012;2:S1.
16. Monnet X, Teboul JL. Passive leg raising: five rules, not a drop of fluid! Crit Care. 2015;19:18.
17. Wilkinson JN, Yates L, Miller A. IV Fluid guidance…don't drown in confusion! Available at: https://criticalcarenorthampton.com/2019/06/21/iv-fluid-guidance-dont-drown-in-confusion/. Accessed 9/8/19.
18. Langer T, Santini A, Scotti E, Van Regenmortel N, Malbrain ML, Caironi P. Intravenous balanced solutions: from physiology to clinical evidence. Anaesthesiol Intensive Ther. 2015;47:s78–88.
19. Marik PE, Malbrain MLNG. The SEP-1 quality mandate may be harmful: how to drown a patient with 30 mL per kg fluid! Anaesthesiol Intensive Ther. 2017;49:323–8.
20. Silversides JA, Perner A, Malbrain MLNG. Liberal versus restrictive fluid therapy in critically ill patients. Intensive Care Med. 2019;45:1440–2.
21. Peeters Y, Lebeer M, Wise R, Malbrain ML. An overview on fluid resuscitation and resuscitation endpoints in burns: past, present and future. Part 2—avoiding complications by using the

right endpoints with a new personalized protocolized approach. Anaesthesiol Intensive Ther. 2015;47:15–26.
22. Hofer CK, Cannesson M. Monitoring fluid responsiveness. Acta Anaesthesiol Taiwanica. 2011;49:59–65.
23. Van der Mullen J, Wise R, Vermeulen G, Moonen PJ, Malbrain MLNG. Assessment of hypovolaemia in critically ill patients. Anaesthesiol Intensive Ther. 2018;50:141–9.

Part V

Hemodynamic Management

14
Update on Right Ventricular Hemodynamic, Echocardiographic and Extra-Cardiac Ultrasound Monitoring

E. J. Couture and A. Y. Denault

14.1 Introduction

In the past 30 years, the importance of right ventricular (RV) function has been increasingly recognized and studied [1]. RV dysfunction has been associated with increased morbidity and mortality in patients suffering from heart failure [2], infiltrative cardiomyopathy [3] and myocardial infarction [4]. The incidence of RV dysfunction after cardiopulmonary bypass (CPB) is 10.9–14.5% in patients with preoperative pulmonary hypertension and is associated with a high mortality rate of 22–88% [5–9]. RV dysfunction has been shown to predict increased postoperative inotrope needs, prolonged mechanical ventilation, prolonged hospital and intensive care unit (ICU) lengths of stay, and increased mortality [5–9]. RV function can be impaired by multiple mechanisms. Acute or acute-on-chronic pressure overload from pulmonary hypertension is an important etiologic factor. RV dysfunction can be precipitated by precapillary sources, such as pulmonary thromboembolism, and postcapillary injury in situations of left heart valvular disease or left ventricular (LV) dysfunction. It can also result from capillary alterations in conditions creating hypoxemia, hypercapnia, acidosis or mechanical compression from elevated positive-pressure mechanical ventilation.

E. J. Couture
Department of Anesthesiology and Intensive Care Medicine Division, Institut Universitaire de Cardiologie et de Pneumologie de Québec, Université Laval, Quebec, QC, Canada

A. Y. Denault (✉)
Department of Anesthesiology and Critical Care Division, Montreal Heart Institute and Centre Hospitalier de l'Université de Montréal, Université de Montréal,
Montreal, QC, Canada
e-mail: andre.denault@umontreal.ca

14.2 Definition of RV Dysfunction and RV Failure

RV dysfunction is generally accepted as a term that encompasses abnormal RV function assessed by echocardiographic or hemodynamic evaluation, regardless of any repercussion on organs. Acute RV failure is generally defined as a state of rapidly progressive systemic congestion from impaired RV filling or RV forward flow [10]. The International Right Heart Failure Foundation Scientific Working Group has defined right heart failure as a clinical syndrome that can be due to an alteration of structure and/or function of the right heart circulatory system that leads to suboptimal delivery of blood flow (high or low) to the pulmonary circulation and/or elevated central venous pressures (CVP)—at rest or with exercise [11]. The definition used by the 6th World Symposium on Pulmonary Hypertension to orient medical management, extracorporeal life support and lung transplantation in patients with right-sided heart failure due to pulmonary hypertension includes a gradation with its severe form characterized by secondary dysfunction of other organs, such as liver, kidneys and gut [12]. The Interagency Registry for Mechanically Assisted Circulatory Support (INTERMACS) defines RV failure as an elevated CVP >16 mmHg and manifestation of elevated CVP including end-organ dysfunction. The definition includes a four-grade classification according to severity (mild, moderate, severe and severe-acute) depending on the duration of inotropic support or the need for RV assist device implantation [13].

14.3 Hemodynamic Parameters

RV failure is the leading cause of death in pulmonary hypertension. The pulmonary artery catheter (PAC) has traditionally been considered the gold standard for pulmonary hypertension and RV function assessment [14]. In addition to the data commonly obtained from the PAC, including CVP, pulmonary artery pressure (PAP), pulmonary artery occlusion pressure (PAOP) and cardiac index (CI), other parameters may be of clinical utility, such as continuous RV pressure monitoring with its waveform analysis, RV function index (RVFI), mean arterial pressure-to-mean pulmonary arterial pressure ratio (MAP/MPAP), RV stroke work index (RVSWI), and pulmonary artery pulsatility index (PAPi) (Table 14.1).

Continuous monitoring of the RV pressure waveform can be done with any PAC equipped with either a RV pacing port or an infusion port [15]. Evaluation of the diastolic component of the RV waveform helps to evaluate adaptation of the right ventricle to the situation of increased PAP (Fig. 14.1). The normal RV diastolic waveform is horizontal with a proto- to end-diastolic gradient typically ≤4 mmHg. This horizontal diastolic waveform is due to the normal RV compliance, which is much higher than for the left ventricle [6, 16].

When RV dysfunction appears, the diastolic component of the waveform will progressively become up-sloping until it looks like a square root (Fig. 14.2a, f, k). Further deterioration of RV function will be associated with equalization of the diastolic RV pressure to diastolic PAP. In severe RV systolic dysfunction, RV *pulsus*

Table 14.1 Right ventricular (RV) function parameters

Index	Description	Findings and rationale
Relative pulmonary pressure	MAP/MPAP	– Normal ≥4 [20] – Independent of preload [20] Correlates with: – Hemodynamic complications after cardiac surgery [20] – Echocardiographic evaluation of IVS curvature [19] – Adverse outcome after liver transplantation [21] – Survival after heart transplantation [22]
Right ventricular function index (RVFI)	sPAP/CI	– Independent risk factor of mortality in critical care patients with pulmonary hypertension if >35 [23] – Increased PAP coupled with reduced RV systolic function is associated with poor prognosis in heart failure [2]
Right ventricular stroke work index (RVSWI)	(MPAP − CVP) × SVI × 0.0136	– Low RVSWI (<250–300 mmHg/ml/m^2) associated with an increased risk of need for RVAD after implantation of a LVAD [24, 50]
Pulmonary arterial pulsatility index (PAPi)	(sPAP − dPAP)/CVP	– Post-chest closure values associated with severe RV failure defined by the need for a RV mechanical support device, inotropic, and/or inhaled pulmonary vasodilator requirements for >14 days [27] – <1.85 provided 94% sensitivity and 81% specificity for identifying RV failure, prolonged inotrope use, or RVAD need after LVAD implantation [30]
Right-to-left filling pressure ratio	CVP/PAOP	– Normal ratio is approximately 0.5, higher values related to RV dysfunction [31, 32] – Ratio >0.63 before LVAD implantation is associated with subsequent RVAD implantation for RV failure [7]
Right ventricular length-force index	TAPSE/sPAP	– <0.36 mm/mmHg associated with unfavorable outcomes in heart failure with both reduced and preserved ejection fraction [33] – Not affected by the severity of LV dysfunction

CI cardiac index, *CVP* central venous pressure, *dPAP* diastolic pulmonary arterial pressure, *IVS* interventricular septal, *LVAD* left ventricular assist device, *MAP* mean systemic arterial pressure, *MPAP* mean pulmonary arterial pressure, *PAP* pulmonary artery pressure, *PAOP* pulmonary artery occlusion pressure, *RVAD* RV assist device, *sPAP* systolic pulmonary arterial pressure, *SVI* stroke volume index calculated as (CI × 1000)/(heart rate), *TAPSE* tricuspid annular plane systolic excursion

tardus and reduction in RV pulse pressure will be observed. In addition, RV outflow tract obstruction can be rapidly diagnosed using RV pressure waveform monitoring [17]. Such obstruction of the RV outflow tract represents a contraindication to the use of inotropes and can often appear after their use [15]. Changes in RV failure will also correlate with changes in CVP waveform. Initially gradual reduction of the X

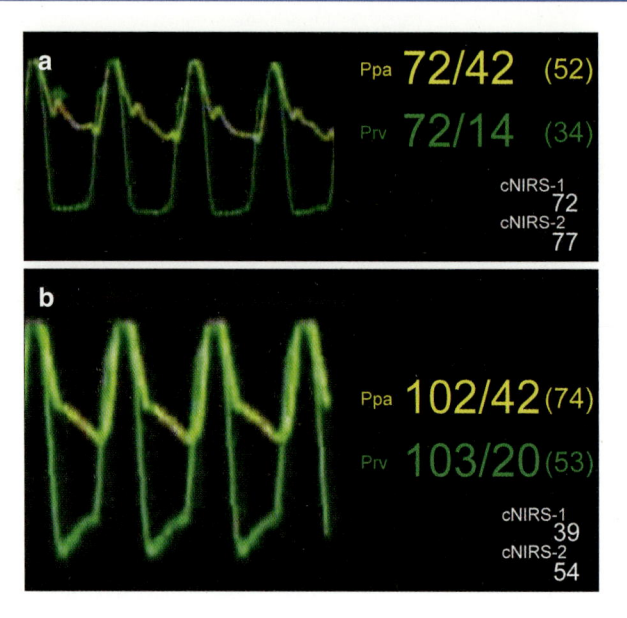

Fig. 14.1 Pulmonary hypertension associated with (**a**) a normal right ventricular pressure waveform (P_{rv}) and normal cerebral near-infrared spectroscopy (cNIRS) value. (**b**) Abnormal P_{rv} waveform with an oblique diastolic slope and reduced cNIRS, indicating abnormal right ventricular-arterial coupling and cerebral hypoperfusion or venous congestions. P_{pa} pulmonary artery pressure (reproduced from [15] with permission)

descent with increase in the V wave and the Y descent will be observed [1] (Fig. 14.2b, g, l). The V wave on the CVP was recently identified as the best predictor of portal venous pulsatility in cardiac surgical patients, which is typically associated with RV dysfunction (see later) [18].

The relative pulmonary pressure defined as the MAP/MPAP ratio is used to describe the severity of pulmonary hypertension in cardiac surgery. By comparing the pulmonary and systemic arterial pressures, it is possible to evaluate the systemic hemodynamic repercussions, the interventricular shift [19] and the degree of functional heart reserve in the face of pulmonary hypertension. In fact, this ratio is significantly lower in patients who encounter hemodynamic complications after cardiac surgery [20]. In a predefined subgroup of patients with pulmonary hypertension, this ratio is independent of the loading conditions, by contrast with MAP and MPAP, which decrease with reduction of preload [20]. Thus, the MAP/MPAP ratio reveals its importance in situations of rapid variation of loading conditions, such as induction prior to tracheal intubation [20]. Also, the MAP/MPAP ratio correlates with the interventricular septal curvature evaluated by transthoracic echocardiography [19], adverse outcome after liver transplantation [21], and survival after heart transplantation [22].

The RVFI is defined as the systolic PAP-to-CI ratio. An increase in this invasive load-adaptability index is an independent risk factor for mortality in critical care patients with pulmonary hypertension [23]. In fact, high systolic PAP due to

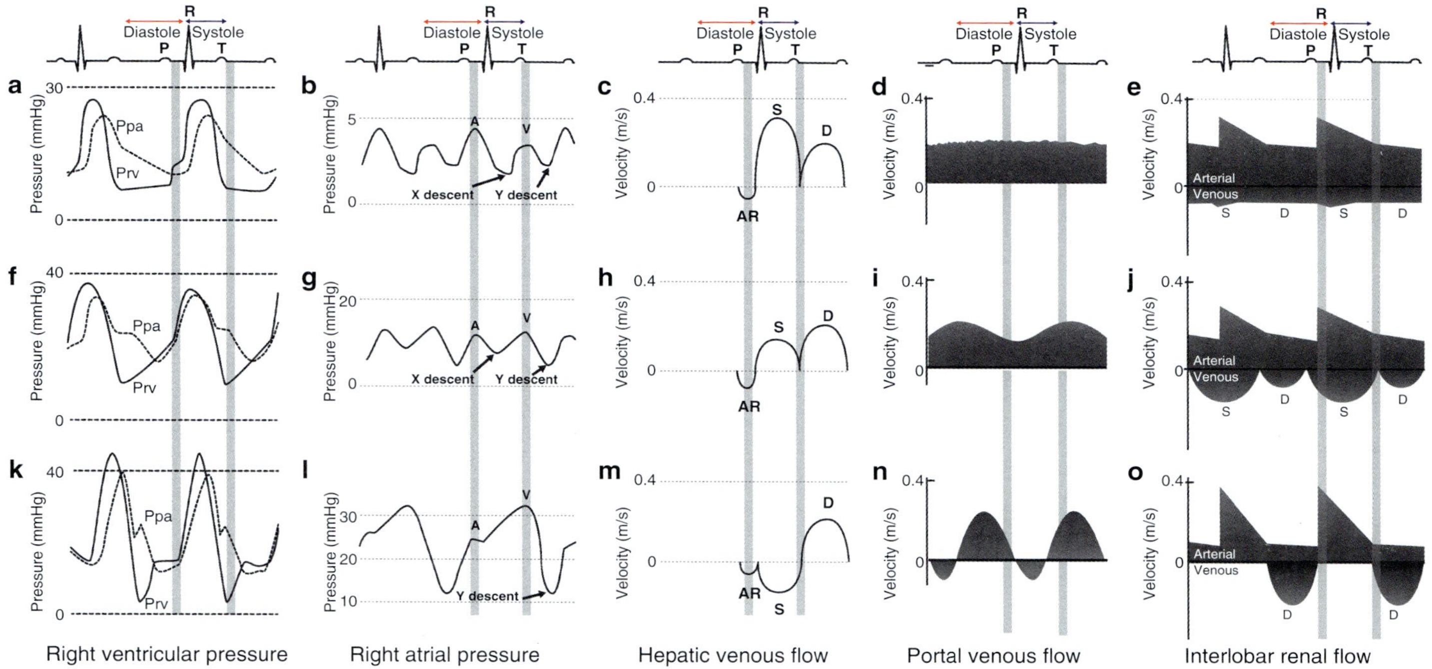

Fig. 14.2 Right ventricular pressure (P_{rv}), right atrial pressure, hepatic venous flow (HVF), portal venous flow, and interlobar arterial and venous renal flow in normal patients (**a–e**). Typical patterns commonly observed in patients with mild (**f–j**) and severe (**k–o**) right ventricular dysfunction. *AR* atrial reversal HVF velocity, *D* diastolic HVF Doppler velocity, P_{pa} pulmonary artery pressure, *S* systolic HVF velocity (reproduced from [15] with permission)

increased pulmonary vascular resistance (PVR) and low CI due to an overt compensatory mechanism of RV adaptability to increase afterload conditions are both epiphenomena of RV failure that can increase the RVFI. Use of the RVFI helps to better evaluate the impact of elevated PAP in patients with preserved RV function and response to medical afterload reduction. In such situations, patients with pulmonary hypertension might respond well with a decrease in PAP due to a decrease in PVR but the reduction in PAP may also reflect progressive RV failure. In this context, very high systolic PAP in the presence of normal CI could present a better prognosis than marginally high systolic PAP in the presence of low CI [2]. Nevertheless, if PVR is low, such as in isolated postcapillary pulmonary hypertension, and RV output is low, the RVFI might not reflect the severity of the situation.

The RVSWI represents the work that the right ventricle must do to move the ejection volume through the pulmonary circulation. It is calculated from the pressure difference between the MPAP and the CVP and the stroke volume index (SVI):

$$SVI = \frac{CI \times 1000}{Heart\ rate}$$

$$RVSWI = (MPAP - CVP) \times SVI \times 0.0136$$

High RVSWI values therefore represent increased myocardial work. A decrease in these values over time may be due to an improvement in pulmonary hemodynamics or progressive RV failure, making its interpretation difficult. High RVSWI values have been associated with increased mortality after lung transplantation, while values <250–300 mmHg/ml/m^2 have been associated with an increased risk for needing a RV assist device after implantation of a LV assist device [24].

The PAPi corresponds to the difference between the systolic PAP and the diastolic PAP or pulse pressure divided by CVP. It links the pressure generated by the right ventricle and its filling pressure [25, 26]:

$$PAPi = \frac{Systolic\ PAP - diastolic\ PAP}{CVP}$$

PAPi takes into consideration the preload, by using CVP as the denominator, against a given afterload, by using the pulmonary artery pulse pressure as the numerator [27, 28]. By using these right heart parameters, characterization of RV contractility is less influenced by disturbances in LV function [26]. The PAPi also has the advantage of being based on values measured continuously in the ICU in patients with a PAC, which enables RV function to be evaluated at short intervals relating to therapeutic interventions. Initially described as a marker of RV failure after acute myocardial infarction [29], the PAPi was strongly correlated with RV function evaluated by echocardiography in patients with inferior myocardial infarction [25]. In these patients, a PAPi <0.9 yielded 100% sensitivity and 98.3% specificity to predict mortality or the need for a RV assist device [25]. Other authors have recently reported an independent association between low PAPi and urgent need for a RV assist device [26], prolonged inotropes (>14 days) [30], or severe RV failure after LV assist device implantation [27].

The ratio between the right and the left ventricular filling pressures can also be used to follow RV function. A disproportionate right atrial pressure elevation relative to PAOP is a marker of RV dysfunction. As the normal right-to-left filling pressure ratio should be around 0.5, a ratio >0.63 has been associated with severe RV failure leading to the need for a RV assist device after LV assist device implantation [7, 31, 32].

The length-force relationship of the right ventricle incorporates hemodynamic monitoring and echocardiographic monitoring. It corresponds to the ratio of the tricuspid annular plane systolic excursion (TAPSE) on systolic PAP. Despite the caveats of TAPSE, it has been shown to be a prognostic factor (<0.36 mm/mmHg) in patients with heart failure with both reduced and preserved ejection fraction as it decreases in non-survivors. Importantly, this ratio is not affected by the severity of LV dysfunction [33].

14.4 Echocardiographic Parameters: 2D, Doppler, Strain, 3D

Long-axis systolic excursion of the lateral aspect of the tricuspid annulus represents an easily recognizable longitudinal movement on echocardiography and may be used as an indicator of RV systolic function. Typically measured in M-mode and corrected for angulation of interrogation, TAPSE is defined as the total excursion of the tricuspid annulus from end diastole to end systole. Normal TAPSE is 20–25 mm with <17 mm suggestive of RV dysfunction and <15 mm being considered significantly depressed [34]. The angle of excursion is toward the cardiac apex, and is slightly greater than normal mitral annular plane excursion [16]. The tricuspid annulus tilts toward the apex, whereas the mitral annulus moves more symmetrically toward the apex, somewhat like a piston, emphasizing the importance of measuring motion at the lateral annulus. Depressed TAPSE measurements suggest depressed RV systolic function from a variety of causes. TAPSE has been correlated to the RV ejection fraction (RVEF). However, it is important to note that TAPSE is angle and load dependent. Also, it reflects only the longitudinal displacement of a single segment of the complex three-dimensional (3D) RV structure.

Volumetric evaluation can be estimated using RV fractional area change (RVFAC) defined as (end-diastolic area − end-systolic area)/end-diastolic area × 100. Diagnosis of RV dysfunction is made by an RVFAC <35% and its severity can be described as mild, moderate, or severe for values of 25–35%, 18–25%, and ≤18%, respectively. However, 2-dimensional (2D) RVFAC from a mid-esophageal four-chamber view using transesophageal echocardiography or from an apical four-chamber views using transthoracic echocardiography does not consider the RV outflow tract volume that corresponds to approximately 20% of the RV volume.

Global assessment of RV function can be made using the RV myocardial performance index (RVMPI) using pulsed wave Doppler or tissue Doppler imaging at the lateral tricuspid annulus. It represents an estimate of both RV systolic and diastolic function. The RVMPI is based on the relationship between ejection and non-ejection work of the heart. The RVMPI is defined as the ratio of isovolumetric time divided by ejection time, or [(isovolumetric relaxation time + isovolumetric contraction time)/(ejection time)]. Presence of RV dysfunction is characterized by a RVMPI >0.43 on pulsed wave Doppler and >0.54 on tissue Doppler imaging [34]. In valvular cardiac surgery, RVMPI is an independent predictor of difficult weaning from CPB, mortality, circulatory failure, duration of hospitalization and ICU stay [35]. This parameter is load dependent and unreliable in situations where right atrial pressure is elevated and RR intervals are irregular, such as atrial fibrillation because of reduced isovolumetric contraction time.

Other regional assessments of RV function include pulsed Doppler or tissue Doppler peak velocity at the tricuspid annulus (S') and RV acceleration during isovolumic contraction. Interrogation of S' by tissue Doppler imaging <9.5 cm/s is a sign of RV dysfunction as it represents the basal lateral wall RV function. RV acceleration during isovolumic contraction is also measured by tissue Doppler imaging at the lateral tricuspid annulus. RV acceleration during isovolumic contraction is defined as the peak isovolumic myocardial velocity divided by time to peak velocity. This parameter is rate dependent and appears to be less load dependent than the RVMPI. Values <2.2 m/s^2 are considered to be related to RV dysfunction. The aspect of the pulmonary artery velocity can also be used as an indicator of increased RV afterload or impedance particularly with reduced acceleration time or when a notched aspect is present [36].

Recently, myocardial strain measured using speckle-tracking echocardiography has gained in popularity as a method to quantify myocardial deformation. Strain (ε), reported as a percentage, describes the extent of myocardial deformation and can be defined as the difference between the initial length (L_0) of a myocardial strip and its stressed length (L) normalized over the initial length (L_0) or as

$$\varepsilon = (L - L_0) / L_0$$

Myocardial strain can be measured using a variety of modalities. Tissue Doppler was the first modality used to assess it in the 1990s, but suffers from angle dependence limitations.

Speckle tracking echocardiography is based on spatial displacement and tracking of the tissue speckles. Speckles are randomly created by interferences between the ultrasound beam and myocardial fibers and the resulting pattern is tracked frame by frame using a statistical algorithm to detect the best-matching areas. Changes in the speckle pattern are assumed to represent movement of the myocardial fibers. The use of speckle-tracking echocardiography to study RV strain is highly feasible and uses an absolute normality cutoff value of >20% (or < -20%) for global longitudinal strain of the right ventricle [34]. In a recent study of 63 patients with non-ischemic cardiomyopathies comparing established echocardiographic parameters for the evaluation of RV function (TAPSE, S', and RVFAC) to those measured using speckle-tracking echocardiography, lateral wall RV longitudinal strain was shown to be the parameter most closely correlated to RVEF measured by cardiac magnetic resonance [37].

Tousignant et al. demonstrated that intraoperative RV global strain measurement using transesophageal echocardiography was feasible in the perioperative setting of cardiac surgery [38]. Others demonstrated that RV strain worsened after CPB [39] but did not study the clinical significance of that echocardiographic finding. Still in the perioperative setting of cardiac surgery, preoperative transthoracic echocardiography evaluation of 2D RV longitudinal strain was a better predictor of mortality after cardiac surgery than RVFAC alone [40]. That study showed that a RVFAC <35% was associated with a greater risk of postoperative mortality, probably because it reflects a severe and advanced form of RV dysfunction with both radial and longitudinal contraction dysfunction. In patients with preserved RVFAC, RV speckle tracking appears to be a sensitive method to identify early RV dysfunction. Abnormal RV longitudinal strain was present in 34% of patients with normal RVFAC. The risk of mortality with abnormal strain was the same as if the patients had RVFAC values <35%. This indicates that RV speckle tracking appears to be a sensitive method to identify early RV dysfunction [40].

The use of 3D echocardiography to evaluate RV end-diastolic and end-systolic volume allows determination of RVEF. A 3D RVEF <45% is highly suggestive of RV dysfunction. End-diastolic volumes >87 ml/m^2 for men and >74 ml/m^2 for women are indicative of RV enlargement. Intraoperative RVEF assessment with 3D transesophageal echocardiography seems to be feasible and reproducible in patients with normal RV function and in patients with a dilated right ventricle without being excessively time consuming [41].

14.5 Extra-Cardiac Echocardiographic Parameters

Echocardiography is crucial to understand the consequences of RV dysfunction. Signs of venous system congestion can be seen through evaluation of flow in the hepatic, portal, and renal systems. Disturbance in liver function assays, creatinine rise, and lactic acidemia are all signs of decreased tissue perfusion pressure that originate from venous congestion as a consequence of progression from RV dysfunction to failure. Echocardiography will be useful to search for signs of venous congestion before their repercussion in biochemical panels appears.

Examination of flow velocity patterns during phases of the cardiac cycle with pulsed wave Doppler can contribute useful information about RV function. Normal Doppler hepatic flow is hepatofugal during systole and diastole with systolic predominance due to downward motion of the tricuspid annulus in ventricular systole resulting in a rapid filling of the right atria. When RV dysfunction occurs, decreased TAPSE will lead to a velocity reduction of the systolic wave. The systolic-to-diastolic ratio will become equal to and subsequently <1. With progression to RV failure the systolic Doppler wave will invert and systolic hepatic flow will become mainly hepatopetal with a negative systolic-to-diastolic velocity ratio (Fig. 14.2c, h, m) [42].

Portal and splenic vein flow can easily be assessed using transthoracic or transesophageal echocardiography, respectively [43]. Assessment of the splenic vein could provide similar information as it drains into the portal vein. Due to its isolation from the systemic circulation by the liver sinusoids and splanchnic capillary bed, venous flow through the portal system is characterized by low velocities

(20 cm/s) and only minimal variations through the cardiac cycle. Appearance of portal pulsatility is a sign of posthepatic portal hypertension (Fig. 14.2d, i, n) and has been reported as a sign of congestive heart failure severity [44] and in cardiac surgical patients it is associated with renal failure, bleeding, reoperation, delirium, and duration of stay in the hospital and in the ICU [18, 45, 46]. The pulsatility fraction can be calculated from the ratio of the difference between systolic and diastolic velocities over the diastolic velocity. Values >50% can be considered abnormal and are called pulsatile portal flow [43]. In severe RV failure, complete absence or reversal of portal flow will be observed [47, 48]. It is important to mention that the portal venous system needs to be free from other causes of portal hypertension, such as cirrhosis and portal thrombosis, to be a reliable marker of RV dysfunction.

Intrarenal hemodynamics will be affected by RV dysfunction as elevated CVP will decrease the arteriovenous perfusion pressure gradient. In normal conditions, venous blood flow in the renal veins is continuous during the cardiac cycle. Elevated CVP and decreased central venous compliance will increase the transmission of systolic and diastolic wave producing a discontinuous biphasic pattern like the pulsed wave Doppler pattern seen in the hepatic veins. Progression of RV dysfunction will transform renal venous flow into a diastolic predominant monophasic discontinuous pattern (Fig. 14.2e, j, o).

The clinical implications of abnormal Doppler intrarenal venous velocity patterns are currently being investigated. Recent studies have shown that abnormal renal venous flow is a predictor of survival in congestive heart failure [49] and a predictor of renal failure after cardiac surgery [45]. Figure 14.2 summarizes respective flow and pressure patterns for RV pressure, right atrial pressure, hepatic venous flow, portal venous flow, and interlobar arterial and venous renal flow in normal patients and in patients with mild and severe RV dysfunction.

14.6 Conclusion

Different modalities are available to evaluate and follow RV function in the acute care setting. Using combined hemodynamic and echographic modalities is helpful to corroborate and strengthen findings in order to rapidly identify RV dysfunction and develop a therapeutic strategy.

References

1. Amsallem M, Kuznetsova T, Hanneman K, Denault A, Haddad F. Right heart imaging in patients with heart failure: a tale of two ventricles. Curr Opin Cardiol. 2016;31:469–82.
2. Ghio S, Gavazzi A, Campana C, et al. Independent and additive prognostic value of right ventricular systolic function and pulmonary artery pressure in patients with chronic heart failure. J Am Coll Cardiol. 2001;37:183–8.
3. Bodez D, Ternacle J, Guellich A, et al. Prognostic value of right ventricular systolic function in cardiac amyloidosis. Amyloid. 2016;23:158–67.
4. Anavekar NS, Skali H, Bourgoun M, et al. Usefulness of right ventricular fractional area change to predict death, heart failure, and stroke following myocardial infarction (from the VALIANT ECHO Study). Am J Cardiol. 2008;101:607–12.

5. Maslow AD, Regan MM, Panzica P, Heindel S, Mashikian J, Comunale ME. Precardiopulmonary bypass right ventricular function is associated with poor outcome after coronary artery bypass grafting in patients with severe left ventricular systolic dysfunction. Anesth Analg. 2002;95:1507–18.
6. Haddad F, Couture P, Tousignant C, Denault A. The right ventricle in cardiac surgery, a perioperative perspective: II. Pathophysiology, clinical importance, and management. Anesth Analg. 2009;108:422–33.
7. Kormos RL, Teuteberg JJ, Pagani FD, et al. Right ventricular failure in patients with the HeartMate II continuous-flow left ventricular assist device: incidence, risk factors, and effect on outcomes. J Thorac Cardiovasc Surg. 2010;139:1316–24.
8. Denault AY, Pearl RG, Michler RE, et al. Tezosentan and right ventricular failure in patients with pulmonary hypertension undergoing cardiac surgery: the TACTICS trial. J Cardiothorac Vasc Anesth. 2013;27:1212–7.
9. Denault AY, Bussieres JS, Arellano R, et al. A multicentre randomized-controlled trial of inhaled milrinone in high-risk cardiac surgical patients. Can J Anesth. 2016;63:1140–53.
10. Harjola VP, Mebazaa A, Celutkiene J, et al. Contemporary management of acute right ventricular failure: a statement from the Heart Failure Association and the Working Group on Pulmonary Circulation and Right Ventricular Function of the European Society of Cardiology. Eur J Heart Fail. 2016;18:226–41.
11. Mehra MR, Park MH, Landzberg MJ, Lala A, Waxman AB, International Right Heart Failure Foundation Scientific Working Group. Right heart failure: toward a common language. J Heart Lung Transplant. 2014;33:123–6.
12. Hoeper MM, Benza RL, Corris P, et al. Intensive care, right ventricular support and lung transplantation in patients with pulmonary hypertension. Eur Respir J. 2019;53:1801906.
13. Amsallem M, Mercier O, Kobayashi Y, Moneghetti K, Haddad F. Forgotten no more: a focused update on the right ventricle in cardiovascular disease. JACC Heart Fail. 2018;6:891–903.
14. Denault AY, Haddad F, Jacobsohn E, et al. Perioperative right ventricular dysfunction. Curr Opin Anaesthesiol. 2013;26:71–81.
15. Raymond M, Gronlykke L, Couture EJ, et al. Perioperative right ventricular pressure monitoring in cardiac surgery. J Cardiothorac Vasc Anesth. 2019;33:1090–104.
16. Haddad F, Couture P, Tousignant C, et al. The right ventricle in cardiac surgery, a perioperative perspective: I. Anatomy, physiology, and assessment. Anesth Analg. 2009;108:407–21.
17. Denault AY, Chaput M, Couture P, Hébert Y, Haddad F, Tardif JC. Dynamic right ventricular outflow tract obstruction in cardiac surgery. J Thorac Cardiovasc Surg. 2006;132:43–9.
18. Eljaiek R, Cavayas YA, Rodrigue E, et al. High postoperative portal venous flow pulsatility indicates right ventricular dysfunction and predicts complications in cardiac surgery patients. Br J Anaesth. 2019;122:206–14.
19. Haddad F, Guihaire J, Skhiri M, et al. Septal curvature is marker of hemodynamic, anatomical, and electromechanical ventricular interdependence in patients with pulmonary arterial hypertension. Echocardiography. 2014;31:699–707.
20. Robitaille A, Denault AY, Couture P, et al. Importance of relative pulmonary hypertension in cardiac surgery: the mean systemic-to-pulmonary artery pressure ratio. J Cardiothorac Vasc Anesth. 2006;20:331–9.
21. Rebel A, Nguyen D, Bauer B, Sloan PA, DiLorenzo A, Hassan ZU. Systemic-to-pulmonary artery pressure ratio as a predictor of patient outcome following liver transplantation. World J Hepatol. 2016;8:1384–91.
22. Bianco JC, Mc Loughlin S, Denault AY, Marenchino RG, Rojas JI, Bonofiglio FC. Heart transplantation in patients >/=60 years: importance of relative pulmonary hypertension and right ventricular failure on midterm survival. J Cardiothorac Vasc Anesth. 2018;32:32–40.
23. Saydain G, Awan A, Manickam P, Kleinow P, Badr S. Pulmonary hypertension an independent risk factor for death in intensive care unit: correlation of hemodynamic factors with mortality. Clin Med Insights Circ Respir Pulm Med. 2015;9:27–33.
24. Fitzpatrick JR 3rd, Frederick JR, Hsu VM, et al. Risk score derived from pre-operative data analysis predicts the need for biventricular mechanical circulatory support. J Heart Lung Transplant. 2008;27:1286–92.

25. Korabathina R, Heffernan KS, Paruchuri V, et al. The pulmonary artery pulsatility index identifies severe right ventricular dysfunction in acute inferior myocardial infarction. Catheter Cardiovasc Interv. 2012;80:593–600.
26. Kang G, Ha R, Banerjee D. Pulmonary artery pulsatility index predicts right ventricular failure after left ventricular assist device implantation. J Heart Lung Transplant. 2016;35:67–73.
27. Gudejko MD, Gebhardt BR, Zahedi F, et al. Intraoperative hemodynamic and echocardiographic measurements associated with severe right ventricular failure after left ventricular assist device implantation. Anesth Analg. 2019;128:25–32.
28. Alfirevic A, Sale S, Soltesz E. Foretelling right ventricular failure after left ventricular assist device implantation: the tale of the pulmonary artery pulsatility index. Anesth Analg. 2019;128:8–10.
29. Lloyd EA, Gersh BJ, Kennelly BM. Hemodynamic spectrum of "dominant" right ventricular infarction in 19 patients. Am J Cardiol. 1981;48:1016–22.
30. Morine KJ, Kiernan MS, Pham DT, Paruchuri V, Denofrio D, Kapur NK. Pulmonary artery pulsatility index is associated with right ventricular failure after left ventricular assist device surgery. J Card Fail. 2016;22:110–6.
31. Drazner MH, Hamilton MA, Fonarow G, et al. Relationship between right and left-sided filling pressures in 1000 patients with advanced heart failure. J Heart Lung Transplant. 1999;18:1126–32.
32. Campbell P, Drazner MH, Kato M, et al. Mismatch of right- and left-sided filling pressures in chronic heart failure. J Card Fail. 2011;17:561–8.
33. Guazzi M, Bandera F, Pelissero G, et al. Tricuspid annular plane systolic excursion and pulmonary arterial systolic pressure relationship in heart failure: an index of right ventricular contractile function and prognosis. Am J Physiol Heart Circ Physiol. 2013;305:H1373–81.
34. Lang RM, Badano LP, Mor-Avi V, et al. Recommendations for cardiac chamber quantification by echocardiography in adults: an update from the American Society of Echocardiography and the European Association of Cardiovascular Imaging. J Am Soc Echocardiogr. 2015;28(1):39. e14.
35. Haddad F, Denault AY, Couture P, et al. Right ventricular myocardial performance index predicts perioperative mortality or circulatory failure in high-risk valvular surgery. J Am Soc Echocardiogr. 2007;20:1065–72.
36. Tousignant C, Van Orman JR. Pulmonary impedance and pulmonary Doppler trace in the perioperative period. Anesth Analg. 2015;121:601–9.
37. Focardi M, Cameli M, Carbone SF, et al. Traditional and innovative echocardiographic parameters for the analysis of right ventricular performance in comparison with cardiac magnetic resonance. Eur Heart J Cardiovasc Imaging. 2015;16:47–52.
38. Tousignant C, Desmet M, Bowry R, Harrington AM, Cruz JD, Mazer CD. Speckle tracking for the intraoperative assessment of right ventricular function: a feasibility study. J Cardiothorac Vasc Anesth. 2010;24:275–9.
39. Duncan AE, Sarwar S, Kateby Kashy B, et al. Early left and right ventricular response to aortic valve replacement. Anesth Analg. 2017;124:406–18.
40. Ternacle J, Berry M, Cognet T, et al. Prognostic value of right ventricular two-dimensional global strain in patients referred for cardiac surgery. J Am Soc Echocardiogr. 2013;26:721–6.
41. Fusini L, Tamborini G, Gripari P, et al. Feasibility of intraoperative three-dimensional transesophageal echocardiography in the evaluation of right ventricular volumes and function in patients undergoing cardiac surgery. J Am Soc Echocardiogr. 2011;24:868–77.
42. Scheinfeld MH, Bilali A, Koenigsberg M. Understanding the spectral Doppler waveform of the hepatic veins in health and disease. Radiographics. 2009;29:2081–98.
43. Denault AY, Beaubien-Souligny W, Elmi-Sarabi M, et al. Clinical significance of portal hypertension diagnosed with bedside ultrasound after cardiac surgery. Anesth Analg. 2017;124:1109–15.
44. Duerinckx AJ, Grant EG, Perrella RR, Szeto A, Tessler FN. The pulsatile portal vein in cases of congestive heart failure: correlation of duplex Doppler findings with right atrial pressures. Radiology. 1990;176:655–8.

45. Beaubien-Souligny W, Benkreira A, Robillard P, et al. Alterations in portal vein flow and intrarenal venous flow are associated with acute kidney injury after cardiac surgery: a prospective observational cohort study. J Am Heart Assoc. 2018;7:e009961.
46. Benkreira A, Beaubien-Souligny W, Mailhot T, et al. Portal hypertension is associated with congestive encephalopathy and delirium after cardiac surgery. Can J Cardiol. 2019;35:1134–41.
47. Tremblay JA, Beaubien-Souligny W, Elmi-Sarabi M, Desjardins G, Denault AY. Point-of-care ultrasonography to assess portal vein pulsatility and the effect of inhaled milrinone and epoprostenol in severe right ventricular failure: a report of 2 cases. A A Case Rep. 2017;9:219–23.
48. Beaubien-Souligny W, Bouchard J, Desjardins G, et al. Extracardiac signs of fluid overload in the critically ill cardiac patient: a focused evaluation using bedside ultrasound. Can J Cardiol. 2017;33:88–100.
49. Iida N, Seo Y, Sai S, et al. Clinical implications of intrarenal hemodynamic evaluation by Doppler ultrasonography in heart failure. JACC Heart Fail. 2016;4:674–82.
50. Fukamachi K, McCarthy PM, Smedira NG, Vargo RL, Starling RC, Young JB. Preoperative risk factors for right ventricular failure after implantable left ventricular assist device insertion. Ann Thorac Surg. 1999;68:2181–4.

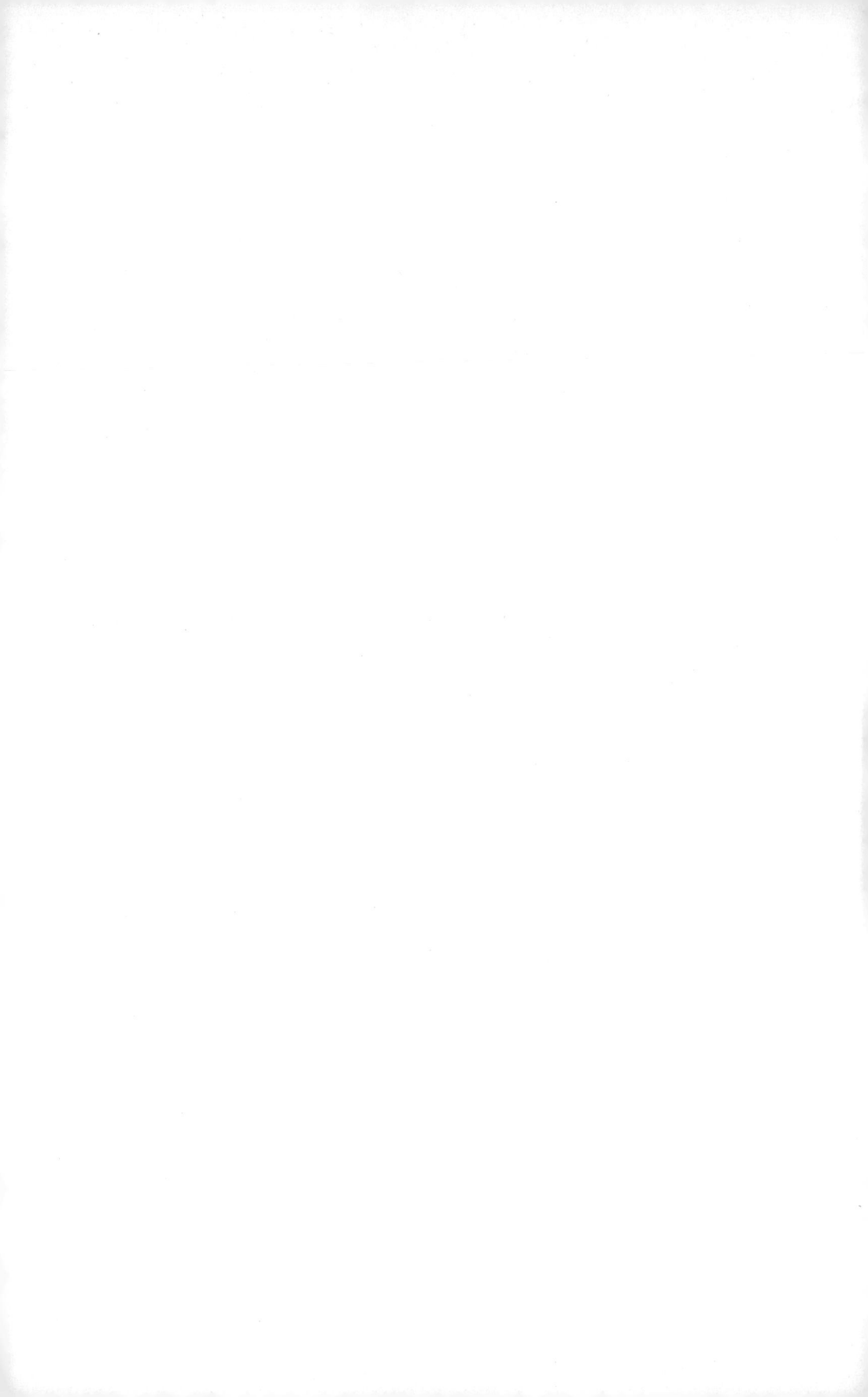

Management of Hypotension: Implications for Noncardiac Surgery and Intensive Care

E. Schneck, B. Saugel, and M. Sander

15.1 Introduction

A patient's hemodynamic status is determined—among multiple other factors—by the blood flow generated by the heart, the blood pressure, and the peripheral vascular resistance. In the last decade, the concept of optimizing blood flow was within the scope of numerous trials on advanced hemodynamic management; simultaneously, evidence for the importance of sufficient blood pressure management was found. It became clear that in surgical and critically ill patients, hypotension is common and associated with adverse outcomes. Despite this knowledge and the evolution of hemodynamic management, hypotension remains a common and challenging problem in perioperative and intensive care medicine. Hypotension is still not universally defined. Even though it is widely accepted that intraoperative hypotension is associated with adverse outcomes, it remains unclear which blood pressure threshold should be maintained to decrease secondary organ dysfunction and eventually to improve postoperative outcomes. Furthermore, alterations in cardiovascular dynamics resulting in hypotension and their changes on therapeutic interventions differ substantially among patients. While surgical patients under general anesthesia mainly suffer from drug-induced vasoplegia, decreased myocardial inotropy, and surgery-induced hypovolemia, critically ill patients face a broad spectrum of hemodynamic alterations. Depending on the underlying disease, damage to the endothelium with consecutive loss of intravascular fluids, hemorrhage, cardiac failure, and

---

E. Schneck · M. Sander (✉)
Department of Anesthesiology, Intensive Care Medicine and Pain Therapy,
University Hospital Giessen, Justus-Liebig University Giessen, UKGM, Giessen, Germany
e-mail: michael.sander@chiru.med.uni-giessen.de

B. Saugel
Department of Anesthesiology, Center of Anesthesiology and Intensive Care Medicine,
University Medical Center Hamburg-Eppendorf, Hamburg, Germany

severe vasoplegia are common causes of hypotension in critically ill patients. Nevertheless, similar diagnostic, prophylactic, and therapeutic approaches to the management of hypotension are used in perioperative and intensive care medicine. Therefore, in this chapter we provide an overview of the assessment and general management of hypotension in patients under general anesthesia during noncardiac surgery as well as in critically ill patients treated in the intensive care unit (ICU).

15.2 Adverse Effects of Hypotension

15.2.1 Intraoperative Hypotension in Noncardiac Surgery

Intraoperative hypotension is common in noncardiac surgery but varies according to the type of surgery, definition, and other patient-related factors. In 2007, Bijker et al. addressed this problem and analyzed 140 different definitions of intraoperative hypotension from 130 studies, including 15,509 patients having noncardiac surgery under general anesthesia [1]. The incidence of intraoperative hypotension varied from 5% to 99%, depending on the chosen definition. As a consequence of the varying but overall high incidence of intraoperative hypotension, two questions arose. First, what is the relevance of intraoperative hypotension, and second, which definition should we use for intraoperative hypotension. To answer the first question, several studies investigated the association between intraoperative hypotension and adverse postoperative outcomes. In noncardiac surgery patients, intraoperative hypotension is associated with cardiovascular complications such as myocardial injury after noncardiac surgery, acute kidney injury (AKI), stroke, and even mortality. The most important studies reporting the association of intraoperative hypotension and postoperative organ failure are shown in Table 15.1.

There is an association between intraoperative hypotension and myocardial injury after noncardiac surgery. Even a short decrease in the mean arterial pressure (MAP ≤60 mmHg) seems to be associated with an increased risk for postoperative myocardial injury after noncardiac surgery and should therefore be avoided [2, 3]. Myocardial injury after noncardiac surgery is defined as an increase in cardiac biomarkers (often troponin T and I) within the first 30 days after noncardiac surgery, independent of the clinical signs of myocardial ischemia or the universal definition of myocardial infarction (MI) [4].

There is also an association between intraoperative hypotension and AKI. It is widely accepted that postoperative renal failure is associated with intraoperative hypotension, but no ultimate threshold has yet been defined [5, 6]. A recent review revealed an increased risk for AKI in the case of a MAP ≤65 mmHg [2]. The association with AKI is strongly dependent on the severity of hypotension and its duration. Even short episodes of intraoperative hypotension (starting from 1 min) are already associated with the occurrence of postoperative AKI [2, 3].

There is no definite evidence for an association between intraoperative hypotension and stroke in noncardiac surgery patients [2]. Patients having cardiac, neuro-,

Table 15.1 Some important studies demonstrating adverse outcomes of intraoperative hypotension in noncardiac surgery

Authors (year of publication)	Study design	Methodological approach	Investigated outcome parameter	Increased risk
Wesselink et al. (2018) [2]	Systematic review of 42 studies	Multivariable logistic regression of various absolute and relative blood pressure thresholds	AKI Myocardial injury Stroke Mortality	Increased risk of AKI and MINS beginning at MAP <80 mmHg for at least 10 min reaching relevance after falling below a MAP of 60 mmHg (even for shorter durations)
Salmasi et al. (2017) [3]	Retrospective cohort analysis of 57,315 patients	Multivariable logistic regression of various absolute and relative blood pressure thresholds	Myocardial injury AKI	MAP ≤65 mmHg or relative threshold of ≥20% progressively related to MINS and AKI
Van Waes et al. (2016) [47]	Prospective cohort study of 890 patients	Four definitions – MAP <60 mmHg – MAP <50 mmHg – Decrease of ≥30% of baseline blood pressure – Decrease of ≥40% of baseline blood pressure	Myocardial injury	A decrease of ≥40% of baseline blood pressure with a cumulative duration of >30 min was associated with myocardial injury
Sun et al. (2015) [5]	Retrospective cohort analysis of 5127 patients	Multivariable logistic regression of exposure-outcome relationship	AKI	Progressive increase in intraoperative hypotension, associated with MAP <60 mmHg for 11–20 min and MAP <55 mmHg for more than 10 min
Monk et al. (2015) [12]	Retrospective cohort analysis of 20,523 patients	Analysis of three definitions: – Population-based thresholds – Absolute thresholds – Relative thresholds	30-day mortality	Increase in 30-day mortality: – Population-based threshold: area under threshold of MAP <49 mmHg for more than 3.9 min – Absolute threshold: MAP <49 mmHg ≥5 min – Relative threshold: decrease of MAP >50% from baseline for ≥5 min

(continued)

Table 15.1 (continued)

Authors (year of publication)	Study design	Methodological approach	Investigated outcome parameter	Increased risk
Walsh et al. (2013) [6]	Retrospective cohort analysis of 33,330 patients	Multivariable logistic regression of exposure-outcome relationship	AKI Myocardial injury	Even short-lasting episodes of intraoperative hypotension <55 mmHg are associated with an increase of AKI and myocardial injury
Bijker et al. (2012) [48]	Case-control study of 48,241 patients	Conditional logistic regression analysis	Stroke	A relative decrease of ≥30% from baseline blood pressure was associated with an increased risk of postoperative stroke

AKI acute kidney injury, *MAP* mean arterial pressure, *MINS* myocardial injury after noncardiac surgery

or carotid surgery are at elevated risk for developing a postoperative stroke and show increased mortality rates compared to stroke patients in the general population [7]. Although several studies have indicated an association of intraoperative hypotension with an increased incidence of stroke, in a recent case-control study of 106,337 patients having general surgery (excluding cardiac, neuro-, and carotid surgical patients), the incidence of stroke was not associated with intraoperative hypotension (defined as MAP ≤70 mmHg) [8]. Furthermore, no relationship between the occurrence of severe intraoperative hypotension (MAP <60 mmHg) and stroke could be identified.

There is no definitive evidence supporting an association of intraoperative hypotension with postoperative cognitive dysfunction (POCD). Due to its association with morbidity, mortality and length of hospital stay, POCD is a major healthcare problem of mainly elderly patients [9]. In 2015, a prospective observational study including 594 patients identified increased blood pressure fluctuations as a risk factor for the development of POCD [10]. However, in a recent randomized control trial, targeted blood pressure management (MAP ≥90% of baseline blood pressure) did not reduce the incidence of POCD compared to more liberal blood pressure management [11].

There is even an association between severe intraoperative hypotension (MAP ≤55 mmHg) and postoperative mortality [2, 6, 12]. For example, a decrease of MAP ≤49 for more than 5 min was associated with a 2.4-fold increase in 30-day mortality in noncardiac surgical patients having general surgery (with the exception of carotid and neurosurgery) [13].

15.2.2 Hypotension in Critically Ill Patients

Hypotension is a major problem in critically ill patients with circulatory shock. With a prevalence of up to 81%, it is a daily challenge for the intensivist [14].

Surprisingly, high-quality prospective studies investigating the consequences of hypotension are rare, resulting in a low quality of evidence. The investigation of critically ill patients is complicated by the high variety of conditions and underlying diseases. Especially in septic patients, profound hypotension is associated with poor outcomes. In a large retrospective analysis, time-weighted adjusted MAP ≤65 mmHg was associated with an increased probability of in-hospital death, AKI and myocardial injury [3]. The only available multicenter randomized trial investigating the influence of using different MAP targets on mortality as a primary outcome did not show a beneficial effect of a MAP target of 80–85 mmHg compared to a MAP target of 65–70 mmHg [15]. Although patients in the high-target group suffered from a higher number of arrhythmias, if they had a history of arterial hypertension they needed less renal replacement therapy (RRT) [15]. The Surviving Sepsis Campaign recommends initially targeting a MAP ≥65 mmHg in patients with septic shock requiring vasopressors, but emphasizes that the target should then be individualized to the patient's condition and pertaining circumstances [16]. The question of whether to aim for a higher blood pressure target in patients with preexisting arterial hypertension remains unanswered.

Even though hypotension in septic shock remains the most investigated condition in critically ill patients, hypotension has also been identified as a significant risk factor for adverse events in other patient cohorts. Already, a decrease in the systolic arterial blood pressure ≤110 mmHg was strongly associated with higher 30-day mortality in patients with penetrating and blunt major trauma [17, 18]. In addition to the underlying conditions, treatment procedures (e.g., tracheal intubation and RRT) and drug adverse effects frequently result in hypotensive episodes [14, 19, 20].

15.3 The Challenge of Defining Hypotension

15.3.1 Defining Intraoperative Hypotension in Noncardiac Surgery

The precise diagnosis of a pathologic condition is the basis of every therapeutic strategy, but in the case of intraoperative hypotension, an ultimate definition is still lacking. From a pathophysiological point of view, significant intraoperative hypotension is defined by its complications, although that does not help in determining the absolute or relative threshold for the individual patient. In a retrospective study that included data from over 33,000 patients, there was an association of intraoperative hypotension with AKI and myocardial injury after noncardiac surgery, even when the blood pressure decreased for only a short duration under an absolute MAP threshold of 55 mmHg [6]. These findings were supported by another retrospective data analysis of 57,315 patients showing an association of a MAP ≤65 mmHg with myocardial injury and AKI after noncardiac surgery [3]. In a meta-analysis, a progressive increase in the risk of postoperative mortality, AKI, and myocardial injury with lower intraoperative BP in noncardiac surgical patients was described, starting at a MAP ≤80 mmHg for more than 10 min. A MAP decrease ≤60 mmHg was associated with a twofold increase in AKI and myocardial injury after noncardiac surgery [2].

Relative thresholds consider conditions such as preexisting arterial hypertension and might therefore display a more individual and physiological approach of defining intraoperative hypotension. Many anesthesiologists refer to the classical teaching opinion that the blood pressure should be kept within 20% of the baseline value. A 20% decrease from baseline MAP was progressively associated with postsurgical AKI and myocardial injury after noncardiac surgery [3]. In another study, a 2.7-fold increase in mortality was described when the blood pressure dropped below 50% of baseline for more than 5 min [13]. However, surprisingly, relative thresholds did not perform better than absolute blood pressure thresholds in large retrospective database studies analyzing large amounts of data in a population-based approach [2, 3].

Relative thresholds are highly dependent on a thorough assessment of preoperative baseline blood pressure [21]. A recent study demonstrated that the pre-induction blood pressure and the mean daytime MAP poorly correlate, and that the pre-induction blood pressure should not be used as a surrogate for the patient's usual baseline blood pressure [22]. Furthermore, the same study showed that the lowest post-induction and intraoperative blood pressures were lower than the lowest nighttime MAPs in the majority of patients, highlighting the relevance of an adequate individual definition of hypotension [22].

In line with those findings, a recent consensus statement from the Perioperative Quality Initiative emphasizes that "ambulatory arterial blood pressure measurement is the optimal method to establish baseline values" [23]. Single preoperative baseline blood pressure values may be used for blood pressure targets when they reflect the patients' usual blood pressure [23]. At the same time, however, the authors stress the problem of a high discrepancy regarding study designs, blood pressure thresholds, and definitions of adverse outcome events in studies investigating intraoperative blood pressure, resulting in a lack of unique blood pressure variables that can be used for risk prediction [23].

15.3.2 Defining Hypotension in the Intensive Care Unit

The broad range of pathophysiologic alterations causing hypotension in critically ill patients makes it almost impossible to define thresholds for hypotension in the ICU. Hypotension is defined as a decrease in MAP ≤65 mmHg by the Surviving Sepsis Campaign. However, in the same context, this guideline also recommends to individualize the thresholds of hypotension in order to take preexisting conditions (e.g., arterial hypertension) into account [16]. This example is representative of the complexity of defining hypotension, even in this one disease entity.

One reasonable approach might be to detect critical blood pressure thresholds that show associations with organ injury. Regarding AKI, evidence hints towards a threshold of MAP ranging from 65 to 70 mmHg since these blood pressure levels were significantly associated with progression to stage 3 oliguric AKI shortly (less than 6 h) after oliguric AKI diagnosis [24]. These findings were supported by the

FINNAKI study, which found that a MAP <73 mmHg was critical for the development of AKI in septic patients [25]. In a retrospective analysis, Maheshwari et al. investigated the risks for AKI, myocardial injury and mortality in septic patients [26]. In that study, the incidence of these complications was already increasing from a MAP <85 mmHg.

Even though myocardial injury is probably highly prevalent, generally the assessment of hypotension-induced myocardial injury has to be evaluated with caution given the heterogeneous sources of elevated cardiac enzymes in critically ill patients. Concerning mortality, a time- and depth-dependent correlation of blood pressure levels starting with a decrease in MAP to <80 mmHg has been shown in patients with distributive shock [27].

Based on the existing evidence, a MAP of at least 65 mmHg should be maintained in critically ill patients, but individual blood pressure thresholds must also be evaluated carefully.

15.4 Individualization of Blood Pressure Measurement

15.4.1 Individual Blood Pressure Targets

The primary objective of hemodynamic management is to maintain adequate organ perfusion and oxygen delivery in order to maintain cellular metabolism. Current guidelines recommend an individualized approach to hemodynamic monitoring, but also strict avoidance of a relative MAP decrease $\geq 20\%$ from baseline or an absolute MAP decline <60 mmHg for cumulatively more than 30 min [28]. However, it has to be considered that the mentioned blood pressure thresholds represent population-based data, which have been shown to be associated with adverse outcomes and do not reflect individual blood pressure thresholds. Therefore, the current guideline underlines the need for individual assessment of the hemodynamic situation, including a blood pressure target.

Several individual factors should be considered to define individual blood pressure targets in surgical and critically ill patients. First, the individual thresholds for the autoregulation of the kidney, brain and abdominal organs cannot at present be investigated and are affected not only by patient condition and hemodynamic management but also by surgical intervention. Second, MAP, as the surrogate parameter for blood inflow, determines not only adequate organ perfusion but also outflow, which can be the central venous or intracranial pressure. Both can be affected by the underlying condition, surgical approach, and patient positioning (e.g., liver and brain surgery). Finally, it should be taken into account that organ perfusion can vary significantly, even in a single patient, without apparent changes in the blood pressure. Therefore, individualized blood pressure targets that consider preexisting diseases (e.g., arterial hypertension, severe hemorrhage), surgical approach (e.g., laparoscopy), and patient positioning (e.g., beach chair) should be defined before treatment, targeted throughout the procedure or ICU stay, and reevaluated continuously. Furthermore, a valid strategy of hemodynamic monitoring and management is needed for the maintenance of adequate blood pressure and flow [29].

15.4.2 Choice of Monitoring

Surgery- and patient-related risk factors dictate the need for continuous or intermittent blood pressure monitoring. While oscillometric measurements lead to blind time spots during which blood pressure fluctuation cannot be detected, continuous blood pressure monitoring is more elaborate. In general, lower risk patients are therefore provided with oscillometric intermittent blood pressure measurement, while continuous blood pressure monitoring is reserved for major surgery or high-risk patients. The beneficial effects of continuous blood pressure monitoring were shown by Meidert et al., who investigated its influence on blood pressure stability in 160 randomized orthopedic patients with a history of chronic hypertension. They showed that continuous blood pressure monitoring led to fewer hypotensive episodes [30]. Regarding blood pressure stability, another randomized controlled trial of 316 moderate- to high-risk patients undergoing general surgery revealed a significant reduction in hypotensive episodes by using continuous noninvasive blood pressure monitoring [31]. However, these studies did not investigate the effect of continuous noninvasive blood pressure monitoring on outcome parameters such as AKI or myocardial injury after noncardiac surgery.

Because of increasing knowledge about the consequences of even short-lasting phases of intraoperative hypotension, the question has been raised whether low-risk patients would also benefit from continuous blood pressure monitoring. Study findings proved a significant reduction in the duration of hypotensive episodes but were unable to show a decrease in postoperative complications [31, 32]. In addition, continuous invasive and noninvasive blood pressure monitoring enables advanced hemodynamic monitoring, such as uncalibrated pulse wave analysis for cardiac output measurements and dynamic preload variables. Interestingly, the current guideline for the cardiovascular assessment and management of patients undergoing noncardiac surgery from the European Society of Anesthesiology gives no recommendation as to when to use invasive blood pressure monitoring. However, it is generally accepted to use invasive blood pressure monitoring in patients having major surgery or in moderate- to high-risk patients [28]. Since invasive arterial access is regularly not justifiable in minor surgery, noninvasive methods can be used as an alternative for continuous blood pressure monitoring. Several different devices for noninvasive advanced hemodynamic monitoring have been introduced in the last few years, but show high variability in accuracy compared to direct arterial monitoring [33]. Furthermore, a benefit from noninvasive, continuous blood pressure monitoring in regard to secondary outcome parameters such as AKI, myocardial injury after noncardiac surgery, or mortality is still lacking.

Noninvasive hemodynamic monitoring methods may exhibit limited measurement performance in critically ill patients. Therefore, the consensus guideline for the hemodynamic monitoring of patients with circulatory shock recommends "that less invasive devices can be used, instead of more invasive devices, only when they have been validated in the context of patients with shock," resulting mostly in the use of methods based on thermodilution and pulse contour analysis [34].

15.5 Management of Hypotension

15.5.1 Goal-Directed Therapy of Intraoperative Hypotension

Since blood pressure and blood flow are indivisible parts of hemodynamic physiology, modern perioperative hemodynamic management relies not only on blood pressure management but also on goal-directed therapy for blood flow (i.e., cardiac output) optimization. Based on the existing evidence, the current guideline of the European Society of Anesthesiology for the cardiovascular assessment and management of patients undergoing noncardiac surgery recommends goal-directed therapy in patients with high cardiac and surgical risk [28]. The benefit of individualized goal-directed therapy compared to standard blood pressure management on outcome variables such as AKI, myocardial injury after noncardiac surgery, and mortality in patients undergoing major abdominal surgery was first shown by the INPRESS study [35]. To date, the INPRESS study remains the only randomized controlled trial to identify a causal relationship between intraoperative hypotension and postoperative organ failure. Goal-directed therapy predefines protocolized hemodynamic treatment goals targeting normal or supranormal levels of oxygen supply and is mainly based on optimization of fluid management and cardiac inotropy. Several different treatment algorithms have been evaluated and shown beneficial effects on patients' perioperative outcomes after noncardiac surgery. Nevertheless, several meta-analyses show conflicting results caused by a high heterogeneity in investigated patient cohorts, types of monitoring, targeted hemodynamic variables, surgical procedures, and overall low risk of bias [36]. In particular, the development of hemodynamic goals might have influenced the results of the meta-analyses because their targets shifted, for example, from supranormal to normal cardiac output.

The Optimisation of Cardiovascular Management to Improve Surgical Outcome (OPTIMISE) trial investigated the value of individualized cardiac output-guided goal-directed therapy in which stroke volume was optimized by fluid challenges and a continuous infusion of dopexamine [37]. Surprisingly, this trial did not show a decrease in mortality in the goal-directed therapy group and demonstrated unwittingly the limits of individualization. Due to the exploitation of the cardiac preload reserve and a fixed infusion of dopexamine, the patients were brought to their individual hemodynamic maximum, rather than to an individualized optimization [29]. Furthermore, the incidence of intraoperative hypotension still remains high, which can be explained by the design of the goal-directed therapy algorithms. Regarding the physiologic goal of maintaining organ perfusion, most goal-directed therapy protocols concentrate on blood flow (in terms of cardiac output) rather than on blood pressure, resulting in a regular occurrence of intraoperative hypotension.

Since intraoperative hypotension is significantly associated with adverse postoperative outcomes, this might influence the results of meta-analyses that investigate the postoperative outcomes following goal-directed therapy. Finally, the timing of goal-directed therapy seems to be crucial for its impact because its positive effect is caused by the prevention and not the treatment of postoperative complications [38].

Overall, the majority of meta-analyses support the beneficial effect of goal-directed therapy in terms of a decrease in postsurgical complications, but less in mortality. In summary, goal-directed therapy represents an effective approach to decrease postoperative morbidity. However, goal-directed therapy has to overcome the conflict of individualized treatment goals on the one hand and protocolized hemodynamic therapy on the other. Therefore, further studies have to identify multimodal treatment algorithms that can reflect the needs of the individual patient.

15.5.2 Goal-Directed Therapy in the Intensive Care Unit

In 2001, River et al. introduced a widely recognized goal-directed therapy protocol for the treatment of patients with septic shock [39]. Even though current studies doubt the effect of this specific protocol, many other goal-directed therapy algorithms have been introduced since then. Analogous to the evolution of perioperative goal-directed therapy, evidence points to an individualized early goal-directed therapy protocol. For example, early treatment algorithms aimed at supranormal targets for oxygen delivery with consecutive elevation of cardiac output in critically ill patients. Because in the early phase septic shock is also associated with hyperdynamic hemodynamics, this approach seems questionable. Then again, septic shock depends crucially on fast, protocolized care that should be initiated as early as possible. Therefore, individualized goal-directed therapy protocols have been proposed for the treatment of the critically ill patient. By contrast, the recently published PRISM meta-analysis showed no beneficial effect of early goal-directed therapy compared to standard therapy in septic shock patients, which was mainly explained with the results of the Protocolized Care for Early Septic Shock (ProCESS), Australasian Resuscitation in Sepsis Evaluation (ARISE), and Protocolised Management in Sepsis (ProMISe) trials [40]. These opposing results are largely explainable with the advances in the early phase of septic shock therapy since the study by Rivers et al. [38]. For example, prior to randomization, study patients had already received 2000–2500 ml of fluid, leading to a lower mortality also in the standard care group compared to the study by Rivers et al. As a result of these findings, the authors postulated that the effect of goal-directed therapy after initial resuscitation was limited and should be carefully evaluated [40]. These findings highlight the importance of early initiation of goal-directed therapy in septic shock patients.

Although the majority of goal-directed therapy studies in critically ill patients include septic patients, some conclusions can be generalized. Especially in severely ill medical patients, early goal-directed therapy protocols may lead to adverse outcomes caused by conflicting disease conditions (e.g., positive signs of volume responsiveness vs. pulmonary edema) that have to be treated using advanced hemodynamic therapy [41]. Therefore, modern hemodynamic management based on goal-directed therapy should target the individual needs in terms of peripheral perfusion and blood pressure, indicating a careful evaluation of fluid responsiveness, general volume status, vasoplegia, and cardiac function.

15.5.3 New Concepts of Goal-Directed Therapy of Intraoperative Hypotension

Hemodynamic algorithms based on the dynamic arterial elastance (Ea_{dyn}), defined as pulse pressure variation divided by stroke volume variation (SVV), are exemplary for modern goal-directed therapy approaches. The Ea_{dyn} does not represent the arterial elastance but rather describes the interaction between pulse pressure and stroke volume over a respiratory cycle. Therefore, it can be used to predict if a patient will increase his/her blood pressure after administration of a fluid bolus. Monge García et al. showed that patients with an $Ea_{dyn} > 0.89$ increased their MAP by more than 15% after a fluid challenge [42]. However, it must be emphasized that in order to use Ea_{dyn} correctly, the patients have to be fluid responsive (SVV >12%). Furthermore, it should not be evaluated without taking the patient's cardiac output into account since it has to be considered as a ventriculo-arterial coupling index that is influenced by vascular and cardiac factors. Overall, Ea_{dyn} can assist in decisions regarding whether a patient needs fluids or vasopressors to overcome hypotension.

By quantifying the peak derivative of left ventricular pressure (LV dP/dt_{max}), another innovative target for treating hypotension has been introduced. LV dP/dt_{max} can be assessed by arterial pulse wave analysis and offers information about cardiac contractility. It has been evaluated thoroughly and has shown good correlation with end-systolic elastance, but it has some limitations [43]. First, it is highly dependent on a solid pulse wave signal. Second, since no normal values are available as a reference, trend values rather than absolute parameters should be used. Finally, it can be affected by other conditions, such as aortic stenosis [44]. However, with respect to the known limitations, the combination of Ea_{dyn} and LV dP/dt_{max} enables an advanced evaluation of the patient's hemodynamic situation, with only one arterial line. For example, a hypotensive patient showing no decrease in LV dP/dt_{max} over time and only a low Ea_{dyn} will most likely need vasopressors. Figure 15.1 shows an example of a goal-directed therapy algorithm based on Ea_{dyn} and LV dP/dt_{max}.

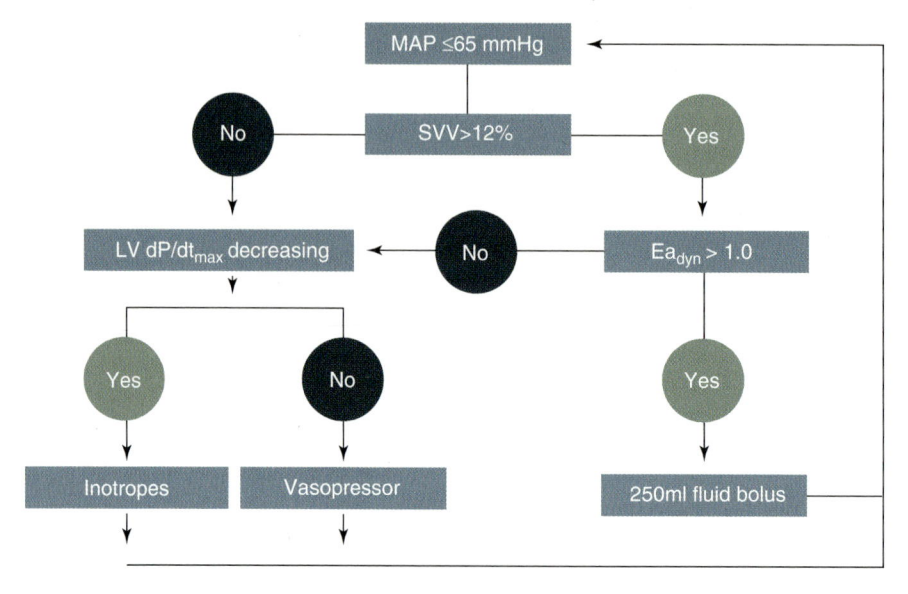

Fig. 15.1 Goal-directed therapy flowchart based on the derivative of left ventricular pressure (LV dP/dt_{max}) and dynamic arterial elastance (Ea$_{dyn}$). *MAP* mean arterial pressure, *SVV* stroke volume variation

15.6 Current Innovation and Future Directions

Current innovations in hemodynamic monitoring have identified potential fields for further development. First, problems in the accuracy of noninvasive monitoring devices have been identified and will be addressed in the future. This may lead to monitoring options beyond the operating room and ICU via an automated connection to the patient's smart devices (e.g., mobile phone, tablet, laptop computer) on the general ward or even at home. This may strengthen the field of baseline blood pressure quantification for the assessment of preoperative blood pressure and influence the development of a relative blood pressure definition of hypotension. Second, since it will be hard (maybe even impossible) to realize a perfect individualized goal-directed therapy algorithm, multimodal algorithms might help to address patients' individual needs. Third, prediction of hypotension may offer new opportunities for the reduction of hypotensive episodes. Innovative methods such as the hypotension prediction index (HPI) are currently being evaluated and show promising results. First described by Hatib et al., the HPI was calculated retrospectively from the data of 25,461 episodes of intraoperative hypotension in 1334 patients and validated in 204 patients suffering from 1923 episodes of intraoperative hypotension [45]. HPI enables prediction of hypotensive events up to 15 min before their occurrence in patients having surgical procedures under general anesthesia and was superior to standard hemodynamic parameters (e.g., MAP or dynamic preload parameters) [46]. Current studies have confirmed the predictive value of HPI, and results from the authors' own studies have shown that combined with a treatment protocol, HPI was able to reduce the number and duration of intraoperative hypotensive episodes (data not yet published).

15.7 Conclusion

Hypotension remains a common problem in the operating room as well as in the ICU and is associated with adverse outcomes. The use of different definitions of hypotension complicates its diagnosis, but both absolute and relative thresholds can be used. Available recommendations emphasize an individual approach of setting thresholds for hypotension in each patient. Use of goal-directed therapy can reduce adverse outcomes in surgical patients and also in those who are critically ill, if started early. Goal-directed treatment protocols should be individualized to each patient's condition and include blood flow and pressure targets.

References

1. Bijker JB, van Klei WA, Kappen TH, van Wolfswinkel L, Moons KGM, Kalkman CJ. Incidence of intraoperative hypotension as a function of the chosen definition: literature definitions applied to a retrospective cohort using automated data collection. Anesthesiology. 2007;107:213–20.
2. Wesselink EM, Kappen TH, Torn HM, Slooter AJC, van Klei WA. Intraoperative hypotension and the risk of postoperative adverse outcomes: a systematic review. Br J Anaesth. 2018;121:706–21.
3. Salmasi V, Maheshwari K, Yang D, et al. Relationship between intraoperative hypotension, defined by either reduction from baseline or absolute thresholds, and acute kidney and myocardial injury after noncardiac surgery: a retrospective cohort analysis. Anesthesiology. 2017;126:47–65.
4. Devereaux PJ, Szczeklik W. Myocardial injury after non-cardiac surgery: diagnosis and management. Eur Heart J. 2019. https://doi.org/10.1093/eurheartj/ehz301 [Epub ahead of print].
5. Sun LY, Wijeysundera DN, Tait GA, Beattie WS. Association of intraoperative hypotension with acute kidney injury after elective noncardiac surgery. Anesthesiology. 2017;123:515–23.
6. Walsh M, Devereaux PJ, Garg AX, et al. Relationship between intraoperative mean arterial pressure and clinical outcomes after noncardiac surgery: toward an empirical definition of hypotension. Anesthesiology. 2013;119:507–15.
7. Ng JLW, Chan MTV, Gelb AW. Perioperative stroke in noncardiac, nonneurosurgical surgery. Anesthesiology. 2011;115:879–90.
8. Hsieh JK, Dalton JE, Yang D, Farag ES, Sessler DI, Kurz AM. The association between mild intraoperative hypotension and stroke in general surgery patients. Anesth Analg. 2016;123:933–9.
9. Scholz AFM, Oldroyd C, McCarthy K, Quinn TJ, Hewitt J. Systematic review and meta-analysis of risk factors for postoperative delirium among older patients undergoing gastrointestinal surgery. Br J Surg. 2016;103:e21–8.
10. Hirsch J, DePalma G, Tsai TT, Sands LP, Leung JM. Impact of intraoperative hypotension and blood pressure fluctuations on early postoperative delirium after non-cardiac surgery. Br J Anaesth. 2015;115:418–26.

11. Langer T, Santini A, Zadek F, et al. Intraoperative hypotension is not associated with postoperative cognitive dysfunction in elderly patients undergoing general anesthesia for surgery: results of a randomized controlled pilot trial. J Clin Anesth. 2019;52:111–8.
12. Monk TG, Bronsert MR, Henderson WG, et al. Association between intraoperative hypotension and hypertension and 30-day postoperative mortality in noncardiac surgery. Anesthesiology. 2015;123:307–19.
13. Monk TG, Saini V, Weldon BC, Sigl JC. Anesthetic management and one-year mortality after noncardiac surgery. Anesth Analg. 2005;100:4–10.
14. Kane-Gill SL, LeBlanc JM, Dasta JF, Devabhakthuni S. A multicenter study of the point prevalence of drug-induced hypotension in the ICU. Crit Care Med. 2014;42:2197–203.
15. Asfar P, Meziani F, Hamel JF, et al. High versus low blood-pressure target in patients with septic shock. N Engl J Med. 2014;370:1583–93.
16. Rhodes A, Evans LE, Alhazzani W, et al. Surviving sepsis campaign: international guidelines for management of sepsis and septic shock: 2016. Intensive Care Med. 2017;43:304–77.
17. Hasler RM, Nüesch E, Jüni P, Bouamra O, Exadaktylos AK, Lecky F. Systolic blood pressure below 110 mmHg is associated with increased mortality in penetrating major trauma patients: multicentre cohort study. Resuscitation. 2012;83:476–81.
18. Hasler RM, Nuesch E, Jüni P, Bouamra O, Exadaktylos AK, Lecky F. Systolic blood pressure below 110 mm Hg is associated with increased mortality in blunt major trauma patients: multicentre cohort study. Resuscitation. 2011;82:1202–7.
19. Smischney NJ, Demirci O, Diedrich DA, et al. Incidence of and risk factors for post-intubation hypotension in the critically ill. Med Sci Monit. 2016;22:346–55.
20. Silversides JA, Pinto R, Kuint R, et al. Fluid balance, intradialytic hypotension, and outcomes in critically ill patients undergoing renal replacement therapy: a cohort study. Crit Care. 2014;18:624.
21. Ard JL, Kendale S. Searching for baseline blood pressure: a comparison of blood pressure at three different care points. J Clin Neurosci. 2016;34:59–62.
22. Saugel B, Reese PC, Sessler DI, et al. Automated ambulatory blood pressure measurements and intraoperative hypotension in patients having noncardiac surgery with general anesthesia: a prospective observational study. Anesthesiology. 2019;131:74–83.
23. Sanders RD, Hughes F, Shaw A, et al. Perioperative quality initiative consensus statement on preoperative blood pressure, risk and outcomes for elective surgery. Br J Anaesth. 2019;122:552–62.
24. Izawa J, Kitamura T, Iwami T, et al. Early-phase cumulative hypotension duration and severe-stage progression in oliguric acute kidney injury with and without sepsis: an observational study. Crit Care. 2016;20:405.
25. Poukkanen M, Wilkman E, Vaara ST, et al. Hemodynamic variables and progression of acute kidney injury in critically ill patients with severe sepsis: data from the prospective observational FINNAKI study. Crit Care. 2013;17:R295.
26. Maheshwari K, Nathanson BH, Munson SH, et al. The relationship between ICU hypotension and in-hospital mortality and morbidity in septic patients. Intensive Care Med. 2018;44:857–67.
27. Vincent JL, Nielsen ND, Shapiro NI, et al. Mean arterial pressure and mortality in patients with distributive shock: a retrospective analysis of the MIMIC-III database. Ann Intensive Care. 2018;8:107.
28. Kristensen SD, Knuuti J, Saraste A, et al. 2014 ESC/ESA Guidelines on non-cardiac surgery: cardiovascular assessment and management: the Joint Task Force on non-cardiac surgery: cardiovascular assessment and management of the European Society of Cardiology (ESC) and the European Society of Anaesth. Eur Heart J. 2014;35:2383–431.
29. Saugel B, Vincent JL, Wagner JY. Personalized hemodynamic management. Curr Opin Crit Care. 2017;23:334–41.
30. Meidert AS, Nold JS, Hornung R, Paulus AC, Zwißler B, Czerner S. The impact of continuous non-invasive arterial blood pressure monitoring on blood pressure stability during general anaesthesia in orthopaedic patients: a randomised trial. Eur J Anaesthesiol. 2017;34:716–22.

31. Maheshwari K, Khanna S, Bajracharya GR, et al. A randomized trial of continuous noninvasive blood pressure monitoring during noncardiac surgery. Anesth Analg. 2018;127:424–31.
32. Rogge DE, Nicklas JY, Haas SA, Reuter DA, Saugel B. Continuous noninvasive arterial pressure monitoring using the vascular unloading technique (CNAP system) in obese patients during laparoscopic bariatric operations. Anesth Analg. 2018;126:454–63.
33. Kim S-H, Lilot M. Accuracy and precision of continuous noninvasive arterial pressure monitoring compared with invasive arterial pressure. Anesthesiology. 2014;120:1080–97.
34. Cecconi M, De Backer D, Antonelli M, et al. Consensus on circulatory shock and hemodynamic monitoring. Task force of the European Society of Intensive Care Medicine. Intensive Care Med. 2014;40:1795–815.
35. Futier E, Lefrant J-Y, Guinot P-G, et al. Effect of individualized vs. standard blood pressure management strategies on postoperative organ dysfunction among high-risk patients undergoing major surgery: a randomized clinical trial. JAMA. 2017;318:1346–57.
36. Kaufmann T, Clement RP, Scheeren TWL, Saugel B, Keus F, van der Horst ICC. Perioperative goal-directed therapy: a systematic review without meta-analysis. Acta Anaesthesiol Scand. 2018;62:1340–55.
37. Gillies MA, Shah ASV, Mullenheim J, et al. Perioperative myocardial injury in patients receiving cardiac output-guided haemodynamic therapy: a substudy of the OPTIMISE Trial. Br J Anaesth. 2015;115:227–33.
38. Saugel B, Michard F, Scheeren TWL. Goal-directed therapy: hit early and personalize! J Clin Monit Comput. 2018;32:375–7.
39. Rivers E, Nguyen B, Havstad S, et al. Early goal-directed therapy in the treatment of severe sepsis and septic shock. N Engl J Med. 2001;345:1368–77.
40. Rowan KM, Angus DC, Bailey M, et al. Early, goal-directed therapy for septic shock—a patient-level meta-analysis. N Engl J Med. 2017;376:2223–34.
41. Kalil AC, Kellum JA. Is early goal-directed therapy harmful to patients with sepsis and high disease severity? Crit Care Med. 2017;45:1265–7.
42. Monge García MI, Gil Cano A, Gracia Romero M. Dynamic arterial elastance to predict arterial pressure response to volume loading in preload-dependent patients. Crit Care. 2011;15:R15.
43. Morimont P, Lambermont B, Desaive T, Janssen N, Chase G, D'Orio V. Arterial dP/dtmax accurately reflects left ventricular contractility during shock when adequate vascular filling is achieved. BMC Cardiovasc Disord. 2012;12:13.
44. Vaquer S, Chemla D, Teboul JL, et al. Influence of changes in ventricular systolic function and loading conditions on pulse contour analysis-derived femoral dP/dtmax. Ann Intensive Care. 2010;9:61.
45. Hatib F, Jian Z, Buddi S, et al. Machine-learning algorithm to predict hypotension based on high-fidelity arterial pressure waveform analysis. Anesthesiology. 2018;129:663–74.
46. Davies SJ, Vistisen ST, Jian Z, Hatib F, Scheeren TWL. Ability of an arterial waveform analysis-derived hypotension prediction index to predict future hypotensive events in surgical patients. Anesth Analg. 2020;130:352–59.
47. Van Waes JAR, Van Klei WA, Wijeysundera DN, Van Wolfswinkel L, Lindsay TF, Beattie WS. Association between intraoperative hypotension and myocardial injury after vascular surgery. Anesthesiology. 2016;124:35–44.
48. Bijker JB, Persoon S, Peelen LM, et al. Intraoperative hypotension and perioperative ischemic stroke after general surgery: a nested case-control study. Anesthesiology. 2012;116:658–64.

Heterogeneity of Cardiovascular Response to Standardized Sepsis Resuscitation

F. Guarracino, P. Bertini, and M. R. Pinsky

16.1 Introduction

The Surviving Sepsis Campaign (SSC) guidelines [1] recommend a hemodynamic optimization strategy to rapidly counteract the impact of sepsis on blood flow in the first few hours after diagnosis. Specifically, the SSC guidelines suggest promptly restoring and ameliorating circulatory shock using early and aggressive volume expansion with crystalloids (30 ml/kg) to achieve a mean arterial pressure (MAP) of at least 65 mmHg. If this initial volume expansion fails to restore MAP, then clinicians are allowed to use vasopressor agents and subsequently inotropic support to achieve this goal. This standardized and mono-dimensional approach to cardiovascular stabilization flies in the face of numerous clinical observations. For example, a large database analysis of patients with septic shock ($n = 3686$) consistently reported that only two-thirds of patients were volume responders [2]. Patients not responding to volume expansion may experience fluid overload, which is in and of itself an independent risk factor for prolonged hospitalization, death, and poor outcome as previously described [3].

16.2 Physiologic Rationale for Resuscitation

The physiologic rationale for initial volume resuscitation in the septic hypotensive patient is not straightforward, although fluid resuscitation is often effective in restoring MAP. The only thing that volume expansion can do is increase circulating blood volume and, by inference, mean systemic pressure (P_{ms}), which is the upstream pressure driving venous return. P_{ms} is a function of the relation between stressed blood volume and vascular compliance. Total blood volume is distributed across the vascular space into volume that does not increase P_{ms}, referred to as unstressed volume, and volume that does cause P_{ms} to increase. Under normal resting conditions, approximately 60–70% of the total circulating blood volume is unstressed volume with a majority of that volume in the splanchnic circulation. Increasing sympathetic tone and exercise decrease splanchnic blood flow distributing more of the blood volume to vascular spaces with lower unstressed volume, thereby increasing P_{ms}. Furthermore, for the associated increase in P_{ms} to increase cardiac output, the right ventricle needs to be volume responsive as manifest by an associated increase in the right atrial pressure to P_{ms} gradient, because venous return can only increase if this gradient increases, the resistance to venous return decreases, or both occur. Finally, in a fluid-responsive septic patient, for MAP to also increase in parallel to the increase in cardiac output, the arterial vasomotor tone must be sufficient to realize an associated increase in pressure to follow the increase in flow. What is unclear is how these processes play out in individual patients presenting with hypotensive sepsis.

Coupled with the effects of sepsis on the systemic circulation is the interaction between left ventricular (LV) pump function and its arterial load, referred to as ventriculoarterial coupling. Ventriculoarterial coupling is characterized by the relation between LV elastance (E_{es}), the primary parameter defining LV contractility, and effective arterial elastance (E_a), a clinical surrogate of LV afterload [4]. The determinants of these LV performance parameters are summarized in Fig. 16.1.

16.3 Clinical Observations

We recently demonstrated in a cohort of 55 septic hypotensive patients that a majority reversed their hypotension in response to volume expansion alone [5]. Since septic shock is defined as hypotension not responsive to volume expansion alone, most patients in our cohort had sepsis but not septic shock. Analyzing the physiologic determinants further, we found that most septic shock patients with hypotension despite volume expansion, owing to loss of arterial tone (i.e., vasoplegia), also displayed significant alterations in ventriculoarterial coupling. The majority of our septic shock patients displayed significant ventriculoarterial uncoupling, with E_a markedly greater than E_{es}. Ventriculoarterial uncoupling markedly decreases LV ejection efficiency and can independently lead to heart failure [4].

In our recent observational study [5] on the effect of therapies on the determinants of cardiovascular status as recommended by the SSC guidelines, we confirmed the efficacy of volume expansion but the results cast light on the lack of

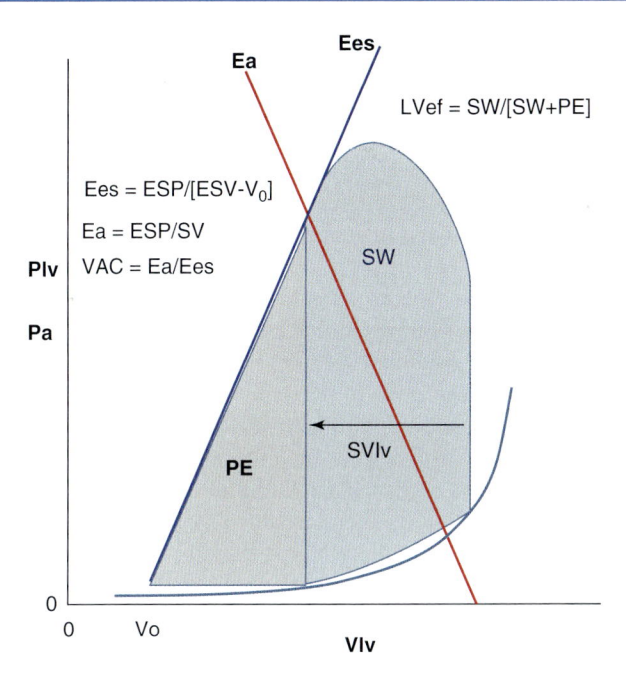

Fig. 16.1 A stylized representation of the relation between left ventricular (LV) pressure (P_{lv}) or arterial pressure (P_a) and LV pressure-volume relations during a cardiac cycle and arterial elastance (E_a) (red line) along with the associated formulae defining end-systolic elastance (E_{es}) (blue line) and E_a. Stroke work (SW) is the area within the LV pressure-volume loop for one cardiac cycle, while the potential energy (PE) is the area sub-served by the E_a and LV end-systolic volume (ESV). LV efficiency (LVef) is the ratio of SW to SW + PE (Reproduced from [5] under a Creative Commons Attribution 4.0 International License)

knowledge about timing and appropriate sequence of hemodynamic resuscitation following volume expansion and vasoactive and inotropic agents. In patients with elevated baseline E_a for example, poor hemodynamic performance was seen after treatment with norepinephrine with less improvement in MAP or cardiac output [5].

In summary, these findings collectively underscore the heterogeneity of cardiovascular responses to a SSC guideline-defined resuscitation protocol in septic patients owing to similarly heterogeneous pathophysiologic states.

In most of our patients, volume expansion was able to restore MAP to >65 mmHg by also increasing cardiac output, E_{es} and P_{ms}, leading to improved energy transfer measurements, such as LV ejection efficiency, ventriculoarterial coupling, and heart efficiency. Interestingly, we documented that volume expansion also increased E_{es}. E_{es} is considered a load-independent measurement of LV contractility. Our observed increase in E_{es} was probably due to the restoration of coronary perfusion pressure demonstrated by MAP increase.

Importantly, we found that individual patient MAP and cardiac output responses to volume expansion were variable, but accurately predicted by baseline pulse pressure variation (PPV), stroke volume variation (SVV) and their ratio, and dynamic elastance (Ea$_{dyn}$), suggesting that fluid resuscitation based on these dynamic measures may be more efficient by resulting in less fluid being given to nonresponders [5]. This is also consistent with prior findings that PPV predicts cardiac output responses to volume expansion in septic patients [6] and that Ea$_{dyn}$ predicted the associated change in MAP in response to changing cardiac output [7]. These data also support the clinical relevance of using functional dynamic measurements to tailor fluid administration in septic patients as recommended by the SSC guidelines [1].

Several studies describe a variable response to norepinephrine in septic shock [8]. In our investigation [5], norepinephrine increased E_a and MAP in most patients but did not achieve a MAP >65 mmHg in the majority and induced ventriculoarterial uncoupling to levels seen prior to resuscitation; it also decreased LV ejection efficiency, which, if sustained, might impair LV performance. These data support the recent observation that sustained use of vasopressors for >6 h in septic shock to maintain a MAP >75 mmHg is associated with increased mortality [9]. Recently, it has been shown in animal studies that norepinephrine can impair LV ejection by increasing the magnitude of arterial pressure reflected waves during ejection, which also becomes manifest as ventriculoarterial uncoupling without increasing coronary perfusion pressure [10]. As was also seen in patients with postoperative vasoplegia [11], we observed that only patients with higher E_{es} and normalized ventriculoarterial coupling increased cardiac output during norepinephrine infusion, presumably because they can tolerate the increased afterload [5].

When dobutamine was added to volume expansion and norepinephrine in a few patients, it restored normal ventriculoarterial coupling and cardiac output, suggesting that inotropic support may improve contractility in septic patients who may be affected by septic cardiomyopathy [12]. These findings have also been reported by others [4, 11, 13]. Analyzing these norepinephrine- and dobutamine-dependent subsets in future investigations may improve our understanding of how vasoactive and inotropic therapies change hemodynamics [8].

16.4 Clinical Relevance

Potentially, the selection of the most appropriate treatment in septic shock patients following initial volume expansion could be ascertained by knowing their E_a, E_{es} and dynamic parameters, such as Ea$_{dyn}$. Similarly, volume expansion should be individualized based on dynamic measures of volume responsiveness.

We suggest that a prospective clinical trial could be conducted to address this specific approach. The criterion for patient recruitment would be the same as for previous investigations, i.e., sepsis with MAP <65 mmHg. Since an initial volume expansion step was beneficial in the majority of patients, it would be the initial treatment but given based on the functional dynamic parameters, PPV and SVV. In patients who do not achieve MAP >65 mmHg after volume expansion, E_a would be measured. If E_a were <2 mmHg/ml, patients would receive norepinephrine aimed at achieving a MAP >65 mmHg. If E_a were ≥2 mmHg/ml, patients would be randomly

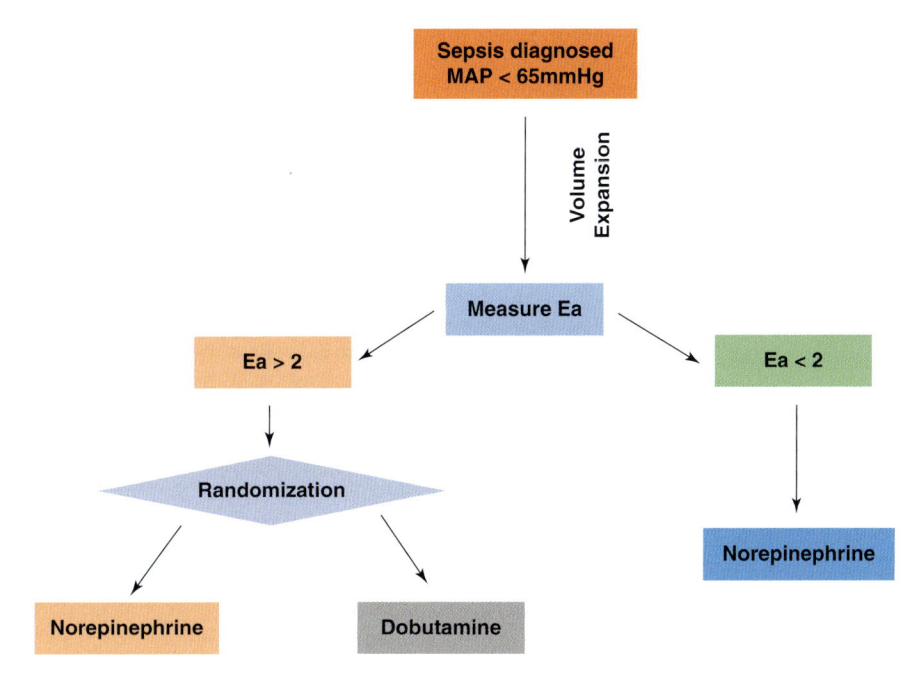

Fig. 16.2 A proposed treatment algorithm to personalize resuscitation in septic patients. E_a arterial elastance

allocated to either norepinephrine or dobutamine (Fig. 16.2) in order to verify the beneficial effect of an early inotropic strategy versus a vasoconstrictive one.

16.5 Conclusion

The determinants of the cardiovascular state collectively called sepsis and septic shock are complex and heterogeneous. The response to resuscitation is also heterogeneous, and thus treatment needs to be individualized to maximize timeliness of appropriate therapies while avoiding volume overload. Prospective clinical trials will help illuminate the optimal strategies, but the principle of individualizing treatment is already valid.

References

1. Rhodes A, Evans LE, Alhazzani W, et al. Surviving sepsis campaign: international guidelines for management of sepsis and septic shock: 2016. Intensive Care Med. 2017;43:304–77.
2. Leisman DE, Doerfler ME, Schneider SM, Masick KD, D'Amore JA, D'Angelo JK. Predictors, prevalence, and outcomes of early crystalloid responsiveness among initially hypotensive patients with sepsis and septic shock. Crit Care Med. 2018;46:189–98.
3. Payen D, de Pont AC, Sakr Y, et al. A positive fluid balance is associated with a worse outcome in patients with acute renal failure. Crit Care. 2008;12:R74.

4. Guarracino F, Ferro B, Morelli A, Bertini P, Baldassarri R, Pinsky MR. Ventriculoarterial decoupling in human septic shock. Crit Care. 2014;18:R80.
5. Guarracino F, Bertini P, Pinsky MR. Cardiovascular determinants of resuscitation from sepsis and septic shock. Crit Care. 2019;23:118.
6. Michard F, Boussat S, Chemla D, et al. Relation between respiratory changes in arterial pulse pressure and fluid responsiveness in septic patients with acute circulatory failure. Am J Respir Crit Care Med. 2000;162:134–8.
7. Monge Garcia MI, Gil Cano A, Gracia Romero M. Dynamic arterial elastance to predict arterial pressure response to volume loading in preload-dependent patients. Crit Care. 2011;15:R15.
8. Levy B, Fritz C, Tahon E, Jacquot A, Auchet T, Kimmoun A. Vasoplegia treatments: the past, the present, and the future. Crit Care. 2018;22:52.
9. Lamontagne F, Day AG, Meade MO, et al. Pooled analysis of higher versus lower blood pressure targets for vasopressor therapy septic and vasodilatory shock. Intensive Care Med. 2018;44:12–21.
10. Monge Garcia MI, Jian Z, Settels JJ, et al. Performance comparison of ventricular and arterial dP/dtmax for assessing left ventricular systolic function during different experimental loading and contractile conditions. Crit Care. 2018;22:325.
11. Guinot PG, Longrois D, Kamel S, Lorne E, Dupont H. Ventriculo-arterial coupling analysis predicts the hemodynamic response to norepinephrine in hypotensive postoperative patients: a prospective observational study. Crit Care Med. 2018;46:e17–25.
12. Rudiger A, Singer M. Mechanisms of sepsis-induced cardiac dysfunction. Crit Care Med. 2007;35:1599–608.
13. Burkhoff D. Pressure-volume loops in clinical research: a contemporary view. J Am Coll Cardiol. 2013;62:1173–6.

Part VI

The Microcirculation

Clinical Relevance of the Endothelial Glycocalyx in Critically Ill Patients

17

D. Astapenko, J. Benes, and V. Cerny

17.1 Introduction

The endothelial glycocalyx has been a subject of extensive experimental and clinical research during the last two decades in several areas of human medicine. Injury to the endothelial glycocalyx plays an important role in the pathophysiology of various acute and chronic conditions. Current evidence on the important role of the endothelial glycocalyx in human health supports the concept of considering the endothelial glycocalyx as a possible therapeutic target in terms of protective modulation of its structure for repair and function restoration as one of the basic conditions for reversal of organ dysfunction or disease. In this chapter, we present an overview of current evidence related to the endothelial glycocalyx and management of critically ill patients.

D. Astapenko
Department of Anaesthesiology and Intensive Care, University Hospital Hradec Kralove, Hradec Kralove, The Czech Republic

Faculty of Medicine in Hradec Kralove, Charles University, Hradec Kralove, The Czech Republic

J. Benes
Department of Anesthesiology and Intensive Care Medicine, University Hospital Plzen, Plzen, The Czech Republic

Faculty of Medicine in Plzen, Charles University, Plzen, The Czech Republic

V. Cerny (✉)
Department of Anaesthesiology and Intensive Care, University Hospital Hradec Kralove, Hradec Kralove, The Czech Republic

Department of Anaesthesiology, Perioperative Medicine and Intensive Care, J.E. Purkinje University, Masaryk Hospital, Usti nad Labem, The Czech Republic
e-mail: vladimir.cerny@kzcr.eu

17.2 Critical Conditions Associated with Injury to the Endothelial Glycocalyx

The endothelial glycocalyx is a fragile structure because of its sugary nature. Critical illness has a significant impact on the endothelial glycocalyx [1]. Damage to the endothelial glycocalyx is linked to dysfunction of the microcirculation [2]: increased filtration, interstitial edema formation, impaired nitric oxide production, coagulopathy, oxidative stress, and loss of immunity surveillance. Sepsis is tightly linked to endothelial glycocalyx damage [3], representing a condition where three factors meet (bacterial enzymes, dysregulated host response, and iatrogenic hypervolemia and hypernatremia due to the fluid resuscitation). Major trauma and surgery induce degradation of the endothelial glycocalyx in several ways. The tissue damage releases markers triggering defense mechanisms and activation of immunity, such as damage-associated molecular patterns (DAMPs) [4]. These markers can degrade the endothelial glycocalyx by enzymatic reaction (mainly matrix metalloproteinases, hyaluronidase, and heparanase). The systemic inflammatory response syndrome ensues that further aggravates the endothelial glycocalyx condition. These changes establish the condition described as traumatic endotheliopathy [5]. Finally, the iatrogenic aspect of endothelial glycocalyx damage takes place as mentioned above. Ischemia–reperfusion syndrome brings uneven damage to the tissues due to the temporary shortage of nutrients and oxygen supply. The endothelial glycocalyx and the microcirculation play a key role in subsequent pathogenesis. Ischemia–reperfusion induces damage to the endothelium, separation from the basal membrane and oxidative stress. Ischemia–reperfusion syndrome is well described as the etiology of endothelial glycocalyx degradation after cardiopulmonary bypass (CPB) [6] as well as in patients after return of spontaneous circulation following cardiopulmonary resuscitation (CPR) [7].

17.3 The Rationale for the Concept of Endothelial Glycocalyx Protection and Repair in the Critically Ill

The endothelial glycocalyx is of utmost importance for the normal function of the microcirculation and its reactivity. The normal function of the endothelial glycocalyx can be maintained only when the balance between disintegration (shedding) and synthesis of its components and integration of its soluble plasma particles exists. The time needed to restore normal thickness of the endothelial glycocalyx was about 20 h in *in vitro* experiments of enzymatic degradation [8] but up to 7 days *in vivo* [9]. Conditions leading to endothelial glycocalyx shedding possibly play an important role in this observation and the presence (or absence) of several growth factors (for example fibroblast growth factor) or enzymes (heparan sulfate biosynthetic enzyme) could hasten or delay the complete recovery. However, the repair process of the endothelial glycocalyx and its determinants have not been clearly identified yet. Therefore, eliminating the cause and preventing further damage is still the cornerstone to restoring the endothelial glycocalyx once the shedding occurs. Moreover, none of the diagnostic possibilities is fast and routine enough to guide therapy. In routine everyday practice, we possibly encounter more patients

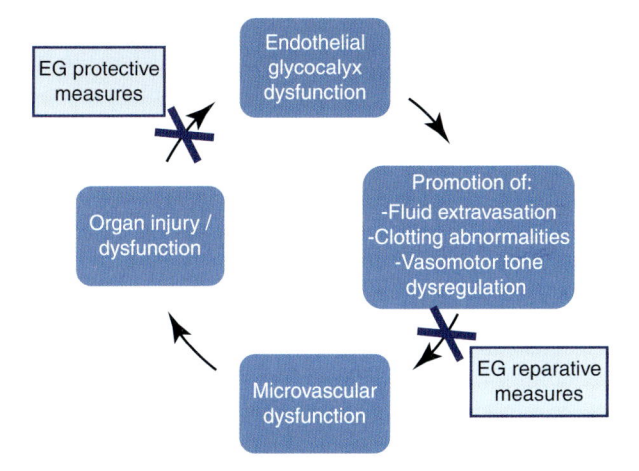

Fig. 17.1 Development of microvascular dysfunction into a vicious cycle and places for therapeutic intervention regarding the endothelial glycocalyx (EG)

with intact (or almost intact) endothelial glycocalyx who undergo different procedures and treatments starting with elective surgery and ending with patients recovering from severe conditions. Because several therapeutic measures (fluid therapy) or frequent conditions (hypertension, hyperglycemia, hypoperfusion) have the potential to induce or promote endothelial glycocalyx damage it is critical to decrease these influences to the absolute minimum (Fig. 17.1).

17.4 Effect of Common Therapeutic Interventions on the Endothelial Glycocalyx

17.4.1 Interventions/Conditions with a Possible Negative Impact

17.4.1.1 Fluid Therapy

Fluid therapy is a natural component of everyday therapy in patients. In critically ill patients and during perioperative care the risks of uncontrolled fluid loading have been demonstrated [10]. Fluid loading is mostly indicated to avoid hypoperfusion—a condition associated with an increase in catecholamine release and ischemia–reperfusion (both conditions negatively affecting the endothelial glycocalyx). Therefore, adequate fluid loading should lead to glycocalyx protection. However, the relationship between the endothelial glycocalyx and fluid therapy is not that straightforward. Under physiologic conditions, the endothelial glycocalyx plays a pivotal role in maintaining endothelium permeability. A revised Starling principle based on a high oncotic endothelial glycocalyx lining with an almost protein-pure sub-glycocalyx seems to be the major determinant of the extravascular fluid shift [11]. If the endothelial glycocalyx is disintegrated for any reason, the endothelial permeability for fluids but also oncotic substances (proteins, e.g., albumin) increases, leading to interstitial edema and promoting the vicious circle (Fig. 17.1). Contrarily, fluid administration itself may lead to damage of the endothelial glycocalyx. Several pathways seem to play a role. Acute hypervolemia leading to secretion of atrial natriuretic peptide (ANP) may be one of these—Chappell et al. demonstrated that ANP may promote endothelial glycocalyx shedding [12]. However, the ANP pathway is possibly not the only pathway—Belavić et al. observed a significant increase in endothelial glycocalyx degradation molecules without a concomitant increase in ANP [13]. Our group has observed an increase in perfused boundary region as monitored via intravital microscopy after fluid administration—a finding corresponding with thinning of the endothelial glycocalyx layer [14]. Interestingly, the effect seems not to be dependent on the reactivity of the systemic circulation (so-called fluid responsiveness) especially in septic patients, supporting the macro-microcirculatory incoherence [15]. Because the luminal part of the endothelial glycocalyx is less dense (sometimes called the endothelial surface layer) [16], acute dilution with crystalloids may change its conformation rather than destroy the endothelial glycocalyx layer as a whole. Rapid reconstitution of the perfused boundary region (within 60–120 min) may point towards this hypothesis (yet untested). The divergent impact of different fluid types on the endothelial glycocalyx may support our finding. Albumin, but not artificial colloids or crystalloids, maintained the endothelial glycocalyx in electron microscopic visualization [17]. Based on this information it seems that an endothelium parallel to the Bellamy "U" curve [18] does exist—limited amounts of fluid leading to hypoperfusion may derange the endothelial glycocalyx as well as fluid loading and/or hypervolemia (though transient); albumin solutions seem to have less impact than other fluids, but this needs to be supported by other evidence.

17.4.1.2 Derangements of Homeostasis

Only limited information exists regarding common derangements of homeostasis and their impact on the endothelial glycocalyx. Hypoperfusion leads to both endothelial glycocalyx damage and lactate production [19] but the causal relationship between lactic acidosis *per se* and endothelial glycocalyx shedding has never been tested. Hyperchloremic acidosis has been coupled with endothelial dysfunction corresponding with endothelial glycocalyx damage [20]. Infusion of hypertonic saline led to a transient increase in the perfused boundary region [21]. Because no difference was observed between groups after osmotherapy using normal (0.9%) and hypertonic (3.2%) saline in another animal study [22] (even though the serum chloride levels did differ significantly), it is questionable to which extent the endothelial glycocalyx changes are due to sodium or chloride levels. Effects of respiratory acidosis (for example in lung-protective ventilation and permissive hypercapnia) or alkalosis have not been studied so far.

17.4.1.3 Anesthesia and Sedation

Volatile anesthetics (especially sevoflurane) have been studied repeatedly for their plausible ischemic preconditioning and protective effect. In several animal studies, sevoflurane was associated with endothelial glycocalyx protection based on glycocalyx disruption molecules [23], leukocyte and platelet adhesion [24], and direct visualization of endothelial glycocalyx fluorescence [25]. By contrast, propofol infusion (even though at supratherapeutic levels) led to endothelial glycocalyx damage and increased permeability in a rat model [26]. However, a recent human study has demonstrated that the endothelial glycocalyx injury induced by lung resection was similar in sevoflurane and propofol anesthesia groups [27]. Moreover, our group has demonstrated that avoiding general anesthesia *per se* may improve the endothelial glycocalyx conditions in patients undergoing elective big joint arthroplasty [28].

17.4.1.4 Organ Support

Contact of the blood with artificial surfaces precipitates activation of the endothelium and endothelial glycocalyx shedding. Damage to the endothelial glycocalyx has been described in dialysis patients [29] although hemodialysis in end-stage kidney disease patients can help to regenerate erythrocyte glycocalyx [30]. In critically ill patients, it is hard to assess whether the hemodialysis or the critical condition itself is responsible for endothelial glycocalyx damage. Our research group has described a significantly increased perfused boundary region in patients admitted to the intensive care unit (ICU) requiring renal replacement therapy (RRT) [31]. We also described no effect of artificial ventilation on the perfused boundary region. Endothelial glycocalyx damage after extracorporeal membrane oxygenation (ECMO) has been well documented [32].

17.4.2 Interventions with a Possible Positive/Reparative Effect

17.4.2.1 Nutritional Support

There are already data on the influence of parenteral nutrition on the endothelial glycocalyx. Our research group has proved a positive impact of lipid infusion on the endothelial glycocalyx (decrease in markers of glycocalyx shedding and nonsignificant increase in the perfused boundary region) in postsurgical patients [33]. On the other hand, parenteral nutrition might produce hyperglycemia if inadequately monitored which has been repeatedly shown to be detrimental for the endothelial glycocalyx even in the short term [34].

17.4.2.2 Blood Products and Anticoagulants

Transfusion of whole blood and/or blood products (including fresh frozen plasma) seems to either help to restore or protect the endothelial glycocalyx during hemorrhage. Torres et al. demonstrated in a set of animal experiments that allogeneic blood products preserve the endothelial glycocalyx better than any other replacement solutions (including artificial colloids and albumin) [35]. Whether this effect is induced by some specific molecule (e.g., sphingosine-1-phosphate) [36] or by natural composition of plasma remains unclear. Use of solvent-detergent-treated frozen plasma was coupled with preserved endothelial glycocalyx, better endothelial function, and better clinical outcomes in the recent VIPER-OCTA trial including patients undergoing emergency thoracic aorta repair [37]. Antithrombin III is a natural component of the endothelial glycocalyx layer as well as other natural heparin-like components (heparin-sulfate, etc.). Pretreatment with antithrombin III reduced syndecan-1 levels in a Wistar rat experiment of endotoxin injury [38] and ischemia–reperfusion [39]. Unfractionated heparin was also demonstrated to be protective against sepsis-induced endothelial glycocalyx shedding [40]. Finally, a Japanese group has recently presented promising results with the use of recombinant thrombomodulin (unpublished data). However, no human studies have been reported so far on this topic. Sulodexide is a sulfurated glycosaminoglycan used as an antithrombotic and endothelium-protective agent in patients with microvascular endotheliopathies. Its positive effect on endothelial glycocalyx repair has recently been demonstrated in patients with diabetes mellitus [41].

17.4.2.3 Corticosteroids

Corticosteroids are extremely potent drugs with multiple immunomodulating properties. Naturally, their effect on the endothelial glycocalyx has been studied. Pretreatment with hydrocortisone prevented endothelial glycocalyx damage in animal experiments of ischemia–reperfusion [42] and models of cardiac arrest [43]. A reduction in metalloproteinase expression and thus its degradative activity on the endothelial glycocalyx was observed in another animal sepsis study using dexamethasone [44]. Whether (and to which extent) the positive results of human studies using corticosteroids in sepsis are partially due to modulation of endothelial glycocalyx injury and repair is unknown.

17.4.2.4 Commonly Used Medications

Antidiabetic Drugs

Vascular injury in diabetic patients is one of the conditions promoting end-organ injury. Damage to the endothelial glycocalyx has been postulated as one of the driving mechanisms. Similarly, dysfunction of the endothelial glycocalyx is probably the first step of arteriosclerotic plate genesis. Only sparse evidence exists about commonly used drugs and even less is known about their use and/or discontinuation in the critically ill. Metformin seems to have some endothelial glycocalyx reparative potential in addition to its antidiabetic effects [45] in animals; human studies are so far lacking.

Statins

The beneficial effect of statins on the endothelial glycocalyx is plausible due to their reduction of reactive oxygen species (and oxidized lipopolysaccharides) [46]. However, their influence on the endothelial glycocalyx has been neglected so far. Only one study observed a positive effect of short-term statin use in patients with familial hypercholesterolemia [47].

Low-Molecular-Weight Heparin

Low-molecular-weight heparin is a cornerstone in deep venous thrombosis prophylaxis in critically ill patients. It is a potential building block of the endothelial glycocalyx to be used for recovery or to stabilize the structure and prevent further glycocalyx shedding [48].

Antimicrobial Therapy

Antimicrobial therapy usually plays a pivotal role in medication in critically ill patients. Antibiotics target receptors within the bacterial glycocalyx, which is of

Table 17.1 Substances to protect or restore the endothelial glycocalyx

Drug/molecule	Patients/model	Effect
Albumin	Guinea pig heart	Decreased fluid extravasation
Low-molecular-weight heparin	Rat mesentery	Mitigation of glycan shedding
Antithrombin	Guinea pig heart	Decreased leukocyte adhesion
Hyaluronic acid and chondroitin sulfate	Hamster cremaster muscle	Reconstitution of the endothelial glycocalyx structure
Metformin	Mouse model of diabetes mellitus	Increased vascular clearance of dextran
Hydrocortisone	Guinea pig heart	Decreased oxidative stress and release of histamine
Methylprednisolone	Neonates undergoing heart surgery	Reduced endothelial glycocalyx shedding
Dexamethasone	Rat model of LPS sepsis	Inhibition of matrix metalloproteinase
Sulodexide	Patients with type II diabetes mellitus	Decreased transcapillary escape rate of albumin
Empagliflozin	*In vitro* model of endothelial glycocalyx in HAAECs	Restoration of endothelial glycocalyx after heparanase III incubation
Sphingosine-1-phosphate	Rat fat-pad endothelial cells	Suppression of metalloproteinase activity
Thrombomodulin	Model of LPS-induced sepsis in mice	Attenuated expression of interleukin-6

LPS lipopolysaccharide, *HAAECs* human abdominal aortic endothelial cells

similar structure to that of the human glycocalyx. Some antibiotics positively modulate the endothelial glycocalyx indirectly by inhibition of enzymatic digestion [49] or inhibition of neutrophil elastase [50]. The overall impact of antibiotics on the human endothelial glycocalyx remains elusive.

17.5 Conclusion

Critically ill patients represent a special population where endothelial glycocalyx damage occurs at a very early stage of their acute illness, likely attributed to the development of organ dysfunction and increased mortality. Involving the endothelial glycocalyx in the complex of mechanisms responsible for developing organ injury and organ dysfunction should become an inseparable part of our clinical thinking.

Protecting the endothelial glycocalyx could therefore be another plausible concept for intensive care medicine in the future. Currently, there is no established specific intervention to prevent endothelial glycocalyx injury despite the fact that several agents have shown promising effects (Table 17.1). The most effective measure to protect the endothelial glycocalyx from injury in clinical practice seems to be to avoid hypervolemia.

References

1. Cerny V, Astapenko D, Brettner F, et al. Targeting the endothelial glycocalyx in acute critical illness as a challenge for clinical and laboratory medicine. Crit Rev Clin Lab Sci. 2017;54:343–57.
2. Iba T, Levy JH. Derangement of the endothelial glycocalyx in sepsis. J Thromb Haemost. 2019;17:283–94.
3. Uchimido R, Schmidt EP, Shapiro NI. The glycocalyx: a novel diagnostic and therapeutic target in sepsis. Crit Care. 2019;23:16.
4. Rahbar E, Cardenas JC, Baimukanova G, et al. Endothelial glycocalyx shedding and vascular permeability in severely injured trauma patients. J Transl Med. 2015;13:117.
5. Johansson PI, Henriksen HH, Stensballe J, et al. Traumatic endotheliopathy: a prospective observational study of 424 severely injured patients. Ann Surg. 2017;265:597–603.
6. Bruegger D, Brettner F, Rossberg I, et al. Acute degradation of the endothelial glycocalyx in infants undergoing cardiac surgical procedures. Ann Thorac Surg. 2015;99:926–31.
7. Grundmann S, Fink K, Rabadzhieva L, et al. Perturbation of the endothelial glycocalyx in post cardiac arrest syndrome. Resuscitation. 2012;83:715–20.
8. Potter DR, Jiang J, Damiano ER. The recovery time course of the endothelial cell glycocalyx in vivo and its implications in vitro. Circ Res. 2009;104:1318–25.
9. Giantsos-Adams KM, Koo AJA, Song S, et al. Heparan sulfate regrowth profiles under laminar shear flow following enzymatic degradation. Cell Mol Bioeng. 2013;6:160–74.
10. Van Regenmortel N, Verbrugghe W, Roelant E, Van den Wyngaert T, Jorens PG. Maintenance fluid therapy and fluid creep impose more significant fluid, sodium, and chloride burdens than resuscitation fluids in critically ill patients: a retrospective study in a tertiary mixed ICU population. Intensive Care Med. 2018;44:409–17.
11. Levick JR, Michel CC. Microvascular fluid exchange and the revised Starling principle. Cardiovasc Res. 2010;87:198–210.
12. Chappell D, Bruegger D, Potzel J, et al. Hypervolemia increases release of atrial natriuretic peptide and shedding of the endothelial glycocalyx. Crit Care. 2014;18:538.
13. Belavić M, Sotošek Tokmadžić V, Fišić E, et al. The effect of various doses of infusion solutions on the endothelial glycocalyx layer in laparoscopic cholecystectomy patients. Minerva Anestesiol. 2018;84:1032–43.
14. Pouska J, Tegl V, Astapenko D, Cerny V, Lehmann C, Benes J. Impact of intravenous fluid challenge infusion time on macrocirculation and endothelial glycocalyx in surgical and critically ill patients. Biomed Res Int. 2018;2018:1–11.
15. Ince C. Hemodynamic coherence and the rationale for monitoring the microcirculation. Crit Care. 2015;19(Suppl 3):S8.
16. Reitsma S, Slaaf DW, Vink H, van Zandvoort MAMJ, oude Egbrink MGA. The endothelial glycocalyx: composition, functions, and visualization. Pflugers Arch. 2007;454:345–59.
17. Jacob M, Bruegger D, Rehm M, Welsch U, Conzen P, Becker BF. Contrasting effects of colloid and crystalloid resuscitation fluids on cardiac vascular permeability. Anesthesiology. 2006;104:1223–31.
18. Bellamy M. Wet, dry or something else? Br J Anaesth. 2006;97:755–7.
19. Annecke T, Fischer J, Hartmann H, et al. Shedding of the coronary endothelial glycocalyx: effects of hypoxia/reoxygenation vs ischaemia/reperfusion. Br J Anaesth. 2011;107:679–86.
20. Lira A, Pinsky MR. Choices in fluid type and volume during resuscitation: impact on patient outcomes. Ann Intensive Care. 2014;4:38.
21. Astapenko D, Dostalova V, Dostalova V, et al. Effect of acute hypernatremia induced by hypertonic saline administration on endothelial glycocalyx in rabbits. Clin Hemorheol Microcirc. 2019;72(1):107–16.
22. Dostalova V, Astapenko D, Dostalova V, et al. The effect of fluid loading and hypertonic saline solution on cortical cerebral microcirculation and glycocalyx integrity. J Neurosurg Anesthesiol. 2019;31:434–43.

23. Annecke T, Chappell D, Chen C, et al. Sevoflurane preserves the endothelial glycocalyx against ischaemia-reperfusion injury. Br J Anaesth. 2010;104:414–21.
24. Chappell D, Heindl B, Jacob M, et al. Sevoflurane reduces leukocyte and platelet adhesion after ischemia-reperfusion by protecting the endothelial glycocalyx. Anesthesiology. 2011;115:483–91.
25. Kazuma S, Tokinaga Y, Kimizuka M, Azumaguchi R, Hamada K, Yamakage M. Sevoflurane promotes regeneration of the endothelial glycocalyx by upregulating sialyltransferase. J Surg Res. 2019;241:40–7.
26. Lin MC, Lin CF, Li CF, Sun DP, Wang LY, Hsing CH. Anesthetic propofol overdose causes vascular hyperpermeability by reducing endothelial glycocalyx and ATP production. Int J Mol Sci. 2015;16:12092–107.
27. Kim HJ, Kim E, Baek SH, et al. Sevoflurane did not show better protective effect on endothelial glycocalyx layer compared to propofol during lung resection surgery with one lung ventilation. J Thorac Dis. 2018;10:1468–75.
28. Astapenko D, Pouska J, Benes J, et al. Neuraxial anesthesia is less harmful to the endothelial glycocalyx during elective joint surgery compared to general anesthesia. Clin Hemorheol Microcirc. 2018;72:11–21.
29. Cornelis T, Broers NJH, Titulaer DCLM, et al. Effects of ultrapure hemodialysis and low molecular weight heparin on the endothelial surface layer. Blood Purif. 2014;38:203–10.
30. Kliche K, Gerth U, Pavenstädt H, Oberleithner H. Recharging red blood cell surface by hemodialysis. Cell Physiol Biochem. 2015;35:1107–15.
31. Astapenko D, Dostál P, Černá Pařízková R, Roman Š, Černý V. Analysis of the sublingual microvascular glycocalyx in critically ill patients – a prospective observational study. Anest Intenziv Med. 2019;30:14–21.
32. Pesonen E, Passov A, Andersson S, et al. Glycocalyx degradation and inflammation in cardiac surgery. J Cardiothorac Vasc Anesth. 2019;33:341–5.
33. Astapenko D, Turek Z, Dostal P, et al. Effect of short-term administration of lipid emulsion on endothelial glycocalyx integrity in ICU patients – a microvascular and biochemical pilot study. Clin Hemorheol Microcirc. 2019;73:329–39.
34. Nieuwdorp M, van Haeften TW, Gouverneur MCLG, et al. Loss of endothelial glycocalyx during acute hyperglycemia coincides with endothelial dysfunction and coagulation activation in vivo. Diabetes. 2006;55:480–6.
35. Torres Filho IP, Torres LN, Salgado C, Dubick MA. Plasma syndecan-1 and heparan sulfate correlate with microvascular glycocalyx degradation in hemorrhaged rats after different resuscitation fluids. Am J Physiol Heart Circ Physiol. 2016;310:H1468–78.
36. Mensah SA, Cheng MJ, Homayoni H, Plouffe BD, Coury AJ, Ebong EE. Regeneration of glycocalyx by heparan sulfate and sphingosine 1-phosphate restores inter-endothelial communication. PLoS One. 2017;12:e0186116.
37. Stensballe J, Ulrich AG, Nilsson JC, et al. Resuscitation of endotheliopathy and bleeding in thoracic aortic dissections. Anesth Analg. 2018;127:920–7.
38. Iba T, Levy JH, Hirota T, et al. Protection of the endothelial glycocalyx by antithrombin in an endotoxin-induced rat model of sepsis. Thromb Res. 2018;171:1–6.
39. Chappell D, Jacob M, Hofmann-Kiefer K, et al. Antithrombin reduces shedding of the endothelial glycocalyx following ischaemia/reperfusion. Cardiovasc Res. 2009;83:388–96.
40. Yini S, Heng Z, Xin A, Xiaochun M. Effect of unfractionated heparin on endothelial glycocalyx in a septic shock model. Acta Anaesthesiol Scand. 2014;59:160–9.
41. Broekhuizen LN, Lemkes BA, Mooij HL, et al. Effect of sulodexide on endothelial glycocalyx and vascular permeability in patients with type 2 diabetes mellitus. Diabetologia. 2010;53:2646–55.
42. Cao RN, Tang L, Xia ZY, Xia R. Endothelial glycocalyx as a potential therapeutic target in organ injuries. Chin Med J. 2019;132:963–75.
43. Zhu J, Li X, Yin J, Hu Y, Gu Y, Pan S. Glycocalyx degradation leads to blood–brain barrier dysfunction and brain edema after asphyxia cardiac arrest in rats. J Cereb Blood Flow Metab. 2018;38:1979–92.

44. Cui N, Wang H, Long Y, Su L, Liu D. Dexamethasone suppressed LPS-induced matrix metalloproteinase and its effect on endothelial glycocalyx shedding. Mediat Inflamm. 2015;2015:1–8.
45. Eskens BJ, Zuurbier CJ, van Haare J, Vink H, van Teeffelen JW. Effects of two weeks of metformin treatment on whole-body glycocalyx barrier properties in db/db mice. Cardiovasc Diabetol. 2013;12:175.
46. Vink H, Constantinescu AA, Spaan JA. Oxidized lipoproteins degrade the endothelial surface layer: implications for platelet-endothelial cell adhesion. Circulation. 2000;101:1500–2.
47. Meuwese MC, Mooij HL, Nieuwdorp M, et al. Partial recovery of the endothelial glycocalyx upon rosuvastatin therapy in patients with heterozygous familial hypercholesterolemia. J Lipid Res. 2009;50:148–53.
48. Lipowsky HH, Lescanic A. Inhibition of inflammation induced shedding of the endothelial glycocalyx with low molecular weight heparin. Microvasc Res. 2017;112:72–8.
49. Lipowsky HH, Lescanic A. The effect of doxycycline on shedding of the glycocalyx due to reactive oxygen species. Microvasc Res. 2013;90:80–5.
50. Carden D, Xiao F, Moak C, Willis BH, Robinson-Jackson S, Alexander S. Neutrophil elastase promotes lung microvascular injury and proteolysis of endothelial cadherins. Am J Phys. 1998;275:H385–92.

Customized Monitoring of the Microcirculation in Patients with a Left Ventricular Assist Device

S. Akin, O. I. Soliman, and C. Ince

18.1 Introduction

Heart failure is a global pandemic affecting at least 26 million people worldwide and is increasing in prevalence. Despite significant advances in therapy and prevention, mortality and morbidity are still high and quality of life remains poor [1]. Alongside, there is increasing demand on heart failure-related healthcare costs from the outpatient clinic to intensive care unit (ICU) admissions due to a greater prevalence of heart failure in an ageing population.

Heart failure impacts perfusion in all organs and compromises central hemodynamics and consequently microvascular perfusion. Previous studies on microcirculation imaging have shown that alterations in the microcirculation have important prognostic value in patients with advanced heart failure (cardiogenic shock) as well as those receiving mechanical circulatory support [2, 3].

S. Akin (✉)
Department of Intensive Care, Haga Teaching Hospital, The Hague, The Netherlands

Department of Cardiology, Thoraxcenter, Unit of Advanced Heart Failure, Heart Transplantation & Mechanical Circulatory Support, Erasmus MC University Medical Centre Rotterdam, Rotterdam, The Netherlands
e-mail: s.akin@hagaziekenhuis.nl

O. I. Soliman
Department of Cardiology, College of Medicine, Nursing and Health Sciences, National University of Ireland Galway, Saolta University Healthcare Group, Galway, Ireland

C. Ince
Intensive Care, Erasmus MC University Medical Centre Rotterdam, Rotterdam, The Netherlands

Acute heart failure and acute decompensated chronic heart failure are increasingly treated using long-term mechanical circulatory support devices, viz. left ventricular assist devices (LVADs) (Fig. 18.1). Technological advances and widespread acceptance of LVADs have improved overall survival and reduced morbidity of patients awaiting or deemed ineligible for heart transplantation. Postoperative care of LVAD patients is typically associated with increased ICU admissions as well as durations of ICU stay. This is due to the characteristically high surgical risk of patients undergoing LVAD as well as the high rate of operative and device-related complications. Anticipation and handling of post-LVAD complications require hemodynamic monitoring as well as possibly adjustment of pump settings. Furthermore, more and more patients with advanced heart failure therapy are eligible for this therapy. Therefore, this new era in advanced heart failure treatment brings increasing needs for monitoring of end-organ function to optimize pump settings and consequently improve cardiac function under mechanical support. Furthermore, there is an unmet need for monitoring of patients with advanced heart failure receiving permanent mechanical circulatory support to detect end-organ perfusion alterations early and possibly avoid rehospitalization. In this chapter, we discuss optimal approaches to microcirculatory monitoring from the ICU to the outpatient clinic in patients with an LVAD.

Fig. 18.1 A left ventricular assist device (LVAD) is implanted in the chest and pumps blood from the left ventricular apex of the heart to the ascending aorta which helps blood flow to the rest of the body. A control unit and battery pack are worn outside the body and are connected to the LVAD through a port in the skin. (1) LVAD (pump), (2) batteries, (3) control unit

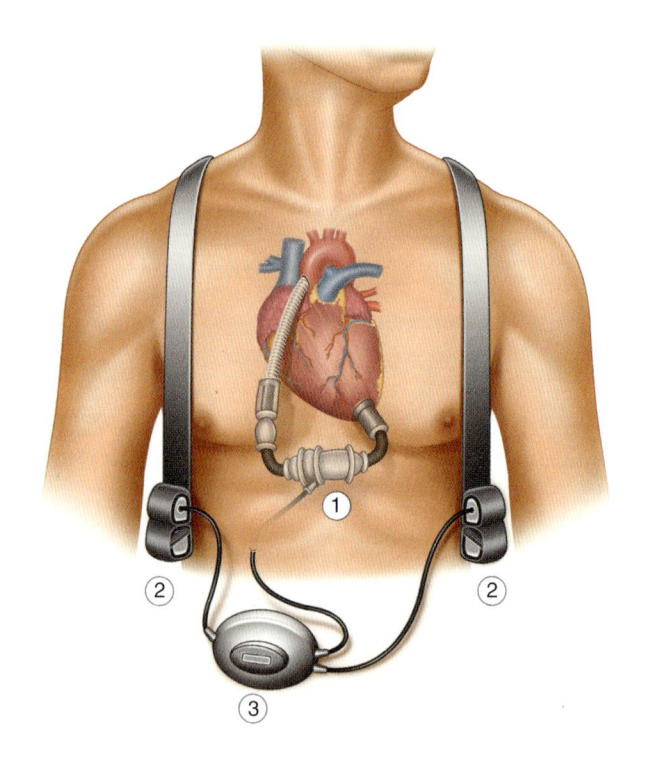

18.2 Microcirculatory Monitoring

The principles of microcirculatory monitoring go back to the early recognition of the clinical relevance of end-organ perfusion in disease states. Bedside microcirculation observation started gaining importance in the 1990s due to the introduction of handheld vital microscopes. Since then, this technology has been in continuous development and can be considered as a potential mainstay hemodynamic monitor to monitor the microcirculation at the bedside [4].

Orthogonal polarized spectral (OPS) and sidestream dark-field (SDF) video microscope imaging devices were introduced for observation of the microcirculation but, due to technical limitations, have remained as research tools. Recently, a novel handheld microscope based on incident dark-field illumination (IDF) has been introduced for clinical use. The Cytocam-IDF (Fig. 18.2) imaging device consists of a pen-like probe incorporating IDF illumination with a set of high-resolution lenses projecting images on to a computer-controlled image sensor synchronized with very short pulsed illumination light [5]. This IDF handheld vital microscope produces high-resolution images showing approximately 30% more capillaries than the previous-generation devices [6]. The hardware of this third-generation device meets the requirements for recently developed automated analysis able to produce functional microcirculatory parameters needed for quantitative identification of microcirculatory alterations in a point-of-care setting required for bedside clinical decision-making, and for optimizing therapy by targeting the normalization of microcirculatory alterations [7].

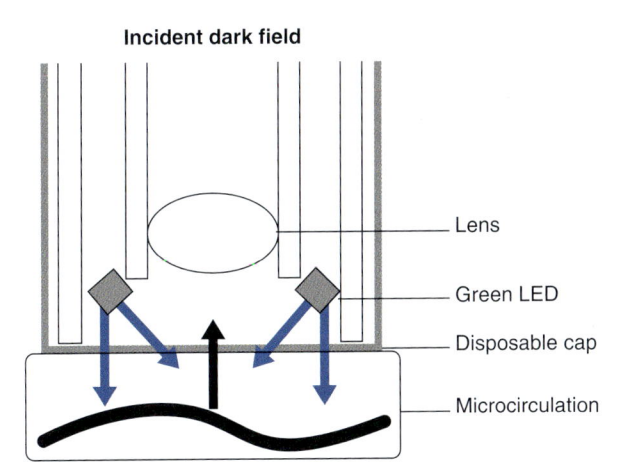

Fig. 18.2 The third-generation Cytocam incident dark-field (IDF) imaging device has a wider field of illumination, a specially designed magnification lens, and a computer-controlled high-resolution image sensor resulting in 30% more capillaries being observed than previous-generation handheld vital microscopy devices. *LED* light-emitting diodes (Adapted from [6] under a Creative Commons Attribution 4.0 International License)

Direct understanding of the functional condition of the microcirculation and interventions to improve tissue perfusion and oxygenation may improve clinical outcomes of the critically ill patients [8–10]. Direct monitoring of the microcirculation by handheld microscopy may provide a more physiological approach than solely monitoring the systemic circulation for clinicians to evaluate the efficacy of therapy and help to assess the presence (or absence) of hemodynamic coherence between the macrocirculation and microcirculation [9].

The clinical approach in critically ill patients is based on resuscitation procedures to correct global hemodynamics, involving the systemic circulation also referred to as the macrocirculation. For resuscitation to be effective there must be a coherent response between the macrocirculation and microcirculation if systemic hemodynamic-driven resuscitation procedures are to be effective in saving end-organ function by correcting tissue perfusion and oxygenation. However, in conditions of inflammation and infection, which often accompany states of shock, vascular regulation and compensatory mechanisms needed to sustain hemodynamic coherence are lost, and the regional circulation and microcirculation remain in shock. These microcirculatory alterations can be observed at the bedside using direct visualization of the sublingual microcirculation.

In early studies, loss of hemodynamic coherence was shown in different states of shock [11, 12]. In patients with mechanical circulatory support, who are missing pulsatility, it has been shown that recovery from shock can be rapidly detected by monitoring the microcirculation [13, 14]. In patients with a continuous-flow LVAD, clinical presentation of complications known to influence end-organ function (e.g., cardiac tamponade, one of the most life-threatening cardiac conditions) remains a challenge. Although it is highly treatable, it can be fatal if not diagnosed timely [10].

Four types of microcirculatory alterations underlying the loss of hemodynamic coherence have been described [9]. These are type 1, heterogeneous microcirculatory flow; type 2, reduced capillary density induced by hemodilution and anemia; type 3, microcirculatory flow reduction caused by vasoconstriction or tamponade; and type 4, tissue edema. Each of these alterations results in oxygen delivery limitation to the tissue cells in patients with heart failure despite the presence of normalized systemic hemodynamic variables. Clinically such patients present with reduced oxygen extraction capacity. In patients with a continuous LVAD, systemic hemodynamic variables, such as blood pressure, are not of prime importance because the LVAD circulation lacks pulsatility. In these patients, microcirculatory imaging provides a potentially interesting alternative to monitor the hemodynamic status of the patient and intervene to optimize LVAD performance. Ultimately, microcirculatory imaging in patients with LVADs can help maximize the oxygen-carrying capacity of the microcirculation to transport oxygen to the tissues and, therefore, help avoid hospitalization of heart failure patients with an LVAD.

18.3 Modern Monitoring of the Macrocirculation in Heart Failure

Heart failure is an emerging epidemic associated with significant morbidity and mortality, impaired quality of life, and high healthcare costs. Despite major advances in pharmacological and device-based therapies, mortality and morbidity remain high. Detection and diagnosis of heart failure are based on clinical signs and symptoms. In advanced heart failure needing LVAD implantation, these symptoms and signs may be lacking. Strategies to diagnose heart failure could be initiated too late because of missed signs and symptoms. Therefore telemonitoring of these patients could be helpful in and out of the hospital.

Modern implantable monitoring devices with wireless remote monitoring of the pulmonary artery pressure (PAP) are available, and in the USA the Cardio Microelectromechanical system (CardioMEMS sensor; Abbott, Sylmar, CA, USA) has been shown to be safe and clinically effective [15]. There were substantial reductions in hospital admissions for acute and chronic heart failure, irrespective of LV pump function, because PAP-guided heart failure management facilitated timely recognition of incipient decompensated heart failure enabling appropriate modification of medical treatment before hospitalization became unavoidable.

European heart failure guidelines are likely to recommend implantation of a CardioMEMS sensor in high-risk patients. Information from this device includes continuous hemodynamic monitoring and patient self-management based on pressure information. Currently, this pressure-guided heart failure management is the only approved (remote) monitoring in heart failure, which will be studied also in LVAD patients to improve clinical outcomes. In general, the target for treatment of heart failure using these devices is to bring the pulmonary pressures back to normal values. Further targets for improving quality of life could be accomplished by management of volume status by early detection of fluid overload, which could lead to optimization of diuretic therapy. Ultimately, avoidance of hospital readmissions in patients with heart failure pre-LVAD insertion and after LVAD implantation should be realized.

18.4 Monitoring the Microcirculation in Patients with a LVAD

In Europe, almost half the patients die within 90 days after LVAD implantation. Early mortality is primarily dominated by multiple organ failure (MOF) followed by sepsis. In contrast, sepsis and cerebrovascular accidents are the primary causes of death beyond 90 days [16].

From implantation, all patients with an LVAD are susceptible to high-risk complications. In two studies, we showed that sublingual measurements of the microcirculation using handheld vital microscopy were useful in the detection of difficult-to-diagnose complications [10, 14].

18.5 Customized Remote Monitoring of the Microcirculation

In this chapter, we have tried to describe microcirculatory monitoring of the advanced heart failure patient with an LVAD. We have based our concepts on earlier research and the large experience gained in microcirculatory monitoring in heart failure patients receiving mechanical circulatory support. This evaluation resulted in our hypothesis that the four types of microcirculatory alteration associated with a loss of hemodynamic coherence could provide a promising model for monitoring of cardiac recovery as well as early identification of potential life-threatening complications. Based on these four types of microcirculatory alterations, we have created a flowchart (Fig. 18.4) for guidance of daily measurements of sublingual microcirculation. As a result the patient with an LVAD can benefit from early detection of cardiac recovery, which can lead to further tests based on echocardiography and right-heart catheterization [22–25] that could lead to optimal treatment.

Identification of the type of alteration would give a corresponding differential diagnosis requiring further targeted clinical investigation. Type 1 abnormalities could identify the need for anti-inflammatory and antibacterial agents to protect the various cellular components of the microcirculation promoting the use of vasoactive medication (e.g., vasodilators). A further possible investigation could be performed using ^{18}F-fluoro-2-deoxyglucose positron-emission tomography/computed tomography (^{18}F-FDG PET/CT) for the diagnosis and management of LVAD-related infections [26].

In type 2 alterations, such as occur in hemodilution, loss of coherence can be corrected by maintaining an adequate hematocrit with appropriate administration of RBCs or diuretic therapy. For further assessment of hemodynamics, echocardiography and further laboratory values could be used for the analysis of anemia and hemodilution. Bleeding complications are very common. Gastrointestinal bleeding especially is a common complication after LVAD implantation, and its risks correlate with longer support time [27].

In type 3 alterations, right-sided heart failure, tamponade, and potential pump thrombosis have to be excluded as soon as possible. By performing a quick bedside echocardiography the need for computed tomography angiography of the thorax can be accelerated. Echocardiography can still be very challenging in patients with LVAD, which influences the apical windows.

Type 4 alterations correspond in general with fluid overload, which could be treated by optimizing heart failure medication, especially using diuretics. However, more life-threatening complications and development of MOF should also be recognized early. In case of severe aortic valve regurgitation, transaortic valve implantation could be considered because aortic regurgitation after LVAD implantation decreases the clinical effectiveness of LVAD therapy [28]. If there are no major complications after intensive investigation of a type 4 alteration, it may be valuable to adjust the LVAD speed settings to see whether there is any benefit for the microcirculation.

In the near future, heart failure nurses will be able to evaluate microcirculatory information from the patient on a remote heart failure station, which could be

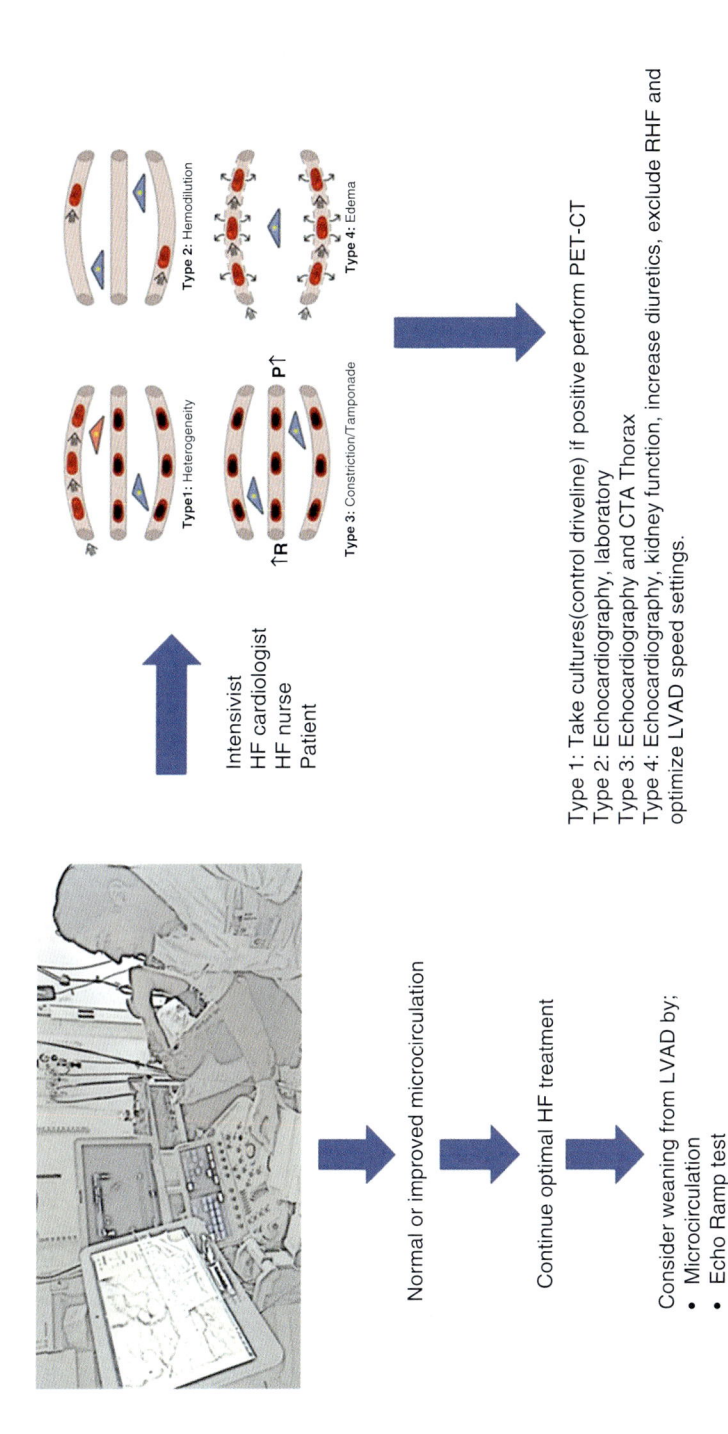

Fig. 18.4 Flowchart for daily microcirculatory assessment at the bedside (intensive care unit (ICU)/high-dependency unit) of patient remote-controlled home monitoring. From ICU to home, the microcirculation could be measured and evaluated by an intensivist, a heart failure (HF) cardiologist, a HF nurse in the hospital, or remotely in the independent patient. *CTA* computed tomography angiography, *LVAD* left ventricular assist device, *PET-CT* positron-emission tomography/computed tomography, *RHF* right-sided heart failure (with permission of the patient and Dr. Akin to use the photo)

directly reviewed by a heart failure cardiologist for treatment options. Telemonitoring could transmit images and videos from handheld vital microscopes used by the patient with minimal artifacts (Fig. 18.4, left upper picture), allowing visualization of the functional condition of not only the right ventricle and the LVAD but also internal organs.

18.6 Conclusion

In this chapter, we have discussed microcirculatory monitoring in clinical and ambulatory patients with an LVAD. We have briefly discussed current modern invasive monitoring devices, such as the CardioMEMS, and described the concepts underlying microcirculatory alterations implemented in short- and long-term monitoring of patients with an LVAD.

We have further described the importance of hemodynamic coherence between the macro- and microcirculations and the importance of monitoring microcirculatory parameters during mechanically generated continuous flow as well as the possibilities of microcirculatory monitoring for early diagnosis of vital complications after implantation of these long-term mechanical circulatory support devices.

With the implantation of an LVAD, survival can be improved. However, months to years after implantation, end-organ recovery can still be limited due to new heart failure occurring by, for example, right heart failure and deteriorating kidney function. Microcirculatory monitoring could be used as a tool for identification of end-organ recovery and persisting functional recovery.

Based on our considerations, we conclude that there is a promising role for customized microcirculatory monitoring of patients with heart failure before and after LVAD implantation, because of the possibility of optimizing medical treatment and preventing early and late complications after LVAD implant.

Acknowledgment We would like to thank Aysima Şenyürek (medical student from the Erasmus MC of Rotterdam) for her help with the creation of Fig. 18.1.

References

1. Savarese G, Lund LH. Global public health burden of heart failure. Card Fail Rev. 2017;3:7–11.
2. den Uil CA, Lagrand WK, van der Ent M, et al. Impaired microcirculation predicts poor outcome of patients with acute myocardial infarction complicated by cardiogenic shock. Eur Heart J. 2010;31:3032–9.
3. den Uil CA, Maat AP, Lagrand WK, et al. Mechanical circulatory support devices improve tissue perfusion in patients with end-stage heart failure or cardiogenic shock. J Heart Lung Transplant. 2009;28:906–11.
4. Ocak I, Kara A, Ince C. Monitoring microcirculation. Best Pract Res Clin Anaesthesiol. 2016;30:407–18.
5. Aykut G, Veenstra G, Scorcella C, Ince C, Boerma C. Cytocam-IDF (incident dark field illumination) imaging for bedside monitoring of the microcirculation. Intensive Care Med Exp. 2015;3:40.

6. van Elteren HA, Ince C, Tibboel D, Reiss IK, de Jonge RC. Cutaneous microcirculation in preterm neonates: comparison between sidestream dark field (SDF) and incident dark field (IDF) imaging. J Clin Monit Comput. 2015;29:543–8.
7. Hilty MP, Guerci P, Ince Y, Toraman F, Ince C. MicroTools enables automated quantification of capillary density and red blood cell velocity in handheld vital microscopy. Commun Biol. 2019;2:217.
8. Kara A, Akin S, Ince C. Monitoring microcirculation in critical illness. Curr Opin Crit Care. 2016;22:444–52.
9. Ince C. Hemodynamic coherence and the rationale for monitoring the microcirculation. Crit Care. 2015;19(Suppl 3):S8.
10. Akin S, Ince C, Den Uil CA, et al. A novel method for early identification of cardiac tamponade in patients with continuous flow left ventricular assist devices by use of sublingual microcirculatory imaging. Eur Heart J. 2018;39(Suppl 1):P5122 (abst).
11. Elbers PW, Ince C. Mechanisms of critical illness—classifying microcirculatory flow abnormalities in distributive shock. Crit Care. 2006;10:221.
12. Ince C, Sinaasappel M. Microcirculatory oxygenation and shunting in sepsis and shock. Crit Care Med. 1999;27:1369–77.
13. Kara A, Akin S, Dos Reis Miranda D, et al. Microcirculatory assessment of patients under VA-ECMO. Crit Care. 2016;20:344.
14. Akin S, Dos Reis Miranda D, Caliskan K, et al. Functional evaluation of sublingual microcirculation indicates successful weaning from VA-ECMO in cardiogenic shock. Crit Care. 2017;21:265.
15. Adamson PB, Abraham WT, Stevenson LW, et al. Pulmonary artery pressure-guided heart failure management reduces 30-day readmissions. Circ Heart Fail. 2016;9:e002600.
16. Akin S, Soliman OII, Muslem R, et al. Preoperative right heart hemodynamics predict right heart failure and early ICU mortality following LVAD implantation. Eur Heart J. 2017;38(Suppl 1):4993 (abst).
17. Reggiori G, Occhipinti G, De Gasperi A, Vincent JL, Piagnerelli M. Early alterations of red blood cell rheology in critically ill patients. Crit Care Med. 2009;37:3041–6.
18. Atasever B, Boer C, Goedhart P, et al. Distinct alterations in sublingual microcirculatory blood flow and hemoglobin oxygenation in on-pump and off-pump coronary artery bypass graft surgery. J Cardiothorac Vasc Anesth. 2011;25:784–90.
19. Dunser MW, Ruokonen E, Pettila V, et al. Association of arterial blood pressure and vasopressor load with septic shock mortality: a post hoc analysis of a multicenter trial. Crit Care. 2009;13:R181.
20. Boerma EC, van der Voort PH, Ince C. Sublingual microcirculatory flow is impaired by the vasopressin-analogue terlipressin in a patient with catecholamine-resistant septic shock. Acta Anaesthesiol Scand. 2005;49:1387–90.
21. Akin S, Soliman OI, Constantinescu AA, et al. Haemolysis as a first sign of thromboembolic event and acute pump thrombosis in patients with the continuous-flow left ventricular assist device HeartMate II. Neth Heart J. 2016;24:134–42.
22. Uriel N, Adatya S, Maly J, et al. Clinical hemodynamic evaluation of patients implanted with a fully magnetically levitated left ventricular assist device (HeartMate 3). J Heart Lung Transplant. 2017;36:28–35.
23. Uriel N, Burkhoff D, Rich JD, et al. Impact of hemodynamic ramp test-guided HVAD speed and medication adjustments on clinical outcomes. Circ Heart Fail. 2019;12:e006067.
24. Uriel N, Morrison KA, Garan AR, et al. Development of a novel echocardiography ramp test for speed optimization and diagnosis of device thrombosis in continuous-flow left ventricular assist devices: the Columbia ramp study. J Am Coll Cardiol. 2012;60:1764–75.
25. Uriel N, Sayer G, Addetia K, et al. Hemodynamic ramp tests in patients with left ventricular assist devices. JACC Heart Fail. 2016;4:208–17.
26. Akin S, Muslem R, Constantinescu AA, et al. 18F-FDG PET/CT in the diagnosis and management of continuous flow left ventricular assist device infections: a case series and review of the literature. ASAIO J. 2018;64:e11–9.

27. Kawabori M, Kurihara C, Critsinelis AC, et al. Gastrointestinal bleeding After HeartMate II or HVAD implantation: incidence, location, etiology, and effect on survival. ASAIO J. 04 Apr 2019; https://doi.org/10.1097/MAT.0000000000000998 [Epub ahead of print].
28. Chung MJ, Ganapathi AM, Vora AN, Schroder JN, Kiefer TL, Hughes GC. Valve-in-ring transcatheter aortic valve replacement after left ventricular assist device therapy. Ann Thorac Surg. 22 Aug 2019; https://doi.org/10.1016/j.athoracsur.2019.06.094 [Epub ahead of print].

Monitoring of the Sublingual Microcirculation at the Bedside: Yes, It Is Possible and Useful

V. Tarazona, A. Harrois, and J. Duranteau

19.1 Introduction

Restoring the microcirculation and tissue oxygenation is the ultimate goal of hemodynamic resuscitation. The purpose of hemodynamic resuscitation should be to prevent tissue hypoperfusion in order to limit organ dysfunction. Unfortunately, the achievement of these goals remains a challenge, because we do not yet have effective monitoring of the microcirculation and tissue oxygenation at the bedside to guide hemodynamic resuscitation. Thus, during shock resuscitation, the goal is to restore the blood pressure and macrovascular oxygen delivery hoping that this will limit tissue hypoxia and organ dysfunction. It is expected that optimization of macrovascular hemodynamic parameters results in an improvement in the microcirculation with restoration of tissue oxygenation. But this hypothesis could be contradicted by the fact that alterations in the microcirculation develop during shock. Indeed, hemorrhagic shock, reperfusion injuries, sepsis, traumatic injuries and inflammation are conditions known to induce microcirculatory alterations, such as viscosity changes, endothelial dysfunction, glycocalyx or erythrocyte alterations, subsequently leading to a loss of the normal physiological relationship between the macro- and microcirculations. In these cases, systemic hemodynamic-driven resuscitation would not be effective in restoring the microcirculation and tissue oxygenation. It is therefore essential to develop microcirculation monitoring tools that provide reliable and clinically relevant microvascular parameters at the bedside.

For several years, handheld vital microscopes (orthogonal polarization spectral imaging [OPS] and sidestream dark-field imaging [SDF] devices) have been used in clinical research to characterize the sublingual microcirculation [1, 2].

V. Tarazona · A. Harrois · J. Duranteau (✉)
Département d'Anesthésie-Réanimation, Hôpitaux Universitaires Paris-Sud, Hôpital de Bicêtre, UMR 942, Le Kremlin-Bicêtre, France
e-mail: jacques.duranteau@aphp.fr

A second consensus on the assessment of the sublingual microcirculation in critically ill patients has been recently published with guidelines for practical use and interpretation of the sublingual microcirculation [3]. Analysis of the sublingual microcirculation has demonstrated that persistent microcirculatory alterations in patients with septic shock were associated with mortality and organ dysfunction despite optimization of the macrocirculation [4–6]. In addition, this approach has made it possible to assess the microvascular response to fluid resuscitation [7, 8], transfusion [9], vasopressors [10] and specific vasodilators [11, 12].

But, are handheld vital microscopes able to provide us with microcirculatory perfusion parameters that can allow us to adapt hemodynamic treatments and improve patient prognosis? To achieve this, handheld vital microscopes must provide clinically relevant parameters, which can be used as markers of severity and which can be used to titrate hemodynamic strategy for more individualized treatment. They must also be easy to use and provide readily interpretable data to ensure adoption by all medical and paramedical staff.

19.2 Sublingual Microvascular Perfusion Parameters

Sublingual videos allow direct visualization of the flow of red blood cells (RBCs) through the capillaries (convective transport of oxygen) and the density of perfused capillaries (diffusive transport of oxygen; also referred to as functional capillary density) in the sublingual microvascular network. The emitted light, corresponding to the wavelength of hemoglobin absorption, displays each erythrocyte in black on a light background. Image acquisition and analysis have to be performed according to international guidelines [3]. The greatest care has to be taken to avoid pressure artifacts. Sequence quality has to be systematically evaluated using the "Microcirculation Image Quality Score" described by Massey and co-workers [13].

Usually four microcirculatory parameters are analyzed:

1. The microvascular flow index (MFI), which is a qualitative evaluation of the microvascular flow: The image is divided into four quadrants, and the predominant type of flow in very small vessels (i.e., diameter less than 20 μm) is assessed in each quadrant using an ordinal score (0 = no flow, 1 = intermittent flow, 2 = sluggish flow, 3 = normal flow). The overall score, called the microvascular flow index, is the sum of each quadrant score divided by the number of quadrants.
2. The percentage of perfused vessels, which is calculated as follows: 100 × (total number of vessels − [no flow + intermittent flow])/total number of vessels.
3. The perfused vessel density (PVD; which can also be referred to as functional capillary density), which is calculated by dividing the area of perfused vessels by the total area of interest.
4. The heterogeneity index, which is calculated as follows: (highest site microvascular flow index − lowest site microvascular flow index) divided by the mean of the microvascular flow index of all sublingual sites.

Microcirculatory images can be analyzed by real-time visual evaluation, off-line manual analysis (e.g., grid based or complete screen based), or off-line software-aided analysis. It is obvious that off-line analysis is very time consuming and is not suitable for clinical intensive care practice. Thus, development of online automatic analysis of microcirculatory images would be a decisive step towards the use of handheld vital microscopes in critically ill patients.

In addition to qualitative evaluation, quantitative evaluation of microcirculatory flow is required for a more precise characterization of the microcirculatory flow patterns in the microvascular network. This enables a better assessment of the heterogeneity of microvascular flows and analysis of the flow-oxygen delivery relationship. Currently, quantitative RBC velocity profiles can be analyzed by space–time diagrams (Automated Vascular Analysis [AVA] software, MicroVision Medical, Amsterdam, The Netherlands) or by averaged perfused speed indicator (CytoCamTools software, CytoCam, Braedius Medical, Huizen, The Netherlands).

19.3 Clinical Relevance of Sublingual Microvascular Perfusion Parameters

The sublingual surface is an easy-access mucosal surface to visualize the microcirculation in the patient, so that handheld vital microscope studies have largely focused on this region. However, what is the evidence that events in the sublingual microcirculation have a relationship to the microcirculations of other critical organs?

Several studies demonstrated that sublingual microcirculatory changes were correlated to gut [14–18] and renal [19, 20] microcirculatory changes. In a large animal model of sepsis, the severity and the time course of microcirculatory changes were similar in sublingual and intestinal microcirculations [14]. Similar results were reported in a sheep model of hemorrhagic shock [17]. de Bruin and co-workers reported in patients undergoing elective gastrointestinal surgery that gut serosal microvascular imaging with a SDF device was similar to sublingual assessment [18]. Recently, Lima and co-workers [20] demonstrated, in a lipopolysaccharide-induced shock model, that the sublingual microcirculation could reflect renal microvascular alterations detected by contrast-enhanced ultrasonography during shock and fluid resuscitation. Thus, the behavior of the sublingual microcirculation is representative of the microcirculation of other organs and especially of vital organs.

Another argument to reinforce the clinical relevance of the sublingual microcirculation is the fact that sublingual microcirculatory perfusion parameters are associated with patient outcome. Indeed, De Backer and co-workers [4] reported that sublingual microvascular parameters were stronger predictors of mortality than global hemodynamic variables and lactate for both early (<24 h) and late (≥24 h) time points. Furthermore, Sakr and co-workers [5] found that survivors were able to restore their sublingual microcirculatory perfusion, whereas non-survivors had persistently impaired sublingual microcirculatory perfusion. More recently, Massey and co-workers [21], in a prospective, formally designed substudy of participants in the Protocolized Care in Early Septic Shock (ProCESS) trial, reported an association between sublingual microcirculatory perfusion parameters at 72 h and mortality. In hemorrhagic shock patients, Tachon and co-workers [22] and Hutchings et al. [23] reported that sublingual microvascular parameters were associated more with increased multiple organ dysfunction syndrome (Sequential Organ Failure Assessment [SOFA score]) than were macrovascular parameters.

Recently, in a prospective observational single-center study in a general intensive care unit (ICU) population (MicroDAIMON study) who had daily sublingual microcirculation assessment from admission to discharge/death, Scorcella and co-workers [24] reported that an abnormal microcirculation at baseline (defined as MFI <2.6) was an independent predictor for mortality (odds ratio 4.594 [1.340–15.754], $p = 0.015$). Additional routine daily microcirculatory monitoring did not reveal extra prognostic information in this study.

Thus, the association between alterations of sublingual microvascular parameters and patient outcomes during the early phase of shock validates the fact that these parameters are clinically relevant for the assessment of patients in shock.

19.4 Titration of Hemodynamic Strategy Using Sublingual Microvascular Perfusion Parameters

The interest in assessment of sublingual microvascular perfusion parameters is not limited to the analysis of the impact of microvascular alterations on patient outcome. This assessment also enables analysis of the microvascular response to the different hemodynamic strategies used. Sublingual microvascular perfusion parameters are dynamic parameters that immediately guide the appropriateness of therapeutic interventions. For example, fluid administration is based on the prediction of preload responsiveness. Dynamic indices, such as pulse pressure variation, detect preload dependence and are used to predict fluid responsiveness. Preload dependence is defined as a state in which increases in right ventricular and/or left ventricular end-diastolic volume result in an increase in stroke volume. Nevertheless, while fluid resuscitation guided by dynamic indices leads to optimization of the macrocirculation, it remains unclear whether it can also improve the microcirculation. Such improvement is dependent on preservation of the microvascular response. Despite an increase in stroke volume, the sublingual microvascular response could be negative due to microvascular alterations and cessation of fluid administration must be considered [7, 8]. Having preload dependence does not give any indication of the state of the microcirculation. The absence of a microvascular response after a fluid challenge should lead to consideration of other therapies such as vasopressors, transfusion, or specific microvascular vasodilators. The presence of a normal sublingual microcirculation before fluid administration may also question the need for fluid administration. More studies are needed to reinforce these statements, but while the microcirculation can be preload dependent when the microcirculation is normally coupled to the macrocirculation, the microcirculation is independent of the macrocirculation when microvascular alterations cause decoupling between the micro- and macrocirculations. Recently, in a prospective observational study, we reported that the occurrence of preload dependence during major abdominal surgery was associated with a decrease in MFI and in PVD (Fig. 19.1) [25]. We observed

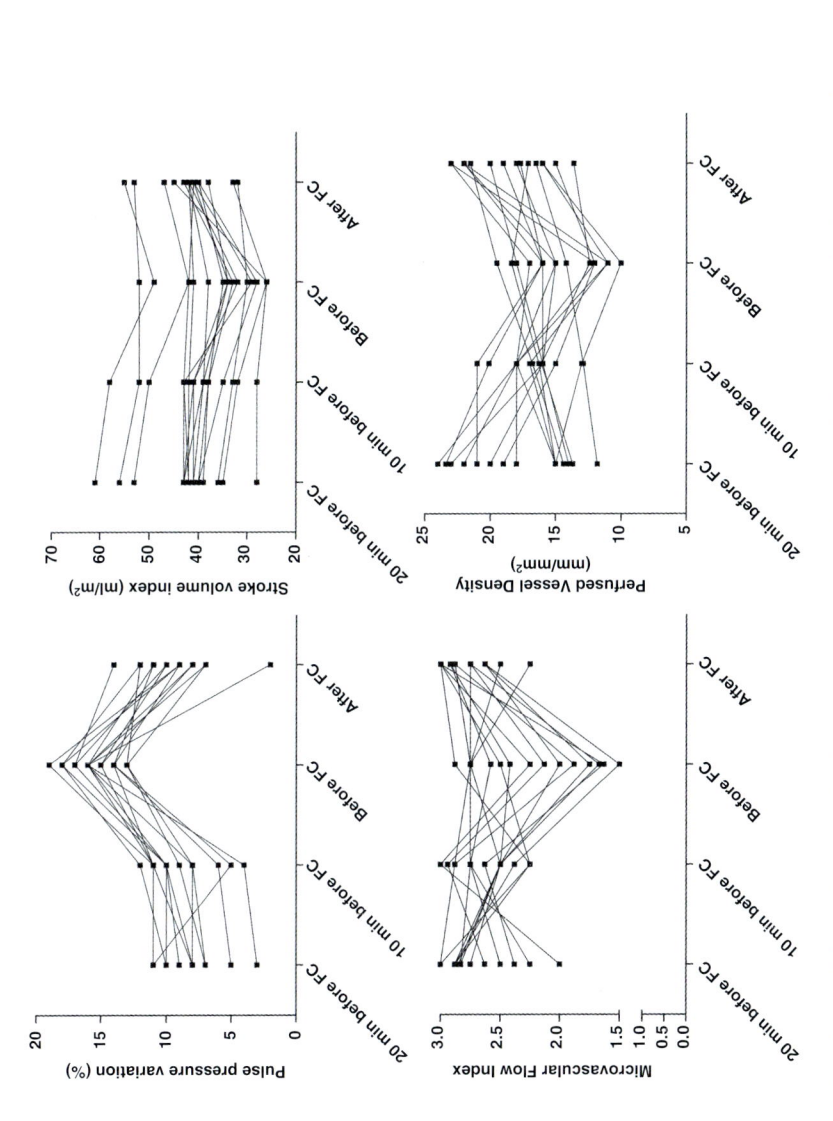

Fig. 19.1 Individual values during abdominal surgery of pulse pressure variation, stroke volume index, microvascular flow index, and perfused vessel density 20 and 10 min before preload dependence, at the time of preload dependence, and after fluid challenge (FC) completion (from [25] with permission)

that fluid administration successfully restored microvascular perfusion. Fluid administration may have corrected an absolute hypovolemia due to a loss of blood volume or relative hypovolemia due to a decrease in venous tone. This should encourage us to correct the preload dependency episodes occurring during surgery to avoid occult microvascular hypoperfusion and microvascular alterations.

To reinforce the fact that assessment of the sublingual microcirculation can be a valuable tool for optimization of microvascular perfusion and personalization of hemodynamic resuscitation, Tanaka and colleagues [9] reported that RBC transfusion improved sublingual microcirculation independently of the macrocirculation and of the hemoglobin level in hemorrhagic shock patients. This positive microcirculatory response to RBC transfusion was not coupled with baseline hemoglobin concentration, the parameter used daily in clinical practice for deciding whether to transfuse RBCs. Only baseline microvascular perfusion parameters predicted the microcirculatory response to RBC transfusion. Of note, most of the patients studied had hemoglobin concentrations within the recommended target hemoglobin concentrations in hemorrhagic shock (7–9 g/dl). This result suggests that RBC transfusion improves microcirculatory perfusion in ways that are not entirely explainable by macrocirculatory effects only. This microcirculatory improvement could involve microvascular local mechanisms in which the erythrocyte could have a central role.

19.5 Sublingual Microvascular Perfusion Parameters at the Bedside

Assuming the clinical relevance of sublingual microvascular parameters, assessment of these parameters is only conceivable if handheld vital microscopes are easy to use and if analysis of the images can be done in real time at the patient's bedside. Several studies have shown that real-time point-of-care assessment by visual inspection of microcirculatory properties at the bedside shows good agreement with off-line evaluation of the microcirculation.

Real-time point-of-care assessment by visual evaluation of the images provides quantitative information on sublingual microvascular perfusion parameters that can detect alterations in microvascular flow and capillary density. Although this evaluation is not accompanied by a detailed quantification of this alteration, it can reveal microvascular alterations and prevent microvascular hypoperfusion being neglected. This approach can be likened to visual evaluation of the left ventricular ejection fraction with echocardiography. Indeed, when a rapid diagnosis is necessary, eyeball evaluation of left ventricular ejection fraction can readily provide an accurate assessment. In addition to the real-time visual evaluation of the images, MFI can be calculated in real time.

Ideally, nurses should be able to perform and interpret the videos to provide real time monitoring. That is why we tested the feasibility of nurses taking bedside measurements of microcirculatory parameters in real time in intensive care patients (MICRONURSE study) [26]. Nurses calculated the MFI score once a 5-s video sequence had been obtained. For assessment of density, the nurse qualitatively evaluated the type of density as poor, normal or rich. Videos initially analyzed by the nurses were given an alphanumeric code to enable delayed off-line analysis by a physician experienced in CytoCam-IDF analysis blinded to all clinical data and nurse real-time MFI values. A real-time bedside qualitative evaluation of MFI and total vessel density by nurses had good agreement with conventional delayed analysis by the physician and was highly sensitive and specific for detecting impaired microvascular flow (MFI <2.5) and low capillary density. These results suggest that real-time point-of-care assessment by visual evaluation could become part of the usual assessment performed by nurses and could be implemented into hemodynamic algorithms in future clinical trials and in regular practice. Naumann and coworkers [27] described a 5-point ordinal scale (the point-of-care microcirculation [POEM] scoring system) of microcirculatory flow and heterogeneity that can be used at the point of care. The authors found minimal inter-user variability amongst healthcare professionals after just 1 h of training and it corresponded well with traditional off-line computer-analyzed parameters.

The development of automatic microcirculatory analysis software systems will be the next step to achieve high-performance quantitative analysis at the patient's bedside and obtain adherence of this monitoring technique by caregivers. Several automatic microcirculatory analysis software systems are being developed. It is also important to work on the analysis of sublingual oxygenation by including analysis of RBC hemoglobin saturation to have a real idea of the oxygen transport in addition to microvascular flow. In addition, characterization of RBC velocities must be more precise because there is no evidence that the relationship between RBC velocity and oxygen transport is linear.

19.6 Impact of Sublingual Microcirculation Monitoring on Patient Outcome

The fact that the analysis of sublingual microcirculation may have an impact on the patient's outcome remains to be proven. For this purpose, we need clinical studies demonstrating that consideration of microvascular sublingual alterations and their treatment can prevent organ failure or mortality during shock or prevent postoperative complications in high-risk patients. In this context, we have started a study to analyze the impact of bedside visual analysis of the sublingual microcirculation in ICU patients in shock (MICROEYE study; ClinicalTrials.gov Identifier: NCT03406598) with the primary outcome to test the ability of visual analysis of the sublingual microcirculation by nurses to predict needs for fluid challenge, vasopressors or transfusion in patients with shock. Studies must also be carried out to determine whether sublingual microcirculation-targeted resuscitation can improve the management of shock patients. Resuscitation protocols similar to the one used by Hernandez et al. [28] (with the capillary refill time, the ANDROMEDA-SHOCK Trial) could be tested using sublingual microcirculation as a target (Fig. 19.2).

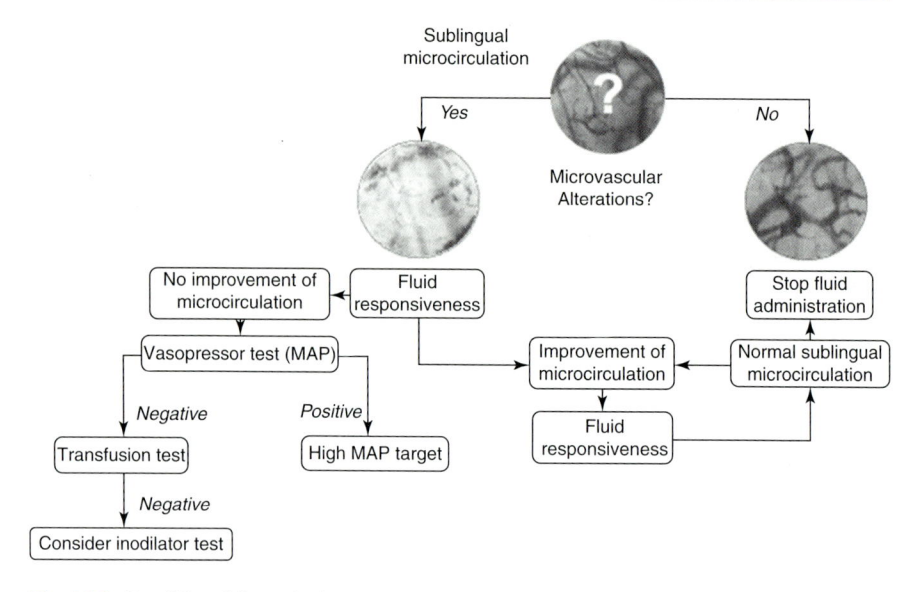

Fig. 19.2 Possible sublingual microcirculation-targeted resuscitation protocol

Monitoring of sublingual microvascular parameters can also add value whenever the static and dynamic macrovascular parameters used to assess preload dependence are unusable (arrhythmia, tidal volume values <8 ml/kg ideal body weight, or spontaneous breathing).

19.7 Conclusion

Restoring the microcirculation and tissue oxygenation is the ultimate goal of hemodynamic resuscitation. Handheld vital microscopes enable direct visualization of the sublingual microcirculation by visualizing RBC flow through the capillaries (convective transport of oxygen) and the density of perfused capillaries (diffusive transport of oxygen). The association between alterations of sublingual microvascular parameters and patient outcomes during shock validates the fact that these parameters are clinically relevant for the assessment of patients in shock. Assessment of sublingual microvascular perfusion parameters at the bedside is only conceivable if handheld vital microscopes are easy to use and if the analysis of the images can be done in real time at the patient's bedside. Ideally, nurses should be able to perform and interpret the videos. Studies have shown that real-time point-of-care assessment by visual inspection of microcirculatory properties at the bedside shows good agreement with off-line evaluation of the microcirculation. The development of automatic microcirculatory analysis software systems will be the next step to obtain high-performance quantitative analysis at the patient's bedside and for caregivers to adhere to this monitoring technique. It is also important to work on an analysis of sublingual oxygenation by including the analysis of the hemoglobin saturation of RBCs. The fact that analysis of the sublingual microcirculation may have an impact on patient outcome remains to be proven. For this purpose, we need clinical studies demonstrating that the consideration of microvascular sublingual alterations and their treatment can prevent organ failure or mortality during shock conditions or prevent postoperative complications in high-risk patients. Monitoring of sublingual microvascular parameters can also add value as additional parameters for the analysis of the preload dependence.

References

1. Verdant C, De Backer D. How monitoring of the microcirculation may help us at the bedside. Curr Opin Crit Care. 2005;11:240–4.
2. De Backer D, Hollenberg S, Boerma C, et al. How to evaluate the microcirculation: report of a round table conference. Crit Care. 2007;11:R101.
3. Ince C, Boerma EC, Cecconi M, et al. Second consensus on the assessment of sublingual microcirculation in critically ill patients: results from a task force of the European Society of Intensive Care Medicine. Intensive Care Med. 2018;44:281–99.
4. De Backer D, Donadello K, Sakr Y, et al. Microcirculatory alterations in patients with severe sepsis: impact of time of assessment and relationship with outcome. Crit Care Med. 2013;41:791–9.
5. Sakr Y, Dubois MJ, De Backer D, Creteur J, Vincent JL. Persistent microcirculatory alterations are associated with organ failure and death in patients with septic shock. Crit Care Med. 2004;32:1825–31.
6. Trzeciak S, McCoy JV, Dellinger RP, Arnold RC, et al. Early increases in microcirculatory perfusion during protocol-directed resuscitation are associated with reduced multi-organ failure at 24 h in patients with sepsis. Intensive Care Med. 2008;34:2210–7.
7. Ospina-Tascon G, Neves AP, Occhipinti G, et al. Effects of fluids on microvascular perfusion in patients with severe sepsis. Intensive Care Med. 2010;36:949–55.
8. Pottecher J, Deruddre S, Teboul JL, et al. Both passive leg raising and intravascular volume expansion improve sublingual microcirculatory perfusion in severe sepsis and septic shock patients. Intensive Care Med. 2010;36:1867–74.
9. Tanaka S, Escudier E, Hamada S, et al. Effect of RBC transfusion on sublingual microcirculation in hemorrhagic shock patients: a pilot study. Crit Care Med. 2017;45:e154–e60.
10. Morelli A, Donati A, Ertmer C, et al. Effects of vasopressinergic receptor agonists on sublingual microcirculation in norepinephrine-dependent septic shock. Crit Care. 2011;15:R217.
11. Boerma EC, Koopmans M, Konijn A, et al. Effects of nitroglycerin on sublingual microcirculatory blood flow in patients with severe sepsis/septic shock after a strict resuscitation protocol: a double-blind randomized placebo controlled trial. Crit Care Med. 2010;38:93–100.
12. Trzeciak S, Glaspey LJ, Dellinger RP, et al. Randomized controlled trial of inhaled nitric oxide for the treatment of microcirculatory dysfunction in patients with sepsis. Crit Care Med. 2014;42:2482–92.
13. Massey MJ, Larochelle E, Najarro G, et al. The microcirculation image quality score: development and preliminary evaluation of a proposed approach to grading quality of image acquisition for bedside videomicroscopy. J Crit Care. 2013;28:913–7.
14. Verdant CL, De Backer D, Bruhn A, et al. Evaluation of sublingual and gut mucosal microcirculation in sepsis: a quantitative analysis. Crit Care Med. 2009;37:2875–81.
15. Pranskunas A, Koopmans M, Koetsier PM, Pilvinis V, Boerma EC. Microcirculatory blood flow as a tool to select ICU patients eligible for fluid therapy. Intensive Care Med. 2013;39:612–9.
16. Jacquet-Lagreze M, Allaouchiche B, Restagno D, et al. Gut and sublingual microvascular effect of esmolol during septic shock in a porcine model. Crit Care. 2015;19:241.

17. Dubin A, Pozo MO, Ferrara G, et al. Systemic and microcirculatory responses to progressive hemorrhage. Intensive Care Med. 2009;35:556–64.
18. de Bruin AF, Kornmann VN, van der Sloot K, et al. Sidestream dark field imaging of the serosal microcirculation during gastrointestinal surgery. Color Dis. 2016;18:O103–10.
19. Sui F, Zheng Y, Li WX, Zhou JL. Renal circulation and microcirculation during intra-abdominal hypertension in a porcine model. Eur Rev Med Pharmacol Sci. 2016;20:452–61.
20. Lima A, van Rooij T, Ergin B, et al. Dynamic contrast-enhanced ultrasound identifies microcirculatory alterations in sepsis-induced acute kidney injury. Crit Care Med. 2018;46:1284–92.
21. Massey MJ, Hou PC, Filbin M, et al. Microcirculatory perfusion disturbances in septic shock: results from the ProCESS trial. Crit Care. 2018;22:308.
22. Tachon G, Harrois A, Tanaka S, et al. Microcirculatory alterations in traumatic hemorrhagic shock. Crit Care Med. 2014;42(6):1433–41.
23. Hutchings SD, Naumann DN, Hopkins P, et al. Microcirculatory impairment is associated with multiple organ dysfunction following traumatic hemorrhagic shock: The MICROSHOCK Study. Crit Care Med. 2018;46:e889–e96.
24. Scorcella C, Damiani E, Domizi R, et al. MicroDAIMON study: microcirculatory DAIly MONitoring in critically ill patients: a prospective observational study. Ann Intensive Care. 2018;8:64.
25. Bouattour K, Teboul JL, Varin L, Vicaut E, Duranteau J. Preload dependence is associated with reduced sublingual microcirculation during major abdominal surgery. Anesthesiology. 2019;130:541–9.
26. Tanaka S, Harrois A, Nicolai C, et al. Qualitative real-time analysis by nurses of sublingual microcirculation in intensive care unit: the MICRONURSE study. Crit Care. 2015;19:388.
27. Naumann DN, Mellis C, Husheer SL, et al. Real-time point of care microcirculatory assessment of shock: design, rationale and application of the point of care microcirculation (POEM) tool. Crit Care. 2016;20:310.
28. Hernandez G, Ospina-Tascon GA, Damiani LP, et al. Effect of a resuscitation strategy targeting peripheral perfusion status vs. serum lactate levels on 28-day mortality among patients with septic shock: the ANDROMEDA-SHOCK randomized clinical trial. JAMA. 2019;32:654–64.

Microcirculation in Patients with Sepsis: From Physiology to Interventions

B. Cantan and I. Martín-Loeches

20.1 Introduction

There are a multitude of reasons why critically ill patients may have reduced cardiac output and perfusion of tissues. Patient survival depends on determining the cause of disease and treating the pathology, as well as supportive care until restoration of normal physiology. Resuscitation guidelines have long been focused on macrohemodynamic variables, such as cardiac output, as well as indirect measures of blood flow and tissue perfusion, such as lactate. In recent years, interest has been developing in the assessment and management of the microcirculation. The microcirculation is the interface between the main oxygen consumers (parenchymal cells in the tissues) and the oxygen supplier (the circulatory system). It serves to deliver nutrients and remove metabolic products in order to support normal tissue function.

For aerobic metabolism to occur there must be a constant delivery of oxygen to cells. Gas exchange occurs in the pulmonary vasculature, oxygenated blood is then circulated systemically via the cardiovascular system, and oxygen diffuses into cells at the level of the microcirculation. It is then used to make cellular adenosine 5′-triphosphate (ATP) through the process of aerobic respiration, primarily through oxidative phosphorylation in the mitochondria.

The microcirculation is a network of small blood vessels (<100 μm diameter), which consists of arterioles, capillaries, and venules. It includes endothelial cells,

---

B. Cantan
Multidisciplinary Intensive Care Research Organization (MICRO), St. James's Hospital, Dublin, Ireland

I. Martín-Loeches (✉)
Multidisciplinary Intensive Care Research Organization (MICRO), St. James's Hospital, Dublin, Ireland

Hospital Clinic, Universidad de Barcelona, CIBERes, Barcelona, Spain
e-mail: lmartinl@tcd.ie

smooth muscle cells (mostly in arterioles), red blood cells (RBCs), leukocytes and platelets [1]. The microcirculation is structured such that every cell has at least one capillary adjacent to it for the purpose of passive diffusion of oxygen from the vasculature into the cell.

The early goals of resuscitation in circulatory shock are to restore global blood flow, oxygen delivery, and organ perfusion pressure with the ultimate aim of improving microcirculatory perfusion and cellular oxygen metabolism. The aim of this chapter is to outline the principles of the microcirculation, microcirculatory dysfunction in sepsis, and therapies to improve microcirculatory function and tissue perfusion.

20.2 Microcirculatory Dysfunction in Sepsis

Sepsis is characterized by macrocirculatory alterations such as relative hypovolemia, a decrease in vascular tone, myocardial depression, and a heterogeneous pattern of blood flow in the microcirculation, as well as the incapacity of cells to extract and adequately use oxygen [1].

Sepsis results in derangements in the microcirculation, with these derangements being most marked in severely ill patients. Clinical and global hemodynamic parameters do not correlate well with microcirculatory perfusion and indeed these microcirculatory abnormalities may persist after the correction of systemic hemodynamic parameters, such as mean arterial pressure (MAP) [2].

The cardiovascular system circulates blood throughout the body but it is the microcirculation in particular that actively and passively regulates the distribution of RBCs and plasma throughout individual organs (Fig. 20.1). In animal models of sepsis, lipopolysaccharide (LPS)-induced microvascular heterogeneity and increased oxygen-diffusion distances affect the distribution of RBCs and oxygen flow within the heart, leading to tissue hypoxia [3]. Endothelial malfunction and rupture of the glycocalyx can lead to microthrombi, capillary leakage, leukocyte rolling, and rouleaux formation [4]. Microcirculatory alterations increase the diffusion distance for oxygen and, due to the heterogeneity of microcirculatory perfusion in sepsis, may promote the development of areas of tissue hypoxia in close proximity to well-oxygenated zones. Improvement of tissue perfusion and oxygenation should be considered the ultimate goal of any resuscitative efforts.

20.3 Hemodynamic Reconciliation in Physiology

Septic shock is a subset of sepsis in which oxygen delivery to cells is insufficient to maintain cellular activity and support organ function. It is associated with a greater risk of mortality than with sepsis alone. It can be clinically identified by a vasopressor requirement to maintain a MAP of ≥ 65 mmHg and serum lactate level <2 mmol/l (18 mg/dl) in the absence of hypovolemia [5]. For resuscitative measures to be effective there must be coherence between the macrocirculation and the

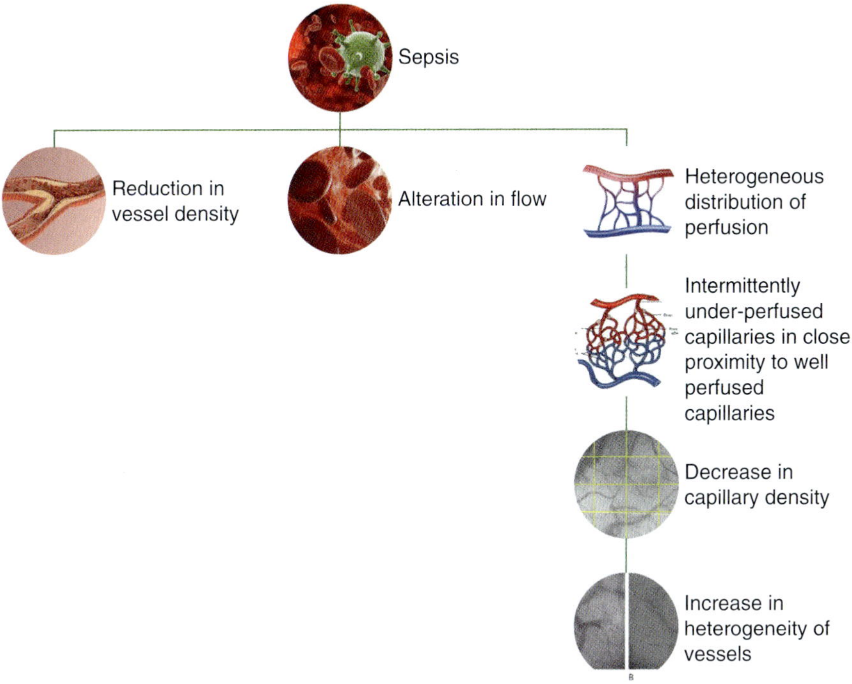

Fig. 20.1 Microcirculatory derangements in sepsis. Derangements are mainly characterized by a reduction in vessel density, alteration in flow, and a heterogeneous distribution of perfusion. Sepsis is associated with intermittently under-perfused capillaries in close proximity to well-perfused capillaries. This causes a decrease in capillary density and increase in heterogeneity of vessels

microcirculation. That is to say, normalization of systemic variables must result in a parallel improvement in perfusion of the microcirculation, oxygenation of parenchymal cells, and restoration of normal cellular activity. In many shock states, tissues can remain hypoperfused even after MAP has been restored.

The potential pathophysiologic mechanisms behind this hemodynamic incoherence during or following resuscitation include unregulated inflammation, cytokine storm, reactive oxygen species, degradation and shedding of the endothelial glycocalyx, endothelial dysfunction and increased permeability, and mitochondrial dysfunction [6].

The persistence of microcirculatory hypoperfusion after restoration of systemic variables has been shown in numerous studies and is associated with worse outcomes. Ince suggested four different types of microcirculatory alterations underlying the loss of hemodynamic coherence [7]:

Type 1 (obstructive): heterogeneous microcirculatory flow in which there are obstructed capillaries next to capillaries with flowing RBCs. Persistence of this type of microcirculatory dysfunction in the presence of normal systemic hemodynamic variables has been associated with adverse outcomes [8]. Increased microcirculatory perfusion during resuscitation is associated with reduced organ failure in septic patients with comparable global hemodynamics [9].

Type 2 (hemodilution/anemic): reduced capillary density induced by hemodilution and anemia, in which dilution of blood causes a loss of RBC-filled capillaries and results in increased diffusion distances between oxygen-carrying RBCs and tissue cells.

Type 3 (hypoperfused): microcirculatory flow reduction caused by vasoconstriction or tamponade in which vasoconstriction of arterial vessels results in microcirculatory ischemia or raised venous pressures inducing microcirculatory tamponade.

Type 4 (distributive): tissue edema caused by capillary leak, which results in increased diffusion distances between the RBCs and tissue cells.

The second consensus on the assessment of the sublingual microcirculation was published in 2018 [10]. It introduced a classification system in order to better characterize microcirculatory alterations other than solely those associated with sepsis. The types of alterations include:

- Type 1: complete stagnated capillaries (circulatory arrest, excessive use of vasopressors)
- Type 2: reduction in the number of flowing capillaries (hemodilution)
- Type 3: stopped-flow vessels are seen next to vessels with flowing cells (sepsis, hemorrhage, and hemodilution)
- Type 4: hyperdynamic flow within capillaries (hemodilution, sepsis)

20.4 The Role of the Endothelium and Coagulation

The normal microcirculation maintains a network of perfused capillaries by autoregulation, which is a regulatory mechanism allowing microcirculatory flow to remain independent of changes in systemic blood pressure (Fig. 20.2). The main component of this autoregulated system is the endothelial cell [1].

The endothelial glycocalyx is a negatively charged, carbohydrate-rich layer, which lines the luminal surface of the vascular endothelium [11]. It consists of proteoglycans, glycoproteins bound with sialic acid, glycosaminoglycans (GAGs), and associated plasma proteins. Proteins such as albumin, fibrinogen, fibronectin, thrombomodulin, antithrombin III, superoxide dismutase, and cell-adhesion molecules all interact with GAGs [12].

The endothelial glycocalyx controls capillary permeability and acts as a barrier [13]. Its negative charge prevents negatively charged proteins such as albumin from passing into the extravascular space, which in turn prevents fluid from passing into the extravascular space. It serves as a barrier to adhesion of leukocytes to the endothelium and indeed shedding of the glycocalyx during activation of endothelial cells may be an essential part of the inflammatory response [14]. It may also serve as a mechanosensor and mediate the release of nitric oxide in response to shear stress

Fig. 20.2 Blood flow and perfusion pressure ratio. Normal microcirculation maintains a network of perfused capillaries by autoregulation, which is a regulatory mechanism allowing microcirculatory flow to stay independent of changes in systemic blood pressure

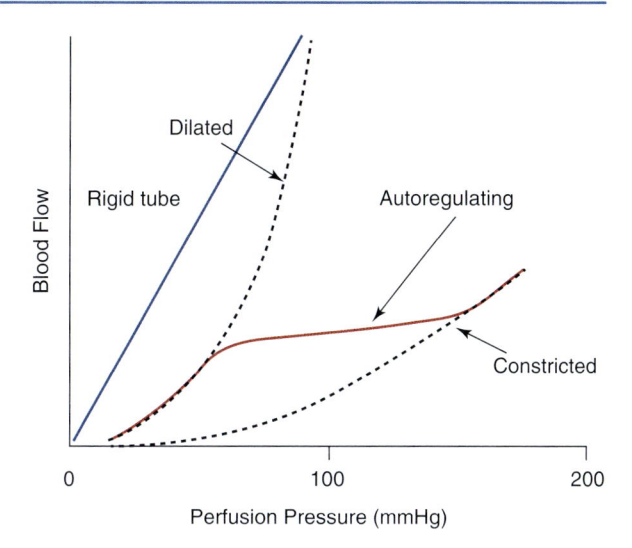

[15]. The permeability of the vascular endothelium is of critical importance in the regulation of fluid homeostasis between the intravascular space and the interstitium and in the regulation of physiological functions of organs [16].

During sepsis, the glycocalyx is degraded by enzymes such as metalloproteinases, heparanase and hyaluronidase, which are activated as part of the inflammatory response [12]. These enzymes are activated in inflammatory states by reactive oxygen species, tumor necrosis factor (TNF)-alpha, and interleukin 1-beta (IL-1β) [17]. Studies have found a significant reduction in the thickness of the glycocalyx in sepsis [18]. Observational studies have found an association between the levels of markers of endothelial damage and the severity of sepsis [19]. This degradation of the glycocalyx leads to vascular hyper-permeability, unregulated vasodilation, microvessel thrombosis, and augmented leukocyte adhesion [12].

Inflammatory-mediated degradation of the glycocalyx may lead to specific organ dysfunction in sepsis, such as acute respiratory distress syndrome (ARDS), acute renal failure, and hepatic dysfunction. Inflammatory cytokines, such as TNF-α, IL-1β, IL-6, and IL-10, have been implicated in the degradation of the glycocalyx [18].

20.5 Assessment of the Microcirculation

20.5.1 Microcirculatory Targets

Macrocirculatory parameters such as MAP are poor predictors of cardiac output. The sympathetic response to stress and neural adaptation tends to initially maintain the MAP in the face of decreasing flow [20]. It is thus a poor indicator in the early assessment of shock. Indeed systemic hemodynamic variables do not indicate the onset of shock but rather indicate the onset of cardiovascular decompensation. Measures of microvascular flow enable the earlier detection of shock (Fig. 20.3).

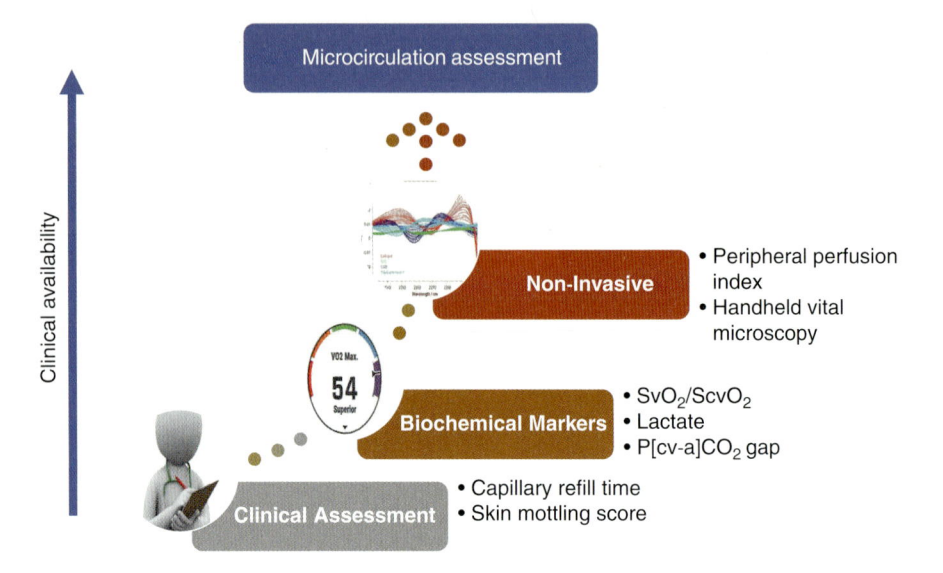

Fig. 20.3 Measures of microvascular assessment classified by their availability in clinical practice. SvO_2 mixed venous oxygen saturation; $ScvO_2$ central venous oxygen saturation; $P[cv\text{-}a]CO_2$ gap central-venous-arterial CO_2 difference

20.5.2 Clinical Assessment

20.5.2.1 Capillary Refill Time

The capillary refill time (CRT) is defined as the time required for a distal capillary bed (i.e., the nail bed) to regain its color after pressure has been applied to cause blanching [21]. Historically the upper limit of normal was quoted to be 2 s; however more recent studies have suggested the upper limit of normal for capillary refill time to be 3.5–4.5 s [22, 23]. It does however vary with factors such as age and temperature, and is subject to inter-observer variability.

Hernandez et al. reported that CRT and central-to-toe temperature difference (Tc-toe) were more significant predictors of successful resuscitation than normalization of metabolic parameters such as central venous oxygen saturation ($ScvO_2$) and central-venous-arterial CO_2 difference ($P[cv\text{-}a]CO_2$ gap). In their study, the presence of normal values of both CRT and Tc-toe at 6 h was independently associated with successful resuscitation [24]. This suggests that noninvasive measures of peripheral perfusion such as CRT and Tc-toe may be used as surrogates for more invasive techniques in the assessment of peripheral perfusion.

Patients with persistently abnormal peripheral perfusion as measured by CRT following initial resuscitation have been shown to have a higher likelihood of developing complications such as organ failure and decreased survival [25].

20.5.2.2 Skin Mottling

Skin mottling is defined as a bluish skin discoloration that typically manifests near the elbows or knees and has a distinct patchy pattern. It is the result of heterogeneic small vessel vasoconstriction and is thought to reflect abnormal skin perfusion [21]. The mottling scoring system (from 0 to 5), based on mottling area extension from the knees to the periphery, is a simple and reliable tool used for the assessment of peripheral perfusion (Fig. 20.4). Higher skin mottling scores have been found to be predictive of mortality in patients admitted to the intensive care unit (ICU) [26].

20.5.3 Biochemical Markers

Biochemical markers are used to indicate global perfusion in both the intensive care and the nonintensive care setting. Mixed venous oxygen saturation (SvO_2), $ScvO_2$, plasma lactate, and $P[cv-a]CO_2$ gap are commonly used measurements for this purpose.

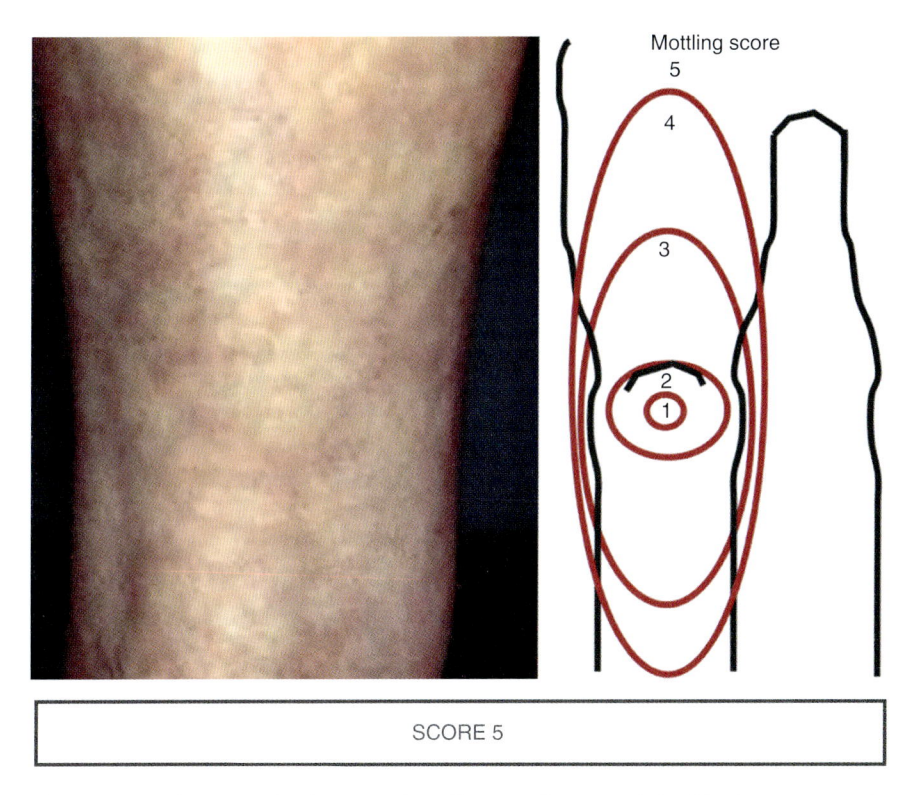

Fig. 20.4 Mottling score showing stage 5 mottling. Mottling score defined by five areas over the knee is developed to evaluate tissue perfusion at bedside

20.5.3.1 SvO₂ and ScvO₂

Using the SvO_2, the Fick equation can be used to calculate the cardiac output [27]:

$$SvO_2 = SaO_2 - (VO_2 / \text{cardiac output} \times Hb \times 1.34)$$

where Hb is the hemoglobin concentration, SaO_2 the arterial oxygen saturation, and VO_2 whole-body O_2 consumption.

When the SaO_2, VO_2, and hemoglobin remain constant, decreasing values of cardiac output result in decreases in SvO_2 secondary to increases in the oxygen extraction rate. Normal values for SvO_2 range from 70% to 75%. The measurement of SvO_2 requires a pulmonary arterial catheter; however, $ScvO_2$ can be obtained from a central venous catheter and although oxygen levels vary slightly it can be used as a surrogate.

20.5.3.2 Lactate

Lactate is perhaps the most commonly used biochemical indicator of resuscitation in sepsis. It is the most easily measurable and interpretable and can be done rapidly with point-of-care testing. In contrast to SvO_2 and $ScvO_2$ it does not require central venous access.

Lactate is a product of anaerobic metabolism and thus indicates inadequate oxygen delivery to or metabolism by the tissues. It is included in the most recent definition of septic shock. The combination of a lactate level >2 mmol/l and vasopressor requirement to maintain MAP >65 mmHg in the absence of hypovolemia has been associated with mortality of >40% [5]. Lactate clearance as a target of resuscitation has been shown to be non-inferior to using $ScvO_2$ monitoring [28].

20.5.3.3 Central-Venous-Arterial CO₂ Difference

The $P[cv-a]CO_2$ gap can be used as an adjunct in the assessment of the macro- and microcirculation. Using a central venous catheter, the $ScvO_2$ can be measured and used as a surrogate for global tissue hypoxia, and the $P[cv-a]CO_2$ gap can be calculated and used as a surrogate for the cardiac index. Persistence of a PCO_2 gap >0.8 kPa (6 mmHg) after 24 h of treatment has been associated with a higher mortality [29].

CO_2 is 20 times more soluble than O_2 and thus as a result is a more sensitive marker of hypoperfusion. Where there is a barrier to O_2 diffusion as a result of hypoperfused or nonfunctional capillaries, CO_2 will still flow into the venous system. In the context of a patient with a $ScvO_2$ >70% and persistently elevated lactate, the PCO_2 gap may be elevated reflecting a barrier to O_2 diffusion at the level of the microcirculation.

20.5.4 Peripheral Perfusion Index

The peripheral perfusion index is based on the analysis of the pulse oximetry signal. It is the ratio between the pulsatile blood flow and non-pulsatile static blood flow in peripheral tissues. It is a noninvasive method that uses the ubiquitous pulse oximeter for its calculation. In a 2002 study by Lima et al. [30], a cutoff of <1.4 was suggested to predict poor peripheral perfusion and a peripheral perfusion index <0.2

predicted ICU mortality in septic patients following resuscitation, with accuracy similar to lactate [31].

20.5.5 Handheld Vital Microscopy

Handheld vital microscopes were introduced clinically in the 1990s and investigations of their use have played a key role in understanding the microcirculation in sepsis. They allow single RBCs to be visualized in the capillaries. The third and most recent generation of handheld vital microscopes is based on a mode of dark-field microscopy called incident dark-field (IDF) imaging. This device gives improved resolution and an increased number of capillaries can be seen in comparison to the previous generation, which was based on sidestream dark-field (SDF) imaging [32].

The most common anatomical location imaged is the sublingual circulation. Microcirculatory abnormalities visualized include increased heterogeneity of perfused vessels, proportion of perfused vessels, total density of small microvessels, and microvascular flow index (MFI) [27]. Currently the clinical relevance of microvascular alterations is expressed in terms of proportion of perfused vessels and MFI [10].

The MFI is used to characterize the velocity of microcirculatory perfusion. The screen is divided into four quadrants. The average flow of RBCs is then calculated and described as absent (0), intermittent (1), sluggish (2), or normal (3) [33]. An MFI <2.6 in combination with tachycardia >90 beats per minute (bpm) has been shown to be an independent risk factor for increased in-hospital mortality [34].

Handheld vital microscopes can also be used to measure the perfused boundary region of the microcirculation, which is calculated as the dimensions of the permeable part of the glycocalyx allowing penetration of circulating RBCs. This provides an index of glycocalyx damage [4]. The perfused boundary region has been shown to be increased in critically ill patients compared with healthy controls reflecting decreased thickness of the endothelial glycocalyx [35]. The perfused boundary region has been shown to be reproducible and have good inter-observer reliability, which makes it a promising tool for guiding resuscitation and decision-making in sepsis.

Monitoring of the microcirculation during resuscitation can help to verify whether interventions have been successful in restoring perfusion and oxygenation of the tissues and in restoring hemodynamic coherence.

20.6 How We Can Modify the Microcirculation in Sepsis

Microvascular perfusion is directly related to the driving pressure (difference between pressure at the entry and exit site of the capillary) and the radius of the vessel (to the fourth power) and inversely related to blood viscosity. Intravenous fluids are a mainstay of supportive care in sepsis and may help to increase microvascular perfusion by increasing the driving pressure, decreasing the blood viscosity, or affecting the interaction between circulating cells and the endothelium [36].

Volume expansion with fluid has been shown to improve microcirculatory perfusion in the early (<24 h) but not in the late (>48 h) phase following the diagnosis of severe sepsis [36]. It is not conclusive yet whether colloids or crystalloids are superior in improving the microcirculation.

Assessment of microcirculatory variables such as MFI may be helpful in determining the need for fluid therapy. A study by Pranskunas et al. [37] examined macrohemodynamic variables, such as oliguria, MAP, $ScvO_2$ and hyperlactatemia, and MFI, as a tool to select ICU patients eligible for fluid therapy. In patients with an MFI of <2.6, fluid therapy resulted in a significant increase in median MFI as well as a reduction in the median number of clinical signs of impaired organ perfusion. In contrast, in patients with an MFI >2.6 at baseline, fluid challenge did not increase the median MFI nor did it result in a reduction in the number of clinical signs of impaired organ perfusion. This suggests that in patients with a normal or near-normal MFI, causes other than microcirculatory flow were to blame for persistent organ dysfunction. Since none of the macrohemodynamic variables were able to discriminate an MFI <2.6, direct assessment of microcirculatory flow may help guide decisions regarding administration of fluids [37].

A study by Hanson et al. [38] looked at liberal fluid resuscitation in severe falciparum malaria. Severity of disease in terms of lactic acidosis correlated with the degree of erythrocyte sequestration as visualized by orthogonal polarized spectroscopy (OPS) rather than hypovolemia. Liberal administration of fluid did little to improve erythrocyte sequestration; however, it did increase the risk of potentially lethal complications of fluid overload and increased capillary permeability. In addition to suggesting against liberal fluid administration in severe falciparum malaria the results also suggest that direct visualization and assessment of the type of microcirculatory dysfunction may guide decisions about whether administration of fluid may be futile and lead to complications rather than resolution.

Further to that, hypervolemia has also been associated with microcirculatory dysfunction and increased degradation of the glycocalyx in sepsis. In a study in patients undergoing on- and off-pump coronary artery bypass surgery, increased levels of atrial natriuretic peptide (ANP) preceded elevation of inflammatory cytokines and shedding of the glycocalyx [39]. Chappell et al. also observed increased levels of ANP and shedding of the glycocalyx in response to volume loading and hypervolemia [40]. ANP has been shown to independently induce shedding of the endothelial glycocalyx in pig hearts as evidenced by increased levels of syndecan-1 and histologically visible degradation of the glycocalyx on electron microscopy. It in turn led to increased vascular permeability [41].

In a study of patients with severe sepsis, high levels of syndecan-1 were associated with the risk of intubation following large-volume fluid resuscitation compared to patients with low levels of syndecan-1. This may reflect the increased vascular permeability following degradation of the glycocalyx leading to increased risk of respiratory failure [42].

Apart from its use as a colloid, albumin may have other beneficial effects on the microcirculation. Sphingosine-1-phosphate (S1P) is an important plasma phospholipid for the maintenance of vascular permeability [43]. S1P suppresses the activity of metalloproteinase, which in turn protects against the loss of syndecan-1 and degradation of the glycocalyx [44]. RBCs are an important source of S1P and albumin may attenuate the degradation of the glycocalyx by acting as a carrier of S1P from RBCs to the endothelium [45].

Transfusion of RBCs has been shown to improve the microcirculation independently of the macrocirculation and the hemoglobin level in hemorrhagic shock patients [46]. A systematic review by Nielsen et al. failed to find a benefit of RBC transfusion in most critically ill patients. However, they identified a number of studies that found that patients with abnormalities in tissue oxygenation or microcirculatory indices do demonstrate improvement following transfusion [47].

Venous vasodilators have been theorized to improve microcirculatory flow by dilating postcapillary venules, thereby increasing capillary flow, and decreasing transcapillary pressure and extravasation into the tissues. In vasoplegic shock, the macrocirculation is vasodilated whilst the microcirculation is vasoconstricted [7]. Studies on the effect of nitroglycerin on the microcirculation in septic shock have yielded conflicting results. Spronk et al. found that it did improve microcirculation [48], whilst Boerma et al. in a larger randomized controlled trial found that it did not improve the microcirculation compared with the placebo group [49]. In this study, both the placebo group and the nitroglycerin group achieved significant improvements in the microcirculation [49]. The median MFI of the nitroglycerin group improved from 1.67 to 2.71, and the placebo group went from 1.42 to 2.71. It may be that other resuscitative efforts were sufficient to improve the MFI to values approaching normal. Nitroglycerin may however be of use in septic shock if its use is decided based on the type of microcirculatory dysfunction and the resuscitation status of the patient, and it is titrated in combination with technologies that can monitor, directly assess, and quantitatively analyze the microcirculation.

Increasing the arterial blood pressure with increasing doses of vasopressors has not been found to improve MFI, proportion of perfused vessels, vessel density, or heterogeneity index [50, 51]. There may be a dissociation between increases in arterial pressure produced by vasopressor agents and improvement in microvascular perfusion and delivery of vital substrates. This is probably due to shunting between postcapillary venules and precapillary arterioles and due to a sustained increase in SvO_2 (as commonly happens in the initial stages of septic shock).

Finally, in critically ill non-bleeding patients, transfusion of fresh frozen plasma (FFP) resulted in a decrease in the levels of syndecan-1 and factor VIII, suggesting an improvement in the endothelium. This was accompanied by, and perhaps a result of, an increase in ADAMTS13 levels and a decrease in von Willebrand factor levels [52].

20.7 Conclusion

The microcirculation is the vital interface at which oxygen is delivered to cells. Without a functioning microcirculation the restoration of aerobic metabolism is impossible. Increased understanding of microcirculatory dysfunction helps to explain the persistence of tissue hypoxia despite restoration of normal macrohemodynamic parameters.

The importance of the microcirculation in critical illness is becoming increasingly clear. With newer and more sophisticated monitoring techniques, the microcirculation can be used to guide resuscitative efforts towards more targeted therapies. In addition to clinical examination and biochemical markers as methods of assessment, handheld vital microscopes allow direct visualization of capillaries and a number of indices and classifications have been developed that show good interobserver reproducibility. As these devices become more widely available they may become routinely used in the management of sepsis and other conditions that affect systemic hemodynamics.

Despite the advances in our understanding of microcirculatory dysfunction there remains a deficit in knowledge regarding how best to treat it. For example, both hypo- and hypervolemia seem to negatively affect the microcirculation and the endothelial glycocalyx, and the type of fluid that is best for restoring perfusion and maintaining endothelial integrity remains to be established. As more clinical studies adopt handheld vital microscopy and investigate treatments based on microcirculatory status we may see that the management of hemodynamics in sepsis becomes more nuanced and individualized.

References

1. Lipińska-Gediga M. Sepsis and septic shock – is a microcirculation a main player? Anaesthesiol Intensive Ther. 2016;48:261–5.
2. Spanos A, Jhanji S, Vivian-Smith A, Harris T, Pearse RM. Early microvascular changes in sepsis and severe sepsis. Shock. 2010;33:387–91.
3. Bateman RM, Tokunaga C, Kareco T, Dorscheid DR, Walley KR. Myocardial hypoxia-inducible HIF-1α, VEGF, and GLUT1 gene expression is associated with microvascular and ICAM-1 heterogeneity during endotoxemia. Am J Physiol Heart Circ Physiol. 2007;293:H448–56.
4. Donati A, Domizi R, Damiani E, Adrario E, Pelaia P, Ince C. From macrohemodynamic to the microcirculation. Crit Care Res Pract. 2013;2013:892710.
5. Weis S, Dickmann P, Pletz MW, Coldewey SM, Gerlach H, Bauer M. Eine neue Definition führt zu neuen Konzepten. Dtsch Arztebl Int. 2017;114:801–10.
6. Kanoore Edul VS, Ince C, Dubin A. What is microcirculatory shock? Curr Opin Crit Care. 2015;21:245–52.
7. Ince C. Hemodynamic coherence and the rationale for monitoring the microcirculation. Crit Care. 2015;19:S8.
8. De Backer D, Donadello K, Sakr Y, et al. Microcirculatory alterations in patients with severe sepsis: impact of time of assessment and relationship with outcome. Crit Care Med. 2013;41:791–9.
9. Trzeciak S, McCoy JV, Dellinger RP, et al. Early increases in microcirculatory perfusion during protocol-directed resuscitation are associated with reduced multi-organ failure at 24 h in patients with sepsis. Intensive Care Med. 2008;34:2210–7.
10. Ince C, Boerma EC, Cecconi M, et al. Second consensus on the assessment of sublingual microcirculation in critically ill patients: results from a task force of the European Society of Intensive Care Medicine. Intensive Care Med. 2018;44:281–99.
11. Reitsma S, Slaaf DW, Vink H, Van Zandvoort MAMJ, Oude Egbrink MGA. The endothelial glycocalyx: composition, functions, and visualization. Pflugers Arch. 2007;454:345–59.
12. Uchimido R, Schmidt EP, Shapiro NI. The glycocalyx: a novel diagnostic and therapeutic target in sepsis. Crit Care. 2019;23:16.

13. Salmon AHJ, Ferguson JK, Burford JL, et al. Loss of the endothelial glycocalyx links albuminuria and vascular dysfunction. J Am Soc Nephrol. 2012;23:1339–50.
14. Mulivor AW, Lipowsky HH. Role of glycocalyx in leukocyte-endothelial cell adhesion. Am J Physiol Heart Circ Physiol. 2002;283:H1282–91.
15. Curry FE, Adamson RH. Endothelial glycocalyx: permeability barrier and mechanosensor. Ann Biomed Eng. 2012;40:828–39.
16. Steinberg BE, Goldenberg NM, Lee WL. Do viral infections mimic bacterial sepsis? The role of microvascular permeability: a review of mechanisms and methods. Antivir Res. 2012;93:2–15.
17. Becker BF, Jacob M, Leipert S, Salmon AHJ, Chappell D. Degradation of the endothelial glycocalyx in clinical settings: searching for the sheddases. Br J Clin Pharmacol. 2015;80:389–402.
18. Wiesinger A, Peters W, Chappell D, et al. Nanomechanics of the endothelial glycocalyx in experimental sepsis. PLoS One. 2013;8:e80905.
19. Anand D, Ray S, Srivastava LM, Bhargava S. Evolution of serum hyaluronan and syndecan levels in prognosis of sepsis patients. Clin Biochem. 2016;49:768–76.
20. Wo CC, Shoemaker WC, Appel PL, Bishop MH, Kram HB, Hardin E. Unreliability of blood pressure and heart rate to evaluate cardiac output in emergency resuscitation and critical illness. Crit Care Med. 1993;21:218–23.
21. Lima A, Bakker J. Clinical assessment of peripheral circulation. Curr Opin Crit Care. 2015;21:226–31.
22. Schriger DL, Baraff L. Defining normal capillary refill: variation with age, sex, and temperature. Ann Emerg Med. 1988;17:932–5.
23. Anderson B, Kelly AM, Kerr D, Clooney M, Jolley D. Impact of patient and environmental factors on capillary refill time in adults. Am J Emerg Med. 2008;26:62–5.
24. Hernandez G, Pedreros C, Veas E, Bruhn A, Romero C, Rovegno M, et al. Evolution of peripheral vs metabolic perfusion parameters during septic shock resuscitation. A clinical-physiologic study. J Crit Care. 2012;27:283–8.
25. Lima A, Jansen TC, Van Bommel J, Ince C, Bakker J. The prognostic value of the subjective assessment of peripheral perfusion in critically ill patients. Crit Care Med. 2009;37:934–8.
26. Dumas G, Lavillegrand JR, Joffre J, et al. Mottling score is a strong predictor of 14-day mortality in septic patients whatever vasopressor doses and other tissue perfusion parameters. Crit Care. 2019;23:211.
27. Huber W, Zanner R, Schneider G, Schmid R, Lahmer T. Assessment of regional perfusion and organ function: less and non-invasive techniques. Front Med. 2019;6:50.
28. Jones AE, Shapiro NI, Trzeciak S, Arnold RC, Claremont HA, Kline JA. Lactate clearance vs central venous oxygen saturation as goals of early sepsis therapy: a randomized clinical trial. JAMA. 2010;303:739–46.
29. Van Beest PA, Lont MC, Holman ND, Loef B, Kuiper MA, Boerma EC. Central venous-arterial pCO2 difference as a tool in resuscitation of septic patients. Intensive Care Med. 2013;39:1034–9.
30. Lima AP, Beelen P, Bakker J. Use of a peripheral perfusion index derived from the pulse oximetry signal as a noninvasive indicator of perfusion. Crit Care Med. 2002;17:1210–13.
31. He HW, Liu DW, Long Y, Wang XT. The peripheral perfusion index and transcutaneous oxygen challenge test are predictive of mortality in septic patients after resuscitation. Crit Care. 2013;17:R116.
32. Hutchings S, Watts S, Kirkman E. The Cytocam video microscope. A new method for visualising the microcirculation using Incident Dark Field technology. Clin Hemorheol Microcirc. 2016;62:261–71.
33. Pozo MO, Kanoore Edul VS, Ince C, Dubin A. Comparison of different methods for the calculation of the microvascular flow index. Crit Care Res Pract. 2012;2012:102483.
34. Vellinga NAR, Boerma EC, Koopmans M, et al. International study on microcirculatory shock occurrence in acutely ill patients. Crit Care Med. 2015;43:48–56.
35. Rovas A, Seidel LM, Vink H, et al. Association of sublingual microcirculation parameters and endothelial glycocalyx dimensions in resuscitated sepsis. Crit Care. 2019;23:260.

36. Ospina-Tascon G, Neves AP, Occhipinti G, Donadello K, Büchele G, Simion D, et al. Effects of fluids on microvascular perfusion in patients with severe sepsis. Intensive Care Med. 2010;36:949–55.
37. Pranskunas A, Koopmans M, Koetsier PM, Pilvinis V, Boerma EC. Microcirculatory blood flow as a tool to select ICU patients eligible for fluid therapy. Intensive Care Med. 2013;39:612–9.
38. Hanson JP, Lam SWK, Mohanty S, Alam S, Pattnaik R, Mahanta KC, et al. Fluid resuscitation of adults with severe falciparum malaria: effects on acid-base status, renal function, and extravascular lung water. Crit Care Med. 2013;41:972–81.
39. Bruegger D, Schwartz L, Chappell D, Jacob M, Rehm M, Vogeser M, et al. Release of atrial natriuretic peptide precedes shedding of the endothelial glycocalyx equally in patients undergoing on-and off-pump coronary artery bypass surgery. Basic Res Cardiol. 2011;106:1111–21.
40. Chappell D, Bruegger D, Potzel J, Jacob M, Brettner F, Vogeser M, et al. Hypervolemia increases release of atrial natriuretic peptide and shedding of the endothelial glycocalyx. Crit Care. 2014;18:1–8.
41. Bruegger D, Jacob M, Rehm M, et al. Atrial natriuretic peptide induces shedding of endothelial glycocalyx in coronary vascular bed of Guinea pig hearts. Am J Physiol Heart Circ Physiol. 2005;289:H1993–9.
42. Puskarich MA, Cornelius DC, Tharp J, Nandi U, Jones AE. Plasma syndecan-1 levels identify a cohort of patients with severe sepsis at high risk for intubation after large-volume intravenous fluid resuscitation. J Crit Care. 2016;36:125–9.
43. Tauseef M, Kini V, Knezevic N, Brannan M, Ramchandaran R, Fyrst H, et al. Activation of sphingosine kinase-1 reverses the increase in lung vascular permeability through sphingosine-1-phosphate receptor signaling in endothelial cells. Circ Res. 2008;103:1164–72.
44. Zeng Y, Adamson RH, Curry FRE, Tarbell JM. Sphingosine-1-phosphate protects endothelial glycocalyx by inhibiting syndecan-1 shedding. Am J Physiol Heart Circ Physiol. 2014;306:H363–72.
45. Adamson RH, Clark JF, Radeva M, Kheirolomoom A, Ferrara KW, Curry FE. Albumin modulates S1P delivery from red blood cells in perfused microvessels: mechanism of the protein effect. Am J Physiol Heart Circ Physiol. 2014;306:H1011–7.
46. Tanaka S, Escudier E, Hamada S, et al. Effect of RBC transfusion on sublingual microcirculation in hemorrhagic shock patients: a pilot study. Crit Care Med. 2017;45:e154–60.
47. Nielsen ND, Martin-Loeches I, Wentowski C. The effects of red blood cell transfusion on tissue oxygenation and the microcirculation in the intensive care unit: a systematic review. Transfus Med Rev. 2017;31:205–22.
48. Spronk PE, Ince C, Gardien MJ, Mathura KR, Oudemans-van Straaten HM, Zandstra DF. Nitroglycerin in septic shock after intravascular volume resuscitation. Lancet. 2002;360:1395–6.
49. Boerma EC, Koopmans M, Konijn A, et al. Effects of nitroglycerin on sublingual microcirculatory blood flow in patients with severe sepsis/septic shock after a strict resuscitation protocol: a double-blind randomized placebo controlled trial. Crit Care Med. 2010;38:93–100.
50. Jhanji S, Stirling S, Patel N, Hinds CJ, Pearse RM. The effect of increasing doses of norepinephrine on tissue oxygenation and microvascular flow in patients with septic shock. Crit Care Med. 2009;37:1961–6.
51. Dubin A, Pozo MO, Casabella CA, et al. Increasing arterial blood pressure with norepinephrine does not improve microcirculatory blood flow: a prospective study. Crit Care. 2009;13:R92.
52. Straat M, Müller MCA, Meijers JCM, et al. Effect of transfusion of fresh frozen plasma on parameters of endothelial condition and inflammatory status in non-bleeding critically ill patients: a prospective substudy of a randomized trial. Crit Care. 2015;19:163.

Part VII

Sepsis

Macrophage Activation Syndrome in Sepsis: Does It Exist and How to Recognize It?

E. J. Giamarellos-Bourboulis and M. G. Netea

21.1 Introduction

Patients with sepsis present with more or less the same constellation of symptoms, which is driven by organ dysfunction. However, the mechanism leading one infection to cause one or more organ dysfunctions is not the same for all patients and presents great variability. In the era of personalized medicine, one promising approach is to be able to recognize the pathogenic mechanism behind every patient with sepsis and deliver treatment targeting the reversal of this mechanism.

Rheumatologists and pediatricians are aware of a rather rare life-threatening disorder called hemophagocytic lymphohistiocytosis (HLH). HLH is driven through a cytokine storm and manifests with fever, hepatobiliary dysfunction, acute renal injury, encephalopathy, cytopenias, and bone marrow hemophagocytosis. HLH may be primary or secondary. Primary HLH is a rare situation and is also known as familial HLH mediated through mutations of the perforin gene [1]. The most common situations of HLH are secondary to malignancy, viral infections, systemic juvenile idiopathic arthritis (sJIA), and systemic lupus erythematosus (SLE). They are also known as macrophage activation syndrome [1].

Repeated clinical and pathophysiological observations have shown that there is a small subset of patients with sepsis who deteriorate rapidly to early mortality, i.e., death in the first 10 days from the start of sepsis, and it has been hypothesized that these patients have features of macrophage activation syndrome. In this chapter, we try to summarize the published evidence for the association of

E. J. Giamarellos-Bourboulis (✉)
4th Department of Internal Medicine, National and Kapodistrian University of Athens, Medical School, Athens, Greece
e-mail: egiamarel@med.uoa.gr

M. G. Netea
Department of Internal Medicine, Center for Infectious Diseases, Radboud University, Nijmegen, The Netherlands

sepsis characterized by rapid deterioration with macrophage activation syndrome. Epidemiology, pathogenesis, and treatment modalities are presented.

21.2 Classification Criteria and Epidemiology

Traditional pathologists consider macrophage activation syndrome only in cases where hemophagocytosis is found in the bone marrow. In a retrospective analysis of bone marrow smears of patients admitted during the years 2013–2016 with clinical suspicion of HLH, among 40 patients who were eventually classified as HLH all presented with signs of hemophagocytosis; only 32% of cases nonclassified as HLH had signs of bone marrow hemophagocytosis [2]. In the same analysis, it was shown that patients with HLH had a greater number of progenitor cell lineages being phagocytosed than patients without HLH [2]. However, this analysis generates one major ambiguity: how can the exact epidemiology of macrophage activation syndrome be assessed and an eventual diagnosis made when bone marrow biopsy is not routinely performed in rapidly deteriorating patients with sepsis and, even when done, imposes delays in intervention because diagnosis is usually slow.

To this end, and taking into consideration that in the above study 32% of patients without HLH had hemophagocytosis, it is considered that in sepsis, fulminant hyperinflammation should be retained for patients with features of macrophage activation syndrome. Patients can be classified as having macrophage activation syndrome or not based on the use of classification scores. The most widely applied criteria, even if not developed for adults, are the HLH-2004 criteria necessitating that a patient meets 5 out of 8 criteria to be classified as macrophage activation syndrome. These criteria are fever, splenomegaly, bicytopenia, hypertriglyceridemia, or hypofibrinogenemia, bone marrow phagocytosis, low or absent natural killer (NK) cell activity, elevated ferritin, and elevated soluble interleukin (IL)-2 receptor [3]. In 2014, the HScore was introduced for the diagnosis of macrophage activation syndrome in adults based on the analysis of patients' records. The HScore provides points for nine variables as follows: 18 points for known immunosuppression; 33 points for fever between 38.4 °C and 39.4 °C and 49 points when above 39.4 °C; 23 points for presence of hepatomegaly or splenomegaly and 38 points when both are present; 24 points for cytopenia of two lineages and 34 points for 3 lineages; 35 points for ferritin between 2000 and 6000 ng/ml and 60 points when >6000 ng/ml; 44 points for triglycerides between 150 and 400 mg/dl and 64 points when >400 mg/dl; 30 points for fibrinogen <250 mg/dl; 30 points for serum aspartate aminotransferase >30 U/l; and 35 points for phagocytosis on bone marrow aspirate [4].

A PubMed search was done using the terms "sepsis" and "macrophage-activation syndrome" from January 2010 to August 2019. A total of 202 publications were retrieved of which eight publications reported classification of macrophage activation syndrome among sepsis patients [5–12]; one publication is a case report [6] and one reports on children [5]. Seven of these studies were retrospective [5–11] and one was prospective [12] in design. A summary of this search is presented in Table 21.1. With the exception of one study in children, the studies in critically ill

Table 21.1 Reported prevalence of macrophage activation syndrome among critically ill patients

Ref.	Age	Critical care condition	Number of pts./pts. screened	Classification criteria	Features of macrophage activation syndrome	Mortality
[5]	Children	↑ferritin + MODS	23/34 (67.5%)	HLH-2004	• ↑ ferritin 100%; cytopenias 96% • ↑TGs 87%; BMH 100%	13% after 28 d
[6]	Adult	*Acinetobacter baumannii* bacteremia	One	HLH-2004	• Cytopenias; ↑TGs; ↑ferritin • BMH	
[7]	Adults	Severe sepsis	43/763 (5.8%)	HBD + DIC	• HBD 100%; DIC 100% • Other features not reported	65%[a] after 28 d
[8]	Adults	Severe sepsis/shock	16	HLH-204	• Ferritin >7000 ng/ml 100% • ↑TGs 100%; cytopenias[b]	37% after 28 d
[9]	Adults	ICU admissions with ferritin >500 ng/ml	9/244 (3.7%)	HLH-204	• ≥2 cytopenias 100% • Ferritin >3000 ng/ml 100% • ↑AST 77.8%; ↑TGs 55.6%	4/9 (44.4%) after 28 d
[10]	Adults	ICU admissions	10/455 (2.2%)	HLH-2004	Not reported for the classified patients	80% after 28 d
[11]	Adults	Presence of SIRS	5/451 (1.1%)	HScore	• Ferritin>6000 ng/ml 80% • ↑AST 100%; ↑TGs 80%	2/5 (40%) after 28 d
[12]	Adults	Infection and SIRS	Cohort A 128/3417 (3.7%) Cohort B 73/1704 (4.3%)	Sepsis-3 criteria + adjusted HScore for lack of bone marrow aspirate ± (both HBD + DIC)	• Ferritin >4420 ng/ml[c] • ↑AST 77.8%; ↑TGs 55.6%	48.9% after 10 d

AST aspartate aminotransferase, *BMH* bone marrow hemophagocytosis, *d* days, *DIC* disseminated intravascular coagulation, *HBD* hepatobiliary dysfunction, *ICU* intensive care unit, *MODS* multiple organ dysfunction syndrome, *pts* patients, *SIRS* systemic inflammatory response syndrome, *TGs* triglycerides
[a]Refers to the 28-day mortality of patients with MAS-treated with placebo
[b]Exact frequency not reported
[c]At that cutoff reported specificity 97.9%, negative predictive value 97.1%

adults shed light on the problem of inability to routinely perform bone marrow aspirates in a large number of patients [9–12]. To this end, all studies classify patients using the HLH-2004 criteria or the HScore with the bone marrow phagocytosis criterion missing. In other terms, it may be more appropriate to refer to these patients as having macrophage activation-like syndrome [12]. The strictest criteria for classification of macrophage activation-like syndrome in sepsis are derived from a Greek study in 5121 patients with infection and systemic inflammatory response syndrome (SIRS) split into two cohorts [12]. Classification into macrophage activation-like syndrome required both criteria as follows:

- Sepsis defined by the Sepsis-3 definitions.
- HScore ≥151 without considering points attributed to bone marrow aspiration for hemophagocytosis OR copresence of hepatobiliary dysfunction and disseminated intravascular coagulation (DIC). Hepatobiliary dysfunction was defined by the presence of at least two of the following: (1) total bilirubin >2.5 mg/dl; (2) aspartate aminotransferase (AST) at least two times higher than the upper normal limit; and (3) international normalized ratio (INR) >1.5. DIC was defined as a DIC Score of the International Society of Thrombosis and Hemostasis (ISTH) ≥5.

As shown in Table 21.1, the frequency of macrophage activation-like syndrome among critically ill patients ranges between 1.1% to 5.8%.

21.3 Pathogenesis

The pathogenesis of secondary HLH is complex. The main hallmark of pathogenesis is the cytokine storm that is stimulated by three main cell types: tissue macrophages, NK cells, and CD8 lymphocytes. Our knowledge of the series of activations taking place in these cells comes from mutations that are described among patients with viral infections that trigger HLH. These mutations show the pathways involved in the pathogenesis of HLH. However, it should be remembered that many patients develop secondary HLH as a result of non-Hodgkin's lymphoma. The mutations associated with non-Hodgkin's lymphoma may affect the complex lymphocyte–histiocyte interaction giving rise to HLH. A common denominator in the pathogenesis is the attenuation of the apoptosis pathway in both NK cells and CD8 lymphocytes due to decrease in perforin. Once these cells are activated, they overproduce interferon-gamma (IFNγ) that stimulates hemophagocytosis in the bone marrow [13], although one recent study in mice reports stimulation of hemophagocytosis in the absence of IFNγ production [14].

Tissue macrophages of patients with sepsis recognize lipopolysaccharide (LPS) through the transmembrane Toll-like receptor (TLR) 4 resulting in the production of pro-inflammatory cytokines. Stimulation of TLR4 leads to excess production of IL-1β that may *per se* further stimulate NK cell activation. Excess production of IL-1β by liver Kupffer cells leads to overproduction of ferritin by hepatocytes. The overproduction of IL-1β is followed by the production of IL-18. Indeed, in an analysis of Greek patients with macrophage activation-like syndrome split into two cohorts, one for derivation and another for validation, the circulating levels of IL-18, IFNγ, IL-6, and sCD163 were greater among patients with hyperferritinemia in both cohorts. CD163 is a scavenger receptor of the hemoglobin–haptoglobin complex on the cell membrane of tissue macrophages. Increased shedding in the circulation of the soluble form sCD163 is an indirect indication of macrophage activation.

Bone marrow biopsies from 10 patients with HLH due to flare-up of an underlying rheumatology condition or due to systemic infection were retrospectively analyzed. Analysis involved histoimmunochemistry of the bone marrow aspirate for H-ferritin, L-ferritin, and CD68 and cytokines. Results were compared with healthy patients and indicated heavy depositions of H-ferritin but not of L-ferritin. H-ferritin/CD68 co-expression was positively correlated with stained cytokines, negatively correlated with circulating platelets and white blood cells, and positively correlated with serum ferritin and serum C-reactive protein (CRP) [15].

However, damage-associated molecular patterns (DAMPs) of the host, such as high mobility group box-1 (HMGB1), may interact with TLR4 of tissue macrophages when released from damaged cells and further stimulate cytokine production. Indeed, in a series of patients with sepsis caused by Gram-negative bacteria, it was found that a late peak of HMGB1 in the circulation taking place 7 days after the initiation of sepsis was accompanied by increased IFNγ and ferritin in the circulation mimicking features of macrophage activation-like syndrome [16]. Synergy was found between a medical history of type 2 diabetes mellitus, chronic heart failure, and chronic renal disease with the occurrence of this late peak in HMGB1 increasing substantially the risk for 28-day mortality. The priming of tissue macrophages of patients with chronic cardiovascular conditions for IL-1β production may explain this synergy [16].

21.4 Diagnostic Biomarkers

Ferritin is the most broadly studied diagnostic biomarker of macrophage activation syndrome in adults with sepsis. Using one derivation cohort of patients with sepsis diagnosed using Sepsis-3 definitions, it was found that serum ferritin >4420 ng/ml may diagnose macrophage activation-like syndrome with 97.9% specificity and 97.1% negative predictive value. The 28-day mortality for patients of the derivation cohort with ferritin >4420 ng/ml was 66.7%; it was 66.0% in the validation cohort. In the same study, a second validation cohort was used consisting of patients hospitalized in the intensive care unit (ICU) of the Karolinska Institute in Sweden who had severe sepsis/septic shock; 28-day mortality for patients with ferritin >4420 ng/ml was 52.9% [12].

Another study reported the diagnostic value of sCD163 in a pediatric population. Sixty-nine children with sepsis were analyzed of whom 23 were classified with secondary HLH using the HLH-2004 classification criteria. CD163 expression was measured by flow cytometry on circulating monocytes and serum sCD163 was measured by enzyme immunosorbent assay. Both monocyte expression of CD163 and sCD163 were significantly greater among children with sepsis and HLH than among children with sepsis without HLH. The diagnostic accuracy was further increased when sCD163 was used in combination with ferritin. However, this study did not report on any specific diagnostic cutoff either of sCD163 or of ferritin [17].

21.5 Management and Future Perspectives

In 2019, recommendations for the management of HLH in adults were published. These recommendations refer specifically to critically ill patients in the ICU. In these patients, it is necessary to try and diagnose the underlying predisposing cause of HLH. When macrophage activation syndrome is developing due to sepsis, then management is supportive and comprises broad-spectrum antimicrobials to combat the infection and organ support. However, no specific treatment targeting the cascade of events leading to macrophage activation syndrome has been reported [18].

Delivering specific therapy for macrophage activation syndrome mandates that this type of treatment should block the rate-limiting step in pathogenesis, i.e., the production of either IL-1β from tissue macrophages or IFNγ by NK cells and CD8 lymphocytes. More than 25 years ago, a double-blind randomized phase 3 clinical trial was conducted in which patients with severe sepsis were allocated to blind intravenous treatment with placebo or anakinra. Anakinra is the recombinant human receptor antagonist of IL-1ra that binds and inactivates both IL-1β and IL-1α. The study primary endpoint was 28-day mortality. The study was prematurely stopped for futility; however, no safety concern was reported with the use of anakinra [19]. In 2016, patients participating in this trial were retrospectively reclassified as having presented features of macrophage activation syndrome or not. No data were available to score for the HLH-2004 criteria or the HScore. As such, classification into macrophage activation syndrome relied on the copresence of hepatobiliary dysfunction and DIC. Hepatobiliary dysfunction was diagnosed by the increase in total bilirubin and AST and DIC by the presence of prolongation of prothrombin/thromboplastin times and decreased platelet count. This retrospective analysis showed that 17 of the 253 patients originally allocated to the placebo group and 26 out of 510 patients originally allocated to the anakinra group had macrophage activation syndrome; 28-day mortality rates were 65% and 25%, respectively ($p = 0.0006$) [7].

These are not the only data studying the efficacy of anakinra in macrophage activation syndrome. Nineteen children with macrophage activation syndrome secondary to sJIA and periodic fever syndromes were studied. Long-term administration of anakinra for 6 months was safe and led to long-term remission of macrophage activation syndrome [20].

In light of the current view of the pathogenesis of sepsis, it may be argued that activation of immune phenomena in sepsis resembles an axis. On the left side of the axis lie patients with single pro-inflammatory sepsis or macrophage activation-like syndrome; on the right side of the axis lie patients with single anti-inflammatory sepsis or sepsis-induced immunosuppression. The patients who lie between these two extremes have mixed pro- and anti-inflammatory characteristics. This concept gave rise to the PROVIDE trial (A Personalized Randomized Trial of Validation and Restoration of Immune Dysfunction in Severe Infections and Sepsis, ClinicalTrials.gov Identifier: NCT03332225). In that trial, patients with septic shock using the Sepsis-3 diagnostic criteria are screened on two consecutive days by measurement

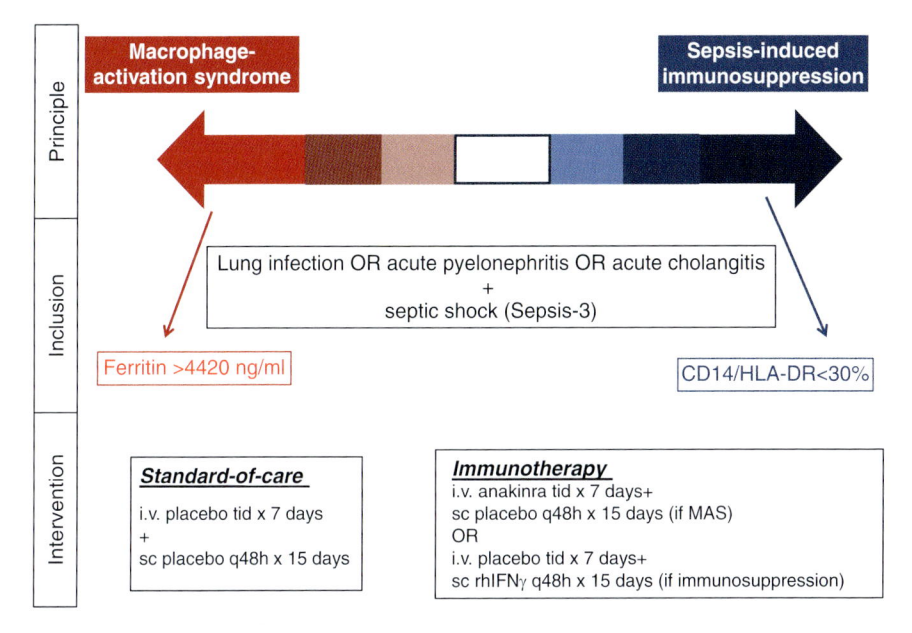

Fig. 21.1 Design of the PROVIDE study (Clinicaltrials.gov Identifier: NCT03332225). *i.v.* intravenous, *MAS* macrophage activation syndrome, *q48h* every other day, *rhIFNγ* recombinant human interferon-gamma, *sc* subcutaneous

of serum ferritin and expression of HLD-DR on CD14-monocytes. Patients with serum ferritin >4420 ng/ml are enrolled as macrophage activation-like syndrome and patients with serum ferritin <4420 ng/ml and CD14/HLA-DR co-expression <30% are enrolled as sepsis-induced immunosuppression. Patients are randomly allocated to the standard-of-care arm of treatment (placebo) or to the immunotherapy arm of treatment. Immunotherapy is delivered double blind and consists of intravenous anakinra three times daily for 7 consecutive days or recombinant human IFNγ every other day for 15 days depending on the diagnosis. The trial has been running since December 2017; trial termination is scheduled for December 2019. The analysis of the PROVIDE study is anticipated to deliver valuable information on (a) the frequency of macrophage activation-like syndrome and sepsis-induced immunosuppression among patients with septic shock and (b) the clinical efficacy of immunotherapy targeting personalized needs. The concept of the PROVIDE study is given schematically in Fig. 21.1.

21.6 Conclusion

The current review showed that in almost 5% of patients with sepsis the mechanism leading to rapid deterioration is dominated purely by pro-inflammatory phenomena or macrophage activation-like syndrome. Diagnosis may rely on the HLH-2004 and the HScore classification systems. However, since routine bone marrow aspirates delay diagnosis, diagnosis may be considerably facilitated by the use of ferritin; concentrations >4420 ng/ml provide almost 98% specificity and negative predictive value for diagnosis. Targeted therapy with anakinra seems the most promising therapeutic option but requires validation in a prospective randomized controlled trial.

References

1. Karakike E, Giamarellos-Bourboulis EJ. Macrophage activation-like syndrome: a distinct entity leading to early death in sepsis. Front Immunol. 2019;10:55.
2. Gars E, Purlington N, Chisholm K, et al. Bone marrow histomorphological criteria can accurately diagnose hemophagocytic lymphohistiocytosis. Haematologica. 2018;103:1635–41.
3. Henter JI, Horne AC, Aricó M, et al. HLH-2004: diagnostic and therapeutic guidelines for hemophagocytic lymphohistiocytosis. Pediatr Blood Cancer. 2007;16:124–31.
4. Fardet L, Galicier L, Lambotte O, et al. Development and validation of the HScore, a score for the diagnosis of reactive hemophagocytic syndrome. Arthritis Rheumatol. 2014;66:2613–20.
5. Demirkol D, Yildizdas D, Bayrakci B, et al. Hyperferritinemia in the critically ill child with secondary hemophagocytic lymphohistiocytosis/sepsis/multiple organ dysfunction syndrome/macrophage activation syndrome: what is the treatment? Crit Care. 2012;16:R52.
6. John TM, Jacob CN, Ittycheria CC, et al. Macrophage activation syndrome following *Acinetobacter baumannii* sepsis. Int J Infect Dis. 2012;16:e223–4.
7. Shakoory B, Carcillo JA, Chatham WW, et al. Interleukin-1 receptor blockade is associated with reduced mortality in sepsis patients with features of macrophage activation syndrome: reanalysis of a prior phase III trial. Crit Care Med. 2016;44:275–81.
8. Kappoor S, Morgan CK, Siddique MA, Gunrupalli KK. Intensive care unit complication and outcomes of adult patients with hemophagocytic lymphohistiocytosis: a retrospective study of 16 cases. World J Crit Care Med. 2018;7:73–83.
9. Lachmann G, Spies C, Schenk T, Brunkhorst F, Balzer F, La Rosée P. Hemophagocytic lymphohistiocytosis: potentially underdiagnosed in intensive care units. Shock. 2018;50:149–55.
10. Meena NK, Sinokrot O, Duggal A, et al. The performance of diagnostic criteria for hemophagocytic lymphohistiocytosis in critically ill patients. J Intensive Care Med. 2019; March 12 https://doi.org/10.1177/0885066619837139, [Epub ahead of print].
11. Gualdoni GA, Hofmann GA, Wohlfarth P, et al. Prevalence and outcome of secondary hemophagocytic lymphohistocytosis among SIRS patients: results from a prospective cohort study. J Clin Med. 2019;8:541.
12. Kyriazopoulou E, Leventogiannis K, Norrby-Teglund A, et al. Macrophage activation-like syndrome: an immunological entity associated with rapid progression to death in sepsis. BMC Med. 2017;15:172.
13. Crayne CB, Albeituini S, Nichols KE, Cron RQ. The immunology of macrophage activation syndrome. Front Immunol. 2019;10:119.
14. Burn TN, Weaver L, Rood JE, et al. Genetic deficiency of IFNγ reveals IFNγ-independent manifestations of murine hemophagocytic lymphohistiocytosis. Arthritis Rheumatol. 2019; August 9, https://doi.org/10.1002/art.41076, [Epub ahead of print].
15. Ruscitti P, Cipriani P, DiBenedetto P, et al. H-ferritin and proinflammatory cytokines are increased in bone marrow of patients affected by macrophage activation syndrome. Clin Exp Immunol. 2017;191:220–8.
16. Karakike E, Adami ME, Lada M, et al. Late peaks of HMGB1 and sepsis outcome: evidence for synergy with chronic inflammatory disorders. Shock. 2019;52:334–9.
17. Cui Y, Xiong X, Ren Y, Wang F, Wnag C, Zhang Y. CD163 as a valuable diagnostic and prognostic biomarker of sepsis-associated hemophagocytic lymphohistiocytosis in critically ill children. Pediatr Blood Cancer. 2019;66:e27909.

18. La Rosée P, Horne AC, Hines M, et al. Recommendations for the management of hemophagocytic lymphohistiocytosis in adults. Blood. 2019;133:2465–77.
19. Opal SM, Fisher CJ Jr, Dhainaut JF, et al. Confirmatory interleukin-1 receptor antagonist trial in severe sepsis: a phase III, randomized, double-blind, placebo-controlled, multicenter trial. Crit Care Med. 1997;25:1115–24.
20. Sönmez HE, Demir S, Bilginer Y, Özen S. Anakinra treatment in macrophage activation syndrome: a single center experience and systemic review of the literature. Clin Rheumatol. 2018;37:3329–35.

Is T Cell Exhaustion a Treatable Trait in Sepsis?

22

M. Fish, C. M. Swanson, and M. Shankar-Hari

22.1 Introduction

Sepsis is defined as life-threatening organ dysfunction caused by dysregulated host responses to infection [1, 2]. Septic shock is defined as a subset of sepsis in which profound circulatory, cellular, and metabolic abnormalities are associated with a greater risk of mortality than with sepsis alone. The global population incidence estimate for hospital-treated sepsis (previously referred to as severe sepsis) in the last decade is 270 (95% CI 176–412) per 100,000 person-years [3]. The incidence of sepsis is increasing and, even with improving trends in outcomes, one in three patients still die in hospital [4, 5]. The number of sepsis survivors discharged from the hospital is also increasing [6]. Importantly, one in six sepsis survivors dies in the first year following hospital discharge [7–9]. Thus, sepsis is associated with a high risk of early and late adverse outcomes (such as mortality) that could be reduced with interventions. Current therapy consists of only supportive treatments and antibiotic therapy; there are no specific interventions that have been proven to reduce sepsis-related deaths. Therefore, therapeutic strategies that improve the prognosis for patients with sepsis are urgently needed.

In the last three decades, more than 200 randomized controlled trials have failed to consistently improve adverse outcomes in sepsis patients. These trials

M. Fish · M. Shankar-Hari (✉)
Peter Gorer Department of Immunobiology, School of Immunology & Microbial Sciences, Faculty of Life Science & Medicine, King's College London, Guy's Hospital, London, UK

Department of Intensive Care Medicine, Guy's and St Thomas' Hospital NHS Foundation Trust, London, UK
e-mail: manu.shankar-hari@kcl.ac.uk

C. M. Swanson
Department of Infectious Diseases, School of Immunology & Microbial Sciences, Faculty of Life Science & Medicine, King's College London, Guy's Hospital, London, UK

share several features [10]. First, candidate interventions were applied globally to a heterogenous population of patients with suspected or proven infection as the likely etiology of acute organ dysfunction [11, 12]. Second, the expected treatment effect of the candidate intervention was often too large. Third, subgroups were often defined *post hoc* and even when defined *a priori*, the expected direction of treatment effect in subgroups was not made explicit at the trial design stage. Thus, the negative results from these trials could be explained by the baseline variability within the sepsis population for the risk of outcome tested [13], the lower than expected attributable risk from sepsis [14], the lower than predicted treatment effect of the candidate intervention, and/or the fact that multiple mechanisms involved in determining outcomes from sepsis are not modified by the candidate intervention [10].

Given these issues, there is a need to identify subpopulations of patients with definite sepsis (practical enrichment), with a greater likelihood to benefit from tested interventions (predictive enrichment) or greater risk of the outcome of interest (prognostic enrichment) [15, 16]. Subpopulations of patients with sepsis who have a well-defined treatment response characteristic and a modifiable biological mechanism are referred to as having a "treatable trait" or "endotype." In this narrative review, we debate whether T cell exhaustion is a treatable trait in sepsis patients, using data primarily from human studies.

22.2 What Is T Cell Exhaustion?

The changes observed in T cell exhaustion are best characterized in cancer and chronic viral infections [17]. While this is currently an area of intense investigation, there are key features at the cellular and molecular level. Exhausted T cells lose their effector function as evidenced by their impaired capacity to produce cytokines (such as tumor necrosis factor [TNF], interferon-gamma [IFNγ], interleukin-2 [IL-2]), impaired cytotoxicity, and impaired proliferation capacity. These effector functions are lost in a hierarchical manner. First, IL-2 production, proliferative capacity, and *ex vivo* cytolytic activity are lost. Next, TNF and IFNγ productions are impaired. Finally, the exhausted cells die due to excessive stimulation.

Exhausted T cells have upregulated cell surface inhibitory molecules referred to as immune checkpoint inhibitors. Immune checkpoints are the inhibitory and stimulatory pathways in immune cells that maintain self-tolerance and regulate the immune responses to danger signals. In exhausted T cells, well studied inhibitory immune checkpoint molecules are upregulated such as programmed death molecule 1 (PD-1), cytotoxic T lymphocyte-associated protein 4 (CTLA-4), lymphocyte-activation gene 3 (LAG-3), T cell immunoglobulin and ITIM domain (TIGIT), T cell immunoglobulin and mucin domain-containing-3 (TIM-3), CD160, and 2B4. Exhausted T cells also have altered metabolic, epigenetic, and transcriptional profiles. They have suppressed glycolytic and mitochondrial metabolism despite mechanistic target of rapamycin (mTOR)-driven upregulation of anabolic pathways and these changes can occur early on in infections [18]. The key epigenetic abnormality in exhausted T cells is the greater chromatin accessibility in exhaustion-specific regions that is fundamentally different from memory T cells. The overall transcriptional program is dysregulated and transcription factors in exhausted T cells that are up- or downregulated include PRDM1/BLIMP1, EOMES, BATF, MAF, NFAT, and TBX21/T-bet.

The key consequence of T cell exhaustion in patients with sepsis is immunosuppression. In healthy people, when T cells are activated they secrete an array of cytokines and chemokines to recruit innate immune cells to sites of infection, enhance their microbicidal activity, help B cell class switch to make antibodies, have *ex vivo* cytolytic activity, and generate T cell subsets including long-lived memory cells [19]. T cell exhaustion impairs pathogen clearance potentially prolonging primary infection, increases the risk of nosocomial infection and reactivation of dormant viruses and potentially increases the duration of sepsis-related organ dysfunction resulting in increased length of hospital stay and increased risk of death (Fig. 22.1).

22.3 There Is Indirect and Direct Evidence for T Cell Exhaustion in Sepsis

Indirect evidence for T cell exhaustion in sepsis comes from pan-leukocyte transcriptome studies [12, 20]. Major changes in the adaptive immune system changes were seen in both these studies. In the study by Davenport and colleagues, a pan-leukocyte transcriptome showed enriched T cell functions of activation, cell death, and apoptosis, with T cell receptor complexes as key upstream regulators [20]. Major alterations in T cell-associated signaling pathways (such as iCOS, CD28, OX40, IL-4, and mTOR), albeit to different degrees depending on the sepsis subphenotype, were also observed by Scicluna and colleagues [12].

Direct evidence for T cell exhaustion comes from the seminal work by Boomer and colleagues [21]. Using splenocytes harvested postmortem from patients with protracted sepsis who died, they analyzed T cell effector functions by assessing cytokine responses to *ex vivo* stimulation with anti-CD3/CD28 beads. They also determined the surface expression of the inhibitory checkpoint molecules PD-1 and CTLA-4 on the splenocytes. This showed that sepsis patients had impaired cytokine production in response to *ex vivo* stimulation and higher expression of these inhibitory immune checkpoint molecules, confirming T cell exhaustion [21]. Other authors have also shown T cell exhaustion in sepsis cohorts, primarily by highlighting the increased expression of inhibitory immune checkpoint molecules on cell surfaces and in serum [22–28]. PD-1 and programmed death-ligand 1 (PD-L1) are upregulated on T and B cells with greater expression found in memory cells compared to naïve cells [22] and higher PD-1 expression is associated with increased risk of death [29]. Abnormalities in PD-1 and PD-L1 pathways are observed for up to 1 year in sepsis survivors [30, 31].

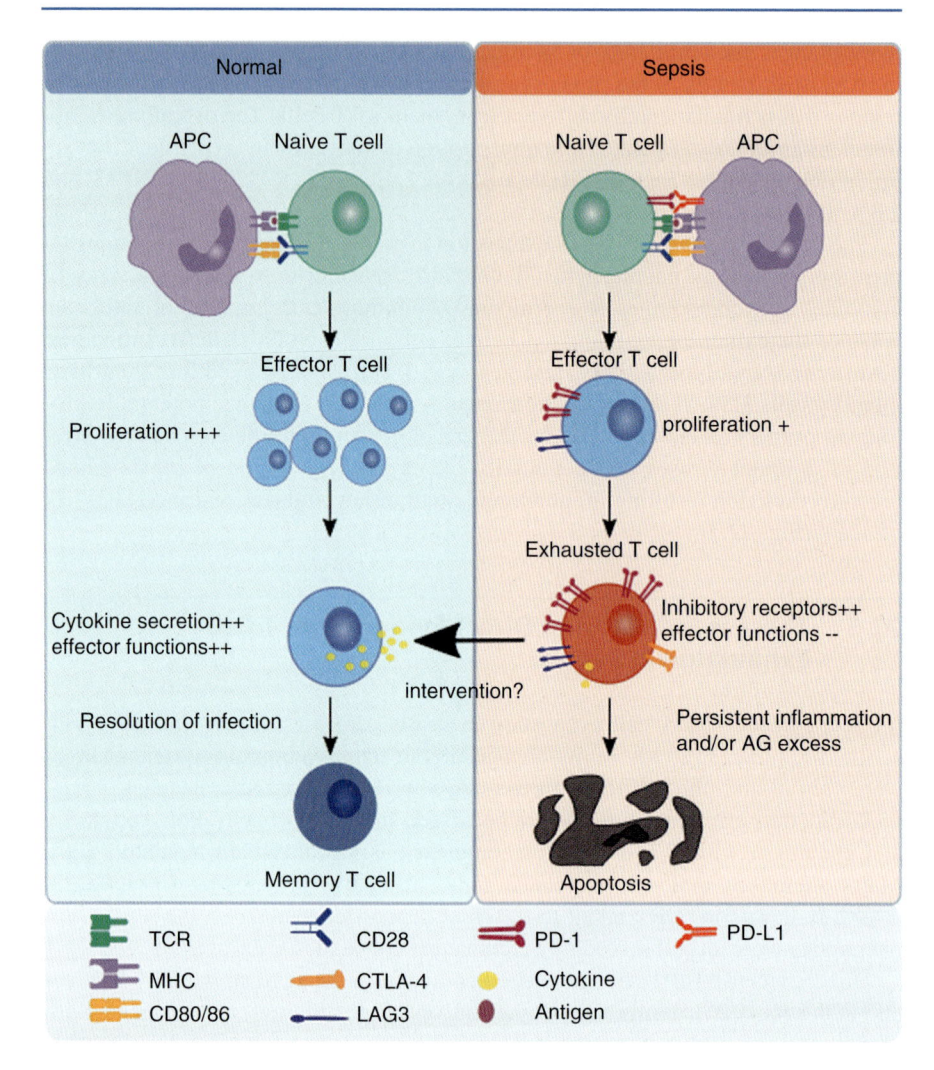

Fig. 22.1 T cell exhaustion in sepsis. During normal infection, naïve T cells are primed and activated through interactions with antigen-presenting cells (APC). Signal transduction is achieved when antigen is recognized through T cell receptors (TCR) and co-stimulation through CD28 and CD80/86 interactions. This allows differentiation into effector cells, which rapidly proliferate and carry out effector functions. Upon successful clearance of antigen, a subset of effector cells differentiates into memory T cells. These cells produce many cytokines, have high survival ability, and can mount rapid recall responses to cognate antigen. During sepsis, persistent inflammation and/or antigen (AG) drives T cell exhaustion promoting immunosuppression. Checkpoint inhibitors, such as programmed death molecule 1 (PD-1) and programmed death-ligand 1 (PD-L1), are upregulated, inhibiting normal T cell functions, such as proliferation. As exhaustion continues, there is an increase in inhibitory receptors (CTLA-4, LAG3), further loss of different effector functions and eventually apoptosis. T cell exhaustion impairs the ability of the adaptive immune to clear pathogen, prolonging primary infection, reactivating dormant viruses, and potentially contributing to secondary infections. Targeting T cell exhaustion through therapies such as anti-PD-1/PD-L1 antibodies may reverse immunosuppression in sepsis and recover T cell function

22.4 T Cell Exhaustion Is Reversible in Cells Isolated from Patients with Sepsis

Patera and colleagues studied leukocyte function before and after passively blocking PD-1 and PD-L1 receptors with antibodies [32]. Leukocytes were obtained from patients with sepsis, non-sepsis critically ill patients and from healthy controls. Patients with sepsis had impaired neutrophil and monocyte function, which correlated with their own PD-L1 expression and with PD-1 expression on CD8+ T cells and natural killer (NK) cells. Interestingly, reduced CD8+ T cell effector functions (such as IFNγ production) were associated with elevated PD-L1 expression in neutrophils. The authors reported that antibodies against PD-1 or PD-L1 restored neutrophil and monocyte function and hypothesized that lymphocyte function was restored [32]. Chang and colleagues also assessed the impact of anti-PD-1 and anti-PD-L1 antibodies in a cohort study involving patients with sepsis and critically ill patients with sepsis [28]. The authors reported that treatment of lymphocytes from sepsis patients with either anti-PD-1 or anti-PD-L1 antibodies reduced lymphocyte apoptosis and restored T cell effector functions, as evidenced by significantly increased IFNγ and IL-2 production [28]. Multidrug-resistant (MDR) bacterial infections are difficult to treat. Thampy and colleagues reported a case series involving 24 sepsis patients who had MDR bacterial infections [33]. These patients had evidence of T cell exhaustion on immunophenotyping. The authors then assessed what proportion of cell secreted IFNγ when treated with IL-7, anti-PD-L1, and OX-40 ligand using the ELISpot method. The best IFNγ response was with IL-7 (62.5%), compared to 41.6% with OX-40 L and 33.3% with anti-PD-L1 [33].

22.5 Case Report of Anti-PD-1 or Anti-PD-L1 Immunotherapy

Fungal infections with mucormycosis are also difficult to treat. A previously healthy 30-year old with polytrauma and burns developed intractable mucormycosis fungal infection, which was preceded by an episode of sepsis. Immunophenotyping revealed low absolute lymphocyte count, low monocyte HLA-DR expression, and increased expression of PD-1 on T cells. Due to the proximity of mucormycosis infection to vascular structures, source control with debridement was not feasible. She was unresponsive to antifungal therapy with liposomal amphotericin-B and posaconazole. The patient made a remarkable recovery following immunotherapy with IFNγ thrice weekly for five doses along with a single 250-mg dose of nivolumab [34].

22.6 Early Phase Randomized Controlled Trials to Reverse T Cell Exhaustion in Sepsis

There have been two recent phase-1 randomized controlled trials assessing the hypothesis that passive immunotherapy with monoclonal anti-PD-L1 antibody (BMS-936559) [35] and anti-PD-1 antibody (nivolumab) [36] may reverse immunosuppression in adult critically ill patients with sepsis and lymphopenia (defined as absolute lymphocyte counts $\leq 1.1 \times 10^3$ cells/µl). Monoclonal anti-PD-L1 (BMS-936559) was administered in escalated doses between 10 mg and 900 mg in 20 sepsis patients and 4 patients were given a placebo. Receptor occupancy of >90% was achieved with the 900 mg dose of BMS-936559 for 28 days after infusion. There was no evidence of drug-induced excess cytokine production, no dose-related increase in adverse events and the immune function improved over 28 days at higher doses of BMS-936559. Monoclonal anti-PD-1 (nivolumab) was administered in two doses of 480 mg in 15 patients and 960 mg in 16 patients with a placebo arm. Receptor occupancy of >90% was achieved with both doses for 28 days after infusion. There was no evidence of drug-induced excess cytokine production, no dose-related increase in adverse events and the immune function improved with both doses [36]. As early phase trials, the key goals for both were to define pharmacokinetics and pharmacodynamics with an emphasis on safety. Sepsis alters the volume of distribution and peak concentrations for most drugs, which was observed in these two trials. It was encouraging to note that there was no cytokine storm for either intervention. Thus, there is a potential opportunity to consider future trials of immune checkpoint inhibitor blocking therapies in adult critically ill patients with sepsis.

Restoring lymphocyte count and function could also be achieved with IL-7. This was tested in a phase-2b placebo-controlled, double-blind, 3-arm randomized controlled trial in 24 sepsis patients with severe lymphopenia (defined as absolute lymphocyte counts $\leq 0.9 \times 10^3$ cells/µl), of recombinant human IL-7 (CYT107) [37]. CYT107 was administered either as low frequency (once weekly) or as high frequency (twice weekly) regimens at a dose of 10 µg/kg body weight, administered intramuscularly, for a duration of 4 weeks. The marked loss of CD4+ and CD8+ immune effector cells was reversed and activation markers of CD4 T cells were increased by CYT107 without an increase in PD-1 expression, implying improvement of impaired lymphocyte function in sepsis patients.

22.7 Designing Future Clinical Trials to Reverse T Cell Exhaustion in Sepsis

The PICO framework (Patient—Intervention—Comparator—Outcome) is a useful structure to discuss this question [38]. In all three early phase trials, the authors enriched the sepsis patient population using low lymphocyte count (lymphopenia). Lymphopenia occurs in nearly 70% of patients with sepsis-related critical illness, with the nadir occurring around three days. This increases the risk of death, with the risk increasing with the severity of lymphopenia, and with persistence of lymphopenia for 3 days or longer [39, 40]. In these early phase trials, lymphopenia is discussed as a prognostic enrichment marker [16] and a marker for presence of immunosuppression. There is no direct evidence to support the notion that lymphopenia is a surrogate for lymphocyte exhaustion and recovery of the lymphocyte count is a marker of immune reconstitution in sepsis patients.

The molecular mechanisms that drive T cell exhaustion in sepsis are poorly understood. Given the major immunological differences between sepsis and cancer or chronic infections, it is essential to understand the molecular basis for T cell exhaustion in sepsis. Predictive enrichment markers need to be identified. The doses for testing for all three interventions in future trials would be the highest tolerated doses in early phase trials. As persistent lymphopenia is a better prognostic enrichment marker with the nadir of lymphocyte count occurring around three days following ICU admission, this may represent a better landmark point for timing of these immunomodulation interventions, as this time point also excludes unmodifiable early deaths. Comparator would be a standard of care, which must be predefined. The outcomes for these interventions could be nosocomial infections or death. It is important to note that attributable risk of death from nosocomial infections may be as low as 15% [41, 42], which will influence sample size considerations. Two potential adverse events to consider with ani-checkpoint inhibitor therapy are cytokine storm and risk of autoimmune reactions. These need to be studied as key adverse events in future trials.

22.8 Conclusion

One facet of immunosuppression in sepsis is T cell exhaustion. This is phenotypically detectable using flow cytometry and is characterized by increased expression of immune checkpoint inhibitory molecules, such as PD-1, LAG-3, and CTLA-4. T cell exhaustion increases the risk of adverse outcomes. Monoclonal antibodies are available against some of these inhibitory molecules and early phase clinical trials suggest that IL-7, anti-PD-1 antibody, and anti-PD-L1 antibody are interventions that should be tested in an enriched sepsis population.

Acknowledgments Dr. Shankar-Hari is supported by the National Institute for Health Research Clinician Scientist Award (CS-2016-16-011). Mr. Fish is supported by the National Institute of Academic Anaesthesia BJA-RCOA PhD Fellowship.

References

1. Singer M, Deutschman CS, Seymour CW, et al. The Third International Consensus Definitions for Sepsis and Septic Shock (Sepsis-3). JAMA. 2016;315:801–10.
2. Shankar-Hari M, Phillips GS, Levy ML, et al. Developing a new definition and assessing new clinical criteria for septic shock: for the Third International Consensus Definitions for Sepsis and Septic Shock (Sepsis-3). JAMA. 2016;315:775–87.
3. Fleischmann C, Scherag A, Adhikari NK, et al. Assessment of global incidence and mortality of hospital-treated sepsis. current estimates and limitations. Am J Respir Crit Care Med. 2016;193:259–72.
4. Kaukonen KM, Bailey M, Suzuki S, Pilcher D, Bellomo R. Mortality related to severe sepsis and septic shock among critically ill patients in Australia and New Zealand, 2000-2012. JAMA. 2014;311:1308–16.
5. Shankar-Hari M, Harrison DA, Rubenfeld GD, Rowan K. Epidemiology of sepsis and septic shock in critical care units: comparison between sepsis-2 and sepsis-3 populations using a national critical care database. Br J Anaesth. 2017;119:626–36.

6. Prescott HC, Angus DC. Enhancing recovery from sepsis: a review. JAMA. 2018;319:62–75.
7. Shankar-Hari M, Ambler M, Mahalingasivam V, Jones A, Rowan K, Rubenfeld GD. Evidence for a causal link between sepsis and long-term mortality: a systematic review of epidemiologic studies. Crit Care. 2016;20:101.
8. Shankar-Hari M, Harrison DA, Ferrando-Vivas P, Rubenfeld GD, Rowan K. Risk factors at index hospitalization associated with longer-term mortality in adult sepsis survivors. JAMA Netw Open. 2019;2:e194900.
9. Prescott HC, Osterholzer JJ, Langa KM, Angus DC, Iwashyna TJ. Late mortality after sepsis: propensity matched cohort study. BMJ. 2016;353:i2375.
10. Marshall JC. Why have clinical trials in sepsis failed? Trends Mol Med. 2014;20:195–203.
11. Shankar-Hari M, Harrison DA, Rowan KM. Differences in impact of definitional elements on mortality precludes international comparisons of sepsis epidemiology—a cohort study illustrating the need for standardized reporting. Crit Care Med. 2016;44:2223–30.
12. Scicluna BP, van Vught LA, Zwinderman AH, et al. Classification of patients with sepsis according to blood genomic endotype: a prospective cohort study. Lancet Respir Med. 2017;5:816–26.
13. Santhakumaran S, Gordon A, Prevost AT, O'Kane C, McAuley DF, Shankar-Hari M. Heterogeneity of treatment effect by baseline risk of mortality in critically ill patients: re-analysis of three recent sepsis and ARDS randomised controlled trials. Crit Care. 2019;23:156.
14. Shankar-Hari M, Harrison DA, Rowan KM, Rubenfeld GD. Estimating attributable fraction of mortality from sepsis to inform clinical trials. J Crit Care. 2018;45:33–9.
15. Prescott HC, Calfee CS, Thompson BT, Angus DC, Liu VX. Toward smarter lumping and smarter splitting: rethinking strategies for sepsis and acute respiratory distress syndrome clinical trial design. Am J Respir Crit Care Med. 2016;194:147–55.
16. Shankar-Hari M, Rubenfeld GD. Population enrichment for critical care trials: phenotypes and differential outcomes. Curr Opin Crit Care. 2019;25:489–97.
17. Pauken KE, Wherry EJ. Overcoming T cell exhaustion in infection and cancer. Trends Immunol. 2015;36:265–76.
18. Bengsch B, Johnson AL, Kurachi M, et al. Bioenergetic insufficiencies due to metabolic alterations regulated by the inhibitory receptor PD-1 are an early driver of CD8(+) t cell exhaustion. Immunity. 2016;45:358–73.
19. van den Broek T, Borghans JAM, van Wijk F. The full spectrum of human naive T cells. Nat Rev Immunol. 2018;18:363–73.
20. Davenport EE, Burnham KL, Radhakrishnan J, et al. Genomic landscape of the individual host response and outcomes in sepsis: a prospective cohort study. Lancet Respir Med. 2016;4:259–71.
21. Boomer JS, To K, Chang KC, et al. Immunosuppression in patients who die of sepsis and multiple organ failure. JAMA. 2011;306:2594–605.
22. Wilson JK, Zhao Y, Singer M, Spencer J, Shankar-Hari M. Lymphocyte subset expression and serum concentrations of PD-1/PD-L1 in sepsis - pilot study. Crit Care. 2018;22:95.
23. Shankar-Hari M, Datta D, Wilson J, et al. Early PREdiction of sepsis using leukocyte surface biomarkers: the ExPRES-sepsis cohort study. Intensive Care Med. 2018;44:1836–48.
24. Niu B, Zhou F, Su Y, Wang L, Xu Y, Yi Z, et al. Different expression characteristics of LAG3 and PD-1 in sepsis and their synergistic effect on T cell exhaustion: a new strategy for immune checkpoint blockade. Front Immunol. 1888;2019:10.
25. Gossez M, Rimmele T, Andrieu T, et al. Proof of concept study of mass cytometry in septic shock patients reveals novel immune alterations. Sci Rep. 2018;8:17296.
26. Boomer JS, Shuherk-Shaffer J, Hotchkiss RS, Green JM. A prospective analysis of lymphocyte phenotype and function over the course of acute sepsis. Crit Care. 2012;16:R112.
27. Spec A, Shindo Y, Burnham CA, et al. T cells from patients with Candida sepsis display a suppressive immunophenotype. Crit Care. 2016;20:15.
28. Chang K, Svabek C, Vazquez-Guillamet C, et al. Targeting the programmed cell death 1: programmed cell death ligand 1 pathway reverses T cell exhaustion in patients with sepsis. Crit Care. 2014;18:R3.

29. Tomino A, Tsuda M, Aoki R, et al. Increased PD-1 expression and altered t cell repertoire diversity predict mortality in patients with septic shock: a preliminary study. PLoS One. 2017;12:e0169653.
30. Riche F, Chousterman BG, Valleur P, Mebazaa A, Launay JM, Gayat E. Protracted immune disorders at one year after ICU discharge in patients with septic shock. Crit Care. 2018;22:42.
31. Yende S, Kellum JA, Talisa VB, et al. Long-term host immune response trajectories among hospitalized patients with sepsis. JAMA Netw Open. 2019;2:e198686.
32. Patera AC, Drewry AM, Chang K, Beiter ER, Osborne D, Hotchkiss RS. Frontline science: defects in immune function in patients with sepsis are associated with PD-1 or PD-L1 expression and can be restored by antibodies targeting PD-1 or PD-L1. J Leukoc Biol. 2016;100:1239–54.
33. Thampy LK, Remy KE, Walton AH, Hong Z, Liu K, Liu R, et al. Restoration of T cell function in multi-drug resistant bacterial sepsis after interleukin-7, anti-PD-L1, and OX-40 administration. PLoS One. 2018;13:e0199497.
34. Grimaldi D, Pradier O, Hotchkiss RS, Vincent JL. Nivolumab plus interferon-gamma in the treatment of intractable mucormycosis. Lancet Infect Dis. 2017;17:18.
35. Hotchkiss RS, Colston E, Yende S, et al. Immune checkpoint inhibition in sepsis: a phase 1b randomized, placebo-controlled, single ascending dose study of antiprogrammed cell death-ligand 1 antibody (BMS-936559). Crit Care Med. 2019;47(5):632–42.
36. Hotchkiss RS, Colston E, Yende S, et al. Immune checkpoint inhibition in sepsis: a Phase 1b randomized study to evaluate the safety, tolerability, pharmacokinetics, and pharmacodynamics of nivolumab. Intensive Care Med. 2019;45:1360–71.
37. Francois B, Jeannet R, Daix T, et al. Interleukin-7 restores lymphocytes in septic shock: the IRIS-7 randomized clinical trial. JCI Insight. 2018;3:e98960.
38. Guyatt GH, Oxman AD, Kunz R, et al. GRADE guidelines: 2. Framing the question and deciding on important outcomes. J Clin Epidemiol. 2011;64:395–400.
39. Shankar-Hari M, Fear D, Lavender P, et al. Activation-associated accelerated apoptosis of memory b cells in critically ill patients with sepsis. Crit Care Med. 2017;45:875–82.
40. Drewry AM, Samra N, Skrupky LP, Fuller BM, Compton SM, Hotchkiss RS. Persistent lymphopenia after diagnosis of sepsis predicts mortality. Shock. 2014;42:383–91.
41. van Vught LA, Klein Klouwenberg PM, Spitoni C, et al. Incidence, risk factors, and attributable mortality of secondary infections in the intensive care unit after admission for sepsis. JAMA. 2016;315:1469–79.
42. Melsen WG, Rovers MM, Groenwold RH, et al. Attributable mortality of ventilator-associated pneumonia: a meta-analysis of individual patient data from randomised prevention studies. Lancet Infect Dis. 2013;13:665–71.

Cell-Free Hemoglobin: A New Therapeutic Target in Sepsis?

L. B. Ware

23.1 Introduction

Sepsis remains one of the most common reasons for intensive care unit (ICU) admission accounting for over 750,000 cases per year in the USA [1]. Although advances in supportive ICU care have improved outcomes for sepsis and other critical illness, mortality for sepsis patients remains high. The lack of pharmacologic therapies for sepsis other than antimicrobials is a major shortcoming of modern ICU care. Similar to other critical illness syndromes, such as acute respiratory distress syndrome (ARDS) and acute kidney injury (AKI), treatments that have been successful in animal models of sepsis have not had efficacy in clinical trials.

As a clinical syndrome, the sepsis definition [2] identifies a heterogeneous group of patients; patients with sepsis have different underlying comorbid conditions, different causative organisms and sites of infection, and differences in host response that contribute to heterogeneous pathobiology. Despite this heterogeneity, most clinical trials in sepsis have relied primarily on identifying patients who meet the clinical definition of sepsis syndrome [2], without any attempt to target trial enrollment based on predicted response to a therapy.

Targeting clinical trial enrollment to patients who are more likely to respond to a specific therapy is termed predictive enrichment [3]. Predictive enrichment has been endorsed by the Food and Drug Administration (FDA) as a valuable approach to clinical trial design [4]. We have identified circulating cell-free hemoglobin as a potential therapeutic target in sepsis. Circulating levels of cell-free hemoglobin could be used to predictively enrich enrollment in clinical trials of agents that target cell-free hemoglobin. In the remainder of this chapter, I will summarize the

L. B. Ware (✉)
Departments of Medicine and Pathology, Microbiology and Immunology, Vanderbilt University School of Medicine, Nashville, TN, USA
e-mail: lorraine.ware@vumc.org

evidence that cell-free hemoglobin is a pathologic mediator of organ dysfunction in sepsis and discuss several therapeutic options for targeting cell-free hemoglobin in sepsis.

23.2 Cell-Free Hemoglobin-Mediated Organ Dysfunction in Sepsis

23.2.1 Cell-Free Hemoglobin Levels in Sepsis

In mammals, the vast majority of hemoglobin is contained within circulating erythrocytes. Any hemoglobin that escapes the confines of the erythrocyte is rapidly scavenged, endocytosed, and degraded such that under normal conditions, cell-free hemoglobin is not detectable in the circulation. A variety of conditions can increase circulating levels of cell-free hemoglobin including acute or chronic hemolytic conditions, infections that directly target red blood cells (RBCs) such as malaria or Babesiosis, left ventricular assist devices (LVADs), and all types of extracorporeal circulation including cardiopulmonary bypass (CPB) and extracorporeal membrane oxygenation (ECMO). Sepsis can also acutely increase levels of circulating cell-free hemoglobin, even in the absence of these known triggers for hemolysis.

Two recent studies have established that critically ill patients with sepsis have elevated levels of plasma cell-free hemoglobin even in the absence of any known hemolytic disorder or the use of extracorporeal circulation and that elevated cell-free hemoglobin is a poor prognosticator in sepsis. In a study of 391 critically ill patients with sepsis, Janz and colleagues [5] reported that 81% of patients had detectable levels of cell-free hemoglobin in the plasma and that higher levels were independently associated with hospital mortality. In a separate cohort of patients with sepsis, Adamzik et al. reported that cell-free hemoglobin levels were independently associated with death [6]. Both of these studies found that even relatively low levels of cell-free hemoglobin in the circulation were associated with poorer outcomes in sepsis. Gross hemolysis, defined as a peripheral blood smear with evidence of RBC fragmentation and a declining hematocrit, was established as an independent predictor of sepsis mortality in patients with polymicrobial bacteremia in 1990 [7].

Mouse studies have also helped to establish that release of cell-free hemoglobin is an important feature of sepsis. Larsen et al. [8] showed that plasma cell-free hemoglobin and free heme levels were elevated in mice rendered septic with cecal ligation and puncture. Administration of additional exogenous free heme greatly enhanced the degree of multiple organ failure and mortality in this model, an effect that was due to Fe-dependent oxidation. Knockout of heme oxygenase-1, an important heme detoxifying enzyme, also enhanced organ dysfunction and mortality in this polymicrobial sepsis model.

Box 23.1 Potential mechanisms of hemolysis in sepsis

Factors that can increase red blood cell (RBC) fragility or decrease deformability
Intercalation of lipopolysaccharide in the RBC membrane
Transfusion of RBCs after prolonged storage
Insufficient glucose supply
Immune-mediated RBC destruction
Complement activation
Transfusion reactions
Factors that can mechanically injure the RBC
Disseminated intravascular coagulation/microangiopathy
Microvascular stasis
Pathogen-mediated RBC injury
Loss of membrane lecithin (*Clostridium perfringens*)
Pore-forming toxins (*Staphylococcus aureus*, *Escherichia coli*, and others)
Direct infection of RBCs (malaria, babesiosis)
Other mechanisms
Induction of RBC apoptosis (eryptosis)

The mechanisms whereby cell-free hemoglobin is elevated in sepsis have not been fully elucidated but are likely multifactorial and variable from patient to patient (Box 23.1) [9]. In addition to factors that can increase RBC fragility in sepsis, RBCs may undergo immune-mediated injury, mechanical injury in the microcirculation or direct injury by pathogens or their toxins. Decrements in the production of scavenging proteins for hemoglobin and heme may also play a role in some patients. In support of this, lower serum haptoglobin and hemopexin levels are associated with worse outcomes in sepsis, particularly in patients with elevated circulating cell-free hemoglobin [10].

23.2.2 Mechanisms of Hemoglobin Toxicity

There are multiple molecular mechanisms whereby cell-free hemoglobin can be injurious (Box 23.2) [11]. These include nitric oxide depletion, damage-associated molecular pattern (DAMP) signaling, and oxidative injury. In addition, hemoglobin breakdown products including heme and free iron may have independent injurious effects. Nitric oxide depletion is thought to be the predominant mechanism leading to vascular disease in patients with chronic hemolytic conditions such as sickle cell disease, but other mechanisms of injury may be relevant as mediators of acute organ dysfunction in sepsis. For example, the oxidative potential of cell-free hemoglobin may be particularly amplified in sepsis. When hemoglobin is constrained to the reducing environment of the RBC, the central heme iron is in the reduced ferrous 2^+ state. Release of cell-free hemoglobin into the extracellular compartment can lead to oxidation of heme iron to the ferric Fe^{3+} state or the highly reactive ferryl Fe^{4+} state [12]. High levels of ambient reactive oxygen species in sepsis can lead to high levels of oxidized Fe^{4+} hemoglobin, which can, in turn, drive lipid peroxidation.

Box 23.2 Mechanisms of hemoglobin toxicity

Reaction with nitric oxide (NO)
Consumes NO leading to vasoconstriction and endothelial dysfunction
Reaction of oxy-hemoglobin with NO generates ferric hemoglobin which can release free heme
Oxidation by peroxides
Generates ferric (Fe^{3+}) and ferryl (Fe^{4+}) hemoglobin and associated globin radicals
Globin radicals can drive lipid and protein peroxidation
Release of free heme from hemoglobin
Heme is a hydrophobic reactive protoporphyrin that can transfer to cell membranes and proteins
Free heme can oxidize low-density lipoprotein, triggering pro-inflammatory, and cytotoxic events
Heme-mediated signaling
Heme can bind Toll-like receptor (TLR)4, triggering pro-inflammatory signaling
Heme inhibits the proteasome
Heme can ligate the nuclear REV-IRB receptor, which regulates circadian rhythm, glucose metabolism, and adipogenesis
Extravascular translocation of hemoglobin
Extracellular hemoglobin forms small (32kD) αβ-chain dimers that can translocate to the vascular wall, kidney, and other tissues

23.2.3 Organ-Specific Effects of Cell-Free Hemoglobin

The acute effects of cell-free hemoglobin on organ function in sepsis have been best studied in the lung. In the isolated perfused human lung, the addition of cell-free hemoglobin to the perfusate at concentrations similar to those observed in sepsis patients increased vascular permeability, leading to pulmonary edema formation (Fig. 23.1) [13]. *In vitro* studies suggest that cell-free hemoglobin has direct effects on pulmonary microvascular endothelial permeability. Cell-free hemoglobin can also injure the lung epithelial barrier. In mice, direct intratracheal instillation of cell-free hemoglobin to target the lung epithelium was sufficient to induce acute lung injury as evidenced by air space inflammation and alveolar–capillary barrier disruption [14]. Direct effects of cell-free hemoglobin were also observed in a mouse lung type II epithelial cell (MLE-12) line; cell-free hemoglobin increased both pro-inflammatory cytokine expression and epithelial paracellular permeability as measured by electrical cell-substrate impedance sensing. Similar pro-inflammatory effects of ferric hemoglobin were reported in human alveolar epithelial cells [15]. Chintagari et al. showed that hemoglobin induced mitochondrial dysfunction and depolarization in cultured alveolar epithelial type I-like cells and that this effect was potentiated by oxidation of the hemoglobin to the ferryl (Fe^{4+}) state [16].

The kidney is also highly susceptible to hemoprotein-mediated injury. In patients with sepsis due to severe malaria, elevation of plasma cell-free hemoglobin was associated with an increased incidence of AKI [17]. Shaver et al. [18] reported that increasing circulating levels of cell-free hemoglobin by administration of intravenous cell-free hemoglobin in a mouse model of polymicrobial intraperitoneal sepsis potentiated AKI as evidenced by decreased glomerular filtration rate (GFR), and increased kidney expression of the kidney injury markers, neutrophil

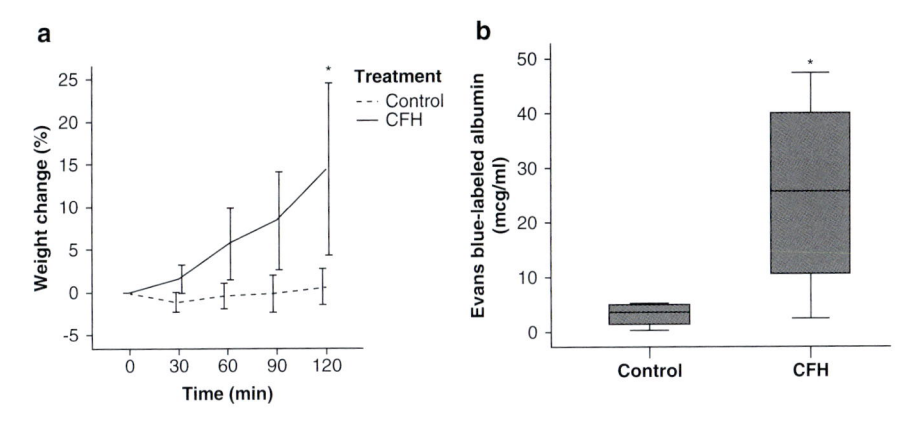

Fig. 23.1 Cell-free hemoglobin (CFH) increased pulmonary edema formation and vascular permeability in *ex vivo* isolated perfused lungs obtained from human organ donors. (**a**) CFH added to the perfusate (100 mg/dl) in the presence of hyperoxia (FiO$_2$ 0.95) results in persistent weight gain over time, indicative of the formation of pulmonary edema, $n = 5$ per group, $*p = 0.047$ versus control. (**b**) CFH increased vascular permeability as evidenced by extravasation of Evans blue labeled albumin into bronchoalveolar lavage fluid, $n = 5$ per group, $*p = 0.027$ versus control at 2 h. Comparisons were made between control and CFH groups by Mann–Whitney U tests (Reproduced from [13] with permission)

gelatinase-associated lipocalin (NGAL) and kidney injury molecule (KIM)-1. Mortality and sepsis severity scores were also increased by intravenous cell-free hemoglobin in that model. Exposure of human tubular epithelial kidney cells to cell-free hemoglobin caused direct cytotoxicity suggesting that cell-free hemoglobin can cause direct renal tubular injury. Tubular injury is a key feature of sepsis-induced AKI [19, 20].

23.3 Targeting Cell-Free Hemoglobin in Sepsis

23.3.1 Overview

Since release of cell-free hemoglobin into the circulation is a common feature of clinical sepsis and has been shown to cause organ dysfunction in experimental models, cell-free hemoglobin represents an important new therapeutic target in sepsis. There are multiple potential approaches to target cell-free hemoglobin in sepsis. Although prevention of the release of cell-free hemoglobin from erythrocytes in sepsis is an attractive upstream target, the mechanisms that promote elevated levels of cell-free hemoglobin in sepsis are likely multifactorial and are not well understood [9]; thus, few interventions have been studied that could prevent cell-free hemoglobin release from erythrocytes. However, strategies that limit RBC transfusion in sepsis may be indirectly beneficial by reducing inadvertent transfusion of cell-free hemoglobin, which is released by degradation of erythrocytes during blood bank storage prior to transfusion and by avoiding hemolysis of transfused erythrocytes. Strategies to increase scavenging of cell-free hemoglobin and to decrease cell-free hemoglobin-mediated oxidation have been the best studied and will be described below.

23.3.2 Haptoglobin

Release of cell-free hemoglobin into the circulation in sepsis can overwhelm endogenous scavenger mechanisms. One approach to reduce circulating levels of cell-free hemoglobin in sepsis is the administration of exogenous scavenger proteins that can bind to cell-free hemoglobin or free heme and promote cellular uptake and degradation. Haptoglobin is the primary endogenous scavenger protein for cell-free hemoglobin. Haptoglobin binds with high affinity to the intact hemoglobin molecule, sequestering cell-free hemoglobin in the intravascular space. Once bound, haptoglobin delivers cell-free hemoglobin to scavenger cells of the reticuloendothelial system via binding to the CD163 receptor. Receptor binding leads to endocytosis of the haptoglobin–hemoglobin complex with subsequent breakdown of the hemoglobin. Although haptoglobin is an acute phase protein in humans, haptoglobin levels are highly variable in sepsis. In a study of 387 patients with sepsis and organ dysfunction, lower haptoglobin levels were independently associated with higher hospital mortality [10]. This finding was most robust in patients with elevated plasma cell-free hemoglobin, suggesting that circulating haptoglobin is critical for limiting the toxicity of cell-free hemoglobin in clinical sepsis.

A number of experimental studies support the therapeutic potential of haptoglobin supplementation in conditions associated with elevated cell-free hemoglobin. In normal guinea pigs and mice, haptoglobin supplementation blocked the toxic effects of transfusion-related cell-free hemoglobin on the heart and kidneys and improved survival [21–23]. In a canine model of severe *Staphylococcus aureus* pneumonia with shock and respiratory failure, purified human haptoglobin administration improved survival, and reduced vasodilatory shock, lung injury scores, and circulating levels of non-transferrin bound iron compared to infusion of human albumin [24]. These findings were accentuated in the setting of superimposed exchange transfusion, which was used to increase circulating cell-free hemoglobin levels, suggesting that the benefit of haptoglobin supplementation was related primarily to improved scavenging of cell-free hemoglobin. Haptoglobin administration was also protective in a neonatal mouse model of necrotizing enterocolitis. In this study, necrotizing enterocolitis was induced by RBC transfusion after premature pups were rendered anemic with serial phlebotomy to mimic the clinical observation that human neonatal necrotizing enterocolitis is associated with antecedent RBC transfusion for anemia and may be mediated in part by increases in cell-free hemoglobin [25].

Purified human haptoglobin has been in commercial use in Japan for the treatment of hemolysis due to extracorporeal circulation, burn injuries, and trauma with massive transfusions since 1985. Data from two small prospective studies and a larger observational study in patients undergoing CPB surgery suggest potential protective effects of exogenous haptoglobin administration on the kidneys but larger prospective trials are needed [26–28]. To date, there have not been any interventional clinical trials of haptoglobin supplementation in humans with sepsis.

23.3.3 Hemopexin

Hemopexin is the endogenous scavenger for the free heme moiety of cell-free hemoglobin. Hemopexin is synthesized by the liver and is normally present in the circulation in high concentrations. Hemopexin has a very high affinity for heme. Once bound to hemopexin, heme is delivered to macrophages of the reticuloendothelial system through the CD91 receptor, preventing the pro-oxidant and pro-inflammatory effects of heme. Heme binding by hemopexin also prevents heme from intercalating in the plasma membrane where it can drive lipid peroxidation [29]. Binding of hemopexin to CD91 leads to internalization of the hemopexin-heme complex with the degradation of heme by heme oxygenase-1 and degradation or recycling of hemopexin.

In humans, normal circulating hemopexin levels are 1–2 mg/ml. In 387 patients with sepsis, the median plasma hemopexin level was only 0.591 mg/ml [10] and lower levels were seen in non-survivors of sepsis across several studies [8, 10, 30]. Low levels of hemopexin and hemopexin-to-heme ratio have also been observed in children with malaria [31].

The therapeutic potential of exogenous hemopexin in sepsis has been explored in animal models. Although hemopexin levels were increased in a variety of mouse models of severe inflammation including endotoxemia, burn wound infection and peritonitis [32], intravenous hemopexin administration reduced pro-inflammatory cytokine expression, nuclear-factor kappa B (NF-κB) activation, acute lung injury, and mortality in a mouse model of sepsis induced by intraperitoneal injection of endotoxin [33]. Hemopexin has not been tested in clinical trials.

23.3.4 Acetaminophen

Acetaminophen has a number of pharmacologic mechanisms, such as inhibition of prostaglandin H_2 synthetase and cyclooxygenase, which are used to treat pain and fever [34, 35]. In addition, it has recently been discovered that acetaminophen at safe, clinically relevant doses can reduce the Fe^{4+} in ferryl cell-free hemoglobin to the less reactive Fe^{3+} form [12, 36, 37]. The specificity of acetaminophen for ferryl cell-free hemoglobin reduction is due to structural similarity between the heme moiety of cell-free hemoglobin and the peroxidase moiety of cyclooxygenase [12]. This unique hemoprotein reductant activity is not present in nonspecific antioxidants such as vitamin E and N-acetyl cysteine at doses that have been studied in clinical sepsis and ARDS [38–40]. Thus, acetaminophen has the potential to target cell-free hemoglobin-mediated organ dysfunction in sepsis where other antioxidants have failed.

In a rat model of AKI due to rhabdomyolysis-induced release of the hemoprotein myoglobin, treatment with acetaminophen before or after rhabdomyolysis induction reduced oxidative injury as measured by F_2-Isoprostanes (a product of lipid peroxidation), and markedly reduced AKI [12]. Acetaminophen also blocked the effects of cell-free hemoglobin on vascular permeability and pulmonary edema formation in the isolated perfused human lung (Fig. 23.2) [13]. In an observational study of 391 sepsis patients [5], clinical use of acetaminophen was independently associated with decreased in-hospital mortality (OR 0.48, 95%CI 0.25–0.91), and lower levels of plasma F_2-Isoprostanes even after accounting for potential confounders; this effect was only evident in patients with elevated plasma cell-free hemoglobin [5]. The protective effect of acetaminophen on cell-free hemoglobin-induced AKI is further supported by a recent observational study [41] in two separate cohorts of pediatric patients undergoing congenital heart surgery, most with the use of CPB. Clinical use of acetaminophen use was independently and dose-dependently associated with less postoperative AKI.

Acetaminophen has also been tested in several small clinical trials that collectively suggest a beneficial effect of acetaminophen on hemoglobin-mediated oxidative injury. In a phase 2a randomized placebo-controlled clinical trial of acetaminophen in 40 patients with severe sepsis and elevated levels of plasma cell-free hemoglobin (measured at enrollment), enteral acetaminophen (1 g every 6 h for 3 days) significantly reduced oxidative injury as measured by plasma F_2-isoprostanes, and AKI as measured by serum creatinine [42]. Acetaminophen also had favorable effects on plasma levels of lipid peroxidation products in two clinical trials in children and adults undergoing cardiac surgery with CPB, a potent inducer of cell-free

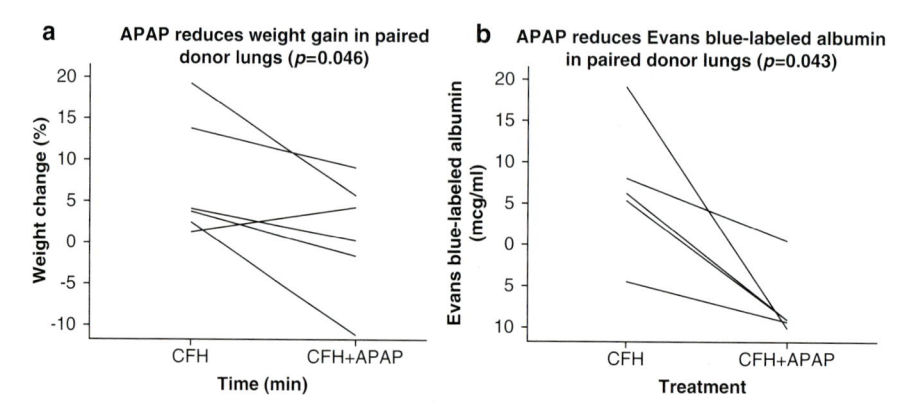

Fig. 23.2 Acetaminophen (APAP), a specific hemoprotein reductant, attenuates microvascular permeability caused by cell-free hemoglobin in isolated perfused human lungs obtained from organ donors. (**a**) *Ex vivo* human isolated perfused lungs inflated with 95% O_2 had less weight gain over time after APAP (15 μg/ml) therapy compared to cell-free hemoglobin (CFH, 100 mg/dl) alone. Each line connects lung weight change for paired donor lungs subjected to CFH and CFH + APAP, *n* = 6 per group, *p* = 0.046 by Wilcoxon rank sum testing. (**b**) Treatment with APAP prevented extravasation of Evans blue-labeled albumin into the airspace, *p* = 0.043 by Wilcoxon rank sum testing (Reproduced from [13] with permission)

hemoglobin release [43, 44]. Finally, a randomized clinical trial in severe falciparum malaria, which causes RBC lysis and high levels of plasma cell-free hemoglobin, also showed a clear beneficial effect of acetaminophen on both lipid peroxidation and AKI [45]. Notably, all of these trials specifically targeted patients with either predicted or measured elevations of cell-free hemoglobin, highlighting the potential for plasma levels of cell-free hemoglobin to be used as a tool for predictive enrichment in clinical trials to target cell-free hemoglobin in sepsis.

23.3.5 Other Potential Therapies

Several other therapeutic agents have the potential to target cell-free hemoglobin-mediated injury in sepsis but are less well studied. Vitamin C (ascorbic acid) has hemoprotein reductant activity and can prevent the increase in endothelial permeability induced by exposure of human endothelial cells to cell-free hemoglobin [46]. Vitamin C has also shown some promise in some clinical trials in sepsis [47] and ARDS, but whether this is related to effects on circulating cell-free hemoglobin is not known. Therapies that target free iron might also be beneficial in the setting of elevated cell-free hemoglobin levels in sepsis.

23.3.6 Current Barriers to Cell-Free Hemoglobin-Targeted Therapeutics

To use circulating cell-free hemoglobin levels as a tool for predictive enrichment of sepsis clinical trials of therapies that target the injurious effects of elevated cell-free hemoglobin, rapid point-of-care measurement of circulating cell-free hemoglobin is needed. Currently, there is no rapid bedside test available for cell-free hemoglobin. Although HemoCue® America markets a point-of-care device that can measure low levels of cell-free hemoglobin (HemoCue® Plasma/Low Hb System), this device is optimized for blood banking rather than measurement of the relatively low levels of plasma cell-free hemoglobin that have been documented in sepsis patients. Although other methods are available for measurement of plasma cell-free hemoglobin, none are rapidly available at the bedside for clinical trial enrollment.

23.4 Conclusion

Sepsis is a heterogeneous clinical syndrome that has defied all attempts to identify effective pharmacologic therapies. A growing body of evidence suggests that an elevated level of circulating cell-free hemoglobin is a feature of some, but not all patients with sepsis. Cell-free hemoglobin can cause tissue injury and organ dysfunction through a variety of injurious mechanisms. The kidney and lung appear to be particularly vulnerable to cell-free hemoglobin-mediated injury. A number of potential therapies to target cell-free hemoglobin in sepsis have been identified including haptoglobin, hemopexin, and acetaminophen. Measurement of cell-free hemoglobin levels at the bedside has the potential to facilitate predictive enrichment for therapeutic trials of these cell-free hemoglobin-targeted therapeutics in sepsis such that only patients with elevated cell-free hemoglobin who would be most likely to benefit would be enrolled. However, rapid, accurate bedside tests for plasma cell-free hemoglobin will need to be developed in order for such trials to move forward.

References

1. Martin GS, Mannino DM, Eaton S, Moss M. The epidemiology of sepsis in the United States from 1979 through 2000. N Engl J Med. 2003;348:1546–54.
2. Singer M, Deutschman CS, Seymour CW, et al. The Third International Consensus Definitions for Sepsis and Septic Shock (Sepsis-3). JAMA. 2016;315:801–10.
3. Prescott HC, Calfee CS, Thompson BT, Angus DC, Liu VX. Toward smarter lumping and smarter splitting: rethinking strategies for sepsis and acute respiratory distress syndrome clinical trial design. Am J Respir Crit Care Med. 2016;194:147–55.
4. US Food and Drug Administration. Enrichment Strategies for Clinical Trials to Support Determination of Effectiveness of Human Drugs and Biological Products: Guidance for Industry. Available at https://www.fda.gov/media/121320/download. Accessed 7 Sept 2019.
5. Janz DR, Bastarache JA, Peterson JF, et al. Association between cell-free hemoglobin, acetaminophen, and mortality in patients with sepsis: an observational study. Crit Care Med. 2013;41:784–90.
6. Adamzik M, Hamburger T, Petrat F, et al. Free hemoglobin concentration in severe sepsis: methods of measurement and prediction of outcome. Crit Care. 2012;16:R125.
7. Cooper GS, Havlir DS, Shlaes DM, Salata RA. Polymicrobial bacteremia in the late 1980s: predictors of outcome and review of the literature. Medicine (Baltimore). 1990;69:114–23.
8. Larsen R, Gozzelino R, Jeney V, et al. A central role for free heme in the pathogenesis of severe sepsis. Sci Transl Med. 2010;2:51ra71.
9. Effenberger-Neidnicht K, Hartmann M. Mechanisms of hemolysis during sepsis. Inflammation. 2018;41:1569–81.
10. Janz DR, Bastarache JA, Sills G, et al. Association between haptoglobin, hemopexin and mortality in adults with sepsis. Crit Care. 2013;17:R272.
11. Schaer DJ, Buehler PW, Alayash AI, Belcher JD, Vercellotti GM. Hemolysis and free hemoglobin revisited: exploring hemoglobin and hemin scavengers as a novel class of therapeutic proteins. Blood. 2013;121:1276–84.
12. Boutaud O, Moore KP, Reeder BJ, et al. Acetaminophen inhibits hemoprotein-catalyzed lipid peroxidation and attenuates rhabdomyolysis-induced renal failure. Proc Natl Acad Sci U S A. 2010;107:2699–704.
13. Shaver CM, Wickersham N, McNeil JB, et al. Cell-free hemoglobin promotes primary graft dysfunction through oxidative lung endothelial injury. JCI Insight. 2018;3:e98546.
14. Shaver CM, Upchurch CP, Janz DR, et al. Cell-free hemoglobin: a novel mediator of acute lung injury. Am J Physiol Lung Cell Mol Physiol. 2016;310:L532–41.
15. Mumby S, Ramakrishnan L, Evans TW, Griffiths MJ, Quinlan GJ. Methemoglobin-induced signaling and chemokine responses in human alveolar epithelial cells. Am J Physiol Lung Cell Mol Physiol. 2014;306:L88–100.
16. Chintagari NR, Jana S, Alayash AI. Oxidized ferric and ferryl forms of hemoglobin trigger mitochondrial dysfunction and injury in alveolar type I cells. Am J Respir Cell Mol Biol. 2016;55:288–98.

17. Plewes K, Kingston HWF, Ghose A, et al. Cell-free hemoglobin mediated oxidative stress is associated with acute kidney injury and renal replacement therapy in severe falciparum malaria: an observational study. BMC Infect Dis. 2017;17:313.
18. Shaver CM, Paul MG, Putz ND, et al. Cell-free hemoglobin augments acute kidney injury during experimental sepsis. Am J Physiol Renal Physiol. 2019;317:F922–9.
19. Alobaidi R, Basu RK, Goldstein SL, Bagshaw SM. Sepsis-associated acute kidney injury. Semin Nephrol. 2015;35:2–11.
20. Zarbock A, Gomez H, Kellum JA. Sepsis-induced acute kidney injury revisited: pathophysiology, prevention and future therapies. Curr Opin Crit Care. 2014;20:588–95.
21. Baek JH, D'Agnillo F, Vallelian F, et al. Hemoglobin-driven pathophysiology is an in vivo consequence of the red blood cell storage lesion that can be attenuated in guinea pigs by haptoglobin therapy. J Clin Invest. 2012;122:1444–58.
22. Baek JH, Zhang X, Williams MC, et al. Extracellular Hb enhances cardiac toxicity in endotoxemic guinea pigs: protective role of haptoglobin. Toxins (Basel). 2014;6:1244–59.
23. Graw JA, Mayeur C, Rosales I, et al. Haptoglobin or hemopexin therapy prevents acute adverse effects of resuscitation after prolonged storage of red cells. Circulation. 2016;134:945–60.
24. Remy KE, Cortes-Puch I, Solomon SB, et al. Haptoglobin improves shock, lung injury, and survival in canine pneumonia. JCI Insight. 2018;3:e123013.
25. MohanKumar K, Namachivayam K, Song T, et al. A murine neonatal model of necrotizing enterocolitis caused by anemia and red blood cell transfusions. Nat Commun. 2019;10:3494.
26. Tanaka K, Kanamori Y, Sato T, et al. Administration of haptoglobin during cardiopulmonary bypass surgery. ASAIO Trans. 1991;37:M482–3.
27. Nomura K, Hashimoto K, Miyamoto N, et al. Hemolytic renal damage during cardiopulmonary bypass and the preventive effect of haptoglobin. Jpn J Cadiovasc Surg. 1993;22:404–8.
28. Kubota K, Egi M, Mizobuchi S. Haptoglobin administration in cardiovascular surgery patients: its association with the risk of postoperative acute kidney injury. Anesth Analg. 2017;124:1771–6.
29. Miller YI, Smith A, Morgan WT, Shaklai N. Role of hemopexin in protection of low-density lipoprotein against hemoglobin-induced oxidation. Biochemistry (Mosc). 1996;35:13112–7.
30. Jung JY, Kwak YH, Kim KS, Kwon WY, Suh GJ. Change of hemopexin level is associated with the severity of sepsis in endotoxemic rat model and the outcome of septic patients. J Crit Care. 2015;30:525–30.
31. Elphinstone RE, Conroy AL, Hawkes M, et al. Alterations in systemic extracellular heme and hemopexin are associated with adverse clinical outcomes in Ugandan children with severe malaria. J Infect Dis. 2016;214:1268–75.
32. Lin T, Maita D, Thundivalappil SR, et al. Hemopexin in severe inflammation and infection: mouse models and human diseases. Crit Care. 2015;19:166.
33. Jung JY, Kwak YH, Chang I, et al. Protective effect of hemopexin on systemic inflammation and acute lung injury in an endotoxemia model. J Surg Res. 2017;212:15–21.
34. Ouellet M, Percival MD. Mechanism of acetaminophen inhibition of cyclooxygenase isoforms. Arch Biochem Biophys. 2001;387:273–80.
35. Anderson BJ. Paracetamol (Acetaminophen): mechanisms of action. Paediatr Anaesth. 2008;18:915–21.
36. Gonzalez-Sanchez MI, Manjabacas MC, Garcia-Carmona F, Valero E. Mechanism of acetaminophen oxidation by the peroxidase-like activity of methemoglobin. Chem Res Toxicol. 2009;22:1841–50.
37. Boutaud O, Roberts LJ 2nd. Mechanism-based therapeutic approaches to rhabdomyolysis-induced renal failure. Free Radic Biol Med. 2011;51:1062–7.
38. Szakmany T, Hauser B, Radermacher P. N-acetylcysteine for sepsis and systemic inflammatory response in adults. Cochrane Database Syst Rev. 2012:CD006616.
39. Roberts LJ 2nd, Oates JA, Linton MF, et al. The relationship between dose of vitamin E and suppression of oxidative stress in humans. Free Radic Biol Med. 2007;43:1388–93.

40. Blumberg JB, Frei B. Why clinical trials of vitamin E and cardiovascular diseases may be fatally flawed. Commentary on "The relationship between dose of vitamin E and suppression of oxidative stress in humans". Free Radic Biol Med. 2007;43:1374–6.
41. Van Driest SL, Jooste EH, Shi Y, et al. Association between early postoperative acetaminophen exposure and acute kidney injury in pediatric patients undergoing cardiac surgery. JAMA Pediatr. 2018;172:655–63.
42. Janz DR, Bastarache JA, Rice TW, et al. Randomized, placebo-controlled trial of acetaminophen for the reduction of oxidative injury in severe sepsis: the Acetaminophen for the Reduction of Oxidative Injury in Severe Sepsis trial. Crit Care Med. 2015;43:534–41.
43. Simpson SA, Zaccagni H, Bichell DP, et al. Acetaminophen attenuates lipid peroxidation in children undergoing cardiopulmonary bypass. Pediatr Crit Care Med. 2014;15:503–10.
44. Billings FT, Petracek MR, Roberts LJ 2nd, Pretorius M. Perioperative intravenous acetaminophen attenuates lipid peroxidation in adults undergoing cardiopulmonary bypass: a randomized clinical trial. PLoS One. 2015;10:e0117625.
45. Plewes K, Kingston HWF, Ghose A, et al. Acetaminophen as a renoprotective adjunctive treatment in patients with severe and moderately severe Falciparum malaria: a randomized, controlled, open-label trial. Clin Infect Dis. 2018;67:991–9.
46. Kuck JL, Bastarache JA, Shaver CM, et al. Ascorbic acid attenuates endothelial permeability triggered by cell-free hemoglobin. Biochem Biophys Res Commun. 2018;495:433–7.
47. Marik PE, Khangoora V, Rivera R, Hooper MH, Catravas J. Hydrocortisone, vitamin c, and thiamine for the treatment of severe sepsis and septic shock: A retrospective before-after study. Chest. 2017;151:1229–38.

Therapeutic Potential of the Gut Microbiota in the Management of Sepsis

M. Bassetti, A. Bandera, and A. Gori

24.1 Introduction

During the last 20 years, the fields of microbiology and infectious diseases have faced a paradigm shift thanks to the discovery of the complex interactions between the host, its immune system, its microbiome, and various pathogens. In fact, the development of various techniques, such as metagenomics, metatranscriptomics, metaproteomics, and metabolomics, has let scientists discover the inner structure of human genetic composition. The human microbiome has been defined as the collective genome of millions of bacteria, viruses, and fungi that exists on every human host. It plays an elegant mutualistic relationship with the human host from birth [1]. Specifically, the human gastrointestinal tract contains trillions of bacteria that compose a complex ecosystem known as the intestinal microbiota that has relevant implications in human health and disease, especially in the hospital setting [2]. Resident microbiota can outcompete pathogens for space, metabolites and nutrients, and can inhibit pathogens with the calibration of the host immune response. Perturbation of these mechanisms is a common starting point for infection, with antibiotic therapy representing the most common cause of microbiome dysregulation [3].

The interaction between sepsis and the microbiome has been defined as an "incompletely understood bi-directional relationship." Some evidence has shown that a diverse and balanced gut microbiota is able to enhance host immunity to both enteric and systemic pathogens and that disturbance of this balance potentially leads to increased susceptibility of sepsis. On the other hand, other studies have shown that the composition of the intestinal microbiota is severely affected by sepsis and its treatment, but the clinical consequences of these disturbances need to be further investigated. In this chapter, we provide an overview of the mechanisms through which gut microbiota can contribute to both susceptibility and outcome of sepsis. We will then describe potential therapeutic effects of interventions on the gut microbiome in the setting of septic and critically ill patients.

24.2 Mechanisms of Dysbiosis in Sepsis

During recent years, resident gut microbial flora has been identified as a key factor in a broad range of functions, such as food digestion, hormone production, and immune system development. Moreover, it has been demonstrated that a condition of disturbance of the gut microbiota, also termed "dysbiosis," can definitely influence host susceptibility to infections.

In general, the gut microbiota consists of three domains of life: bacteria, archaea, and eukarya. The human gut microbiota has a large variety of bacterial species—around 200 dominant species and 1000 non-dominant species—and they vary across individuals. The diversity within an individual's microbiota is known as alpha diversity, whereas different composition between individuals is called beta diversity. Four phyla represent most of the microbiota members: *Bacteroidetes*, *Firmicutes*, *Actinobacteria*, and *Proteobacteria*, the former and the latter accounting for more than 90% of the bacterial population of the colon. The bacteroidetes phylum is composed of Gram-negative, rod-shaped bacteria that digest complex polysaccharides with the release of volatile short-chain fatty acids that regulate intestinal epithelial cell growth as well as differentiation and stimulation of the immune system. The *Firmicutes* phylum is composed mainly of Gram-positive bacteria that can form endospores (*Clostridia* class). These bacteria release butyrate, promoting intestinal epithelial health and inducing colonic T regulatory cells. However, these phyla contain clinically relevant members such as *Bacteroides fragilis*, *Clostridium perfringens*, *Clostridium difficile*, *Enterococcus* spp., and *Streptococcus* spp. that can cause sepsis and fatal outcome during intestinal dysbiosis [2]. As the composition of the gut microbiota is specific for each person, dysbiosis can be interpreted as a relative change in the composition of an individual's commensal microbiota compared with others in the community, which can be loss of beneficial microbiota, increased pathogenic microbiota or decreased microbiota variety. Several mechanisms presenting during gut barrier dysfunction can be considered both a result and a cause of sepsis development: the increased permeability of gut mucosa, tissue edema, reduced perfusion, dysregulation of tissue coagulation, shift in the gut microbiome, apoptotic damage to the mucosal epithelia, and bacterial translocation. Gut mucosal perfusion is reduced during sepsis, which produces destruction of the

24 Therapeutic Potential of the Gut Microbiota in the Management of Sepsis

Box 24.1 Glossary of terms

Microbiome	Collective genome of millions of bacteria, viruses, and fungi that exists on every human host
Microbiota	The totality of microbial genomes in a definite host or organ
Pathobiome	The dysregulation between diverse resident bacterial populations in the gut
Dysbiosis	Condition of disturbance of gut microbiota
Metagenomics	The study of the collective genomes of a given community of microorganisms
Metabolomics	The study of the total small metabolites present in a given environment
Alpha diversity	The diversity within an individual's microbiota
Beta diversity	Different composition of microbiota between individuals
Prebiotics	Nutrients that favor the growth and predominance of beneficial microbes and their inherent functions
Probiotics	Live microorganisms which, when administered in adequate amounts, confer a health benefit on the host
Synbiotics	Combination of probiotics and prebiotics

Adapted from [9]

mucosal barrier and increased permeability [4]. Transmigration of bacteria and endotoxin can induce relevant systemic effects, inducing an immune response in the local gut-associated lymphoid tissue (GALT), which in turn activates Toll-like receptor (TLR)4 and priming neutrophils, causing remote lung injury, explaining the appearance of acute respiratory distress syndrome (ARDS) during sepsis [5]. The dysregulation between diverse resident bacterial populations in the gut can lead to a "pathobiome" that finally dysregulates the immune system [6] (Box 24.1). Indeed, in critically ill patients, hypoxic injury, disrupted epithelial permeability, altered gut motility, and treatment with vasopressors, parenteral nutrition, and opioids facilitate the expansion of pathobionts, including multidrug-resistant (MDR) bacteria [7]. Commonly, the gut microbiome of septic intensive care unit (ICU) patients demonstrates a loss of microbial richness and diversity, dominance of a single taxon (often a potential pathogen), and loss of site specificity with isolation of the same organism at multiple sites [8]. The duration of ICU dysbiosis, the clinical impact of dysbiosis, and phenotypes of critically ill patients more prone to develop it are all aspects that need to be clarified.

24.3 Dysbiosis as a Potential Risk Factor for Sepsis

It is generally assumed that sepsis mortality is due to an immunologic disorder, where the causative pathogen is considered irrelevant once the deregulated immune response has begun [10]. As a healthy gut microbiota has been demonstrated to have protective effects on the host and to prevent colonization with MDR bacteria, several researchers have hypothesized that shifts in microbiota composition potentially predispose patients to a state of immunosuppression and thus increase the risk of sepsis.

In an animal model of mice fed with an obesogenic Western diet, a diet high in fat and sucrose and low in fiber, it has been recently demonstrated that they become susceptible to lethal sepsis with multiple organ damage after exposure to antibiotics and an otherwise-recoverable sterile surgical injury. Analysis of the gut microbiota in this model demonstrated that the Western diet alone led to loss of *Bacteroidetes*, increased *Proteobacteria*, and had evidence of antibiotic resistance development even before antibiotics were administered. In this elegant work, it was clearly shown how the selective pressures of diet, antibiotic exposure, and surgical injury can converge on the microbiome, resulting in lethal sepsis and organ damage without the introduction of an exogenous pathogen [11].

A similar recent study conducted by Napier and colleagues, while confirming the effect of Western diet on disease state and outcomes of a lipopolysaccharide (LPS)-driven sepsis model, found that this relationship was independent of the microbiome. Indeed, they demonstrated that Western diet-fed mice had higher baseline inflammation and signs of sepsis-associated immunoparalysis compared with mice fed with standard fiber-rich chow. Western diet mice also had an increased frequency of neutrophils, some with an "aged" phenotype, in the blood during sepsis compared with standard fiber-rich mice. Importantly, they found that the Western diet-dependent increase in sepsis severity and higher mortality was independent of the microbiome, suggesting that the diet may be directly regulating the innate immune system through an unknown mechanism [12].

This preclinical observation has been confirmed by some limited clinical studies in which patients who developed sepsis showed an altered microbiota pattern at baseline. In a recent study, differences in the gut microbiota and plasma LPS level were evaluated in 32 patients who underwent splenectomy and 42 healthy individuals. The splenectomy group was divided into three subgroups according to the length of their postoperative time. Significant differences were observed in gut microbiota composition measured by 16s rRNA gene sequencing with regard to the relative bacterial abundances of 2 phyla, 7 families, and 15 genera. The LPS level was significantly higher in the splenectomy group than in healthy controls and was negatively associated with five bacterial families with low abundance in the splenectomy group. Interestingly, the degree of gut microbiota alteration increased with the length of the postoperative time [13]. Similarly, a seminal study showed that patients undergoing allogeneic bone marrow transplantation who developed antibiotic-induced dysbiosis had a five- to ninefold increased risk of bloodstream infection and sepsis [14]. These observations were confirmed by a retrospective cohort study including over 10,000 elderly patients in the United States and showing that dysbiosis was associated with a more than threefold increased incidence of a subsequent hospitalization for sepsis [15]. Expanding on these findings, Baggs et al. recently showed that exposure to longer durations of antibiotics, additional classes of antibiotics and broader-spectrum antibiotics during hospitalization were each associated with dose-dependent increases in the risk of subsequent sepsis. This association was not found for other causes of hospital readmissions, suggesting that the association between antibiotic exposure and subsequent sepsis is related to microbiome depletion, not to severity of illness [16].

Accumulating evidences thus indicate that gut microbiota disruption may increase the risk of sepsis; future innovations focused on restoring or protecting the gut microbiota from disruption might become a possible approach for preventing sepsis, especially in fragile populations.

24.4 The Gut Microbiota as a Predictor of Clinical Outcome in Sepsis

The transition of a microbiome into a pathobiome has also been hypothesized to be a driver of severe outcome and mortality from sepsis, at least in part by the ability of invading bacteria to act as antigens and thus modulate the host immune response.

In animal models, the effect of the gut microbiome on sepsis outcome has been clearly demonstrated by different studies. In a well-designed recent study, sepsis evolution was analyzed in genetically identical, age- and sex-matched mice obtained from different vendors and subjected to cecal ligation and puncture (CLP), the most frequently used model of sepsis [17]. Beta diversity of the microbiome measured from feces of mice coming from two different laboratories demonstrated significant differences and, more importantly, mice from the first lab had significantly higher mortality following CLP, as compared to mice from the second lab (90% vs. 53%). Differences were also found in immune phenotypes in splenic or Peyer's patch lymphocytes. To verify if the differences in the microbiome were responsible for the different outcomes, mice were co-housed for 3 weeks, after which they assumed a similar microbiota composition. Interestingly, co-housed mice had similar survival regardless of their vendor of origin and differences in immune phenotype disappeared. This elegant experiment clearly shows that the microbiome plays a crucial role in survival from and in the host immune response to sepsis, representing a potential target for therapeutic intervention.

Clinical studies also confirmed the observation that outcome of sepsis could be influenced by gut microbiota disruption. In the ICU setting, Shimizu et al. quantitatively measured changes in gut microbiota in patients with systemic inflammatory response syndrome (SIRS). These patients had 100–10,000 times fewer total anaerobes, including *Bifidobacterium* and *Lactobacillus*, and 100 times more *Staphylococcus* bacteria compared with healthy volunteers. An important finding of this study was that the dominant factors associated with mortality and septic complications were the numbers of total obligate anaerobes [6]. To evaluate the effect of dynamics of the gut microbiome, a single-center study prospectively analyzed 12 ICU patients and showed that changes in the gut microbiota can be associated with patient prognosis [18]. Indeed, the proportions of *Bacteroidetes* and *Firmicutes* significantly changed during the stay in the ICU, and "extreme changes" in the *Bacteroides/Firmicutes* ratio were observed in almost all the patients with a poor prognosis, suggesting a correlation between alteration in gut microbiota composition and sepsis outcome [18].

The gut has been also hypothesized to be "the motor" of multiple organ dysfunction syndrome (MODS), as reviewed by Klingensmith and Coopersmith [19]. Indeed, evidence from models of murine sepsis and from human patients with ARDS has shown that the lung microbiota is enriched by bacteria translocating from the gut. Importantly, the presence of these bacteria, such as *Bacteroides* spp, is associated with the grade of systemic and local inflammation [20]. Moreover, preliminary studies performed in mice and in patients dying from sepsis suggest that microbial translocation from the gut can be related to neuro-inflammation in sepsis [21]. All these observations provide evidence that dysbiosis observed during sepsis could potentially contribute to worsening inflammation and consequently severe clinical outcome. However, well-designed human clinical studies are still needed as our current knowledge of the consequences of ICU-related dysbiosis in clinical practice is limited.

24.5 Modulation of the Microbiota as Potential Therapeutic Immunonutrition

Probiotics are considered as living microorganisms, which, in adequate amounts, can induce health benefits to the human host. Among them, the genera *Lactobacillus* and *Bifidobacterium* are the most widely used. Probiotics have been increasingly applied and studied in different clinical applications. Probiotics have been hypothesized to reduce the risk of disease through competition for binding locus and nutrients with pathogens, producing bacteriocins to kill pathogens, synthesizing IgA to support immune responses and reducing inflammation. Prebiotics are defined as a non-digestible food ingredient that beneficially impacts the host by stimulating the growth and/or activity of a limited number of bacterial species in the gut. Synbiotics are composed of probiotics and prebiotics.

In the context of sepsis models and ICU patients, probiotics have been studied and evaluated in terms of sepsis evolution and subsequent outcome. A study by Chen and coauthors reported that prophylactic administration of a probiotic bacterial species in a septic mouse model effectively reduced mortality [22]. More recently, a study conducted on a model of septic mice specifically demonstrated that after the onset of sepsis, there was an appearance of opportunistic gut pathogens such as *Staphylococcaceae* and *Enterococcaceae* and a disappearance of beneficial *Prevotellaceae* [23]. Relative abundance of potentially pathogenic commensals was associated with more severe immune responses during sepsis, demonstrated by higher peripheral pro-inflammatory cytokine levels, gut epithelial cell apoptosis, and disruption of tight junctions. Interestingly, in animals pre-treated with *Lactobacillus rhamnosus* GG, opportunistic pathogens decreased or even disappeared, while beneficial bacteria, such as *Verrucomicrobiaceae*, increased, promoting inhibition of gut epithelial cell apoptosis and tight junction formation. Moreover, in a novel *in vitro* gut model to study *Candida* pathogenicity, the introduction of a microbiota of antagonistic lactobacilli emerged as a significant factor for protection against *C. albicans*-induced necrotic damage, with a time-, dose-, and species-dependent protective effect of probiotics against *C. albicans*-induced cytotoxicity [24].

Use of prebiotics/probiotics/synbiotics in clinical ICU studies has been evaluated in many small studies in different populations (summarized in Table 24.1): (1) to prevent infections, especially in the context of postoperative and mechanically

Table 24.1 Immunonutrition in critically ill patients: clinical settings, outcomes, and research gaps

Clinical settings	Products	Outcomes	Research gaps
Mechanically ventilated patients	Probiotics Synbiotics	Incidence of VAP	Choice of probiotics/synbiotics; dosing and route of administration VAP definition Adverse effects evaluation Paucity of data on the effect on MDR colonization
Elective surgery/trauma	Probiotics Synbiotics	Incidence of postoperative/post-traumatic infections	Paucity of data on microbiota before surgery Choice of probiotics/synbiotics; dosing and route of administration Adverse effects evaluation
Pre-term infants	Probiotics Synbiotics	Incidence of sepsis Incidence of necrotizing enterocolitis	Impact of type of feeding (mother's milk, donor milk, formula) Evaluation of impact of human milk oligosaccharides on microbiome Choice of single probiotic strain versus multiple strains To address the risk of probiotic-related sepsis and transmission of antibiotic resistance To address the risk of cross-colonization or cross-contamination
ICU patients	Probiotics Synbiotics	Incidence of new infections Mortality ICU length stay	Choice of probiotics/synbiotics; dosing and route of administration To address short- and long-term effects on gut microbiome To address candidate populations and timing of administration

VAP ventilator-associated pneumonia, *MDR* multidrug resistant, *ICU* intensive care unit

ventilated patients; (2) to improve outcome of sepsis; (3) to restore gut commensals after sepsis to reduce late infections and subsequent mortality.

Administration of probiotics and synbiotics had been demonstrated to reduce infectious complications, and meta-analyses suggest that probiotics are safe and effective at preventing infection in both postoperative and mechanically ventilated patients [25, 26]. However, various concerns have been raised regarding the type and optimal dose of probiotic therapy, as well as the small size of the individual studies. Morrow et al., in the most rigorous study, reported that the incidence of ventilator-associated pneumonia (VAP) in patients treated with *L. rhamnosus* GG was significantly lower than in controls (19.1% vs. 40.0%) in 138 ICU patients. Moreover, probiotic administration significantly reduced oropharyngeal and gastric colonization by pathogenic species [27]. However, other clinical reports showed no significant difference in the occurrence of VAP in the ICU [28]. In a recent randomized controlled study, the effect of prophylactic synbiotics on gut microbiota and on the incidence of infectious complications including enteritis, VAP, and bacteremia was evaluated in mechanically ventilated patients with sepsis. Seventy-two patients completed the trial, of whom 35 patients received synbiotics and 37 patients did not. In the synbiotics group, the incidence of enteritis and the incidence of VAP were significantly lower compared to controls. The incidence of bacteremia and mortality, however, did not differ significantly between the two groups [29]. Currently, we are waiting for the results of a large randomized placebo-controlled study [30] aimed to determine the effect of *L. rhamnosus* GG on the incidence of VAP and other clinically important outcomes (*C. difficile* infection, secondary infections, diarrhea) in critically ill mechanically ventilated patients (Clinicaltrials.gov Identifier: NCT02462590).

Several studies have assessed the role of probiotics in other populations, such as pre-term and underweight children, finding no differences in sepsis incidence and mortality, indicating that the potential effects of microbiota restoration are not uniformly conserved across populations and settings [31, 32]. Interestingly, a recent randomized, double-blind, placebo-controlled trial testing an oral synbiotic preparation (*Lactobacillus plantarum* plus a fructooligosaccharide) in healthy, term-neonates in India was interrupted early because of a reduction of 40% in death and sepsis in the treatment arm [33].

The last frontier in the context of immunonutrition is the development of next-generation probiotics able to selectively inhibit specific pathogens, such as *C. difficile* and MDR bacteria, in order to administer a target population that would support colonization resistance and prevent infections and sepsis [34].

24.6 Fecal Microbiota Transplantation

Fecal microbiota transplantation (FMT) consists of administering fecal material from a healthy donor into the intestinal tract of a patient with an altered gut microbiota to restore its functions. Clinician interest in this treatment was renewed in 2013 with publication of the results of a randomized controlled trial showing the substantial superiority of FMT over standard care in the treatment of recurrent *C. difficile* infections [35]. Based on the absolute number of introduced bacteria, FMT is thought to be the most powerful immunomodulatory tool. In animal models, FMT alone is capable of restoring bacterial communities in cecal crypts, which act as a reservoir of commensal bacteria to restore the intestinal epithelium. Crypts are also crucial in protecting intestinal stem cells and in preservation of immunological pathways by enhancing the expression of nod-like and Toll-like receptors. Depletion of commensal organisms in crypts enhances pathogen proliferation, which can result in severe inflammation and disruption of homeostasis. Another potential advantage of FMT is that, along with the transfer of bacterial communities, other products (short-chain fatty acids, bile acids, eukaryotic, and prokaryotic viruses) are introduced to the intestinal ecosystem, leading to a complete restoration of homeostasis [36].

The rationale for use of FMT in critical illness is fascinating and promising. However, its application in clinical practice among ICU patients is unexplored. We believe that FMT can have a potential role in critical patients in two directions: (1) restoration of ICU-associated dysbiosis and (2) implementation of gut decolonization of MDR organisms. In fact, the introduction of a high burden of commensal bacteria may reverse resistant pathobiont dominance and even decrease the antibiotic resistance genes present in the microbiome (resistome) [37]. However, only five cases have been described in which FMT has been employed to address disruption of the microbiota in the ICU. All these cases showed that treatment with FMT led to a successful reversal of dysbiosis, with subsequent improvement in outcome. In addition, some cases noted a steep decrease in inflammatory mediators and normalized Th1/Th2 and Th1/Th17 ratios following FMT. Apart from difficulties with extrapolating the data derived from these case reports to the general ICU population, we are far from obtaining conclusive evidence that restoration of dysbiosis by FMT in critical illness is beneficial. However, given the promising results of FMT learned from *C. difficile* treatment experience, clinical trials are needed to implement a microbiota-targeted approach.

Colonization with MDR bacteria is a leading cause of sepsis complications especially among vulnerable ICU patients [38]. The use of FMT for this purpose has been evaluated in different case series, retrospective and prospective studies, highlighting that this approach can be feasible safe and effective [39]. Results cannot be easily analyzed because of the high risk of bias in smaller studies, but in a recent review that considered only studies with low and moderate risk of bias, an eradication rate between 37.5% and 87.5% was described [40]. However, results of different studies cannot be conclusive because of different patient populations (with the most commonly organisms isolated pre-FMT being carbapenem-resistant *Enterobacteriaceae* [CRE], vancomycin-resistant *Enterococci* [VRE], and extended-spectrum β-lactamase [ESBL]-producing bacteria, and also *Pseudomonas*, methicillin-resistant *S. aureus* [MRSA], and *Acinetobacter*, and differences in route of administration, choice of donors, and length of follow-up [39]. Recently, a randomized controlled trial has been completed showing that patients given nonabsorbable oral antibiotics followed by FMT had a slight decrease in ESBL and CRE colonization compared with control patients, although without reaching statistical significance. The unfavorable results are potentially due to the study design (two different routes of FMT in the interventional group and contemporary antibiotic administration may have influenced carriage in the interventional group) and early trial termination [41]. However, it is important to note that so far none of the published studies has been conducted in ICU patients. Until now, only one pilot study is ongoing among ICU patients with a prevision of enrollment of 10 mechanically ventilated patients with MDR colonization (Clinicaltrials.gov Identifier: NCT03350178).

Various concerns specific to ICU patients have been raised in addition to other unanswered questions regarding FMT itself (e.g., transmission of pathogens, dose, route, and long-term safety), as well as several practical aspects that need to be investigated. First, we do not know which candidate population of septic patients is best and what the correct timing of FMT administration is in relation to antibiotic use because of the risk of nullifying the effects of transplantation.

A microbiota suspension as a fecal filtrate transfer (FFT) seems to maintain the ability to stimulate host responses via pattern recognition receptors enabling ecologic niches to be modified for outgrowth of existing beneficial bacteria or even successful novel colonization [42]. This characteristic, together with a possibility to create a capsule, can increase the chances of successful FMT application even during antibiotic treatment, reducing also the potential risk of instillation of large bacterial burdens among immunocompromised patients.

Furthermore, more experience is crucial to evaluate what is the best route of administration (colonoscopy or enema vs nasogastric tract) and use of autologous vs heterologous transplantation. Colonoscopy or enema are the most commonly used methods of stool delivery. A randomized study found that FMT using the nasogastric tract was less effective than colonoscopy [43]. Expert opinion tends to favor colonoscopy because of its ability to visualize the entire colon and to deliver larger amounts of stool near the affected pathological segment of the bowel [44]. Moreover, non-inferiority of capsule use over colonoscopy was demonstrated in a randomized study [45].

Finally, the use of autologous vs heterologous FMT needs to be clarified because autologous FMT can have a higher potential application in the ICU setting among patients receiving solid or hematopoietic transplant in an attempt to prevent infections after a period of dysbiosis.

In conclusion, we believe that the potential benefits from FMT (regarding the control of MDR bacteria and *C. difficile* infection) justify the investigation of this promising approach in ICU patients.

24.7 Conclusion and Future Perspectives

Despite the impressive achievement that has been made in knowledge of the microbiome, there is still a huge gap about the microorganisms that reside outside the gut and interactions of bacteria with viruses, archeae, helminths, fungi, and protozoa, which influence each other and in turn regulate the host. In the context of critically ill septic patients, we need large human cohort studies that document microbiota composition, prior to, during and after an episode of sepsis in order to identify protective commensals and microbiota potentially associated with increased susceptibility and worse outcome.

At the same time, new treatment opportunities are gaining space in clinical practice, including the addition of a probiotic, or by tailoring microbiome therapy and selecting specific commensal repletion that could target a specific infectious disease. In this setting, human studies and randomized clinical trials are challenging but still fundamental in order to translate basic research into innovative paradigms.

References

1. Harris VC, Haak BW, Boele van Hensbroek M, et al. The intestinal microbiome in infectious diseases: the clinical relevance of a rapidly emerging field. Open Forum Infect Dis. 2017;4:3.
2. Kim S, Covington A, Pamer EG. The intestinal microbiota: antibiotics, colonization resistance, and enteric pathogens. Immunol Rev. 2017;279:90–105.

3. Buffie CG, Pamer EG. Microbiota-mediated colonization resistance against intestinal pathogens. Nat Rev Immunol. 2013;13:790–801.
4. Hausser F, Chakraborty S, Halbgebauer R, et al. Challenge to the intestinal mucosa during sepsis. Front Immunol. 2019;10:891.
5. Dickson RP, Pamer EG, Newstead MV, et al. Enrichment of the lung microbiome with the gut bacteria in sepsis and the acute respiratory distress syndrome. Nat Microbiol. 2016;1:16113.
6. Shimizu K, Ogura H, Hamasaki T, et al. Altered gut flora are associated with septic complications and death in critically ill patients with systemic inflammatory response syndrome. Dig Dis Sci. 2011;56:1171–7.
7. Donskey CJ. Antibiotic regimens and intestinal colonization with antibiotic-resistant Gram-negative bacilli. Clin Infect Dis. 2006;43:S62–9.
8. Yeh A, Rogers MB, Firek B, et al. Dysbiosis across multiple body sites in critically ill adult surgical patients. Shock. 2016;46:649–54.
9. Akram K, Sweeney DA. The microbiome of the critically ill patient. Curr Opin Crit Care. 2018;24:49–54.
10. Alverdy JC, Krezalek MA. Collapse of the microbiome, emergence of the pathobiome and the immunopathology of sepsis. Crit Care Med. 2017;45:337–47.
11. Hyoju SK, Zaborin A, Keskey R, et al. Mice fed an obesogenic western diet, administered antibiotics, and subjected to a sterile surgical procedure develop lethal septicemia with multidrug resistant pathobionts. mBio. 2019;10:e00903–19.
12. Napier BA, Andres-Terre M, Massis LM, et al. Western diet regulates immune status and the response to LPS-driven sepsis independent of diet-associated microbiome. Proc Natl Acad Sci U S A. 2019;116:3688–94.
13. Zhu H, Liu S, Li S, et al. Altered gut microbiota after traumatic splenectomy is associated with endotoxemia. Emerg Microbes Infect. 2018;7:1–10.
14. Taur Y, Xavier JB, Lipuma L, et al. Intestinal domination and the risk of bacteremia in patients undergoing allogeneic hematopoietic stem cell transplantation. Clin Infect Dis. 2012;55:905–14.
15. Prescott HC, Dickson RP, Rogers MA, et al. Hospitalization type and subsequent severe sepsis. Am J Respir Crit Care Med. 2015;192:581–8.
16. Baggs J, Jernigan JA, Halpin AL, et al. Risk of subsequent sepsis within 90 days after hospital stay by type of antibiotic exposure. Clin Infect Dis. 2018;66:1004–12.
17. Fay KT, Klingensmith NJ, Chen CW, et al. The gut microbiome alters immunophenotype and survival from sepsis. FASEB J. 2019;33:11258–69.
18. Ojima M, Motooka D, Shimizu K, et al. Metagenomic analysis reveals dynamic changes of whole gut microbiota in the acute phase of intensive care unit patients. Dig Dis Sci. 2016;61:1628–34.
19. Klingensmith NJ, Coopersmith CM. The gut as the motor of multiple organ dysfunction in critical illness. Crit Care Clin. 2016;32:203–12.
20. Dickson RP, Singer BH, Newstead MW, et al. Enrichment of the lung microbiome with gut bacteria in sepsis and the acute respiratory distress syndrome. Nat Microbiol. 2016;1:16113.
21. Singer BH, Dickson RP, Denstaedt SJ, et al. Bacterial dissemination to the brain in sepsis. Am J Respir Crit Care Med. 2018;197:747–56.
22. Chen L, Xu K, Gui Q, et al. Probiotic pre-administration reduces mortality in a mouse model of cecal ligation and puncture-induced sepsis. Exp Ther Med. 2016;12:1836–42.
23. Chen L, Li H, Li J, et al. Lactobacillus rhamnosus GC treatment improves intestinal permeability and modulates microbiota dysbiosis in an experimental model of sepsis. Int J Mol Med. 2019;43:1139–48.
24. Graf K, Last A, Gratz R, et al. Keeping Candida commensal—How lactobacilli antagonize pathogenicity of Candida albicans in an in vitro gut model. Dis Model Mech. 2019;14:dmm039719.
25. Manzanares W, Lemieux M, Langlois PL, Wischmeyer PE. Probiotic and synbiotic therapy in critical illness: a systematic review and meta-analysis. Crit Care. 2016;20:262.

26. Kasatpibal N, Whitney JD, Saokaew S, Kengkla K, Heitkemper MM, Apisarnthanarak A. Effectiveness of probiotic, prebiotic, and synbiotic therapies in reducing postoperative complications: a systematic review and network meta-analysis. Clin Infect Dis. 2017;64:S153–60.
27. Morrow LE, Kollef MH, Casale TB. Probiotic prophylaxis of ventilator-associated pneumonia: a blinded, randomized, controlled trial. Am J Respir Crit Care Med. 2010;182:1058–64.
28. Knight DJ, Gardiner D, Banks A, et al. Effect of synbiotic therapy on the incidence of ventilator associated pneumonia in critically ill patients: a randomised, double-blind, placebo- controlled trial. Intensive Care Med. 2009;35:854–61.
29. Shimizu K, Yamada T, Ogura H, et al. Synbiotics modulate gut microbiota and reduce enteritis and ventilator-associated pneumonia in patients with sepsis: a randomized controlled trial. Crit Care. 2018;22:239.
30. Johnstone J, Heels-Ansdell D, Thabane L, et al. For the PROSPECT Investigators and the Canadian Critical Care Trials Group. Evaluating probiotics for the prevention of ventilator-associated pneumonia: a randomised placebo-controlled multicentre trial protocol and statistical analysis plan for PROSPECT. BMJ Open. 2019;e025228:9.
31. Jacobs SE, Tobin JM, Opie GF, et al. Probiotic effects on late-onset sepsis in very preterm infants: a randomized controlled trial. Pediatrics. 2013;132:1055–62.
32. Costeloe K, Hardy P, Juszczak E, Wilks M, Millar MR. Bifidobacterium breve BBG-001 in very preterm infants: a randomised controlled phase 3 trial. Lancet. 2016;387:649–60.
33. Panigrahi P, Parida S, Nanda NC, et al. A randomized synbiotic trial to prevent sepsis among infants in rural India. Nature. 2017;548:407–12.
34. Pamer EG. Resurrecting the intestinal microbiota to combat antibiotic-resistant pathogens. Science. 2016;352:535–8.
35. Kelly CR, Ihunnah C, Fisher M, et al. Fecal microbiota transplant for treatment of Clostridium difficile infection in immunocompromised patients. Am J Gastroenterol. 2014;109:1065–71.
36. Van Nood E, Speelman P, Nieuwdorp M, et al. Fecal microbiota transplantation: facts and controversies. Curr Opin Gastroenterol. 2014;30:34–9.
37. Li Q, Wang C, Tang C, et al. Successful treatment of severe sepsis and diarrhea after vagotomy utilizing fecal microbiota transplantation: a case report. Crit Care. 2015;19:37.
38. Wang Z, Qin RR, Huang L, et al. Risk factors for carbapenem-resistant *Klebsiella pneumoniae* infection and mortality of *Klebsiella pneumoniae* infection. Chin Med J. 2018;131:56–62.
39. Gargiullo L, Del Chierico F, D'Argenio P, et al. Gut microbiota modulation for multidrug resistant organism decolonization: present and future perspectives. Front Microbiol. 1704;2019:10.
40. Saha S, Tariq R, Tosh PK, et al. Faecal microbiota transplantation for eradicating carriage of multidrug resistant organisms: a systematic review. Clin Microbiol Infect. 2019;25:958–61.
41. Huttner BD, De Lastours V, Wassenberg M, et al. A 5-day course of oral antibiotics followed by faecal transplantation to eradicate carriage of multidrug-resistant Enterobacteriaceae: a randomized clinical trial. Clin Microbiol Infect. 2019;25:830–8.
42. Ott SJ, Waetzig GH, Rehman A. Efficacy of sterile fecal filtrate transfer for treating patients with Clostrodium difficile infection. Gastroenterology. 2017;152:799–811.
43. Gundacker ND, Tamhane A, Walker JB, et al. Comparative effectiveness of faecal microbiota transplant by route of administration. J Hosp Infect. 2017;96:349–52.
44. Ramai D, Zakhia K, Ofosu A, et al. Fecal microbiota transplantation: donor relation, fresh or frozen, delivery methods, cost effectiveness. Ann Gastroenterol. 2019;32:30–8.
45. Kao D, Roach B, Silva M, et al. Effect of oral capsule- vs colonoscopy-delivered fecal microbiota transplantation on recurrent Clostridium difficile infection: a randomized clinical trial. JAMA. 2017;318:1985–93.

Part VIII
Bleeding and Transfusion

Blood Transfusion Practice During Extracorporeal Membrane Oxygenation: Rationale and Modern Approaches to Management

C. Agerstrand, B. Bromberger, and D. Brodie

25.1 Introduction

The use of extracorporeal membrane oxygenation (ECMO) to support patients with severe respiratory, cardiac, or combined cardiopulmonary failure has dramatically increased in little more than a decade [1]. Advancements in ECMO circuit technology, coupled with the encouraging global experience with ECMO during the 2009 influenza A (H1N1) pandemic and the publication of the Efficacy and Economic Assessment of Conventional Ventilatory Support versus Extracorporeal Membrane Oxygenation for Severe Adult Respiratory Failure (CESAR) trial, largely drove this increase, resulting in widespread adoption of ECMO as a support technology for numerous cardiopulmonary conditions [1–3]. Though not positive in the traditional sense, the recently published ECMO to Rescue Lung Injury in Severe Acute Respiratory Distress Syndrome (EOLIA) trial showed favorable results in the group randomized to ECMO [4]. A subsequent *post hoc* Bayesian analysis confirmed a high probability of benefit, as well as the encouraging safety profile seen in EOLIA, and has resulted in a greater acceptance of ECMO by the critical care community in general [5]. A subsequent meta-analysis of studies of ECMO for the acute respiratory distress syndrome (ARDS) also confirmed a mortality benefit at 60 days [6]. Venoarterial ECMO has been shown to have a survival benefit in both cardiogenic shock and cardiac arrest [7]. An evidence-based approach to management of patients receiving ECMO has not been able to keep pace with this enthusiasm for and

---

C. Agerstrand (✉) · D. Brodie
Division of Pulmonary, Allergy, and Critical Care Medicine, Department of Medicine, Columbia University Vagelos College of Physicians and Surgeons/NewYork-Presbyterian Hospital, New York, NY, USA
e-mail: ca2264@cumc.columbia.edu

B. Bromberger
Department of Surgery, Columbia University Vagelos College of Physicians and Surgeons/NewYork-Presbyterian Hospital, New York, NY, USA

© Springer Nature Switzerland AG 2020
J.-L. Vincent (ed.), *Annual Update in Intensive Care and Emergency Medicine 2020*, Annual Update in Intensive Care and Emergency Medicine, https://doi.org/10.1007/978-3-030-37323-8_25

increased utilization of this advanced and resource-intensive technology, however. As such, the optimal management of patients receiving ECMO largely remains unknown, and contemporary practice has been predominantly experience-driven. This has resulted in highly variable approaches to patient management and areas of significant controversy within the ECMO and critical care communities; one such area of controversy is the approach to blood transfusions in ECMO-supported patients.

25.2 ECMO Physiology

ECMO is a form of temporary mechanical circulatory support that works by supplanting the function of the injured heart, lungs, or both in the setting of acute injury in order to bridge patients to recovery, or in acute on chronic failure as a bridge to transplantation or durable mechanical cardiac support. The primary purpose of ECMO is to augment the total systemic tissue oxygen delivery, with the circuit contribution being a product of the effective ECMO blood flow and the oxygen content of the arterialized blood. As hemoglobin concentration is a primary contributor to oxygen content, at a given effective blood flow, a higher hemoglobin achieves greater systemic oxygen delivery.

During ECMO, blood is withdrawn from the venous system via a catheter inserted in a central vein, pumped through a gas exchange device known as an oxygenator, and returned to the venous or arterial system, depending on ECMO configuration (Fig. 25.1). The oxygenator is fed with a continuous supply of oxygen-rich sweep gas that is separated from the blood by a semipermeable membrane across which diffusion-mediated gas exchange occurs so that the blood exiting the oxygenator is well oxygenated and low in carbon dioxide.

In venovenous ECMO, the well-oxygenated blood is returned to a central vein and passes through the heart and lungs before being delivered systemically, functioning in series with the patient's native cardiopulmonary system. Thus, ECMO-related systemic oxygen delivery is dependent on both the proportion of central venous blood effectively oxygenated by the ECMO circuit and native cardiac output. Venovenous ECMO can therefore be used to support patients with severe hypoxemic or hypercapneic respiratory failure, such as in cases of severe forms of ARDS, status asthmaticus, or as a bridge to lung transplantation [4, 8, 9].

In contrast, venoarterial ECMO provides hemodynamic and partial respiratory support, as the well-oxygenated blood is reinfused into the arterial system, bypassing the heart and thereby obviating its need to meet the entirety of physiologic demand. Venoarterial ECMO is used to treat patients with acute decompensated heart failure, acute myocardial infarction with cardiogenic shock, refractory ventricular arrhythmias, severe acute myocarditis, and as extracorporeal cardiopulmonary resuscitation (ECPR), in which ECMO is initiated during cardiac arrest in an attempt to restore systemic oxygen delivery during ongoing resuscitative efforts, among other indications related to cardiogenic shock [7, 10, 11].

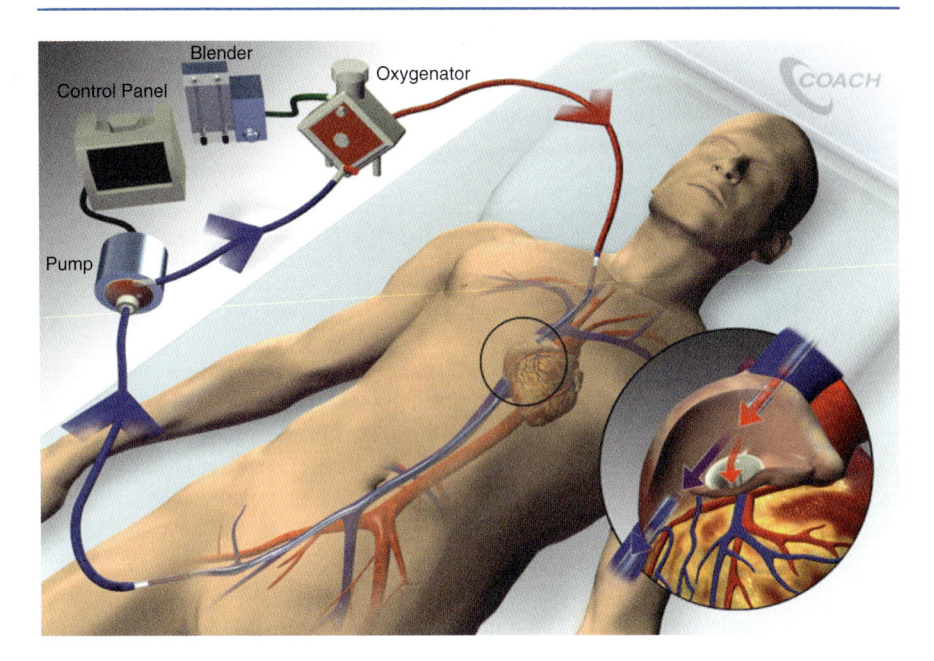

Fig. 25.1 Dual-site venovenous extracorporeal membrane oxygenation (ECMO) (Figure from collectedmed.com)

25.3 Blood Loss During ECMO

Bleeding is the most common complication of both venovenous and venoarterial ECMO and may be severe. Bleeding is reported in 27–61% of ECMO-supported patients in recent studies, with up to 71% of deaths attributed to bleeding complications, although definitions of what constitutes bleeding vary throughout the literature [2, 4, 12, 13]. According to the Extracorporeal Life Support Organization, which maintains a registry of patients supported with ECMO at more than 300 centers worldwide, the most common sites of bleeding are cannulation and surgical sites [14] and may be affected by cannulation strategy and patient age. Several factors make patients supported with ECMO at risk of bleeding, including the use of continuous anticoagulation typically required, platelet and coagulation factor consumption by the ECMO circuit, and the effects of critical illness.

Once nearly universal, significant blood loss and bleeding during ECMO have decreased in the modern era due to several factors. Enhanced biocompatibility of modern ECMO circuits, cannula and tubing, transition from a roller to centrifugal pump system, and circuit simplification have reduced clinically significant hemolysis, disseminated intravascular coagulation (DIC), as well as thrombotic propensity, the latter of which has permitted use of low-dose anticoagulation compared to the higher doses once required. In addition, modern approaches to anticoagulation monitoring, with transition in adult patients from activated clotting time to activated partial thromboplastin time and anti-factor Xa levels, have allowed for a more accurate assessment of coagulation status [4, 15, 16]. Finally, the improved safety profile of ECMO has allowed for more parsimonious phlebotomy than was once typical, with a minimization of iatrogenic blood loss [17, 18].

25.4 Blood Transfusions in Critically Ill Patients

The value of a higher hemoglobin results from its impact on oxygen delivery. However, the potential benefit of a higher hemoglobin level may not occur when transfusions are required to achieve it. Multiple clinical studies have demonstrated an association between transfusions and worsened outcomes in critically ill patients, including worsening ARDS, volume overload, transfusion-related acute lung injury, risk of infection, and death [19–24]. It is the number of packed red blood cell (RBC) transfusions and not baseline hemoglobin that has been associated with increased mortality [20, 25]. Even small numbers of transfusions (as low as 1–2 units of packed RBCs) have been associated with worsened clinical outcomes in a dose-dependent manner [23]. The potential for these potentially discretionary units of packed RBCs to impact clinical outcomes raises concern about the risk versus benefit of their administration [23].

One of the most cited studies evaluating the hemoglobin threshold at which transfusions should be administered is the Transfusion Requirements in Critical Care (TRICC) trial, a multicenter trial that randomized patients to a restrictive (hemoglobin trigger <7.0 g/dl) or a liberal (hemoglobin trigger <10.0 g/dl) transfusion strategy. The trial demonstrated a significant decrease in mortality in the restrictive group, specifically among patients younger than 55 years and an Acute Physiology and Chronic Health Evaluation (APACHE) II score of less than 20 [19]. Based on available evidence, the American Association of Blood Banks recommends the use of a restrictive transfusion strategy with a hemoglobin transfusion trigger of 7.0 g/dl in hemodynamically stable patients [26]. Comparable outcomes between a restrictive (hemoglobin trigger <7.0 g/dl) versus liberal (hemoglobin trigger <9.0 g/dl) transfusion strategy have also been found in patients with septic shock, even when leukoreduced blood was transfused [27]. A similarly restrictive transfusion trigger of <8.0 g/dl is recommended for patients with cardiovascular disease [26, 28]. Notably, the lack of evidence as opposed to differences in clinical outcomes may explain the variable recommendations between groups [26].

25.5 Effect of Transfused Blood

The mechanisms of transfusion-related organ dysfunction are not fully understood. Storage duration has been implicated as a factor, as metabolic and structural alterations occur in packed RBCs over time [29]. These changes may impair functioning *in vivo* and include depletion of 2,3-diphosphoglycerate, which results in increased oxygen binding to hemoglobin and impaired tissue oxygen uptake; reduced adenosine triphosphate (ATP) and increased oxidative stress, which lead to conformational changes and impaired microcirculatory flow in the lungs and other organs; and increased plasma-free hemoglobin, which may cause vasoconstriction and intravascular thrombosis [29–31].

Conflicting evidence exists as to the impact of RBC age on clinical outcomes. Studies have shown deleterious effects including impaired tissue oxygenation in blood transfused after longer duration of storage [31]. However, several multicenter randomized trials have subsequently failed to show a difference in outcomes such as infection, organ dysfunction, and mortality between patients treated with fresh versus standard-issue packed RBCs, although the standard blood used in these trials varied between approximately 2–3 weeks in age [32, 33]. It is unclear if comparisons with packed RBCs transfused at the extreme end of storage (42 days) would produce similar outcomes.

The effect of transfused blood during ECMO is largely unknown, but a small study of ECMO-supported pediatric patients did not suggest that storage duration impacted tissue oxygenation or clinical biomarkers [34]. Notably, there was also minimal change in patient biomarkers such as mixed venous oxygen saturation, serum lactate levels, and cerebral oximetry pre- and posttransfusion, raising questions as to the clinical impact of transfusion, particularly in the setting of ECMO [34]. In contrast, a small, but well-designed study of adults supported with venovenous ECMO demonstrated that transfusion of packed RBCs increased apparent oxygen content and delivery, and ECMO blood flow could be reduced 20% further following transfusion [35].

25.6 Current Approach to Transfusion During ECMO

The benefit of maintaining a high hemoglobin level with blood transfusions must be weighed against the risks of transfused blood. The optimal transfusion threshold in patients receiving ECMO has not been established. Historically, due to the importance of hemoglobin in determining oxygen content and the fact that ECMO is often utilized when native oxygen delivery is inadequate, packed RBC transfusion rates are known to be high and transfusion to a normal hematocrit of greater than 40% has been recommended [36]. Even modern multicenter studies have reported a median of 1500 ml (IQR 400-2990) to 1800 ml (IQR 904–3750) of blood administered over the duration of ECMO support for severe ARDS [2, 13].

Both transfusion rates and quantities have decreased in the modern ECMO era due to several factors. Along with decreased hemolysis and bleeding complications, there has been a trend toward a decreased transfusion trigger in ECMO [4, 17, 37]. A decreased transfusion trigger is due, in part, to literature in other critically ill patients, which supports use of a lower transfusion trigger and tolerance of a moderate degree of anemia [19]. In addition, adequate systemic oxygen delivery may also be achieved with the use of modern circuits that more safely allow for a higher ECMO blood flow compared to older ECMO technology, permitting tolerance of a lower hemoglobin. Maintaining a blood flow rate to cardiac output ratio greater than

60% achieved adequate systemic oxygenation in a well-conducted physiologic study (arterial oxygen saturation [SaO_2] > 90% or a PaO_2 > 60 mmHg) (35).

There are no randomized trials comparing restrictive versus liberal transfusion triggers in ECMO-supported patients. However, the multicenter EOLIA trial strongly encouraged a transfusion trigger of 7–8 g/dl of hemoglobin, while transfusion to a hemoglobin of 10 g/dl was permitted in the setting of refractory and persistent hypoxemia [4]. Furthermore, excellent clinical outcomes using restrictive approaches to packed RBC transfusions (hemoglobin trigger < 7.0 g/dl) have been reported in severely hypoxemic ARDS patients [17, 38]. Mean or median hemoglobin was 8.3 g/dl in these studies [17, 38]. In one of these studies, which included 38 patients with ARDS supported with venovenous ECMO, survival was 74% despite a median pre-ECMO PaO_2 to fraction of inspired oxygen (FiO_2) ratio of 53 mmHg and high severity of illness scores [17]. The restrictive transfusion trigger was combined with a low-dose anticoagulation strategy, conservative approach to phlebotomy, and reinfusion of circuit blood at the time of decannulation in order to encompass a blood conservation strategy. This multifactorial approach resulted in a median of 1 unit of packed RBCs transfused over the duration of the ECMO run, equaling 0.11 U/day of ECMO support, while approximately 40% of patients never required transfusion [17].

The recently published TRAIN-ECMO survey of nearly 450 ECMO practitioners sought to characterize global transfusion practices during venovenous ECMO and showed that approximately 46% of respondents used a pre-defined hemoglobin trigger for transfusion [37]. The average hemoglobin trigger was higher in ECMO patients than for other critically ill patients (9.1 versus 8.3 g/dl, $p < 0.01$) and was without significant geographic variation. Notably, a lower hemoglobin trigger was associated with more institutional ECMO experience. Centers with more than 24 cases annually had an average hemoglobin trigger of 8.4 g/dl compared to a trigger of 9.6 mg/dl in centers with fewer than 12 cases ($p < 0.01$) and were more likely to use a protocolized approach to transfusion. Parameters such as hematocrit, pre-oxygenator saturation, hemodynamic status, and lactate were also considered by respondents contemplating transfusion, though their utility for triggers of transfusion in venovenous ECMO is unclear and significant variation in practice exists [37].

Robust data regarding bleeding complications, transfusion, and hemoglobin levels in patients supported with venoarterial ECMO is generally lacking [7]. However, transfusion rates in adult venoarterial ECMO have been reported with similar frequency as in venovenous ECMO [39, 40]. Optimal hemoglobin may vary based on the etiology of the underlying disease, as hyperoxia has been associated with worsened neurologic outcomes and mortality, particularly in post-cardiac arrest patients [41, 42].

25.7 Future Directions

Where do we go from here? A better understanding of transfusion practices during venovenous and venoarterial ECMO is needed. An ongoing prospective multicenter observational study on transfusion practice in venovenous ECMO patients

(PROTECMO) study seeks to describe blood product usage, bleeding, and anticoagulation strategies in an attempt to add clarity and better define contemporary ECMO practices and complications (ClinicalTrials.gov Identifier: NCT03815773). A similar study of blood management during ECMO for cardiac support (OBLEX) seeks to characterize practices in patients receiving venoarterial ECMO for heart failure (ClinicalTrials.gov Identifier: NCT03714048).

In addition to defining contemporary management practices, prospective and randomized trials are needed comparing restrictive and liberal transfusion strategies in ECMO patients. Inclusion of the varying patient populations supported with ECMO is key, as optimal transfusion targets may vary with ECMO configuration and underlying disease. For example, the optimal transfusion trigger for a patient in cardiogenic shock supported with venoarterial ECMO likely differs from that of a well-supported patient awaiting lung transplantation, who may be better served at a hemoglobin below 7.0 g/dl if it avoids the risk of allosensitization associated with transfusion. Multiparameter modeling that incorporates indicators of global and regional hypoperfusion may better define the threshold for transfusion for a variety of patient populations [37].

Understanding the impact of ECMO on regional blood flow may also help predict oxygen delivery and uptake during varying physiologic states. Cerebral autoregulation, as determined by neuroimaging, cerebral blood flow, and cerebral oximetry may be affected during ECMO and by manipulation of ECMO circuit blood flow, although the impact is unclear [43, 44]. Evaluation of microcirculatory function shows promise in assessing tissue level hypoxia and may help target optimal oxygen delivery. Alterations in the microcirculation have been associated with increased mortality, including in patients supported with venoarterial ECMO with normalized hemodynamics [45–47]. Broader understanding of microcirculatory function and the potential impact of ECMO is an intriguing area of study that requires additional investigation.

25.8 Conclusion

ECMO is a potentially life-saving technology that has altered the treatment paradigm for patients with advanced cardiopulmonary failure. However, despite its potential benefits, ECMO is resource-intensive and lacks standardization of evidence-supported management practices in many key areas, including the approach to transfusion. A restrictive approach to transfusion is well supported in other critically ill patients and may extend to some populations of patients receiving ECMO. While the risks of transfused blood must be balanced against potential for augmented systemic oxygen delivery, contemporary literature suggests favorable outcomes in even severely hypoxemic patients with ARDS managed with a restrictive approach to transfusion. Consideration of global and regional markers of hypoxia and improved understanding of the impact of ECMO on the microcirculation may help better define optimal transfusion management in patients receiving venovenous or venoarterial ECMO.

References

1. Brodie D, Slutsky AS, Combes A. Extracorporeal life support for adults with respiratory failure and related indications: a review. JAMA. 2019;322:557–68.
2. Davies A, Jones D, Bailey M, et al. Extracorporeal membrane oxygenation for 2009 influenza A (H1N1) acute respiratory distress syndrome. JAMA. 2009;302:1888–95.
3. Peek GJ, Mugford M, Tiruvoipati R, et al. Efficacy and economic assessment of conventional ventilatory support versus extracorporeal membrane oxygenation for severe adult respiratory failure (CESAR): a multicentre randomised controlled trial. Lancet. 2009;374:1351–63.
4. Combes A, Hajage D, Capellier G, et al. Extracorporeal membrane oxygenation for severe acute respiratory distress syndrome. N Engl J Med. 2018;378:1965–75.
5. Goligher EC, Tomlinson G, Hajage D, et al. Extracorporeal membrane oxygenation for severe acute respiratory distress syndrome and posterior probability of mortality benefit in a post hoc bayesian analysis of a randomized clinical trial. JAMA. 2018;320:2251–9.
6. Munshi L, Walkey A, Goligher E, Pham T, Uleryk EM, Fan E. Venovenous extracorporeal membrane oxygenation for acute respiratory distress syndrome: a systematic review and meta-analysis. Lancet Respir Med. 2019;7:163–72.
7. Ouweneel DM, Schotborgh JV, Limpens J, et al. Extracorporeal life support during cardiac arrest and cardiogenic shock: a systematic review and meta-analysis. Intensive Care Med. 2016;42:1922–34.
8. Brenner K, Abrams D, Agerstrand C, Brodie D. Extracorporeal carbon dioxide removal for refractory status asthmaticus: experience in distinct exacerbation phenotypes. Perfusion. 2014;29:26–8.
9. Biscotti M, Gannon WD, Agerstrand C, et al. Awake extracorporeal membrane oxygenation as bridge to lung transplantation: a 9-year experience. Ann Thorac Surg. 2017;104:412–9.
10. Chen B, Chang YM. CPR with assisted extracorporeal life support. Lancet. 2008;372:1879.
11. Keebler ME, Haddad EV, Choi CW, et al. Venoarterial extracorporeal membrane oxygenation in cardiogenic shock. JACC Heart Fail. 2018;6:503–16.
12. Burrell AJC, Bennett V, Serra AL, et al. Venoarterial extracorporeal membrane oxygenation: a systematic review of selection criteria, outcome measures and definitions of complications. J Crit Care. 2019;53:32–7.
13. Patroniti N, Zangrillo A, Pappalardo F, et al. The Italian ECMO network experience during the 2009 influenza A (H1N1) pandemic: preparation for severe respiratory emergency outbreaks. Intensive Care Med. 2011;37:1447–57.
14. Extracorporeal Life Support Organization. ECLS registry report, international summary. Available at https://www.elso.org/Portals/0/Files/Reports/2019/International%20Summary%20January%202019.pdf. Accessed 3/1/20.
15. Atallah S, Liebl M, Fitousis K, Bostan F, Masud F. Evaluation of the activated clotting time and activated partial thromboplastin time for the monitoring of heparin in adult extracorporeal membrane oxygenation patients. Perfusion. 2014;29:456–61.
16. Price EA, Jin J, Nguyen HM, Krishnan G, Bowen R, Zehnder JL. Discordant aPTT and anti-Xa values and outcomes in hospitalized patients treated with intravenous unfractionated heparin. Ann Pharmacother. 2013;47:151–8.
17. Agerstrand C, Burkart K, Baldwin M, et al. Conservative blood transfusion strategies are effective for the management of adult patients with severe acute respiratory distress syndrome requiring extracorporeal membrane oxygenation. Am J Respir Crit Care Med. 2011;183:A1655 (abst).
18. Yu JS, Barbaro RP, Granoski DA, et al. Prospective side by side comparison of outcomes and complications with a simple versus intensive anticoagulation monitoring strategy in pediatric extracorporeal life support patients. Pediatr Crit Care Med. 2017;18:1055–62.
19. Hebert PC, Wells G, Blajchman MA, et al. A multicenter, randomized, controlled clinical trial of transfusion requirements in critical care. Transfusion Requirements in Critical Care Investigators, Canadian Critical Care Trials Group. N Engl J Med. 1999;340:409–17.

20. Vincent JL, Baron JF, Reinhart K, et al. Anemia and blood transfusion in critically ill patients. JAMA. 2002;288:1499–507.
21. Ferraris VA, Davenport DL, Saha SP, Bernard A, Austin PC, Zwischenberger JB. Intraoperative transfusion of small amounts of blood heralds worse postoperative outcome in patients having noncardiac thoracic operations. Ann Thorac Surg. 2011;91:1674–80.
22. Shorr AF, Duh MS, Kelly KM, Kollef MH. Red blood cell transfusion and ventilator-associated pneumonia: a potential link? Crit Care Med. 2004;32:666–74.
23. Carson JL, Terrin ML, Noveck H, et al. Liberal or restrictive transfusion in high-risk patients after hip surgery. N Engl J Med. 2011;365:2453–62.
24. Marik PE, Corwin HL. Acute lung injury following blood transfusion: expanding the definition. Crit Care Med. 2008;36:3080–4.
25. Corwin HL, Gettinger A, Pearl RG, et al. The CRIT Study: anemia and blood transfusion in the critically ill – current clinical practice in the United States. Crit Care Med. 2004;32:39–52.
26. Carson JL, Guyatt G, Heddle NM, Grossman BJ, Cohn CS, Fung MK, et al. Clinical Practice Guidelines From the AABB: red blood cell transfusion thresholds and storage. JAMA. 2016;316:2025–35.
27. Holst LB, Haase N, Wetterslev J, et al. Transfusion requirements in septic shock (TRISS) trial—comparing the effects and safety of liberal versus restrictive red blood cell transfusion in septic shock patients in the ICU: protocol for a randomised controlled trial. Trials. 2013;14:150.
28. Mueller MM, Van Remoortel H, et al. Patient blood management: recommendations from the 2018 Frankfurt Consensus Conference. JAMA. 2019;321:983–97.
29. Tinmouth A, Fergusson D, Yee IC, Hébert PC. Clinical consequences of red cell storage in the critically ill. Transfusion. 2006;46:2014–27.
30. Lelubre C, Vincent JL. Red blood cell transfusion in the critically ill patient. Ann Intensive Care. 2011;1:43.
31. Kiraly LN, Underwood S, Differding JA, Schreiber MA. Transfusion of aged packed red blood cells results in decreased tissue oxygenation in critically injured trauma patients. J Trauma. 2009;67:29–32.
32. Fergusson DA, Hebert P, Hogan DL, et al. Effect of fresh red blood cell transfusions on clinical outcomes in premature, very low-birth-weight infants: the ARIPI randomized trial. JAMA. 2012;308:1443–51.
33. Lacroix J, Hebert PC, Fergusson DA, et al. Age of transfused blood in critically ill adults. N Engl J Med. 2015;372:1410–8.
34. Datta S, Chang S, Jackson NJ, Ziman A, Federman M. Impact of age of packed RBC transfusion on oxygenation in patients receiving extracorporeal membrane oxygenation. Pediatr Crit Care Med. 2019;20:841–6.
35. Schmidt M, Tachon G, Devilliers C, et al. Blood oxygenation and decarboxylation determinants during venovenous ECMO for respiratory failure in adults. Intensive Care Med. 2013;39:838–46.
36. Winkler AM. Transfusion management during extracorporeal support. In: Brogan T, Lequier L, Lorusso R, MacLaren G, Peek G, editors. Extracorporeal life support: the ELSO red book. 5th ed. Ann Arbor: Extracorporeal Life Support Organization; 2017. p. 108.
37. Martucci G, Grasselli G, Tanaka K, et al. Hemoglobin trigger and approach to red blood cell transfusions during veno-venous extracorporeal membrane oxygenation: the international TRAIN-ECMO survey. Perfusion. 2019;34(1_suppl):39–48.
38. Voelker MT, Busch T, Bercker S, Fichtner F, Kaisers UX, Laudi S. Restrictive transfusion practice during extracorporeal membrane oxygenation therapy for severe acute respiratory distress syndrome. Artif Organs. 2015;39:374–8.
39. Guimbretiere G, Anselmi A, Roisne A, et al. Prognostic impact of blood product transfusion in VA and VV ECMO. Perfusion. 2019;34:246–53.
40. Kon ZN, Bittle GJ, Pasrija C, et al. Venovenous versus venoarterial extracorporeal membrane oxygenation for adult patients with acute respiratory distress syndrome requiring precannulation hemodynamic support: a review of the ELSO Registry. Ann Thorac Surg. 2017;104:645–9.

41. Sznycer-Taub NR, Lowery R, Yu S, Owens ST, Hirsch-Romano JC, Owens GE. Hyperoxia is associated with poor outcomes in pediatric cardiac patients supported on venoarterial extracorporeal membrane oxygenation. Pediatr Crit Care Med. 2016;17:350–8.
42. Kilgannon JH, Jones AE, Parrillo JE, et al. Relationship between supranormal oxygen tension and outcome after resuscitation from cardiac arrest. Circulation. 2011;123:2717–22.
43. Ingyinn M, Rais-Bahrami K, Viswanathan M, Short BL. Altered cerebrovascular responses after exposure to venoarterial extracorporeal membrane oxygenation: role of the nitric oxide pathway. Pediatr Crit Care Med. 2006;7:368–73.
44. Kazmi SO, Sivakumar S, Karakitsos D, Alharthy A, Lazaridis C. Cerebral pathophysiology in extracorporeal membrane oxygenation: pitfalls in daily clinical management. Crit Care Res Pract. 2018;2018:3237810.
45. Kara A, Akin S, Dos Reis Miranda D, et al. Microcirculatory assessment of patients under VA-ECMO. Crit Care (London, England). 2016;20:344.
46. Sakr Y, Dubois MJ, De Backer D, Creteur J, Vincent JL. Persistent microcirculatory alterations are associated with organ failure and death in patients with septic shock. Crit Care Med. 2004;32:1825–31.
47. van Genderen ME, Lima A, Akkerhuis M, Bakker J, van Bommel J. Persistent peripheral and microcirculatory perfusion alterations after out-of-hospital cardiac arrest are associated with poor survival. Crit Care Med. 2012;40:2287–94.

The Use of Frozen Platelets for the Treatment of Bleeding

26

D. J. B. Kleinveld, N. P. Juffermans, and F. Noorman

26.1 Introduction

Platelet products are stored at room temperature, with a current shelf life of 5–7 days, after which products need to be discarded. This limited storage duration of platelets poses an obvious challenge for ensuring a continuous supply by blood banks, in particular in austere settings and in case of massive transfusion. Due to high waste, smaller hospitals may not be able to justify having full-time availability of platelet products. Cryopreservation of platelet products provides a solution for supply and will resolve waste of overdue products. For decades, frozen platelets have been used by the Dutch military during operations abroad. However, widespread use of frozen platelets has not been implemented, which is presumably due to the observed changes of the platelets following the process of cryopreservation and thawing. After thawing and resuspension, frozen platelets become highly activated [1]. They appear swollen and damaged [2], associated with impaired aggregation and

D. J. B. Kleinveld
Department of Intensive Care Medicine, Amsterdam UMC, Location AMC,
Amsterdam, The Netherlands

Laboratory of Experimental Intensive Care and Anesthesiology, Amsterdam UMC, Location AMC, Amsterdam, The Netherlands

Department of Trauma Surgery, Amsterdam UMC, Location AMC,
Amsterdam, The Netherlands

N. P. Juffermans (✉)
Department of Intensive Care Medicine, Amsterdam UMC, Location AMC,
Amsterdam, The Netherlands

Laboratory of Experimental Intensive Care and Anesthesiology, Amsterdam UMC, Location AMC, Amsterdam, The Netherlands
e-mail: n.p.juffermans@amsterdamumc.nl

F. Noorman
Military Blood Bank, Utrecht, The Netherlands

adhesion in *in vitro* testing [3]. Autologous transfusion of thawed frozen platelet products in volunteers yields a lower recovery rate when compared to liquid platelets [2]. Together, these changes have caused concern about the efficacy of frozen platelets. However, a low recovery rate does not correlate with a low hemostatic potential of platelets. In contrast, the cryopreservation process may even enhance some processes of the coagulation reaction. This may be due to activation of the platelets, resulting in increased extracellular vesicle content, which contributes to the coagulation process. Enhanced coagulation ability is also suggested by results of several small trials in patients undergoing cardiac surgery who were treated with frozen platelets [4, 5].

Frozen platelets thus affect coagulation differently than normal (liquid) stored platelets. If the use of frozen platelets is superior in enhancing hemostasis, we may start to think about the possibility of a differential use of platelet products for specific indications, such as the use of frozen platelets for active bleeding and the use of liquid-stored platelets for the correction of thrombocytopenia. Prior to such an approach, it should be established what the effect of frozen platelets is on hemostasis, as well as whether frozen platelets are safe. Use of frozen platelets may possibly increase the risk of thromboembolic events or have other side effects, such as fueling an inflammatory response. In this chapter, we will summarize the effect of the freeze-thawing cycle on the platelets, with associated functional changes *in vitro* and *in vivo*, providing a rationale for the use of frozen platelets as a hemostatic agent in bleeding. The experience with frozen platelets in the military setting worldwide is also described, as well as the data from trials in several patient populations.

26.2 Manufacture of Frozen Platelets

Throughout history, many different methods of freezing and different additive solutions have been used to cryopreserve platelet products. Nowadays, these efforts have led to a stable frozen platelet product in which platelets are frozen concentrated in 5–6% dimethylsulfoxide (DMSO). The frozen platelets are stored at −80 °C for as long as 2 years. When needed, these frozen platelets are thawed and resuspended in plasma and directly administered to the patient. This manufacturing process has several implications for the function of frozen-thawed and resuspended platelets.

26.3 The Impact of Freeze-thawing on Platelets

26.3.1 Morphology

The morphology of platelets depends on their activation status [6]. Freshly drawn platelets have a discoid shape, but shape changes occur very rapidly following collection [7]. Platelets transform from discs into spheres during room temperature storage in plasma. Discs refract light differently from spheres or aggregates. The motion of disc-shaped platelets is also different from that of spheres in solution, which depends on their size and the density of the solution. The freezing and thawing of platelets result in morphology changes due to damage to the platelets, with approximately 75% platelet recovery after resuspension. Loss of membrane integrity is partially prevented when 5–6% DMSO is added to the storage solution prior to freezing, which stabilizes the cytoskeleton and platelet membrane [8]. Frozen platelets protected with 5–6% DMSO survive their freeze-thaw cycle. Morphology changes can be measured with the Kunicki morphological scoring system [9], the "swirling" test [10] and the Thrombolux technology [11, 12]. Due to changes in morphology and the large amount of extracellular vesicles, freeze-thawed platelets show less swirling, a lower Kunicki score, and a lower Thrombolux score when compared to normal stored platelets [13]. The morphological differences between normal stored platelets and frozen platelets are shown in Fig. 26.1. Collectively, these changes suggest an activated phenotype.

Fig. 26.1 Morphology of standard stored and frozen platelets. Phase contrast microscopy of glutaraldehyde fixed normal stored (upper) and freeze-thawed platelets (lower). Black square indicates a length of 5.0 μm

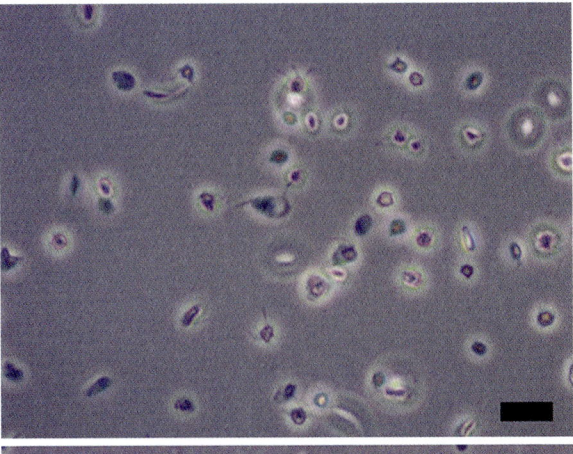

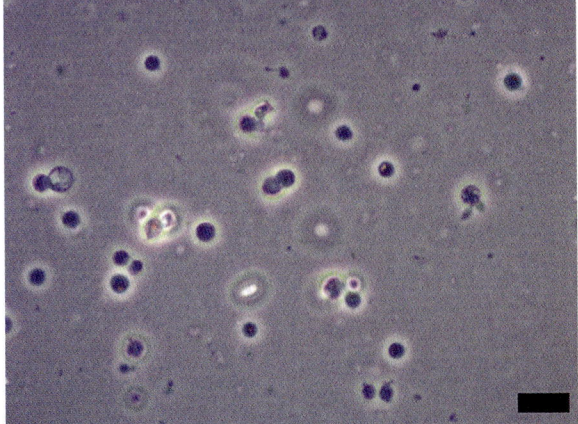

26.3.2 Activation Status

The addition of the cryoprotectant DMSO reduces damage to platelet membranes caused by the freeze-thawing [8]. However, even with DMSO added, freeze-thawed platelets still have an activated phenotype, as evidenced by a higher expression of P-selectin (CD62P), which is due to exocytosed platelet alpha granules [14], although there are large differences across studies using different production facilities [2, 15]. During post-thaw storage, P-selectin expression increases even further [16]. P-selectin plays a role in the recruitment and aggregation of platelets at areas of vascular injury. Thereby, an activated platelet state could contribute to enhanced coagulation.

26.3.3 Externalization of Phosphatidylserine and Extracellular Vesicle Shedding

In addition to upregulated exocytosis of P-selectin to the outer platelet membrane, intracellular calcium levels are higher in frozen platelets compared to liquid-stored platelets [17]. Higher levels of intracellular calcium levels are thought to induce phosphatidylserine externalization, leading to a more negative charge of the outer membrane, resulting in a loss of asymmetry in the platelet shape. Phosphatidylserine exposure is essential for connection of coagulation factor complexes (e.g., tenase and thrombinase), which are necessary for thrombin generation [18]. Furthermore, higher intracellular calcium levels in frozen platelets are associated with greater release of extracellular vesicles [19]. Extracellular vesicles, including microparticles and exosomes, are phospholipid-enclosed vesicles of less than 750 nm, the diameter of which is often 100-fold smaller than the cell. Extracellular vesicles are released by platelets upon activation. Estimates of extracellular vesicle content in freeze-thawed platelet concentrates differ between detection methods and experimental settings [12]. When the same detection method is used, the amount of extracellular vesicle content varies between 15% and 40% of the platelet population. Following freeze-thawing, approximately 15 times more extracellular vesicles are present when compared to pre-freeze levels. As extracellular vesicles are budding off from the activated platelet, phosphatidylserine is also abundantly expressed on platelet-derived extracellular vesicles, possibly enhancing the coagulation process.

26.4 The Impact of Freeze-Thawing on *In Vitro* Functional Coagulation Processes

26.4.1 Aggregation of Platelets

Aggregation of activated platelets is enhanced by von Willebrand factor and by fibrinogen. The expression of glycoprotein (GP)2b3a, which is the receptor both for von Willebrand factor and for fibrinogen, is not affected by the freezing procedure.

Freezing partially activates GP2b3a, leading to decreased PAC-1 binding, and thrombin receptor activating peptide (TRAP)-stimulated PAC-1 binding is lower compared to liquid-stored platelets [3, 16, 17, 20, 21]. Although different results between production sites have been reported, it appears that GP1b expression (which is the von Willebrand receptor) is also reduced in all or a subpopulation of frozen platelets. These GP1b-reduced platelets have decreased PAC-1 binding [22]. Also, lower GP1b receptor expression correlates with reduced aggregation responses [3]. Thereby, frozen platelets appear to have a reduced aggregation capacity *in vitro* when compared to fresh liquid-stored platelets [3, 22]. However, other facilitators of platelet aggregation, such as thromboxane, are found in higher levels in frozen platelets units when compared to normal stored platelets [16].

26.4.2 Thrombin Generation

Although *in vitro* aggregation is diminished in frozen platelets compared to liquid-stored platelets, thrombin-generating potential is enhanced in frozen platelets. As mentioned earlier, frozen platelets and their platelet-derived extracellular vesicles have increased expression of phosphatidylserine. As phosphatidylserine is able to bind coagulation factors V and X and is essential for connection of coagulation factor complexes [22], a higher phosphatidylserine expression is associated with earlier and more abundant thrombin generation [1, 14].

26.4.3 Viscoelastic Tests

All studies that have used viscoelastic tests, such as thromboelastography (TEG) and rotational thromboelastometry (ROTEM), in the characterization of their frozen platelets show the same results: frozen platelets have shorter clotting times compared to liquid platelets, indicating faster initiation of clotting, whereas clot strength is reduced. In Fig. 26.2, a representative figure of the kaolin TEG traces of normal liquid-stored platelets, frozen platelets, and plasma is shown. The reduction in clotting time with frozen platelets is from 8 to 5 min in kaolin TEG R-time in different studies, which relates to an approximately 38% reduction in the clotting time [1, 15]. The shorter clotting times are highly correlated with a higher thrombin-generating capacity of frozen platelets, which is related to the high proportion of phosphatidylserine-positive platelets and phosphatidylserine-positive platelet-derived extracellular vesicles [1]. A reduction in clot strength (maximum amplitude [MA] in TEG or maximum clot firmness [MCF] in ROTEM) of frozen platelets is correlated to lower GP1b expression on platelets, whereas extracellular vesicles do not contribute to clot strength in viscoelastic tests [21]. Thereby, frozen platelets seem to induce faster clotting than liquid-stored platelets, with an overall lower clot strength. These results underline the *in vitro* tests: a shorter clotting time correlates with increased thrombin-generating potential, and a lower clot strength correlates with decreased platelet aggregation.

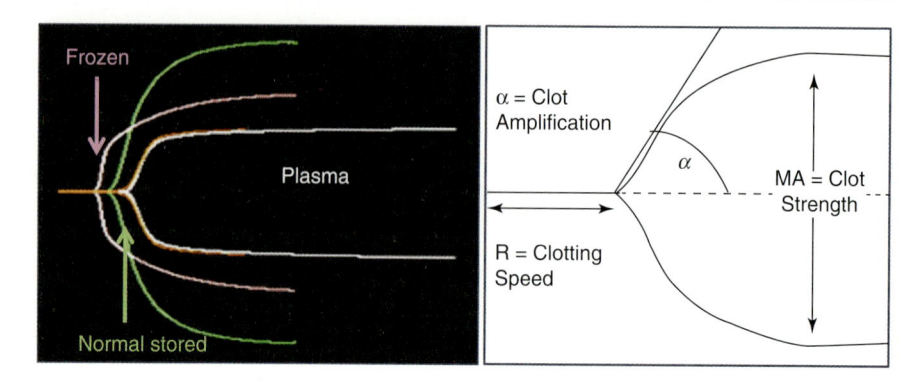

Fig. 26.2 Thromboelastography (TEG) traces of normal stored and frozen platelets. Typical TEG results of frozen and normal stored platelets with shortened R-time and reduced maximum amplitude (MA). Green trace = fresh platelet product, pink trace = frozen platelet product, and white trace = plasma

26.4.4 Flow Coagulation Models

In flow models, platelets flow over coated surfaces or vascular segments under different sheer rates. These models can be used to study factors that influence platelet margination to the vessel wall under different experimental conditions [23, 24]. The production process of frozen platelets did not result in an altered fibrin deposition in a flow model, suggesting that frozen platelets adequately stimulate fibrin formation [3, 25]. In another experiment using a flow model, frozen platelets resulted in the same amount of fibrin deposition compared to liquid-stored platelets [26]. As frozen platelets have decreased GP1b receptor expression and decreased platelet binding, it is possible that the increased concentration of extracellular vesicles accounts for the equivalent fibrin formation of frozen platelets in flow models. It is likely that compared to full-size platelets, the smaller extracellular vesicles can more easily interact with the vessel wall and initiate fibrin formation. In line with this thought, in a flow model, platelet-derived extracellular vesicles were shown to bind to immobilized collagen, fibrinogen, and von Willebrand factor, with increased thrombin production [3]. These data were further confirmed in a rodent model of mechanical vascular endothelial wall injury, in which infusion of platelet-derived labeled extracellular vesicles was associated with increased extracellular vesicle adherence to a damaged endothelial wall [27].

Taking the *in vitro* coagulation data together, frozen platelets show increased activation of coagulation, decreased aggregation, and increased thrombin-generating potential compared to liquid-stored platelets. In flow models, functional fibrin disposition is not different.

26.5 Clearance of Frozen Platelets

Most *in vitro* evaluations of platelets have limited value in prediction of *in vivo* functioning [28]. Frozen platelets have been studied in dogs [29, 30], rabbits [31], mice [32], and baboons [33]. Following transfusion in baboons, frozen platelets show faster clearance compared to fresh platelets, which depends on GP1b expression. The entire subpopulation of frozen platelets with reduced GP1b expressed was cleared from the circulation within 5 min, whereas 48% of the subpopulation of frozen platelets with normal GP1b expression had a 1–2 h survival, and a total lifespan similar to normal stored platelets (slightly less than 6 days) [22]. Phosphatidylserine and P-selectin mediate the endocytosis of platelet-derived extracellular vesicles by endothelial cells *in vitro* [34]. Platelet-derived extracellular vesicles are cleared fast from the circulation. A half-life of 5–6 h has been determined in thrombocytopenic patients for liquid-stored platelet-derived extracellular vesicles [35]. As frozen platelet-derived extracellular vesicles contain more surface markers than normal stored platelet extracellular vesicles, the half-life of frozen platelet-derived extracellular vesicles might be even faster.

26.6 Efficacy of Frozen Platelets in Experimental *In Vivo* Settings

Despite the more rapid clearance of frozen platelets following transfusion, the efficacy of the platelets to stop bleeding may be enhanced. In baboons treated with aspirin ($n = 5$), transfusion of frozen platelets, but not of 72-h liquid-stored platelets, reduced bleeding times. Frozen platelets also increased the levels of thromboxane in these baboons [36]. These findings are further supported by older trials in human volunteers ($n = 42$) pretreated with 650 mg of aspirin who received autologous platelet transfusion with different storage methods (groups varied from 8 to 12 volunteers). In these volunteers, bleeding times were reduced following transfusion with frozen platelets, but not after transfusion of normal stored platelets [37]. These data were reproduced by two other trials in healthy volunteers with aspirin pretreatment, in which frozen platelets were able to significantly reduce bleeding times [38, 39].

26.7 Experience with Frozen Platelets in the Military Setting

The technique to cryopreserve platelets was developed by the US Navy in the 1970s. In 2001, the Dutch Military Blood Bank adopted a modified platelet freezing method [40], including the use of thawed AB plasma instead of saline to resuspend the platelets after thawing. The Dutch military implemented and used this product for the first time in April 2002 during the ongoing war in Bosnia [41]. To date, the Netherlands military is still the only defense organization that uses frozen blood products in the treatment of bleeding trauma patients during operations abroad [42,

43]. The frozen platelets produced by the Dutch Military Blood Bank are available in Dutch medical treatment facilities as well as in some treatment facilities of coalition forces during mutual operations abroad. Between 2002 and 2019, 1055 bleeding patients were transfused with frozen blood products, including 356 patients who received 1152 frozen platelet products. These patients received a median of 2 [IQR 1–4] frozen platelet units per patient. Only two mild transfusion reactions (urticaria) have so far been observed, in two patients after transfusion of a unit of frozen platelets. These mild transfusion reactions are relatively low compared to the transfusion reaction rate reported with liquid-stored platelets (4–5 reactions per 1000 platelet products) in the Netherlands in 2017.

In the treatment facility of Tarin Kowt during the Afghanistan war (2006–2010), frozen platelets were the only platelet source available for the treatment of bleeding trauma patients. In Tarin Kowt, the use of a massive transfusion protocol was introduced. This introduction led to a higher use of plasma (median 4–6 units) and frozen platelet products (median 2–3 units) compared to the pre-protocol period. After introduction of the massive transfusion protocol, in-hospital mortality of massively (>5 red blood cell units/24 h) transfused trauma patients decreased from 44% to 14%, despite higher injury scores. Mortality was similar compared to the mortality of trauma patients in civilian and military trauma care who were treated with similar transfusion protocols but containing liquid-stored platelets [43]. These data suggest that the use of frozen platelets is effective and safe in military casualty care. The experience with Dutch frozen platelets during military operations [41, 43] has motivated many countries to learn the procedure from the Dutch military blood bank and start studying and producing frozen platelets [14, 42, 44, 45]. The Dutch military is currently preparing for a clinical non-inferiority trial to compare the efficacy of frozen platelets to normal stored platelets in the Netherlands in trauma and vascular surgery patients.

26.8 Clinical Trials with Frozen Platelets

26.8.1 Correction of Thrombocytopenia

Most of the earlier trials with frozen platelets were done in oncology patients with thrombocytopenia. In the trials prior to 2013 in oncology patients, product recovery was lower, and survival of frozen platelets following transfusion was similar to that of normal stored liquid platelets. However, frozen platelets were superior in reducing bleeding times and preventing bleeding events in these patient groups [46]. More recently, a multicenter dose-escalation randomized trial was performed in patients with (hematologic) malignancies with thrombocytopenia. Patients were randomized to receive either normal stored or different doses (0.5, 1, 2, or 3 units) of frozen platelets. In total, 28 patients were randomized. Of these, 24 received different doses of frozen platelets and 4 patients normal stored platelets. Platelet count increment was approximately six times lower in patients receiving frozen products compared to those receiving standard platelet products, which is in line with previous trials. In this trial, no bleeding episodes occurred and no thrombotic events were recorded. Also, no serious adverse events related to frozen platelet transfusion were observed. Minor reactions occurred in three patients treated with frozen platelets, varying from mild chills and fever to DMSO skin odor. In the four patients treated with normal stored platelets, no adverse events were observed [47].

26.8.2 Treatment of Bleeding

Recently, a case-control study was conducted in hemorrhaging polytrauma patients (n = 46), of whom 25 patients received frozen products. There were no differences in the amount of blood products in patients treated with normal stored platelets compared to frozen platelet-treated patients. A lower posttransfusion platelet count (41.5×10^9 vs. 97×10^9 /l) was seen in patients treated with frozen platelets compared to those in the normal stored platelet group.

In a recent pilot clinical trial, 121 elective cardiac surgery patients were randomized to receive either cryopreserved platelets or standard products for perioperative surgical bleeding (CLIP-1 trial) [5]. The trial randomized 121 patients; however, only 41 patients received the allocated treatment. In the remaining patients, platelet transfusion was not clinically indicated. Patients randomized to frozen products had a lower platelet count posttransfusion compared to those randomized to normal stored products (112 vs. 150×10^9/l, $p = 0.02$). However, frozen platelets were associated with a reduction in bleeding complications compared to normal stored platelets, although not reaching statistical significance (30.4% vs. 55.6% of patients, $p = 0.1$). Patients received a median of 2 units of frozen platelets or 1 unit of liquid-stored platelets. An explanation of the difference in volumes of platelet transfusion between the arms might be that physicians were targeting platelet increments, which are lower with frozen platelets compared to normal stored platelets. Interestingly, in the CLIP-1 trial, more patients ($n = 23$) allocated to frozen platelets were transfused with fresh frozen plasma (FFP) compared to patients randomized to normal stored platelets. Patients who received FFP received an equal dose (median 2 units). The finding of more FFP transfusions in patients treated with frozen platelets was contradictory to an earlier trial in cardiac surgery patients [4]. In this trial, 73 patients undergoing cardiac surgery were randomized to frozen platelets or normal stored platelets. Frozen platelets were associated with less blood loss and less transfusion product use compared to normal stored platelets, including FFP [4]. The reason for this discrepancy between the two largest trials on cryopreserved platelets in cardiac surgery is unclear.

26.9 Safety of Frozen Platelets

Frozen platelets may have inflammatory properties, as they contain more soluble P-selectin, produce more chemokine ligand 5 (CCL5) compared to fresh liquid platelets, and have a lower level of soluble CD40 ligand [15]. The elevated levels of soluble P-selectin suggest more platelet activation. CCL5 is a chemotactic molecule involved in the activation of T cells and natural killer cells. Soluble CD40 ligand can activate endothelial cells. In addition, frozen platelets are phagocytosed by macrophages, also generating an inflammatory response. This response is evidenced by increased release of tumor necrosis factor (TNF)-α, interleukin (IL)-1β, and transforming growth factor (TGF)-β compared to normal stored platelets and additionally increased IL-6 compared to fresh stored platelets [48]. Recently, in a mouse model of volume-controlled hemorrhage, transfusion of frozen platelets was associated with higher concentrations of pro-inflammatory cytokines in the liver compared to transfusion of liquid-stored platelets [32]. By contrast, following incubation with dendritic cells, an immunosuppressive effect of frozen platelet incubation was observed, as shown by decreased levels of pro-inflammatory cytokines compared to no transfusion controls [49]. However, to date, no serious adverse events have been reported in the various trials in oncology patients and the more recent trials of bleeding patients. As mentioned earlier, in the military experience, only two mild (urticarial) reactions were observed in 356 patients treated with frozen products [32].

Thus, when translating the *in vitro* data to the clinical situation, the evidence of an augmented inflammatory response after transfusion of cryopreserved platelets is limited [46]. This may be due to the rapid clearance of the freeze-thawed platelets and their derived extracellular vesicles. It should be noted however that prospective studies on complications are lacking.

26.10 Toward Specification of Platelet Products for Differential Use

Thawed and resuspended frozen platelets appear to be activated, with diminished aggregation properties, but with increased thrombin-generation potential. Lower clotting times in viscoelastic testing suggest faster clot initiation. In bleeding patients, frozen platelets seem promising due to these early hemostatic capacities. Frozen platelets are cleared more rapidly from the circulation. However, when bleeding has stopped, increased clearance of the transfused platelets may not be harmful to the patient and perhaps even beneficial. Conversely, given the superior survival rate, fresh liquid-stored platelets probably remain the product of choice for correction of thrombocytopenia. However, storage at room temperature for days may negatively influence platelet survival times in these products. When platelet survival is key, data suggest fresh normal stored platelets should be transfused.

26.11 Conclusion

In conclusion, data on the early hemostatic activity and use of cryopreserved platelets in initial clinical trials in bleeding patients are promising. Future directions should focus on verifying the results from previous trials in different subpopulations of massively bleeding civilian patients. Active screening for adverse events remains warranted in these trials.

References

1. Johnson L, Coorey CP, Marks DC. The hemostatic activity of cryopreserved platelets is mediated by phosphatidylserine-expressing platelets and platelet microparticles. Transfusion. 2014;54:1917–26.
2. Dumont LJ, Cancelas JA, Dumont DF, et al. A randomized controlled trial evaluating recovery and survival of 6% dimethyl sulfoxide-frozen autologous platelets in healthy volunteers. Transfusion. 2013;53:128–37.
3. Six KR, Delabie W, Devreese KMJ, et al. Comparison between manufacturing sites shows differential adhesion, activation, and GPIbalpha expression of cryopreserved platelets. Transfusion. 2018;58:2645–56.
4. Khuri SF, Healey N, MacGregor H, et al. Comparison of the effects of transfusions of cryopreserved and liquid-preserved platelets on hemostasis and blood loss after cardiopulmonary bypass. J Thorac Cardiovasc Surg. 1999;117:172–83.
5. Reade MC, Marks DC, Bellomo R, et al. A randomized, controlled pilot clinical trial of cryopreserved platelets for perioperative surgical bleeding: the CLIP-I trial. Transfusion. 2019;59:2794–804.
6. Frojmovic MM, Milton JG. Human platelet size, shape, and related functions in health and disease. Physiol Rev. 1982;62:185–261.
7. Fijnheer R, Pietersz RN, de Korte D, Roos D. Monitoring of platelet morphology during storage of platelet concentrates. Transfusion. 1989;29:36–40.
8. Reid TJ, LaRussa VF, Esteban G, et al. Cooling and freezing damage platelet membrane integrity. Cryobiology. 1999;38:209–24.
9. Fijnheer R, Pietersz RN, de Korte D, et al. Platelet activation during preparation of platelet concentrates: a comparison of the platelet-rich plasma and the buffy coat methods. Transfusion. 1990;30:634–8.
10. Bertolini F, Murphy S. A multicenter inspection of the swirling phenomenon in platelet concentrates prepared in routine practice. Biomedical Excellence for Safer Transfusion (BEST) Working Party of the International Society of Blood Transfusion. Transfusion. 1996;36:128–32.
11. Maurer-Spurej E, Brown K, Labrie A, Marziali A, Glatter O. Portable dynamic light scattering instrument and method for the measurement of blood platelet suspensions. Phys Med Biol. 2006;51:3747–58.
12. Maurer-Spurej E, Larsen R, Labrie A, Heaton A, Chipperfield K. Microparticle content of platelet concentrates is predicted by donor microparticles and is altered by production methods and stress. Transfus Apher Sci. 2016;55:35–43.
13. Raynel S, Padula MP, Marks DC, Johnson L. Cryopreservation alters the membrane and cytoskeletal protein profile of platelet microparticles. Transfusion. 2015;55:2422–32.
14. Hornsey VS, McMillan L, Morrison A, Drummond O, Macgregor IR, Prowse CV. Freezing of buffy coat-derived, leukoreduced platelet concentrates in 6 percent dimethyl sulfoxide. Transfusion. 2008;48:2508–14.
15. Crimmins D, Flanagan P, Charlewood R, Ruggiero K. In vitro comparison between gamma-irradiated cryopreserved and Day 7 liquid-stored buffy coat-derived platelet components. Transfusion. 2016;56:2799–807.
16. Johnson L, Reade MC, Hyland RA, Tan S, Marks DC. In vitro comparison of cryopreserved and liquid platelets: potential clinical implications. Transfusion. 2015;55:838–47.
17. Waters L, Padula MP, Marks DC, Johnson L. Cryopreserved platelets demonstrate reduced activation responses and impaired signaling after agonist stimulation. Transfusion. 2017;57:2845–57.
18. Schoenwaelder SM, Yuan Y, Josefsson EC, et al. Two distinct pathways regulate platelet phosphatidylserine exposure and procoagulant function. Blood. 2009;114:663–6.
19. Tegegn TZ, De Paoli SH, Orecna M, et al. Characterization of procoagulant extracellular vesicles and platelet membrane disintegration in DMSO-cryopreserved platelets. J Extracell Vesicles. 2016;5:30422.

20. Meinke S, Wikman A, Gryfelt G, et al. Cryopreservation of buffy coat-derived platelet concentrates photochemically treated with amotosalen and UVA light. Transfusion. 2018;58:2657–68.
21. Waters L, Padula MP, Marks DC, Johnson L. Cryopreservation of UVC pathogen-inactivated platelets. Transfusion. 2019;59:2093–102.
22. Barnard MR, MacGregor H, Ragno G, et al. Fresh, liquid-preserved, and cryopreserved platelets: adhesive surface receptors and membrane procoagulant activity. Transfusion. 1999;39:880–8.
23. de Witt SM, Swieringa F, Cavill R, et al. Identification of platelet function defects by multiparameter assessment of thrombus formation. Nat Commun. 2014;5:4257.
24. van Geffen JP, Brouns SLN, Batista J, et al. High-throughput elucidation of thrombus formation reveals sources of platelet function variability. Haematologica. 2019;104:1256–67.
25. Six KR, Devloo R, Compernolle V, Feys HB. Impact of cold storage on platelets treated with Intercept pathogen inactivation. Transfusion. 2019;59:2662–71.
26. Cid J, Escolar G, Galan A, et al. In vitro evaluation of the hemostatic effectiveness of cryopreserved platelets. Transfusion. 2016;56:580–6.
27. Keuren JF, Magdeleyns EJ, Bennaghmouch A, Bevers EM, Curvers J, Lindhout T. Microparticles adhere to collagen type I, fibrinogen, von Willebrand factor and surface immobilised platelets at physiological shear rates. Br J Haematol. 2007;138:527–33.
28. Marks DC, Johnson L. Assays for phenotypic and functional characterization of cryopreserved platelets. Platelets. 2019;30:48–55.
29. Valeri CR, Feingold H, Melaragno AJ, Vecchione JJ. Cryopreservation of dog platelets with dimethyl sulfoxide: therapeutic effectiveness of cryopreserved platelets in the treatment of thrombocytopenic dogs, and the effect of platelet storage at −80 degrees C. Cryobiology. 1986;23:387–94.
30. Callan MB, Appleman EH, Sachais BS. Canine platelet transfusions. J Vet Emerg Crit Care (San Antonio). 2009;19:401–15.
31. Rothwell SW, Maglasang P, Reid TJ, Gorogias M, Krishnamurti C. Correlation of in vivo and in vitro functions of fresh and stored human platelets. Transfusion. 2000;40:988–93.
32. Zhao J, Sun Z, You G, et al. Transfusion of cryopreserved platelets exacerbates inflammatory liver and lung injury in a mice model of hemorrhage. J Trauma Acute Care Surg. 2018;85:327–33.
33. Valeri CR, Ragno G. The survival and function of baboon red blood cells, platelets, and plasma proteins: a review of the experience from 1972 to 2002 at the Naval Blood Research Laboratory, Boston, Massachusetts. Transfusion. 2006;46(8 Suppl):1S–42S.
34. Ma R, Xie R, Yu C, et al. Phosphatidylserine-mediated platelet clearance by endothelium decreases platelet aggregates and procoagulant activity in sepsis. Sci Rep. 2017;7:4978.
35. Rank A, Nieuwland R, Delker R, et al. Cellular origin of platelet-derived microparticles in vivo. Thromb Res. 2010;126:e255–9.
36. Valeri CR, Giorgio A, Macgregor H, Ragno G. Circulation and distribution of autotransfused fresh, liquid-preserved and cryopreserved baboon platelets. Vox Sang. 2002;83:347–51.
37. Valeri CR. Hemostatic effectiveness of liquid-preserved and previously frozen human platelets. N Engl J Med. 1974;290:353–8.
38. Spector JI, Yarmala JA, Marchionni LD, Emerson CP, Valeri CR. Viability and function of platelets frozen at 2 to 3 C per minute with 4 or 6 per cent DMSO and stored at −80 C for 8 months. Transfusion. 1977;17:8–15.
39. Vecchione JJ, Melaragno AJ, Hollander A, Defina S, Emerson CP, Valeri CR. Circulation and function of human platelets isolated from units of CPDA-1, CPDA-2, and CPDA-3 anticoagulated blood and frozen with DMSO. Transfusion. 1982;22:206–9.
40. Valeri CR, Ragno G, Khuri S. Freezing human platelets with 6 percent dimethyl sulfoxide with removal of the supernatant solution before freezing and storage at −80 degrees C without postthaw processing. Transfusion. 2005;45:1890–8.
41. Lelkens CC, Koning JG, de Kort B, Floot IB, Noorman F. Experiences with frozen blood products in the Netherlands military. Transfus Apher Sci. 2006;34:289–98.

42. Cohn CS, Dumont LJ, Lozano M, et al. Vox Sanguinis International Forum on platelet cryopreservation: Summary. Vox Sang. 2017;112:684–8.
43. Noorman F, van Dongen TT, Plat MJ, Badloe JF, Hess JR, Hoencamp R. Transfusion: −80 degrees C frozen blood products are safe and effective in military casualty care. PLoS One. 2016;11:e0168401.
44. Johnson LN, Winter KM, Reid S, Hartkopf-Theis T, Marks DC. Cryopreservation of buffy-coat-derived platelet concentrates in dimethyl sulfoxide and platelet additive solution. Cryobiology. 2011;62:100–6.
45. Bohonek M, Kutac D, Landova L, et al. The use of cryopreserved platelets in the treatment of polytraumatic patients and patients with massive bleeding. Transfusion. 2019;59:1474–8.
46. Slichter SJ, Jones M, Ransom J, et al. Review of in vivo studies of dimethyl sulfoxide cryopreserved platelets. Transfus Med Rev. 2014;28:212–25.
47. Slichter SJ, Dumont LJ, Cancelas JA, et al. Safety and efficacy of cryopreserved platelets in bleeding patients with thrombocytopenia. Transfusion. 2018;58:2129–38.
48. Zhao J, Xu B, Chen G, et al. Cryopreserved platelets augment the inflammatory response: role of phosphatidylserine- and P-selectin-mediated platelet phagocytosis in macrophages. Transfusion. 2019;59:1799–808.
49. Ki KK, Johnson L, Faddy HM, Flower RL, Marks DC, Dean MM. Immunomodulatory effect of cryopreserved platelets: altered BDCA3(+) dendritic cell maturation and activation in vitro. Transfusion. 2017;57:2878–87.

Viscoelastic Assay-Guided Hemostatic Therapy in Perioperative and Critical Care

G. E. Iapichino, E. Costantini, and M. Cecconi

27.1 Introduction

Major bleeding and associated coagulopathy (either endogenous or pharmacological) complicate the course of a considerable proportion of invasive surgical procedures as well as different critical care settings. In addition, hemorrhage is the leading cause of potentially preventable deaths after traumatic injury [1]. Following the introduction of damage control principles in trauma care, treatment of severe bleeding has shifted from resuscitation with large volumes of crystalloids and colloids aiming at quasi-normal arterial pressure to permissive hypotension, crystalloid restriction, and early delivery of blood products in fixed ratios [2]. During the last three decades, viscoelastic tests such as thromboelastography (TEG) and thromboelastometry (ROTEM) have gained substantial attention for their ability to depict all phases of the coagulation process in a more timely and logistically convenient manner compared to standard coagulation tests. Furthermore, standard coagulation tests were designed to monitor anticoagulant therapy and evidence for their use to guide treatment with procoagulants is lacking [3]. By contrast, viscoelastic tests rapidly identify patients at risk of massive transfusion [4] and enable therapy to be customized according to the individual hemostatic deficit. The use of goal-directed protocols [5] is associated with faster time to hemostasis and reduction of blood product use, and such strategies are now integrated in both the European guideline on management of major bleeding following trauma and the European Society of

---

G. E. Iapichino · E. Costantini
Department of Anesthesia and Intensive Care Medicine, Humanitas Clinical and Research Center—IRCCS, Rozzano, Italy

M. Cecconi (✉)
Department of Anesthesia and Intensive Care Medicine, Humanitas Clinical and Research Center—IRCCS, Rozzano, Italy

Department of Biomedical Sciences, Humanitas University, Milan, Italy
e-mail: maurizio.cecconi@hunimed.eu

Anesthesiology guidelines on the management of severe perioperative bleeding [6, 7]. Nowadays, viscoelastic tests are part of the point-of-care laboratory of an increasing number of operating rooms and intensive care units (ICUs) worldwide and their application is expanding to other aspects of hemostasis, such as thromboembolic risk prediction, identification of patients with disseminated intravascular coagulation (DIC), anticoagulation monitoring during extracorporeal membrane oxygenation (ECMO), and monitoring of the newer oral anticoagulants. The aim of this chapter is to review the literature regarding the applications of viscoelastic tests in guiding hemostatic therapies in different clinical scenarios.

27.2 Viscoelastic Tests

Viscoelastic tests are coagulation assays performed on whole blood; they require less pre-analytic manipulations compared to standard coagulation tests (i.e., centrifugation to obtain platelet-free plasma) and provide better approximation of hemostasis as it occurs *in vivo*. The two most commonly used devices are TEG and ROTEM. In the TEG 5000, derived from the first experimental devices by Hartert in the early 1950s, 360 μl of whole blood are placed in a plastic cup with a pin on a torsion wire suspended in it. The cup then oscillates around the vertical axis through a total angle of 4.75°. As coagulation progresses and the viscoelastic strength of the clot increases, more rotation torque is transmitted to the pin and detected by the electromagnetic transducer. The signal is then interpreted by the software and depicted as the TEG tracing. Conversely, in the ROTEM *delta*, the pin oscillates while the cup is held in place and the pin encounters increasing resistance with increasing clot strength. In each assay, various activators can be added to the blood to better assess different portions of the clotting cascade and discriminate between the contribution of fibrinogen and platelets to clot strength (Table 27.1 and Fig. 27.1). The viscoelastic tracing shows time on the *x* axis (in minutes or seconds depending on the device and activator used) and amplitude in millimeters on the *y* axis as a measure of clot strength. In recent years both producers came up with revised products: the new generation ROTEM *sigma* kept the same viscoelastic mechanism as the previous *delta* platform but using a completely automated system based on a viscoelastic cartridge with four adjacent cups for four simultaneous tests. The new generation TEG 6S, on the other hand, changed mechanism of viscoelasticity measurement (the sample is exposed to a fixed vibration frequency and through light-emitting diode [LED] illumination a detector measures up/down motion of the blood meniscus) and is based on microfluidic cartridges designed for simultaneous assays.

27.3 Major Trauma and Trauma-Induced Coagulopathy

Acute hemorrhage often complicates the course of severely injured patients and is the leading cause of potentially preventable deaths after trauma [1]. Clinical and laboratory coagulopathy ensues very early after trauma, driven by a mix of

Table 27.1 Assay tests and activators

Assay name		Reagents		
TEG	ROTEM	TEG	ROTEM	Rationale
Native	NATEM	No reagents[a]	$CaCl_2$	Very sensitive to any endogenous activator such as tissue factor-expression but slower results
Kaolin	INTEM	Kaolin	$CaCl_2$ + ellagic acid	Coagulation activated by contact phase to assess intrinsic pathway
Heparinase	HEPTEM	Kaolin + heparinase	$CaCl_2$ + ellagic acid + heparinase	Detection of heparin or heparinoid effect by comparison with kaolin TEG or INTEM
RapidTEG		Kaolin + tissue factor		Rapid assessment of coagulation through activation of both intrinsic and extrinsic pathways
	EXTEM		$CaCl_2$ + tissue factor	Assessment of extrinsic pathway through tissue factor–factor VII activation
Functional fibrinogen	FIBTEM	Tissue factor + abciximab	$CaCl_2$ + tissue factor + cytochalasin D	Incorporates a platelet inhibitor to asses fibrin contribution to clot strength
	APTEM		$CaCl_2$ + tissue factor + tranexamic acid	Incorporates antifibrinolytic drugs to discriminate between fibrinolysis and normal clot retraction
	ECATEM		$CaCl_2$ + ecarin	Detection of direct thrombin inhibitors (hirudin, bivalirudin, argatroban, dabigatran)

$CaCl_2$ calcium chloride
[a]The TEG® 5000 provides analysis of whole blood and citrated whole blood; the newer version, TEG® 6S, uses only citrated whole blood. Whenever citrated whole blood is used, $CaCl_2$ is incorporated into the reagents

hypoperfusion, endothelial injury, activation of the protein C pathway, and innate immunity [8]. Coagulopathic trauma patients have greater odds of dying, higher transfusion requirements, and longer hospital stays [9]. It is therefore not surprising that the application of viscoelastic tests in this setting has increased exponentially over the last decades. Viscoelastic tests can rapidly detect coagulopathy and hyperfibrinolysis after admission in the trauma bay with a significantly shorter turnaround compared to conventional laboratory tests [10]. The ability of viscoelastic tests to identify coagulopathy and predict massive transfusion was demonstrated by a prospective international multicenter cohort study on 808 patients: a FIBTEM clot

EXTEM/Kaolin TEG	FIBTEM/Functional Fibrinogen TEG	Diagnosis
		Normal tracing
		Low Platelets
		Low Fibrinogen
INTEM/Kaolin TEG	HEPTEM/Heparinase TEG	
		Heparin effect
EXTEM/Kaolin TEG	APTEM	
		Hyperfibrinolysis

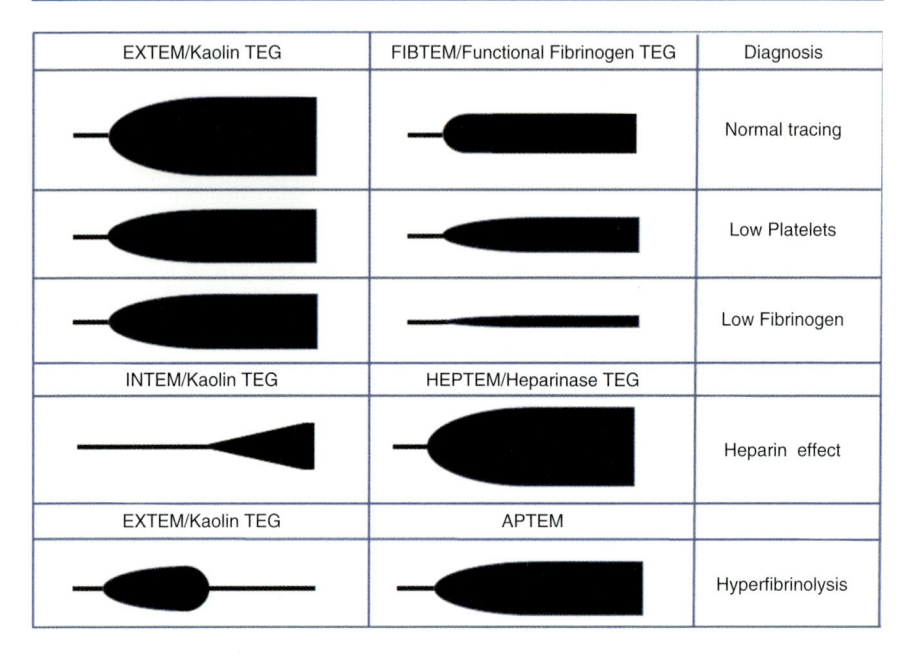

Fig. 27.1 Normal and pathological viscoelastic tracings. Viscoelastic tracing using extrinsic or intrinsic activators of coagulation is depicted in the left column. In the middle column are depicted tracings obtained with extrinsic or intrinsic activators plus other additives that block platelet function (FIBTEM/functional fibrinogen TEG), neutralize heparin (HEPTEM/heparinase TEG), or inhibit fibrinolysis (APTEM). The third column shows the interpretation of the viscoelastic tracings

amplitude at 5 min (A5) ≤8 mm detected coagulopathy in 67.5% of patients, and a FIBTEM A5 cutoff value ≤9 mm predicted massive transfusion in 77.5%. Similarly, an EXTEM A5 cutoff value ≤40 mm predicted massive transfusion in 72.7% of patients [11]. One of the hallmarks of trauma-induced coagulopathy is hyperfibrinolysis: it is a direct consequence of both tissue injury and shock, and is in part mediated by the consumption of plasminogen activator inhibitor-1 by activated protein C [8]. Viscoelastic tests can detect hyperfibrinolysis as reduced clot stability over time, but caution is warranted to distinguish pathological reduction in clot firmness from normal, low-grade clot retraction occurring in the late phase of the test and depending on platelet function. In a retrospective analysis of severe trauma patients presenting hyperfibrinolysis at ROTEM®, Schöchl and colleagues identified three different patterns of hyperfibrinolysis (fulminant: complete clot lysis within 30 min from start of the test; intermediate: complete lysis between 30 and 60 min; late: clot lysis after 60 min) [12]. The presence of hyperfibrinolysis was associated with significant mortality, with no survivors in the fulminant hyperfibrinolysis group. Other studies in the literature have reported on the incidence of hyperfibrinolysis detected by TEG (ranging from 2.5% to 7.2%) and its contribution to mortality in trauma patients [13]. More recently, Moore and colleagues investigated defective fibrinolysis, defined as fibrinolysis shutdown and diagnosed with a TEG lysis ≤0.9% at 30 min, in a cohort of 180 severely injured patients [14]. They found that fibrinolysis shutdown was frequent (63% of the patients) and associated with higher mortality compared to physiologic fibrinolysis. Those results, however, were questioned in a later retrospective study by Gomez-Builes and colleagues in a cohort of 550 trauma patients [15]. In their ROTEM®-based study, the authors defined shutdown as a value of maximum lysis <3.5%; the incidence of shutdown at admission was 25.6% and, despite a higher injury severity score and greater need for blood transfusions, it was not associated with mortality, suggesting that it could represent an appropriate physiologic response to life-threatening trauma. TEG and ROTEM are therefore able to quickly identify patients at risk from massive transfusion and to discriminate the predominant phenotype of coagulopathy, providing clinicians with critical data for decision-making.

Evidence of effectiveness of viscoelastic tests in reducing transfusion requirements, healthcare costs, and complication rates is increasing [16–18]. In the trauma setting, the first report of benefit from a viscoelastic test-guided algorithm was published by Schöchl and colleagues, who demonstrated favorable survival rates as compared to predicted trauma and injury severity score (TRISS) mortality (24.4% vs. 33.7%; $p = 0.032$) in a retrospective analysis of 131 patients treated with a ROTEM-guided algorithm [19]. In their pre-post cohort study published in 2015, Nardi and colleagues assessed the impact of early ROTEM-based coagulation support on blood product consumption, mortality, and treatment costs [20]. They compared two matched cohorts of patients (median ISS 32.9 vs. 33.6) before and after the introduction of a coagulation support protocol based on the early delivery of 4 units of packed red blood cells (RBCs) and 2 g of fibrinogen concentrate followed by ROTEM-guided transfusions. The authors found marked reduction in blood product consumption, reaching statistical significance for fresh frozen plasma (FFP) and platelet concentrates, and a non-significant trend toward a reduction in early and 28-day mortality. The overall costs for transfusion and coagulation support (including point-of-care tests) decreased by 23% between 2011 and 2013. One year later, Gonzalez and colleagues published their single-center randomized controlled trial comparing goal-directed hemostatic resuscitation using TEG versus standard coagulation tests [21]. In their trial, all patients enrolled (131 patients, 56 in the TEG group, 55 in standard coagulation tests group) received an initial transfusion of 4 units of RBCs and 2 units of FFP upon activation of the massive transfusion protocol. After the initial transfusion, patients followed an algorithm based either on standard coagulation tests (international normalized ratio [INR], platelet count, fibrinogen level, and D-dimer) or on rapid-TEG. Twenty-eight-day mortality was greater in the standard coagulation test group compared to the TEG group (36.4% vs. 19.6%, $p = 0.032$). The two groups did not differ in terms of RBC transfusions, but the TEG group received less FFP, platelets, and cryoprecipitate at selected time points. Finally, in 2017, Innerhofer and colleagues prospectively compared the efficacy of ROTEM-guided administration of coagulation factor concentrates (fibrinogen, factor XIII, and four-factor PCC) versus plasma transfusion to treat traumatic coagulopathy and to stop bleeding [22]. Trauma patients with ISS >15 and signs of coagulopathy were randomized to either 15 ml/kg of FFP (48 patients) or coagulation factor concentrate therapy (predominantly fibrinogen) guided by ROTEM (52 patients). After the second round of therapy according to each protocol (FFP vs. factor concentrates) and in case of treatment failure (persisting coagulopathic bleeding or pathological ROTEM results), rescue therapy was initiated with crossover of the protocols. The trial was stopped early as the preplanned interim analysis showed a significant difference in treatment failure combined with an increased risk of massive transfusion in patients in the FFP group. Indeed, FFP failed to correct coagulopathy in 52% of patients compared to only 4% of patients in the ROTEM-guided group. Furthermore, massive transfusion rate (12% vs. 30%; $p = 0.042$) and number of days on hemofiltration (11.0 vs. 27.0; $p = 0.038$) were lower in the ROTEM-guided group. Further high-quality evidence on the use of viscoelastic tests to guide hemostatic resuscitation after severe trauma will be provided soon from three ongoing randomized clinical trials: two single-center studies (STATA trial—Clinicaltrials.gov Identifier: NCT02416817; VISCOTRAUMA trial—Clinicaltrials.gov Identifier: NCT03380767) and one multicenter study (iTACTIC trial—Clinicaltrials.gov Identifier: NCT02593877).

27.4 Cardiovascular Surgery

The contribution of viscoelastic tests to perioperative hemostasis management in cardiac surgery has been extensively studied in past years. Many retrospective, observational, before and after studies as well as randomized controlled studies have pointed toward a benefit of viscoelastic test-guided algorithms compared to standard care in reducing time to diagnosis of coagulopathy, allogeneic blood component transfusions, surgical re-explorations, thromboembolic events, and incidence of postoperative kidney failure. It is worth noting that, compared to other clinical settings, the use of perioperative antiplatelet drugs is more frequent in cardiac surgery and point-of-care tests of platelet function are commonly integrated with viscoelastic results in algorithms of hemostasis management. A systematic review and cost-effectiveness analysis in the cardiac surgery setting found that viscoelastic tests were cost-saving and more effective than standard coagulation tests, with the greatest saving per-patient for TEG (£79) followed by ROTEM (£43) [17]. The authors confirmed previous findings of a significant reduction in RBC transfusions [RR 0.88, 95% confidence interval (CI) 0.80–0.96; six studies], platelet transfusions (RR 0.72, 95% CI 0.58–0.89; six studies), and FFP transfusions (RR 0.47, 95% CI 0.35–0.65; five studies); however, clinical outcomes did not differ significantly between groups. Deppe and colleagues recently published a meta-analysis of 17 studies (9 randomized controlled trials and 8 observational studies) [18]. For patients allocated to viscoelastic test algorithms, they confirmed decreased odds to receive allogeneic blood products (OR 0.63, 95% CI 0.56–0.71; $p < 0.00001$) and re-exploration due to postoperative bleeding (OR 0.56, 95% CI 0.45–0.71; $p < 0.00001$), and reduced incidence of acute kidney injury (AKI; OR 0.77, 95% CI 0.61–0.98; $p = 0.0278$) and thromboembolic events (OR 0.44, 95% CI 0.28–0.70; $p = 0.0006$). A subsequent meta-analysis, including a large multicenter stepped-wedge cluster randomized controlled study on 7402 patients, concluded that evidence to support use of viscoelastic testing in cardiac surgery is weak because TEG- or ROTEM-guided algorithms for management of coagulopathic hemorrhage had no effect on clinically sound outcomes such as mortality, stroke, emergency re-exploration, or ICU length of stay [23]. Nevertheless, the 2017 joint guidelines from the European Association for Cardio-Thoracic Surgery and European Association for Cardiothoracic Anesthesiology suggest considering viscoelastic test-based algorithms for the bleeding patient to reduce the number of transfusions (Class IIa, level B) [24].

27.5 Liver Disease, Hepatic Surgery, and Transplantation

The coagulopathy of end-stage liver disease, once diagnosed by prolongation of conventional coagulation tests and thought to expose patients to an increased tendency to bleed, results from complex derangements in both anti- and procoagulant processes and involves humoral and cell-based hemostasis. Patients with cirrhosis are now believed to have a "rebalanced" coagulation system because decreased levels of procoagulants are accompanied by decreased levels of naturally occurring anticoagulants. This new balance, however, may be easily shifted toward bleeding or thrombosis by underlying or ensuing clinical conditions as well as invasive procedures. Prothrombin time (PT) and activated partial thromboplastin time (aPTT) are unsuitable in this setting as they only measure reduced procoagulant factor concentrations, missing the simultaneous drop in anticoagulants. Viscoelastic tests are not hindered by conventional test limits and have been increasingly applied in liver disease and liver surgery since the early 1990s. Two studies investigated the ability of ROTEM to predict transfusion requirements during liver transplantation and in the postoperative period. In their retrospective study on 100 patients, Fayed and colleagues examined the correlation of preoperative ROTEM results with intraoperative transfusion requirements and demonstrated that prolonged preoperative EXTEM clotting time was an independent predictor for RBC and FFP transfusions [25]. Similarly, Dötsch and colleagues retrospectively analyzed data from 243 patients undergoing liver transplantation to evaluate whether ROTEM or standard coagulation tests obtained at ICU admission could predict the occurrence of bleeding requiring relaparotomy or transfusion of three or more packed RBC units within 48 h [26]. Patients were treated with an evidence-based ROTEM-guided transfusion algorithm intraoperatively and in the ICU, and the overall incidence of bleeding was 12.3%; aPTT (area under the curve [AUC] 0.69 [0.63–0.75]), PT (0.62 [0.56–0.69]), EXTEM clotting time (0.68 [0.62–0.74]), and FIBTEM A10 (0.64 [0.57–0.70]) were significantly associated with major postoperative bleeding, with FIBTEM being a better predictor of postoperative bleeding compared to plasma fibrinogen concentration. Viscoelastic tests not only predict bleeding but may also help in the prediction of thrombotic complications after liver transplantation. A retrospective analysis of 828 liver transplant patients revealed an incidence of hepatic artery thrombosis of 9.5% (79 patients); the maximum amplitude on preoperative TEG was significantly higher in patients diagnosed with early hepatic artery thrombosis compared to those without (71.2 mm vs. 57.9 mm; $p < 0.0001$). Receiver operating characteristic analysis with the cutoff value for maximum amplitude of 65 mm or greater returned an AUC of 0.75 ($p < 0.001$) predicting early hepatic artery thrombosis with a sensitivity of 70% [27].

Viscoelastic test-guided management of invasive procedures in cirrhotic patients and of bleeding during liver surgery has been investigated in recent years by several retrospective and prospective studies. As in cardiac surgery, the bulk of the literature suggests a role for viscoelastic-guided protocols to reduce allogeneic blood product exposure along with postoperative complications but without significant improvements in mortality. For the sake of the present review, it is worth reporting the results of two pragmatic studies. De Pietri and colleagues, in their prospective, open-label randomized controlled study, randomized 60 consecutive cirrhotic patients with coagulopathy (INR > 1.8 and/or platelet count <50 × 10^9/l) scheduled to undergo an invasive procedure to receive blood products according to either standard coagulation tests or TEG results [28]. All subjects in the standard coagulation test group received blood products vs. only five in the TEG group (100% vs. 16.7%, $p < 0.0001$). Post-procedural bleeding occurred in only one subject in the conventional test group; numbers of packed RBC transfusions were comparable in both groups. Leon-Justel and colleagues prospectively evaluated the institution of a point-of-care hemostasis management strategy in 200 consecutive liver transplant patients [29]. They compared the first 100 patients (before cohort) with the next 100 patients (after cohort) and found that a ROTEM-guided transfusion algorithm reduced the rate of transfusion of packed RBCs, FFP, and platelets, resulting in an increased rate of transfusion-free transplants from 5% to 24% ($p < 0.001$), a reduction of massive transfusion from 13% to 2% ($p = 0.005$), and a concomitant reduction in postoperative complications [29].

27.6 Postpartum Hemorrhage

Despite the decline in mortality due to improvements in obstetric and anesthetic management, hemorrhage remains the most frequent cause of major morbidity in the obstetric population leading to postpartum hysterectomies and ICU admissions. Severe obstetric hemorrhage is often associated with coagulopathy of dramatic onset, the severity of which varies depending on the cause: dilution of the circulating volume with non-hemostatic fluids, consumption of coagulation factors, and fibrinogen and fibrinolytic cascade disturbances to mention a few. Importantly, during normal pregnancy, there is an increase in coagulation factors, a decrease in naturally occurring anticoagulants, and an increase in platelet reactivity, inducing a procoagulant milieu (detected by viscoelastic assays [30]), which allows most cases of postpartum hemorrhage to be well tolerated without the need for administration of allogeneic blood products. On the other hand, low plasma fibrinogen is associated with increased risk of progression to severe postpartum hemorrhage. The utility of viscoelastic tests in the prediction of severity of bleeding episode and need for transfusions was investigated by Collins and colleagues in a prospective cohort study of 347 women with estimated blood loss of at least 1 liter [31]. The authors found that FIBTEM A5 and plasma fibrinogen had similarly improved diagnostic ability for larger hemorrhage volumes and prediction of transfusion of 4 or more RBC units (AUC 0.78 for both FIBTEM A5 and fibrinogen); FIBTEM results, however, were available much sooner compared to laboratory fibrinogen levels. The same group, in a later multicenter study, randomized women with ongoing postpartum hemorrhage and a FIBTEM A5 ≤15 mm to receive either fibrinogen concentrate or placebo [32]. The study was negative: fibrinogen concentrate therapy was not associated with fewer transfusions, but the pre-specified subgroup analyses suggested that fibrinogen replacement may be beneficial in case of lower FIBTEM A5 (≤12 mm). More recently, McNamara and colleagues reported the results of an observational study following the introduction of a ROTEM-guided fibrinogen concentrate-based algorithm to treat coagulopathy in major obstetric hemorrhage [33]. In the 4-year study period, 893 women had an estimated blood loss exceeding 1500 ml (defined as major hemorrhage), 203 of whom exhibited a FIBTEM A5 ≤12 mm. The authors compared clinical outcomes and transfusions of those 203 patients with 52 patients with the same criteria over a 12-month pre-intervention period. In the algorithm group, there was a significant reduction in the number of units ($p < 0.0001$) and total volume of blood products transfused ($p = 0.0007$), with a reduction in transfusion-associated circulatory overload ($p = 0.002$). Reduction of FFP transfusion explains the significant reduction in overall allogeneic transfusions; the use of fibrinogen concentrates to treat coagulopathy instead of FFP is likely to be responsible for the improvement in clinical outcome (and elimination of the incidence of transfusion-associated circulatory overload). Again, viscoelastic test-guided algorithms facilitate rapid and precise diagnosis of coagulopathy and also diagnosis of absence of coagulopathy, avoiding unnecessary blood product transfusion.

27.7 Venous Thromboembolism

In addition to their role in the management of coagulopathies, viscoelastic tests can detect hypercoagulability and help in the prediction of thrombotic complications. Trauma patients often arrive at the emergency department in a hypocoagulable or normocoagulable state, but, within 5 days, over half of the patients progress to hypercoagulability and are at increased risk of deep vein thrombosis, as shown in a retrospective analysis of prospectively collected data on 898 trauma patients [34]. Furthermore, hypercoagulable TEG results at admission predicted subsequent venous thromboembolism in two large cohorts of trauma patients [35, 36]: Brill and colleagues, in their prospective cohort study on 684 patients, found hypercoagulable TEG (reaction time below, angle above, or maximum amplitude above reference ranges) to be independently associated with deep vein thrombosis at multivariate analysis, with an odds ratio of 2.41 (95% confidence interval, 1.11–5.24; $p = 0.026$) [35]; similarly, Cotton and colleagues found maximal amplitude >72 mm on the admission TEG to predict pulmonary embolism risk with an odds ratio of almost 6.0 (5.8, 95% confidence interval 2.86–11-78; $p < 0.0001$). Maximal amplitude cutoff >72 mm alone had a sensitivity of 49% and specificity of 87% for pulmonary embolism prediction [36].

In the ICU setting, an Australian group enrolled patients with suspected coagulopathy (PT >1.5 and/or aPTT >40 s and/or platelet count <150 × 10^9/l) and higher perceived risk of bleeding and performed a TEG analysis within 48 h from admission [37]. At follow-up, 15.8% of the 215 patients enrolled developed symptomatic thromboembolism; most patients had normal or increased clot strength at TEG analysis (despite abnormal standard coagulation tests) and several TEG parameters suggested hypercoagulability in those who subsequently developed thromboembolism. Additionally, a viscoelastic-based algorithm to adjust low-molecular-weight heparin (LMWH) in ICU patients was compared to standard fixed dosing in two recent randomized controlled studies [38, 39]. Together, the two studies enrolled 235 trauma and general surgery patients admitted to the ICU. In the TEG-based group the targeted value of the change in reaction time (reaction time without heparinase - reaction time with heparinase) was 1–2 min in one study [38] and >1.4 min in the other [39], and LMWH dose was titrated accordingly. In both studies, the proportion of patients in the treatment groups achieving the target change in reaction time was low (10.4% in the study by Connelly and colleagues [38] and 12% in the study by Harr and colleagues [39]), and there were no differences in thromboembolic events between the treatment and control groups.

27.8 Sepsis and Septic Shock

Given the complexity and number of interconnections between the inflammatory and hemostatic systems, it is no surprise that coagulation disturbances are frequent in patients with sepsis and associated with increased mortality [40]. Due to their ability to depict bed-sided whole blood coagulation potential, viscoelastic tests are privileged tests in the assessment of patients with septic shock in the ICU. In their prospective study on 50 septic patients, Ostrowski and colleagues found that patients with hypocoagulable kaolin-activated TEG at admission (maximal amplitude <51 mm) had higher Sequential Organ Failure Assessment (SOFA) scores and DIC scores compared with hypercoagulable patients and higher 28-day mortality compared with normocoagulable patients (all $p < 0.05$) [40]. Those results were confirmed by a retrospective analysis on the data from 260 patients from a randomized controlled trial of hetastarch resuscitation in sepsis [41]. The authors performed a Cox regression analysis with time-dependent covariates and joint modeling techniques including TEG variables at admission and daily in the ICU and clinical data such as bleeding and mortality. They found that deterioration toward hypocoagulability (or hypercoagulability) in any TEG variable significantly increased (or decreased) the risk of death compared with normocoagulability. The impact of fibrinolysis derangement on the outcome of septic patients was analyzed in two studies using TEG and ROTEM, respectively [42, 43]. Both studies prospectively enrolled patients with sepsis or septic shock admitted to the ICU: Panigada and colleagues performed a modified kaolin TEG test with the addition of urokinase to better assess fibrinolysis; their analysis revealed a greater impairment of fibrinolysis in septic patients ($n = 40$) compared to healthy individuals ($n = 40$), and the lysis at 30 min parameter predicted mortality at ICU discharge (OR 0.95, 95% CI 0.93–0.98, $p = 0.003$) in univariate logistic regression [42]. Similarly, Prakash and colleagues enrolled 70 septic patients followed with ROTEM analysis, standard coagulation tests and other parameters at admission and daily for 72 h [43]. Impaired fibrinolysis on ROTEM was correlated with severity of organ failure in septic patients at presentation. By contrast, improvement in sepsis-related organ failure was strongly associated with an early increase in fibrinolysis as reflected by an increase in maximum lysis. Aside from the described prognostic ability, the implications for viscoelastic-guided therapeutic intervention in sepsis are still unknown.

27.9 Extracorporeal Membrane Oxygenation

Choice of anticoagulant, degree of anticoagulation, and its monitoring during ECMO are highly debated topics in the literature. While many centers rely on multiple coagulation tests to follow the course of ECMO patients, the evidence for viscoelastic tests to guide bleeding and anticoagulation in this setting is scarce. Reduced clot firmness at EXTEM and FIBTEM was significantly associated with severe bleeding in a retrospective study of 24 ECMO patients and 23 patients with a ventricular assist device [44]; conversely, no association between TEG variables and bleeding was found in a retrospective study on 32 patients on venovenous ECMO, although 46% of the kaolin TEG analyses showed considerable heparin effect [45]. The same group recently published a pilot randomized controlled trial on the safety and feasibility of a TEG-based protocol to guide anticoagulation during venovenous ECMO as compared with an aPTT-based protocol [46]. The patients allocated to the TEG group compared to the aPTT group received less heparin (11.7 vs. 15.7 units/kg/h, $p = 0.03$), had a trend toward fewer bleeding events (47.6% vs. 71.4%, $p = 0.21$), and experienced the same number of thrombotic events (19% vs. 19%, $p = 1$).

27.10 Conclusion

Viscoelastic tests have become an essential part of hemostatic assessment in a wide range of clinical scenarios spanning from the emergency setting through elective surgery to the ICU. Coagulation management guided by algorithms incorporating viscoelastic tests has been shown to be effective in reducing bleeding, transfusion requirements, complication rates, and healthcare costs. The role of viscoelastic tests in improving important clinical endpoints, however, is currently supported by limited and low-quality evidence. Moreover, further research on the optimal transfusion triggers and targets using viscoelastic tests may facilitate clinical practice and result in improved patient safety.

References

1. Holcomb JB, del Junco DJ, Fox EE, et al. The prospective, observational, multicenter, major trauma transfusion (PROMMTT) study: comparative effectiveness of a time-varying treatment with competing risks. JAMA Surg. 2013;148:127–36.
2. Bogert JN, Harvin JA, Cotton BA. Damage control resuscitation. J Intensive Care Med. 2016;31:177–86.
3. Haas T, Fries D, Tanaka KA, Asmis L, Curry NS, Schöchl H. Usefulness of standard plasma coagulation tests in the management of perioperative coagulopathic bleeding: is there any evidence? Br J Anaesth. 2015;114:217–24.
4. Song JG, Jeong SM, Jun IG, Lee HM, Hwang GS. Five-minute parameter of thromboelastometry is sufficient to detect thrombocytopenia and hypofibrinogenaemia in patients undergoing liver transplantation. Br J Anaesth. 2014;112:290–7.
5. Schöchl H, Maegele M, Voelckel W. Fixed ratio versus goal-directed therapy in trauma. Curr Opin Anaesthesiol. 2016;29:234–44.
6. Spahn DR, Bouillon B, Cerny V, et al. The European guideline on management of major bleeding and coagulopathy following trauma: fifth edition. Crit Care. 2019;23:98.
7. Kozek-Langenecker SA, Ahmed AB, Afshari A, et al. Management of severe perioperative bleeding: guidelines from the European Society of Anaesthesiology: First update 2016. Eur J Anaesthesiol. 2017;34:332–95.
8. Brohi K, Cohen MJ, Ganter MT, et al. Acute coagulopathy of trauma: hypoperfusion induces systemic anticoagulation and hyperfibrinolysis. J Trauma. 2008;64:1211–7.
9. Maegele M, Lefering R, Yucel N, et al. Early coagulopathy in multiple injury: an analysis from the German Trauma Registry on 8724 patients. Injury. 2007;38:298–304.
10. Schöchl H, Cotton B, Inaba K, et al. FIBTEM provides early prediction of massive transfusion in trauma. Crit Care. 2011;15:R265.
11. Hagemo JS, Christiaans SC, Stanworth SJ, et al. Detection of acute traumatic coagulopathy and massive transfusion requirements by means of rotational thromboelastometry: an international prospective validation study. Crit Care. 2015;19:97.
12. Schöchl H, Frietsch T, Pavelka M, Jámbor C. Hyperfibrinolysis after major trauma: differential diagnosis of lysis patterns and prognostic value of thrombelastometry. J Trauma. 2009;67:125–31.
13. Carroll RC, Craft RM, Langdon RJ, et al. Early evaluation of acute traumatic coagulopathy by thrombelastography. Transl Res. 2009;154:34–9.
14. Moore HB, Moore EE, Gonzalez E, et al. Hyperfibrinolysis, physiologic fibrinolysis, and fibrinolysis shutdown: the spectrum of postinjury fibrinolysis and relevance to antifibrinolytic therapy. J Trauma Acute Care Surg. 2014;77:811–7.
15. Gomez-Builes JC, Acuna SA, Nascimento B, Madotto F, Rizoli SB. Harmful or physiologic: diagnosing fibrinolysis shutdown in a trauma cohort with rotational thromboelastometry. Anesth Analg. 2018;127:840–9.
16. Wikkelsø A, Wetterslev J, Møller AM, Afshari A. Thromboelastography (TEG) or thromboelastometry (ROTEM) to monitor haemostatic treatment versus usual care in adults or children with bleeding. Cochrane Database Syst Rev. 2016;CD007871.
17. Whiting P, Al M, Westwood M, et al. Viscoelastic point-of-care testing to assist with the diagnosis, management and monitoring of haemostasis: a systematic review and cost-effectiveness analysis. Health Technol Assess. 2015;19:1–228.
18. Deppe AC, Weber C, Zimmermann J, et al. Point-of-care thromboelastography/thromboelastometry-based coagulation management in cardiac surgery: a meta-analysis of 8332 patients. J Surg Res. 2016;203:424–33.
19. Schöchl H, Nienaber U, Hofer G, et al. Goal-directed coagulation management of major trauma patients using thromboelastometry-guided administration of fibrinogen concentrate and prothrombin complex concentrate. Crit Care. 2010;14:R55.

20. Nardi G, Agostini V, Rondinelli B, et al. Trauma-induced coagulopathy: impact of the early coagulation support protocol on blood product consumption, mortality and costs. Crit Care. 2015;19:83.
21. Gonzalez E, Moore EE, Moore HB, et al. Goal-directed hemostatic resuscitation of trauma-induced coagulopathy: a pragmatic randomized clinical trial comparing a viscoelastic assay to conventional coagulation assays. Ann Surg. 2016;263:1051–9.
22. Innerhofer P, Fries D, Mittermayr M, et al. Reversal of trauma-induced coagulopathy using first-line coagulation factor concentrates or fresh frozen plasma (RETIC): a single-centre, parallel-group, open-label, randomised trial. Lancet Haematol. 2017;4:e258–71.
23. Serraino GF, Murphy GJ. Routine use of viscoelastic blood tests for diagnosis and treatment of coagulopathic bleeding in cardiac surgery: updated systematic review and meta-analysis. Br J Anaesth. 2017;118:823–33.
24. Pagano D, Milojevic M, Meesters MI, et al. 2017 EACTS/EACTA Guidelines on patient blood management for adult cardiac surgery. Eur J Cardiothorac Surg. 2018;53:79–111.
25. Fayed N, Mourad W, Yassen K, Görlinger K. Preoperative thromboelastometry as a predictor of transfusion requirements during adult living donor liver transplantation. Transfus Med Hemother. 2015;42:99–108.
26. Dötsch TM, Dirkmann D, Bezinover D, et al. Assessment of standard laboratory tests and rotational thromboelastometry for the prediction of postoperative bleeding in liver transplantation. Br J Anaesth. 2017;119:402–10.
27. Zahr Eldeen F, Roll GR, Derosas C, et al. Preoperative thromboelastography as a sensitive tool predicting those at risk of developing early hepatic artery thrombosis after adult liver transplantation. Transplantation. 2016;100:2382–90.
28. De Pietri L, Bianchini M, Montalti R, et al. Thrombelastography-guided blood product use before invasive procedures in cirrhosis with severe coagulopathy: a randomized, controlled trial. Hepatology. 2016;63:566–73.
29. Leon-Justel A, Noval-Padillo JA, Alvarez-Rios AI, et al. Point-of-care haemostasis monitoring during liver transplantation reduces transfusion requirements and improves patient outcome. Clin Chim Acta. 2015;446:277–83.
30. Sharma SK, Philip J, Wiley J. Thromboelastographic changes in healthy parturients and postpartum women. Anesth Analg. 1997;85:94–8.
31. Collins PW, Lilley G, Bruynseels D, et al. Fibrin-based clot formation as an early and rapid biomarker for progression of postpartum hemorrhage: a prospective study. Blood. 2014;124:1727–36.
32. Collins PW, Cannings-John R, Bruynseels D, et al. Viscoelastometric-guided early fibrinogen concentrate replacement during postpartum haemorrhage: OBS2, a double-blind randomized controlled trial. Br J Anaesth. 2017;119:411–21.
33. McNamara H, Kenyon C, Smith R, Mallaiah S, Barclay P. Four years' experience of ROTEM-guided algorithm for treatment of coagulopathy in obstetric haemorrhage. Anaesthesia. 2019;74:984–91.
34. Sumislawski JJ, Kornblith LZ, Conroy AS, Callcut RA, Cohen MJ. Dynamic coagulability after injury: Is delaying venous thromboembolism chemoprophylaxis worth the wait? J Trauma Acute Care Surg. 2018;85:907–14.
35. Brill JB, Badiee J, Zander AL, et al. The rate of deep vein thrombosis doubles in trauma patients with hypercoagulable thromboelastography. J Trauma Acute Care Surg. 2017;83:413–9.
36. Cotton BA, Minei KM, Radwan ZA, et al. Admission rapid thrombelastography predicts development of pulmonary embolism in trauma patients. J Trauma Acute Care Surg. 2012;72:1470–5.
37. Harahsheh Y, Duff OC, Ho KM. Thromboelastography predicts thromboembolism in critically ill coagulopathic patients. Crit Care Med. 2019;47:826–32.
38. Connelly CR, Van PY, Hart KD, et al. Thrombelastography-based dosing of enoxaparin for thromboprophylaxis in trauma and surgical patients: a randomized clinical trial. JAMA Surg. 2016;151:e162069.

39. Harr JN, Moore EE, Chin TL, et al. Platelets are dominant contributors to hypercoagulability after injury. J Trauma Acute Care Surg. 2013;74:756–65.
40. Ostrowski SR, Windeløv NA, Ibsen M, Haase N, Perner A, Johansson PI. Consecutive thrombelastography clot strength profiles in patients with severe sepsis and their association with 28-day mortality: a prospective study. J Crit Care. 2013;28:317.e1–11.
41. Haase N, Ostrowski SR, Wetterslev J, et al. Thromboelastography in patients with severe sepsis: a prospective cohort study. Intensive Care Med. 2015;41:77–85.
42. Panigada M, Zacchetti L, L'Acqua C. Assessment of fibrinolysis in sepsis patients with urokinase modified thromboelastography. PLoS One. 2015;10:e0136463.
43. Prakash S, Verghese S, Roxby D, Dixon D, Bihari S, Bersten A. Changes in fibrinolysis and severity of organ failure in sepsis: a prospective observational study using point-of-care test – ROTEM. J Crit Care. 2015;30:264–70.
44. Laine A, Niemi T, Suojaranta-Ylinen R, et al. Decreased maximum clot firmness in rotational thromboelastometry (ROTEM®) is associated with bleeding during extracorporeal mechanical circulatory support. Perfusion. 2016;31:625–33.
45. Panigada M, Iapichino G, L'Acqua C, et al. Prevalence of "flat-line" thromboelastography during extracorporeal membrane oxygenation for respiratory failure in adults. ASAIO J. 2016;62:302–9.
46. Panigada M, Iapichino GE, Brioni M, et al. Thromboelastography-based anticoagulation management during extracorporeal membrane oxygenation: a safety and feasibility pilot study. Ann Intensive Care. 2018;8:7.

Extracorporeal Filter and Circuit Patency: A Personalized Approach to Anticoagulation

S. Romagnoli, Z. Ricci, and C. Ronco

28.1 Introduction

Acute kidney injury (AKI) occurs in about 50% of all critically ill patients admitted to the intensive care unit (ICU), and 10–20% of them require renal replacement therapy (RRT) [1]. In patients with hemodynamic instability and shock, continuous RRT (CRRT) is preferred over intermittent hemodialysis [2]. In order to deliver the prescribed therapy minimizing the downtime, extracorporeal circuit and filter patency has to be effectively obtained. Early extracorporeal circuit and filter clotting is a frustrating experience that reduces treatment efficacy and increases bedside workload and costs. Until recently, the most common approach to extracorporeal circuit and filter anticoagulation was based on the infusion of unfractionated heparin (UFH) [2]. Although generally infused into the circuit, UFH infusion generally leads to systemic anticoagulation, with an increased risk of bleeding, especially in critically ill patients and surgical patients who may have impaired hemostasis independently of heparin administration. In view of this and other potential

---

S. Romagnoli
Department of Health Science, University of Florence, Azienda Ospedaliero-Universitaria Careggi-Florence, Florence, Italy

Department of Anesthesiology and Intensive Care, Azienda Ospedaliero-Universitaria Careggi-Florence, Florence, Italy

Z. Ricci
Department of Cardiology and Cardiac Surgery, Pediatric Cardiac Intensive Care Unit, Bambino Gesù Children's Hospital, IRCCS-Rome, Rome, Italy

C. Ronco (✉)
International Renal Research Institute of Vicenza, Vicenza, Italy

Department of Nephrology, Dialysis and Transplantation and International Renal Research Institute of Vicenza, San Bortolo Hospital, Vicenza, Italy

Department of Medicine, University of Padova, Padua, Italy
e-mail: cronco@goldnet.it

complications (e.g., heparin-induced thrombocytopenia [HIT]), alternative modalities of anticoagulation during CRRT have gained popularity in recent years and have somehow changed the way CRRT is prescribed and delivered.

28.2 Systemic Strategies

28.2.1 Unfractionated and Low-Molecular-Weight Heparin

Heparin increases antithrombin (AT) activity on factors Xa, IIa, IXa, Xia, and XIIa. During CRRT, heparin can (theoretically) be infused directly to the patient (dedicated external line) or into the extracorporeal circuit via a dedicated internal line. The latter approach is recommended since, logically, the highest heparin concentration is reached at the prefilter site and thus at the location where the coagulation system is activated. In many centers, systemic heparin anticoagulation is the standard modality for CRRT. Heparin administration implies low costs, good drug availability, easy monitoring with activated prothrombin time (aPTT), and the possibility of administering an antagonist (protamine). However, systemic heparin anticoagulation has some adverse effects that are contributing to its replacement with alternative techniques: increased bleeding risks (e.g., secondary to sepsis-associated thrombocytopenia and/or coagulopathy; major surgery, hepatectomy; trauma), HIT, and ineffective anticoagulation due to heparin resistance [3]. Bleeding occurs in 5–40% of patients undergoing CRRT with systemic heparin anticoagulation [3–8], and this risk appears higher than with regional citrate anticoagulation [3, 9] (Fig. 28.1).

The complex of heparin and platelet factor 4 leads to the production of autoantibodies that are at the basis of HIT. The antibody-platelet binding leads to platelet

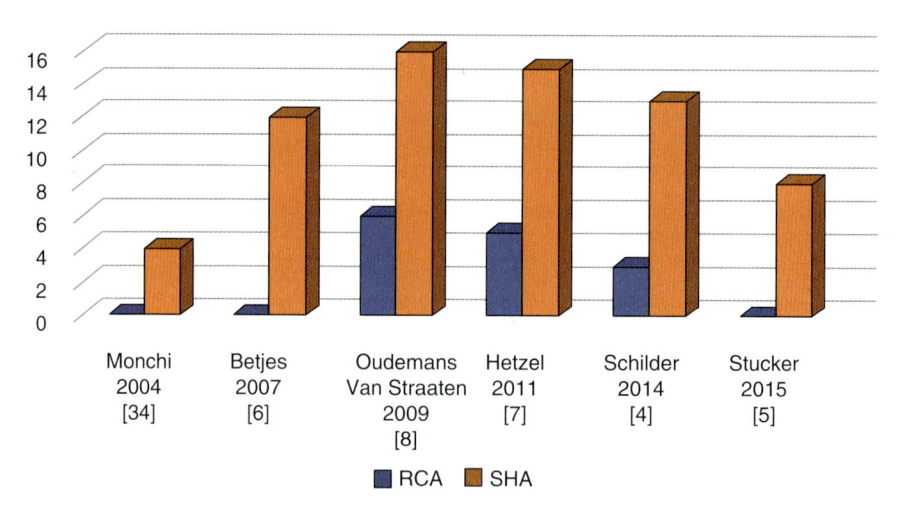

Fig. 28.1 Bleeding complications (% of patients) with regional citrate anticoagulation (RCA) or systemic heparin anticoagulation (SHA)

activation, causing potentially life-threatening thrombosis or thromboembolism. HIT is not a rare phenomenon and patients who receive unfractionated heparin for 7–10 days are at the highest risk with an incidence of 1–3% after cardiac surgery [10]. Logically, many studies have demonstrated a higher incidence of HIT during systemic heparin anticoagulation than with regional citrate anticoagulation [4, 5, 11].

In some patients, UFH infusion is not able to maintain sufficient anticoagulation and or the dose of UFH has to be increased in order to achieve the same aPTT level. This form of "resistance" can be related to different phenomena: insufficient AT concentration (AT should be measured in patients undergoing systemic heparin anticoagulation-CRRT) due to congenital deficit (rare) [12], decrease due to clinical conditions (e.g., chronic, acute or acute-on-chronic liver failure, bleeding, consumption). Heparin resistance may occur independently from AT concentration: heparin can be bound by a number of molecules including platelet factor 4, collagen, growth factors, elastase, and factor VIII [12, 13].

A potential alternative to UFH is low-molecular-weight heparin (LMWH) that can be suggested because of a lower incidence of HIT, less platelet activation, less inactivation by platelet factor-4, greater and more consistent bioavailability, and no metabolic adverse effects. Many disadvantages limit the widespread use of LMWH as an anticoagulation strategy for CRRT: (1) LMWH is eliminated via the kidneys and in case of renal failure its biological half-life is prolonged causing a risk of accumulation [14]; (2) CRRT only partially removes LMWH [15]; monitoring of the effect of LMWH requires the measurement of anti-Xa-activity (expensive and not available in all centers) [16]; (3) due to the difficulty in evaluating its concentration, LMWH cannot be completely antagonized by protamine. Few data can be found in the literature comparing LMWH and UFH. One randomized controlled study dates back more than 10 years [17]: enoxaparin showed difference in bleeding events compared to UFH, but anti-Xa-activity was tested every day and enoxaparin adjusted accordingly. Interestingly, the filter lifespan was longer in the LMWH group versus UFH (31 vs. 22 h, respectively; $p < 0.017$) [17]. Due to the paucity of data available on LMWH as an anticoagulant during CRRT, a final recommendation for or against its use cannot be made. Probably LMWH could be considered as a second-line anticoagulant after systemic heparin anticoagulation, when adverse effects, such as resistance or inadequate anticoagulation, are observed with UFH.

28.2.2 Direct Thrombin Inhibitors

Two techniques are available as potential alternatives to UFH or LMWH: hirudine and argatroban. Recombinant hirudin, a direct inhibitor of factor IIa (thrombin), can be used in cases of HIT. Since hirudin is eliminated by the kidneys, its half-life can be prolonged from 1 to 2 h to over 50 h in case of renal insufficiency [18]. The molecule cannot be eliminated via hemofiltration (molecular weight is about 7000 Da) and no antidote exists. Its effect can be measured using the ecarin clotting time, which is not available in all the hospitals. Filter lives are shorter in comparison with other techniques and bleeding complications more frequent [18]. Argatroban, another factor IIa inhibitor, is a 500 Da molecule derived from L-arginine and metabolized in the liver [19]. With a half-life of 45 min, its anticoagulant effect decreases 2–4 h after cessation of continuous infusion [20]. Argatroban is licensed for use in HIT. There are few data available in the literature. In a prospective study of 30 patients with HIT, argatroban was used as anticoagulant during continuous veno-venous hemodialysis (CVVHD). Only two patients developed minor bleeding and no patient developed severe bleeding. Ninety-eight percent of the extracorporeal filters ran for at least 24 h [21]. In conclusion, in case of HIT and/or extracorporeal circuit and filter thrombosis, when regional citrate anticoagulation is not available or not deemed to prevent clotting [22], argatroban could be the anticoagulant of choice. Interestingly, repeated and unexplained filter clotting during CRRT under regional citrate anticoagulation should encourage clinicians to exclude HIT [22].

28.3 Regional Strategies

28.3.1 Regional Citrate Anticoagulation

Techniques aimed to manage the coagulation in the extracorporeal circuit without affecting systemic coagulation (regional anticoagulation), although theoretically more complex to deliver, have been considered and significantly developed in recent years. Indeed, regional citrate anticoagulation has been demonstrated to prolong filter life and decrease the rate of complications, downtime, and costs compared with heparin [23] and is now recommended as the first-line anticoagulation strategy for CRRT in patients without contraindications [2]. This regional technique is based on the reversible chelation of ionized calcium, a cofactor of many steps in the clotting cascade, in the extracorporeal circuit and filter. In order to optimize the anticoagulant effect, citrate is infused proximally to the vascular access by means of the pre-dilution line (Fig. 28.2). The application of regional

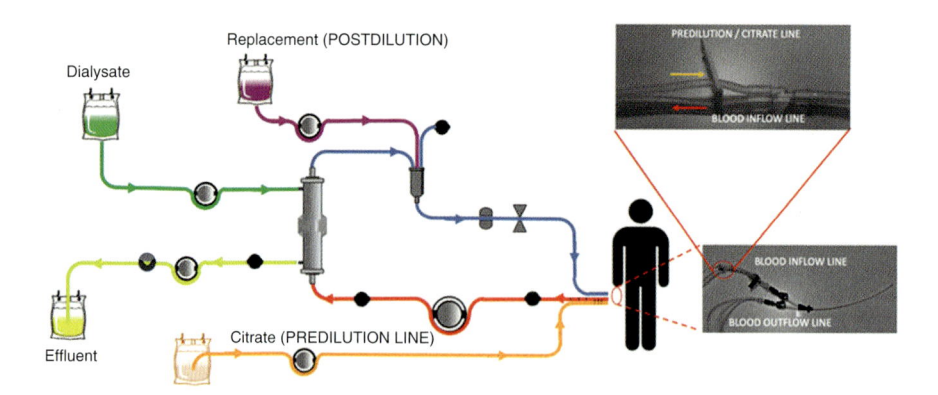

Fig. 28.2 Continuous renal replacement therapy (CRRT) circuit with citrate regional anticoagulation

citrate anticoagulation requires particularly dedicated protocols, knowledge of the biochemical mechanisms underpinning this particular technique of anticoagulation and specific training of both medical and nursing staff.

In this section, some "advanced" aspects of citrate anticoagulation strategy will be summarized. Clinicians aware of the basic concepts of regional citrate anticoagulation could take advantage of specific aspects of regional citrate anticoagulation to better personalize the strategy to individual patients.

28.3.1.1 Citrate Infusion Rate and Citrate Load

The infusion rate of citrate and the patient's resultant citrate load depend on the following:

- The prescribed citrate/blood flow (Q_B) ratio: the citrate infusion depends on the dose of citrate (in mmol) the operator decides to infuse per liter of blood flow (Q_B)—mmol (citrate) per 1 (blood). Companies suggest starting with an initial dose of 3 or 4 mmol of citrate per liter of blood. The target range of ionized calcium in the circuit is 0.25–0.35 mmol/l (slightly variable in the literature) [24, 25]. An ionized calcium of <0.2 mmol/l prevents activation of coagulation cascades and platelets. The infusion rate of the citrate solution is modified according to the ionized calcium concentration sampled from the outflow line (Fig. 28.3). In modern CRRT machines, the citrate administration rate is electronically coupled with blood flow.
- The blood flow rate—citrate administration is coupled with the blood pump. Since a citrate dose/Q_B ratio is set by the operator and modifiable at any time,

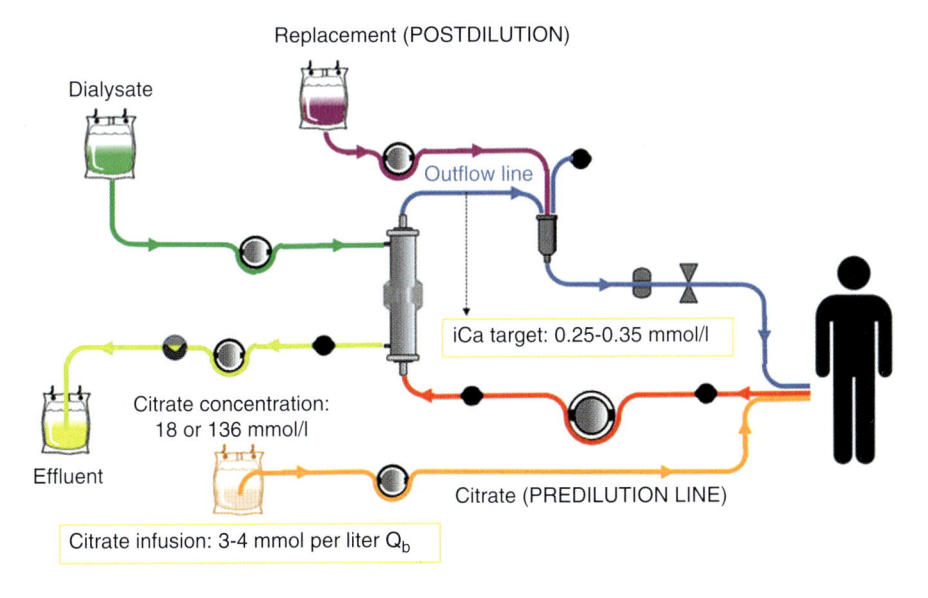

Fig. 28.3 Continuous renal replacement therapy (CRRT) circuit with citrate regional anticoagulation. Ionized calcium (iCa) sampling site and citrate solution infusion scheme

Table 28.1 Metabolic derangements during regional citrate anticoagulation

Clinical condition	Risks	Metabolic derangement	Interventions[a]
• Liver dysfunction • Hypoxemia • Shock	Citrate accumulation	• Metabolic acidosis • Decreased iCa • ↑ Ca/iCa • Hyperlactatemia	• Alternative anticoagulation strategy • ↓Citrate load: ↓Q_B; ↓citrate/Q_B ratio (depending on iCa in the post-filter) • ↑CCC elimination: ↑Q_D in CVVHD, CVVHDF; ↑Q_R^{POST} in CVVH, CVVHDF • Supply calcium
• Normal liver and mitochondrial function (A)	Citrate overload	• Metabolic alkalosis (citrate metabolism + increase in SID due to sodium load) • No increase in Ca/iCa • iCa normal	• ↓Citrate load: ↓Q_B; ↓citrate/Q_B ratio (depending on iCa in the post-filter) • ↑ CCC elimination: ↑Q_D in CVVHD, CVVHDF; ↑Q_R^{POST} in CVVH, CVVHDF • Supply calcium
• Normal liver and mitochondrial function (B)	Insufficient citrate load	• Metabolic acidosis (source could be AKI)—insufficient compensation with buffers coming from citrate metabolism • No increase in Ca/iCa	• ↑ Citrate load: ↑Q_B; ↑citrate/Q_B ratio (depending on iCa in the post-filter) • ↓CCC elimination: decrease Q_D in CVVHD, CVVHDF; decrease Q_R^{POST} in CVVH, CVVHDF

AKI acute kidney injury, *Ca* calcium, *CVVH* continuous veno-venous hemofiltration, *CVVHD* continuous veno-venous hemodialysis, *CVVHDF* continuous veno-venous hemodiafiltration, *CCC* calcium-citrate complex, *iCa* ionized calcium, Q_B blood flow: dialysate flow, Q_R^{POST} replacement flow in post-dilution, *SID* strong ion difference
[a]Interventions depend on the actual situation (e.g., machine setting—Q_B, Q_D, Q_R^{POST}, post-filter iCa)

depending on the ionized calcium concentration in the outflow line, the higher the Q_B, the higher the citrate infusion into the extracorporeal circuit.
- Concentration of the citrate solution used: two main solutions are commonly used. A diluted solution (e.g., 18 mmol of citrate per l of solution; bags of 5 l) or a concentrated solution (e.g., 136 mmol of citrate per l of solution; bags of 2 l). Once the dose is prescribed and the Q_B set, the citrate solution used will depend on the concentration. By changing the concentration, the total amount of citrate infused into the extracorporeal circuit does not change; what will change will be the flow of the solution infused into the inflow line via the pre-dilution line.

Importantly, the citrate–calcium complex has a molecular weight of 298 Da, high hydrosolubility (due to the negative charge of a free carboxylate radical) and a sieving coefficient of 1 [25]. Thus, up to 50% or 30–60% of the infused citrate–calcium complexes are removed via the hemofilter during the first passage (Table 28.1).

Consequently, depending on the prescription, the citrate–calcium complexes can be actively removed in the effluent flow (Q_{EFF}). By increasing the CRRT dose, dialysate flow (Q_D), and/or an increase in replacement flow (Q_R^{POST}), more citrate–calcium complexes will be filtered into the Q_{EFF} leaving the extracorporeal circuit and eventually reducing the citrate load.

Depending on the removal rate of citrate–calcium complexes, some degree of hypocalcemia (and hypomagnesemia) will occur and to avoid a negative calcium balance an infusion of calcium is recommended and a mandatory step in any protocol specifically dedicated to regional citrate anticoagulation (calcium chloride must be infused either in the outflow line—via a dedicated line and pump—or directly through a separate central line). Clinical signs of hypocalcemia in humans appear below a level of 0.8 mmol/l of plasma ionized calcium [26]. The citrate–calcium complexes that are not filtered into the Q_{EFF} enter the systemic circulation (citrate load). In conditions of normal perfusion and oxygenation, citrate–calcium complexes dissociate and under physiological conditions, citrate's half-life is approximately 5 min [25]. The citrate is metabolized via the Krebs's cycle (a mitochondrial metabolic pathway involved in the chemical conversion of carbohydrates, fats, and proteins to generate adenosine triphosphate [ATP]), being an intermediate in aerobic organisms, mostly in liver cells and also in the skeletal muscle and in the renal cortex releasing sodium as well as calcium ions [25–27] (Fig. 28.4). Even though solutes containing citrate vary in concentration, the actual citrate delivery rate to the CRRT extracorporeal circuit ranges from 17 to 45 mmol/h [28].

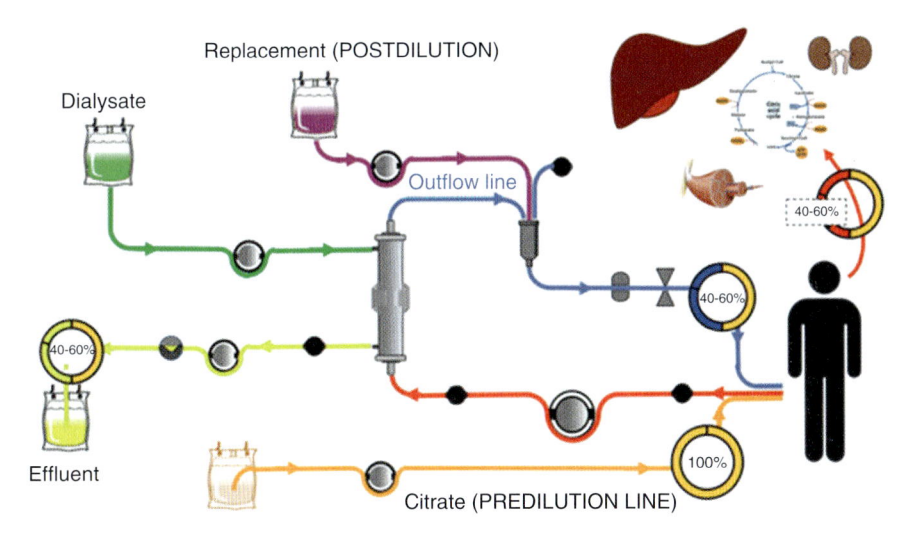

Fig. 28.4 Citrate kinetics: about half of citrate load is excreted with the effluent and the remaining part is returned to the patient and eventually metabolized by the Krebs cycle

28.3.1.2 Acid Base Disorders and Citrate Load Management

Within its metabolic pathway, one molecule of citrate yields energy (2.48 kJ [593 cal]/mmol citrate) [29] and three molecules of bicarbonate represent a consistent source of bases. Metabolic alkalosis can result during regional citrate anticoagulation from two different pathways: (a) citrate solutions have a high sodium content (three Na^+ for one citrate molecule); trisodium citrate [$Na_3C_3H_5O(COO)_3$] is a rich source of sodium that may increase the plasma strong ion difference leading to increase in pH; (b) bicarbonate results from the metabolism of citrate as trisodium citrate can react with carbonic acid to form sodium bicarbonate (Table 28.1). Therefore, when citrate is regularly metabolized, regional citrate anticoagulation may be associated with metabolic alkalosis. Nevertheless, AKI and, more generally, critical illness are frequently associated with metabolic acidosis, and the buffer supplementation provided by citrate in terms of bicarbonates could be desirable.

In case of metabolic alkalosis, the operator may modify the CRRT prescription in different ways choosing one or a combination of the following possibilities:

- By increasing the CRRT dose (Q_D and/or Q_R^{POST}), more citrate–calcium complexes will be eliminated in the Q_{EFF} reducing the citrate load to the patient.
- By reducing the citrate dose/Q_B ratio, less citrate will be infused into the extracorporeal circuit.
- By reducing Q_B, less citrate will be infused into the extracorporeal circuit.

In clinical practice, the choice that the operator applies will depend on patient condition: ionized calcium concentration in the outflow line (post-filter), Q_B, prescribed dose, etc.

Limited Q_B, aimed at a minimum citrate load administration, is usually recommended during regional citrate anticoagulation, and most protocols using diffusive modes (CVVHD) would recommend Q_B between 80 and 150 ml/min [25].

In case of metabolic acidosis, it is very important to distinguish citrate accumulation (acidosis due to impaired citrate metabolism) from AKI-related metabolic acidosis. In fact, citrate ($C_6H_5O_7$) is an organic weak acid and circulating citrate–calcium complexes ($C_6H_5O_7 = Ca^{++}$) might lead to (potential) plasma acidification that in normal conditions is negligible due to their rapid clearance from the blood (about 5 min). Nevertheless, when citrate catabolism is markedly impaired, citrate–calcium complexes accumulate leading to citrate accumulation that may further worsen any previously existing metabolic acidosis. When a validated protocol is correctly applied, citrate accumulation is unlikely to occur [30]. Citrate accumulation must be promptly diagnosed and in the absence of a specific assay, it can only be suspected by an increased total calcium/ionized calcium ratio > 2.5 when both total and ionized calcium are measured in mmol/l (or > 10 if total calcium is measured in mg/dl) [25, 28] (Fig. 28.5). The accumulation of citrate in a patient's blood leads to a decrease in the systemic ionized calcium concentration, whereas the bound fraction of calcium rises because the calcium infused to correct the low ionized calcium binds to citrate. Consequently, there is a disproportional increase in total Ca, but

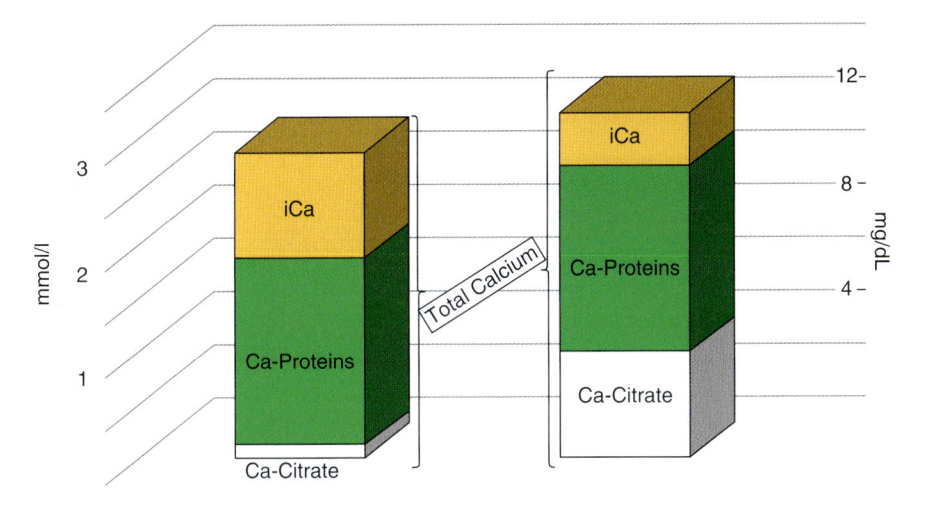

Fig. 28.5 When citrate is not metabolized (e.g., severe liver failure, shock): (1) the total serum Ca concentration appears to increase; (2) ionized calcium (iCa) falls due to the increase in Ca–citrate complexes; (3) the "calcium gap" (Ca–iCa) increases

ionized calcium remains low. The calcium gap (total calcium—ionized calcium) and the total calcium/ionized calcium ratio increases. Worsening metabolic acidosis and hypocalcemia leading to systolic myocardial dysfunction and vasodilatation could be additional findings.

It is hard to identify those patients who are unable to tolerate the citrate load *a priori*, but some categories of patients should be considered at risk: acute liver failure or acute-on-chronic liver failure (not an absolute contraindication for regional citrate anticoagulation), circulatory shock with impairment of the Krebs cycle, intoxications causing mitochondrial blockage. Serum lactate concentration may help to appraise this risk since hyperlactatemia is a common finding in these conditions. Nevertheless, it has to be noted that hyperlactatemia *per se* is not a contraindication for regional citrate anticoagulation.

In general, to minimize citrate accumulation, a few rules can help:

- Identify high-risk patients for reduced citrate clearance (liver failure, shock, intoxications) and decide whether a different anticoagulation strategy should be provided or a modified regional citrate anticoagulation protocol (e.g., accepting higher intra-filter ionized calcium levels by delivering a reduced citrate load).
- Use limited Q_B (to limit citrate administration): since during convective modalities (continuous veno-venous hemofiltration [CVVH]) a low Q_B is associated with high filtration rate (to increase citrate–calcium complex clearance), and early membrane clogging, using diluted citrate solutions delivered in pre-dilution (Q_R^{PRE}), may help to minimize this issue. On the other hand, in diffusive modes (CVVHD), low blood flow (>80 ml/min) may still provide adequate blood purification since Q_D is not restricted by filtration fraction and high flux membranes allow high clearance of citrate–calcium complexes.

- Increase Q_D and/or Q_R^{POST}, depending on the prescribed modality, to increase citrate removal.

In case of metabolic acidosis and a total calcium/ionized calcium ratio < 2.5, an increase in Q_B should be sufficient to compensate the clinical picture. In fact, an increase in Q_B will be followed by an increase in citrate infusion and, therefore, bicarbonate production and release into the circulation. Alternatively, or in association, a decrease in Q_D and/or a decrease in Q_R^{POST} should reduce the filtration of citrate–calcium complexes in the Q_{EFF} increasing the amount of citrate metabolized to bicarbonate. It is important to consider that in case of reduction of a filter's clearance capacity (e.g., progressive clogging), a decrease in citrate–calcium complex elimination may occur. In such situations, it is important to promptly replace the filter to avoid excessive citrate administration and underdialysis.

28.3.1.3 Regional Citrate Anticoagulation and Outcomes

Until now, evidence of a reduction in mortality with regional citrate anticoagulation compared to systemic anticoagulation is still lacking, but a prospective randomized controlled trial (RCT) comparing regional citrate anticoagulation with systemic heparin anticoagulation and targeting >1000 patients is currently being executed (Clinicaltrials.gov Identifier: NCT02669589). In the meantime, a prolonged filter lifetime is the most evident positive outcome related to the use of regional citrate anticoagulation as shown by multiple studies [23]: (1) with regional citrate anticoagulation, 17% of all circuits run up to 72 h, but none of those with systemic heparin anticoagulation; (2) clotting is the cause for discontinuation of therapy in 80% of systems using heparin and in 30% of those using regional citrate anticoagulation; (3) the mean hemofilter lifespan/benchmark is about 15–20 h during systemic heparin anticoagulation versus 60 h with regional citrate anticoagulation.

The protocol published by Morgera and collaborators in 2009 gives clear recommendations to adapt the citrate dose following measurement of ionized calcium in the circuit [31]. The same group, in an observational prospective study analyzing 100 filters in 75 patients treated with a CRRT dose of 45 ml/kg/h, showed a mean filter running time of 78 h [32]. Interestingly, 51 circuits had to be replaced because of extended filter running time (96 h), 33 for reasons not related to RRT (62 h), and only 13 due to filter clotting (58 h) [32]. Additional interesting results were as follows: (1) the mean dose during the first 72 h was 49 ml/kg/h; (2) acid–base status after 72 h was well controlled in 62% of patients, metabolic alkalosis occurred in 29%, and metabolic acidosis in 9% and in only 1 patient treatment was stopped because of citrate accumulation; (3) no bleeding complications occurred even if the selected population was deemed at high bleeding risk [32].

28.3.1.4 Patients at High Risk of Bleeding

Recently, results from an RCT designed to compare CVVH with regional citrate anticoagulation and with no anticoagulation in patients with a high risk of bleeding (admitted to the ICU after major surgery) were published [33]. Fifty-six patients were equally allocated into the regional citrate anticoagulation or no anticoagulation group. Compared to the no anticoagulation group, the regional citrate anticoagulation group had fewer transfusions of packed red blood cells (RBCs) and platelets and a longer filter lifespan. The authors concluded that regional citrate anticoagulation used in CVVH is a safe and effective modality to deliver RRT to patients with an elevated risk profile for bleeding complications. Among the first studies exploring bleeding as a complication of regional citrate anticoagulation, one crossover RCT was published in 2004 [34]. Patients received systemic heparin or regional citrate anticoagulation and those who needed a second CVVH run received the other study medication in a cross-over design until the fourth circuit. Forty-nine circuits were analyzed and major bleeding only occurred during heparin anticoagulation [34]. Morabito and collaborators evaluated 33 cardiac surgery patients who were switched from hemofiltration with no anticoagulation or systemic heparin to regional citrate anticoagulation (using a 12 mmol/l citrate solution). Interestingly, the transition to regional citrate anticoagulation significantly reduced transfusion requirements by more than 50% compared to both systemic heparin and no anticoagulation [35]. Moreover, regional citrate anticoagulation-CVVH filter life (about 50 h) was significantly longer ($p < 0.0001$) when compared with heparin (30 h) or no anticoagulation (25 h) [35].

28.3.1.5 Patients with Liver Failure

Patients with liver failure are one of the categories at higher risk for citrate accumulation, and liver dysfunction or failure was originally considered a contraindication for regional citrate anticoagulation because early clinical observations had raised concerns about the safety and efficacy of regional citrate anticoagulation in these patients [3]. However, in patients with liver dysfunction, coagulation is often impaired and even if the bleeding risk is high (e.g., major liver surgery; major surgery in patients with cirrhosis; shock in trauma), the extracorporeal circuit and filter undergo frequent clotting due to a tendency of these patients to have increased clotting [36]. Thus, patients with impaired liver function might particularly benefit from regional citrate anticoagulation versus systemic heparin anticoagulation.

In 2015, Slowinski and collaborators published a multicenter, prospective, observational study, which included 133 patients (48 with normal liver function—bilirubin <2 mg/dl, 43 with mild liver dysfunction—bilirubin 2–7 mg/dl, and 42 with severe liver dysfunction—bilirubin >7 mg/dl) who were treated with regional citrate anticoagulation during CVVHD [37]. Metabolic imbalance was the main focus of the trial. The frequency of safety endpoints [acidosis or alkalosis (pH $\leq$7.2 or $\geq$7.55, respectively)] in the three patient strata did not differ and severe acidosis, the most feared complication, was found in 13, 16, and 14% in normal, mild, and severe liver dysfunction groups, respectively ($p = 0.95$). Only 3 patients showed signs of impaired citrate metabolism. Overall filter patency was 49% at 72 h and after eliminating for interruption of the treatment due to non-clotting causes, estimated 72-h filter survival was 96%. Recently, a systematic review [38], which included 10 studies and 1241 patients with liver failure, concluded that regional citrate anticoagulation can be considered safe in liver failure patients undergoing CRRT, yielding a favorable filter lifespan (55 h). Specifically, the pooled rate of citrate accumulation was 12% and the bleeding rate was 5%. No significant increase in serum citrate was observed at the end of CRRT. Compared with non-liver failure patients, the liver failure patients showed no significant difference in the pH, serum lactate level, or total calcium/ionized calcium ratio during CRRT.

Since liver failure patients represent a category at risk for metabolic derangements, a close monitoring for citrate accumulation is mandatory (but this is also true for all patients undergoing regional citrate anticoagulation).

28.3.1.6 Hypoxemic Patients

A vast majority of patients are admitted to the ICU with cellular hypoxia due to circulatory and or respiratory failure. The metabolic pathway of citrate is oxygen dependent, and severe hypoxemia or inability to bring oxygen to the cells might impair this cycle and citrate metabolism. Nonetheless, there are very few data in the literature regarding regional citrate anticoagulation in patients with cellular hypoxia. A small study including 10 severely hypoxemic patients (PaO_2 < 60 mmHg) concluded that regional citrate anticoagulation can be safely used in patients with hepatic function impairment but may induce acidosis and a decline in serum ionized calcium when used with hypoxemic patients [39]. Hence, hypoxemia should be acknowledged as an important risk factor for citrate accumulation and possibly alternative anticoagulation strategies should be considered. Larger trials are currently awaited to confirm this biologically plausible observation.

In conclusion, understanding of citrate "kinetics" may help the clinician correctly manage regional citrate anticoagulation in any clinical condition. In case of acid–base disorder, clinicians should be able to distinguish citrate overload (metabolic alkalosis) from accumulation (elevated total calcium/ionized calcium ratio, increase need for calcium replacement, and worsening of acidosis). If an initial regional citrate anticoagulation strategy is delivered and eventually stopped due to an emerging contraindication or strategy failure, a switch to an alternative modality should be promptly considered, even within the context of the same CRRT session (e.g., stop regional citrate anticoagulation and start systemic heparin anticoagulation, a possibility that is commonly allowed by third- and fourth-generation machines).

28.3.2 Regional Heparin–Protamine Anticoagulation

In this strategy, UFH is infused into the inflow line of the extracorporeal circuit, while protamine is infused into the outflow line to neutralize the anticoagulant effect of AT. aPTT must be measured in the circuit and in the systemic circulation [40]. This strategy is not recommended by the Kidney Disease Improving Global Outcomes (KDIGO) guidelines: "It is cumbersome and difficult to titrate because heparin has a much longer half-life than protamine, inducing a risk of rebound. In addition, it exposes the patient to the side-effects of both heparin (mainly the risk of

HIT) and protamine (mainly anaphylaxis, platelet dysfunction, hypotension, and pulmonary vasoconstriction with right ventricular failure) and is therefore not recommended" [2]. Even if regional heparin–protamine anticoagulation, in comparison with the other techniques, is more complex and associated with a high risk of adverse effects [13], it can be considered when heparin dosage is increased due to repeated filter clotting and excessively short extracorporeal filter life, regional citrate anticoagulation is unavailable or contraindicated, and UFH in excess may expose the patient to unacceptable bleeding risk. Clinicians applying regional heparin–protamine anticoagulation should be aware that this technique has to be limited to skilled centers and continued for short periods.

28.4 No Anticoagulation Strategies

The KDIGO guidelines recommend that regional citrate anticoagulation should be the first choice for CRRT in a patient without contraindications for citrate and in patients with a high bleeding risk rather than no anticoagulation. In the ICU, some patients should avoid heparin because of bleeding risk and citrate for contraindications. RRT can be done without anticoagulation, but some aspects should be considered in order to avoid very early clotting of the extracorporeal circuit and filter.

28.4.1 Determinants of Clotting Risk: Vascular Access, Circuit, Modality

The most frequent clotting sites are the venous access (vascular catheter), the hemofilter, and the venous air trap [41]. In particular, the vascular access, sometimes neglected, should be considered a sort of "Achille's heel" for CRRT performance and coagulation since a well-functioning vascular access is a key factor to avoid premature failure of the extracorporeal circuit. In fact, catheter malfunction eventually leads to intermittent stasis of blood flow, which promotes clotting and subsequent circuit failure. Site of insertion, catheter length, and size and shape all represent key aspects to carefully consider as soon as the physician has decided that RRT is needed. Inadequate Q_B has been demonstrated to contribute to circuit failure [42]. Recommended sites of vascular access placement are the right internal jugular vein (with the tip in the right atrium) or femoral vein (with a length > 24 cm). A catheter size around 11.5–12 Fr is also strongly suggested [2, 43, 44]. The subclavian position should be avoided given the high risk of kinking, the potential for subclavian stenosis [45], and inherent risks (pneumothorax, bleeding) [2]. Intrathoracic sites should be avoided in case of high intrathoracic pressures and, similarly, intra-abdominal sites should be avoided in case of intra-abdominal hypertension. Catheters with side holes are discouraged because turbulent flow initiates clotting and contact of the holes with the vessel wall can arrest flow, thereby activating clotting. Short-term catheters for CRRT are made largely of polyurethane or silicone. The first are stiffer, more traumatic for the vessel wall, easier to place, and with a larger inner lumen. The second are more flexible, less traumatic, less easy to place and with a narrower inner lumen (thicker wall).

The bio-incompatibility of the membrane surface sustains a complex activation of tissue factor, leukocytes, and platelets, favoring clotting [46]. To reduce the thrombogenicity of the membrane, surface coating with substances such as heparin or polyethyleneimine has been applied (e.g., Oxiris membrane by Baxter, Cleveland, MS, USA). However, the use of polyethyleneimine-coated membranes has not been demonstrated to prolong circuit lifespan during CVVH without anticoagulation in the critically ill population [47]. Similarly, the use of heparin in the priming solution (a common procedure applied while setting up the machine) did not reduce thrombogenicity of the membrane in continuous veno-venous hemodiafiltration (CVVHDF) [48].

In air trap chambers, the contact of blood with air may favor clotting. The addition of a continuous flow of water may significantly reduce the risk. For example, giving post-dilution fluids into the chamber can create a fluid layer on top of the blood level, possibly reducing clot development.

Hemodialysis is associated with a longer circuit life than hemofiltration [49]. During CVVH (basic solute transport mechanism is convection), hemoconcentration eventually occurs, promoting clotting because of higher concentrations of cells and coagulation factors in the filter. To reduce hemoconcentration, a blood filtration fraction (filtrate/Q_B) <0.15–0.20 is recommended and since higher blood flows are crucial to keep filtration fraction low, vascular access is key [42]. In order to reduce hemoconcentration, pre-dilution (the fluid lost by ultrafiltration is replaced before the filter) clearly represents a non-pharmacologic measure for clotting prevention. Some studies have demonstrated a longer filter lifespan with pre-dilution [50]. A recent RCT was designed to determine whether Q_B influences circuit life in CRRT: 96 patients were randomized at 150 or 250 ml/min in CVVH or CVVHD (50% pre-dilution in CVVH and 100% post-dilution in CVVHD; vascular catheter 13.5 Fr). The authors found no difference in extracorporeal circuit and filter lifespan: 462 circuits showed a median life for the first circuit (clotted) of 9 h (150 ml/min) vs 10 h (250 ml/min); $p = 0.37$. It should be underlined that patients at risk of bleeding received no anticoagulation, and regional heparin–protamine anticoagulation was delivered in the others. Although the external validity of this study can be questioned due to extremely low extracorporeal circuit lives, the important message here is that Q_B could be inadequate both with excessively low rates (presumably favoring hemoconcentration and coagulation processes) and with excessively high rates (likely due to shear stress at resistance points). Not only should anticoagulation be tailored to patients during CRRT but also many other aspects such as vascular access performance and an optimally coupled Q_B.

Finally, training and education for staff has a direct relationship to success and therefore circuit life. Machine "troubleshooting" alarms, recognizing access failure and correct use of anticoagulation (non-pharmacologic and pharmacologic), are the key areas for education and training.

28.5 Conclusion

When a clinician has decided that CRRT is indicated, the choice of the anticoagulation strategy is crucial to guarantee the optimal delivery of dialysis therapy. In patients without absolute contraindications, regional citrate anticoagulation is strongly recommended as it is safe, and effective for both extracorporeal circuit patency and bleeding complications. Regional citrate anticoagulation must be safely managed by an adequately trained staff according to precise protocols, including any deviation for specific patients. When impaired citrate metabolism and accumulation risks are significant (severe liver failure, hypoxemia, shock), UFH may represent a second-line approach. In case of HIT, argatroban could be considered if regional citrate anticoagulation is not efficient. Alternative techniques include LMWH, hirudin, and regional heparin–protamine anticoagulation, which are probably not recommended as routine practice but could be considered in very specific situations.

References

1. Hoste EAJ, Bagshaw SM, Bellomo R, et al. Epidemiology of acute kidney injury in critically ill patients: the multinational AKI-EPI study. Intensive Care Med. 2015;41:1411–23.
2. Kidney Disease Improving Global Outcomes. Kidney disease improving global outcomes (KDIGO) clinical practice guideline for acute kidney injury. Kidney Int Suppl. 2012;2:1–138.
3. Brandenburger T, Dimski T, Slowinski T, et al. Renal replacement therapy and anticoagulation. Best Pract Res Clin Anaesthesiol. 2017;31:387–401.
4. Schilder L, Nurmohamed SA, Bosch FH, et al. Citrate anticoagulation versus systemic heparinisation in continuous venovenous hemofiltration in critically ill patients with acute kidney injury: a multi-center randomized clinical trial. Crit Care. 2014;18:1–9.
5. Stucker F, Ponte B, Tataw J, et al. Efficacy and safety of citrate-based anticoagulation compared to heparin in patients with acute kidney injury requiring continuous renal replacement therapy: a randomized controlled trial. Crit Care. 2015;19:1–9.
6. Betjes MGH, van Oosterom D, van Agteren M, et al. Regional citrate versus heparin anticoagulation during venovenous hemofiltration in patients at low risk for bleeding: similar hemofilter survival but significantly less bleeding. J Nephrol. 2007;20:602–8.
7. Hetzel GR, Schmitz M, Wissing H, et al. Regional citrate versus systemic heparin for anticoagulation in critically ill patients on continuous venovenous haemofiltration: a prospective randomized multicentre trial. Nephrol Dial Transplant. 2011;26:232–9.
8. Oudemans-Van Straaten HM, Bosman RJ, Koopmans M, et al. Citrate anticoagulation for continuous venovenous hemofiltration. Crit Care Med. 2009;37:545–52.
9. Liu C, Mao Z, Kang H, et al. Regional citrate versus heparin anticoagulation for continuous renal replacement therapy in critically ill patients: a meta-analysis with trial sequential analysis of randomized controlled trials. Crit Care. 2016;20:1–13.
10. Arepally GM. Heparin-induced thrombocytopenia. Blood. 2017;129:2864–72.
11. Gattas DJ, Rajbhandari D, Bradford C, et al. A randomized controlled trial of regional citrate versus regional heparin anticoagulation for continuous renal replacement therapy in critically ill adults. Crit Care Med. 2015;43:1622–9.
12. Tait RC, Walker ID, Reitsma PH, et al. Prevalence of antithrombin deficiency in the healthy population. Br J Haematol. 1994;87:106–12.
13. Thota R, Ganti AK, Subbiah S. Apparent heparin resistance in a patient with infective endocarditis secondary to elevated factor VIII levels. J Thromb Thrombolysis. 2012;34:132–4.

14. Frydman A. Low-molecular-weight heparins: an overview of their pharmacodynamics, pharmacokinetics and metabolism in humans. Haemostasis. 1996;26(Suppl):24–38.
15. Straaten O, Wester JPJ, Leyte A. Hemostasis during low molecular weight heparin anticoagulation for continuous venovenous hemofiltration: a randomized cross-over trial comparing two hemofiltration rates. Crit Care. 2009;13:R139.
16. Oudemans-van Straaten HM, Wester JPJ, De Pont ACJM, et al. Anticoagulation strategies in continuous renal replacement therapy: can the choice be evidence based? Intensive Care Med. 2006;32:188–202.
17. Joannidis M, Kountchev J, Rauchenzauner M, et al. Enoxaparin vs. unfractionated heparin for anticoagulation during continuous veno-venous hemofiltration: a randomized controlled crossover study. Intensive Care Med. 2007;33:1571–9.
18. Hein OV, Von Heymann C, Diehl T, et al. Intermittent hirudin versus continuous heparin for anticoagulation in continuous renal replacement therapy. Ren Fail. 2004;26:297–303.
19. Koster A, Fischer KG, Harder S, et al. The direct thrombin inhibitor argatroban: a review of its use in patients with and without HIT. Biol Targets Ther. 2007;1:105–12.
20. Di Nisio M, Middeldorp S, Büller H. Direct thrombin inhibitors. N Engl J Med. 2005;353:1028–40.
21. Link A, Girndt M, Selejan S, et al. Argatroban for anticoagulation in continuous renal replacement therapy. Crit Care Med. 2009;37:105–10.
22. Lehner GF, Schöpf M, Harler U, et al. Repeated premature hemofilter clotting during regional citrate anticoagulation as indicator of heparin induced thrombocytopenia. Blood Purif. 2014;38:127–30.
23. Bai M, Zhou M, He L, et al. Citrate versus heparin anticoagulation for continuous renal replacement therapy: an updated meta-analysis of RCTs. Intensive Care Med. 2015;41:2098–110.
24. Ataullakhanov F, Pohilko A, Sinauridze E, et al. Calcium threshold in human plasma clotting kinetics. Thromb Res. 1994;75:383–94.
25. Schneider AG, Journois D, Rimmelé T. Complications of regional citrate anticoagulation: accumulation or overload? Crit Care. 2017;21:1–7.
26. Monchi M. Citrate pathophysiology and metabolism. Transfus Apher Sci. 2017;56:28–30.
27. Ricci D, Panicali L, Facchini MG, Mancini E. Citrate anticoagulation during continuous renal replacement therapy. Contrib Nephrol. 2017;190:19–30.
28. Davenport A, Tolwani A. Citrate anticoagulation for continuous renal replacement therapy (CRRT) in patients with acute kidney injury admitted to the intensive care unit. NDT Plus. 2009;2:439–47.
29. New AM, Nystrom EM, Frazee E, et al. Continuous renal replacement therapy: a potential source of calories in the critically ill. Am J Clin Nutr. 2017;105:1559–63.
30. Khadzhynov D, Schelter C, Lieker I, et al. Incidence and outcome of metabolic disarrangements consistent with citrate accumulation in critically ill patients undergoing continuous venovenous hemodialysis with regional citrate anticoagulation. J Crit Care. 2014;29:265–71.
31. Morgera S, Schneider M, Slowinski T, et al. A safe citrate anticoagulation protocol with variable treatment efficacy and excellent control of the acid-base status. Crit Care Med. 2009;37:2018–24.
32. Kalb R, Kram R, Morgera S, et al. Regional citrate anticoagulation for high volume continuous venovenous hemodialysis in surgical patients with high bleeding risk. Ther Apher Dial. 2013;17:202–12.
33. Gao J, Wang F, Wang Y, et al. A mode of CVVH with regional citrate anticoagulation compared to no anticoagulation for acute kidney injury patients at high risk of bleeding. Sci Rep. 2019;9:1–10.
34. Monchi M, Berghmans D, Ledoux D, et al. Citrate vs. heparin for anticoagulation in continuous venovenous hemofiltration: a prospective randomized study. Intensive Care Med. 2004;30:260–5.
35. Morabito S, Pistolesi V, Tritapepe L, et al. Regional citrate anticoagulation in cardiac surgery patients at high risk of bleeding: a continuous veno-venous hemofiltration protocol with a low concentration citrate solution. Crit Care. 2012;16:R111.

36. Habib M, Roberts LN, Patel RK, et al. Evidence of rebalanced coagulation in acute liver injury and acute liver failure as measured by thrombin generation. Liver Int. 2014;34:672–8.
37. Slowinski T, Morgera S, Joannidis M, et al. Safety and efficacy of regional citrate anticoagulation in continuous venovenous hemodialysis in the presence of liver failure: The Liver Citrate Anticoagulation Threshold (L-CAT) observational study. Crit Care. 2015;19:1–11.
38. Zhang W, Bai M, Yu Y, et al. Safety and efficacy of regional citrate anticoagulation for continuous renal replacement therapy in liver failure patients: a systematic review and meta-analysis. Crit Care. 2019;23:1–11.
39. Gong D, Ji D, Xu B, et al. Regional citrate anticoagulation in critically ill patients during continuous blood purification. Chin Med J. 2003;116:360–3.
40. Tolwani AJ, Wille KM. Anticoagulation for continuous renal replacement therapy. Semin Dial. 2009;22:141–5.
41. Oudemans-Van Straaten HM. Hemostasis and thrombosis in continuous renal replacement treatment. Semin Thromb Hemost. 2015;41:91–8.
42. Baldwin I, Bellomo R, Koch B. Blood flow reductions during continuous renal replacement therapy and circuit life. Intensive Care Med. 2004;30:2074–9.
43. Huriaux L, Costille P, Quintard H, et al. Haemodialysis catheters in the intensive care unit. Anaesth Crit Care Pain Med. 2017;36:313–9.
44. Parienti J-J, Mégarbane B, Fischer MO, et al. Catheter dysfunction and dialysis performance according to vascular access among 736 critically ill adults requiring renal replacement therapy: a randomized controlled study. Crit Care Med. 2010;38:1118–25.
45. Schillinger F, Schillinger D, Montagnac R, et al. Post catheterisation vein stenosis in haemodialysis: comparative angiographic study of 50 subclavian and 50 internal jugular accesses. Nephrol Dial Transplant. 1991;6:722–4.
46. Joannidis M, Oudemans-van Straaten HM. Clinical review: patency of the circuit in continuous renal replacement therapy. Crit Care. 2007;11:1–10.
47. Schetz M, Van Cromphaut S, Dubois J, et al. Does the surface-treated AN69 membrane prolong filter survival in CRRT without anticoagulation? Intensive Care Med. 2012;38:1818–25.
48. Opatrný K, Polanská K, Krouželký A, Vít L, Novák I, Kasal E. The effect of heparin rinse on the biocompatibility of continuous veno-venous hemodiafiltration. Int J Artif Organs. 2002;25:520–8.
49. Ricci Z, Romagnoli S, Ronco C. Acute kidney injury: to dialyse or to filter? Nephrol Dial Transplant. 2019; Feb 18 https://doi.org/10.1093/ndt/gfz022. [Epub ahead of print].
50. Uchino S, Bellomo R, Morimatsu H, et al. Continuous renal replacement therapy: a worldwide practice survey: The Beginning and Ending Supportive Therapy for the Kidney (B.E.S.T. Kidney) Investigators. Intensive Care Med. 2007;33:1563–70.

Part IX

Prehospital Intervention

29
Prehospital Resuscitation with Low Titer O+ Whole Blood by Civilian EMS Teams: Rationale and Evolving Strategies for Use

P. E. Pepe, J. P. Roach, and C. J. Winckler

29.1 Introduction: Civilian Setting Resuscitation Strategies for Bleeding over the Past Half Century

For the Life of all flesh, is the blood thereof. (Leviticus 17:14, the Bible)

Most modern out-of-hospital emergency medical services (EMS) systems, as we have come to recognize them today, were established in the 1960s and 1970s when a cadre of intrepid physicians ventured into the streets and later published their successful experiences with lifesaving approaches to managing acute coronary syndromes, trauma care, and cardiopulmonary arrest on-scene [1–3]. These lifesaving reports helped to propel the widespread adoption of EMS systems and the concomitant introduction of specially trained (non-physician) emergency medical technicians called "paramedics" in many parts of the globe [1–5]. In addition, nursing personnel also ventured into the realm of on-scene emergency response, particularly in the arena of air medical services, often retrieving trauma patients in non-urban, distant settings.

P. E. Pepe (✉)
Dallas County EMS and Public Safety Operations, Fire Marshal's Office, Dallas, TX, USA

The Broward Sheriff's Office Department of Fire Rescue and Air Rescue,
Fort Lauderdale, FL, USA
e-mail: Paul_Pepe@sheriff.org

J. P. Roach
The Broward Sheriff's Office Department of Fire Rescue and Air Rescue,
Fort Lauderdale, FL, USA

C. J. Winckler
The City of San Antonio Fire Department Emergency Medical Services,
San Antonio, TX, USA

Departments of Emergency Health Science and Emergency Medicine, The University of Texas Health Science Center, San Antonio, TX, USA

By the early 1980s, the standard of care for hypotensive trauma patients, be it blunt or penetrating injury, was the application of the pneumatic anti-shock garment and the infusion of intravenous isotonic fluids, generally crystalloids [6–8]. These interventions were provided for the purposes of restoring a "normalized" blood pressure with an intent to "re-perfuse the tissues" [6–8].

These adopted practices had their roots in elegant laboratory experiments that demonstrated the value of infusing crystalloid-like fluids, along with blood, to mitigate mortality after large (life-threatening) volumes of blood had been removed from the study animals [9, 10]. Subsequently, the evolution of prehospital EMS and air medical rescue programs facilitated the ability to bring these interventions to patients as early as possible. In turn, almost all systems of prehospital trauma care began immediate infusion of isotonic crystalloid fluids such as lactated Ringer's solution, normal saline, or modified products such as PlasmaLyte or Normosol either on-scene or en-route to a trauma center. In certain venues, intravenous resuscitation for hypotensive trauma patients included other intravascular volume-restoring interventions including colloids such as albumin and hypertonic saline–dextran infusions [11]. While innumerable arguments soon ensued regarding which product was superlative to the others, the very early prehospital administration of non-hematologic intravenous fluids became a seemingly universal standard of care in most trauma care systems by the 1980s.

In the mid-1980s and early 1990s, however, clinical trials were conducted that appeared to refute the value of the pneumatic anti-shock garment as well as prehospital fluid resuscitation. Ironically, this inability to confirm a survival advantage was particularly applicable to their use for penetrating truncal injuries, a condition in which the main cause of death was usually related to internal hemorrhage [7, 8]. Not only were both prehospital interventions of no apparent advantage, but there were also inferences and observed trends that mortality might even be higher with these interventions, even though they did raise blood pressure [7, 8].

Later, in the 1990s, new experimental models sought to examine internal hemorrhage that was uncontrollable prior to its operative intervention [12–16]. These laboratory studies demonstrated that isotonic and hypertonic intravenous fluid infusions prior to bleeding control were indeed detrimental. The original 1950–60s animal models of fluid infusions that showed improved outcomes with intravenous crystalloid fluids largely involved scenarios in which the animal's blood was removed in large volumes. However, there was no longer an ongoing loss of blood after the large volume blood removal [9, 10]. In other words, they were mimicking scenarios in which bleeding would have been controlled prior to intravascular volume infusion. Those original studies also generally included a certain degree of restoration of whole blood along with the crystalloids [9, 10].

In the subsequent uncontrolled bleeding models that demonstrated a detrimental effect, it was shown directly that early infusions of fluids that were not blood-based generally created multiple problems including hydraulic acceleration of hemorrhage and a dislodging of early soft clots that had not yet had a fibrinous transformation [12–16]. There was also dilution of clotting factors, but at the time, that association with detrimental outcomes was simply considered an inferential factor [8].

Nevertheless, the notion to restore patients to normotensive status, particularly those with head injuries, remained a persistent practice, even well into the early 2000s [6, 17, 18]. The focus remained on expediting mechanical bleeding control (surgical hemostasis) at a trauma center, be it for intracranial, intrathoracic, or intra-abdominal bleeding. However, while more judicious with their infusions, clinicians still sought to maintain a degree of hemodynamic support in the preoperative phase with intravenous fluids, be they colloids or crystalloids.

29.2 The Recent Evolution of Non-Mechanical Bleeding Control Interventions

Vanguard work largely coming out of the U.S. military experience in the Middle East during the 2000s, not only focused on the application of tourniquets for external hemorrhage control but also clot-stimulating dressings and other forms of mechanical bleeding control. While the clot-forming dressings implied a form of non-mechanical intervention, they were still used in the prehospital setting for large wounds and accompanied direct compression of the hemorrhage site.

Based on that same military experience as well as other clinical trials primarily based on the European continent, the concept of non-mechanical bleeding control began to evolve quite strongly. For example, the CRASH-2 trial supported the use of tranexamic acid early on after injury [19]. The tranexamic acid was used presumably to enhance intravascular clotting non-mechanically. However, the overall mechanism of action remained unclear, and it was also shown that delayed infusion was associated with worse outcomes [19]. Nevertheless, those early tranexamic acid trauma studies did begin to indicate that very early interventions to enhance clotting would become important adjuncts in the preoperative management of trauma patients.

Concurrently, other pivotal publications further enhanced that line of thinking and fostered the notion of so-called damage control resuscitation in which case-controlled study outcomes appeared to be much better with the infusion of red blood cells (RBCs) and plasma in more of a 1:1 ratio versus the more traditional 8:1 ratio [20]. Later the addition of platelets, creating a triplet damage control resuscitation strategy of 1:1:1 (cells:plasma:platelets), evolved and eventually spread into the civilian population [21].

More recently, the concept of just providing early plasma infusion alone as in the prehospital setting has been independently associated with improved outcomes [22]. In addition, early results from studies of soldiers with traumatic brain injury (TBI) indicate a lifesaving effect of tranexamic acid in that setting [23], and early reports from other unpublished studies may indicate that the early infusion of 2 g tranexamic acid may be superior to only 1 g initially followed by a second gram infused slowly over the next few hours.

These evolving data help to further drive a renewed focus on infusing products that might induce non-mechanical bleeding control in the prehospital setting. The CRASH-3 trial (tranexamic acid for TBI) has now been published, further reinforcing the focus on these concepts [24]. As will be discussed in the next section, it has also stimulated a movement away from using intravenous fluids that are not blood-based (e.g., crystalloid/colloid) and a focus more toward the use of plasma and whole blood as a form of "remote damage control" resuscitation [25–28].

29.3 The Detrimental Effects of Isotonic/Hypertonic Fluid Infusions

Evolving experimental work has now demonstrated that non-hematological fluid infusions have deleterious effects beyond the hydraulic acceleration of hemorrhage and the dislodging of early soft clot formation. More recently, it has been demonstrated that such intravenous fluids, can be detrimental to the glycocalyx, the important coating over the vascular endothelium [25, 26, 29].

The glycocalyx is a "fuzzy" layer of glycoproteins and sugar moieties located on the external side of the plasma membrane of most cell types. The composition of the glycocalyx, which can be altered in disease states and with non-blood component fluid infusions, influences numerous properties of the cell membrane, including coagulation, cell–cell recognition, and the cell's interface with the microenvironment. Experimentally, its erosion along the vascular endothelium can lead to leaking capillaries, corrupted platelet function, dysfunctional coagulation, and subsequent risk for multiple organ failure [25, 26, 29]. Therefore, like heart failure or kidney failure, "blood failure" can occur in the face of severe hemorrhage as manifested by oxygen debt (acidosis), platelet dysfunction, coagulopathy, and an "endotheliopathy."

Recent evidence suggests that blood products, including both whole blood and plasma, help to maintain the integrity of the glycocalyx, protect its properties and its ability to form clots and also promote other forms of non-mechanical hemostasis, whereas crystalloids disrupt it [25, 26, 29]. Recent clinical studies support the lifesaving effect of early on-scene plasma infusion, and follow-up studies confirm that the addition of RBCs to plasma enhance that effect [22, 30]. These findings indicate that the original demonstration of potential harm from colloids/crystalloids is related to more than just the simple dilution of the clotting factors and the accompanying factors of hydraulic acceleration of bleeding and soft clot disruption. There are also potential detrimental effects from infusion of fluids at ambient temperatures and numerous other physiological sequelae.

Even if infusion of traditional crystalloid and colloid fluids is discouraged, there are remaining challenges in terms of infusing products that maintain the glycocalyx and other critical factors that mitigate bleeding and subsequent complications. A recent study in an urban setting (Denver) showed no distinct advantage to the particular type of plasma product that was studied [31]. However, that neutral result might be because of the short distances to the trauma center or the time to prepare the product for infusion [31]. While they can be maintained on ambulances for much longer periods, freeze-dried products may also have their limitations, and

Table 29.1 Comparison of component blood products versus whole blood

	Component therapy	Whole blood
Composition	1 unit of packed red blood cells + 1 unit of platelets + 1 unit of fresh frozen plasma + 1 unit of cryoprecipitate	1 unit of low titer O+ whole blood
Volume and temperature	680 ml and cold	500 ml and warm
Hematocrit	29%	38–50%
Platelet count	80 K	150–400 K
Coagulation factors	65% of initial concentration	100%
Fibrinogen	1000 mg	1000 mg

storage of fresh frozen plasma (FFP) still requires thawing and its shelf-life is limited.

With the evolution of using blood products and particularly 1:1:1 damage control resuscitation in hospital, the thought might be to consider the same in the prehospital setting, but storage of those blood products would be unfeasible [27, 28]. It would be very expensive to continue to maintain these products at all times, even on helicopters, let alone ground ambulances. This is exacerbated by the very short half-life of stored platelets (e.g., 3–5 days) and even fresh plasma after thawing (e.g., 5 days). In addition, infusion of all these individual components is not an easy task and infusion of whole blood would not only make more sense logistically (one versus multiple infusions that need to be checked and verified), but it is actually more effective in terms of longevity of platelet counts, clotting functions (Table 29.1), and perhaps even outcomes [32]. In fact, the 1:1:1 approach was actually a secondary strategy that came about in the early 2000s when whole blood products were in short supply. The original intent was always to use blood in the field.

However, on the surface, use of whole blood brings its own challenges in terms of prevalent misconceptions. Even though portable devices are now available that can rapidly warm refrigerated whole blood in a matter of minutes, many clinicians, wary of the risk of transfusion reactions, believe that whole blood cannot be used before blood-typing and crossmatching are accomplished. Nevertheless, as discussed in the next section, there may be a solution to those concerns.

29.4 The Rationale for Prehospital Use of Low Titer O+ Whole Blood

While O-negative whole blood has traditionally been called the "universal donor" because of its lack of A, B, and Rh antigens, it is only found in about 8% of the U.S. population (i.e., about 4% of males) and may be less than 3% worldwide. Therefore, blood banks and decision-making clinicians prefer to protect the use of O-negative for the benefit of certain cancer patients, neonates, and women of childbearing age.

In contrast, O-positive blood constitutes the blood line for about 40% of the U.S. population and likely more elsewhere. Recent evidence suggests that a very large proportion of persons with O-positive blood may have very low titers of A and B antibodies and, specifically, not enough to create an immediate hemolytic or life-threatening negative transfusion reaction. The latest available data suggest that transfusion reactions are very rare when using O+ low titer whole blood in which the IgM or IgG anti-A and anti-B titers are less than 256 [27, 28]. While many other venues are using titers <128, most are beginning to use blood with titers of <256 [27, 28].

In fact, military experience and records from over half a million transfusions now indicate that using donor blood with O+ titers <1000 may be safe as another type of "universal donor" and that as many as 60–70% of persons with O+ blood would fall into that low titer category [33–35]. This constitutes roughly a third of the population. Until recently, O+ men (about 20% of the general U.S. population) have preferably been used as low titer O+ blood donor targets because, compared to men, there is a lower proportion of women with eligible low titer O+ blood. A significant percentage of women also have human leukocyte antigen (HLA) which may predispose the recipient to the risk of another complication, namely a rare but finite risk for transfusion-associated lung injury (TRALI). Nevertheless, the level of HLA correlates with the number of past pregnancies and thus some predictors exist to anticipate its presence. In essence, there are many women with the potential to safely donate low titer O+ whole blood, creating another excellent source for donors. In addition, the risk for creating TRALI would again be so much lower than the high risk of dying from the severe hemorrhage that indicated the transfusion in the first place.

The latest data indicate that the civilian risk of mild hemolytic transfusion reactions due to plasma-incompatible transfusions, using titer-screened donors, is approximately 1:80,000 [27, 28, 35–37]. Therefore, infusion of low titer O+ whole blood can be performed with relative confidence. In addition, with fewer donor exposures than currently occur with the multiple component transfusions (such as the typical 1:1:1 massive transfusion protocols), this enhances the safety profile [35–37].

In terms of isoimmunization and Rh type, the traditional concern is hemolytic disease of the fetus and newborn in women of childbearing age. But recent studies now indicate that this concern is largely mitigated by the immunosuppression of trauma patients and by the administration of anti-D immune globulin to those women receiving the whole blood (i.e., RhIg) [38–40]. Therefore, women of childbearing age who receive Rh+ packed cells or low titer O+ whole blood should be evaluated for RhIg administration candidacy and obstetric and pathology consultation within 24 h. Nevertheless, their risk of having fetal complications is so far outweighed by the lifesaving need that would indicate infusion of the blood [27, 28]. In San Antonio, for example, among 124 patients receiving massive transfusion over a 30-month period, only 26 were women and only 18 of those were of childbearing age. More than half of those women (10/18) died [40]. Furthermore, the one woman of childbearing age who was found to have a D-negative blood type was actually one of the mass transfusion survivors.

The ability to provide whole blood without having to obtain prior typing and crossmatching creates a scenario in which prehospital administration of whole blood may not only be feasible but actually preferred for those who are likely to be exsanguinating. Based on the prior discussion, whole blood would be more feasible and expeditious than mixed component therapy. It is also more effective, and its potential longevity is much greater [27, 28, 32–34]. For all those reasons, the rationale for using low titer O+ whole blood is fairly clear. However, additional challenges remain: (1) finding and obtaining adequate sources of the blood; (2) sustaining and managing its effectiveness to prevent waste of the donated blood; (3) appropriate triggers for infusing the blood; (4) appropriate equipment and related training; (5) sustainable funding; and (6) strategic distribution of the stored blood among the response teams who would be providing the transfusions. In the following section, several strategies for implementation will be described for consideration by those contemplating prehospital use of whole blood, particularly those considering ground ambulance use.

29.5 Some Current Experiences with Implementation of Prehospital Whole Blood

Several EMS systems and air medical rescue programs have now successfully implemented the prehospital use of low titer O+ whole blood including the City of San Antonio Fire Department in San Antonio, Texas and the Broward County Sheriff's Office Department of Fire Rescue in Broward County, Florida. Other civilian and military programs globally have already incurred far more experience with the use of whole blood in the prehospital setting and some of the strategies used by these two agencies for implementation reflect lessons learned, good and bad, from that experience. Nevertheless, as the San Antonio Fire Department and Broward County Sheriff's Office Department of Fire Rescue are the bases of operations for the authors, the following discussion is provided to present two different but current parallel examples of this kind of initiative currently in evolution.

29.5.1 Source of the EMS System Blood Supply

While the Broward County teams currently obtain their blood supply through a commercial agency, San Antonio has a very unique, special model. The city is fortunate to be the home of a longstanding military medical research complex with veteran military trauma researchers who have led many of the advances in trauma care over the past two decades including application of tourniquets, damage control resuscitation, and the use of whole blood in resuscitation. The military medical complex includes a military-staffed trauma center, and there is also a collaborating major university-affiliated trauma center that serves the San Antonio civilian population, which has advanced much of the current work in whole blood resuscitation.

In their efforts to implement a civilian trauma resuscitation system that sustains a substantive supply of whole blood for use in the prehospital setting at the "point of injury," a collaboration was constructed between that university-affiliated trauma hospital and the State of Texas regional trauma advisory council for South Texas (STRAC). In turn, that collaboration helped to create a blood donation program called "Brothers in Arms" funded by a San Antonio Medical Foundation grant. This program, developed and managed by the affiliated South Texas Blood and Tissue Center (STBTC), identifies men with low titer O+ blood types. Those identified are subsequently asked to volunteer to participate in the program. A large source of donors now actually includes many of the EMS rescuers and firefighters who eventually provide the medical rescue and transfusions in the prehospital setting.

Using safe intervals between blood donations from the individuals involved as well as the other usual safeguards and best practices in testing blood donations, "Brothers in Arms" and the affiliated blood bank program itself is quite a unique endeavor, and represents a whole new service line in the San Antonio area as it includes specialized equipment for whole blood retrieval and preservation, testing, packaging and distribution directly to the involved EMS units or stations.

29.5.2 Deciding How to Distribute the Blood Supply

In collaboration with local trauma center teams, the San Antonio Fire Department team identified various areas of the city of San Antonio from where the highest volumes of patients with life-threatening hemorrhage had originated [27]. For example, they determined areas of the city where patients who later received multiple transfusions in-hospital were retrieved and, in turn, used EMS response vehicles covering those areas of the city as the targets for storing and utilizing the blood product [27]. Among several dozen EMS response units in the city, 8 of the units, each staffed with paramedics, were chosen to carry the blood in the initial round of evaluation.

In the case of Broward County Sheriff's Office Department of Fire Rescue, they have now developed a specialized air rescue program to deliver the blood due to the expansive and complex geography in their EMS response jurisdiction and the ensuing concern for extensive delays transporting the severely bleeding patient to the closest trauma center. While they are currently planning a move to add whole blood onto the ground units as well, the air rescue program is the current focus for the new program.

In San Antonio, each of the 8 units assigned was provided with just one 500-ml standard container of whole blood for transfusion. The blood was kept in a portable cooler that maintains the blood at 0 to 6 °C (Credo ProMed^R, Pelican BioThermal, LLC, Plymouth, MN, USA) and is monitored for any breach of temperature control. Broward County uses a different cooler (BloodBoxx^R by Thermal Logistics Solutions, Combat Medical, Harrisburg, NC, USA) at 0–4 °C with automated monitoring for temperature breaches.

The carried unit of whole blood is considered to be fully transfusable and effective for several weeks. The blood can be maintained in a viable state for up to

Fig. 29.1 Low titer O+ whole blood in the out-of-hospital setting. Whole blood can now be stored and maintained for significant periods of time on ambulances (photo courtesy of the Broward County Sheriff, Broward County, Florida, USA)

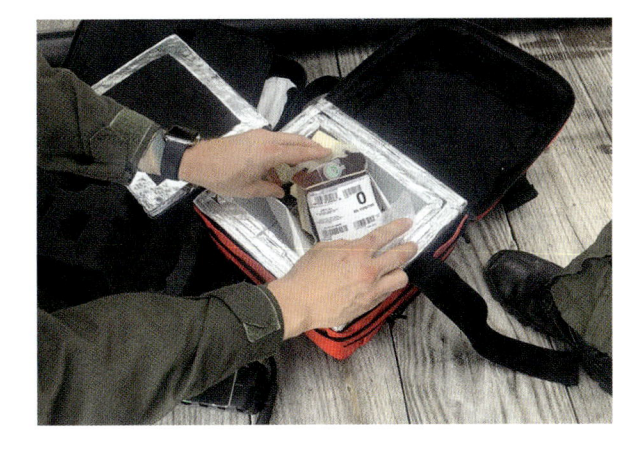

21 days at 1–6 °C in the anticoagulant, citrate–phosphate–dextrose, or for 35 days at 1–6 °C in citrate–phosphate–dextrose–adenine substrate [27, 28] (Fig. 29.1). However, to preempt the possibility of wasting any blood unused by EMS, the blood in San Antonio is rotated back every 14 days to the civilian trauma center (and other area medical centers) for the usual in-hospital transfusions. Experience to date from the San Antonio Fire Department is that 75% of the blood is used prehospital and over 200 patients were treated in the first year of operation. With 8 EMS response units carrying the blood, this translates into about 6 units being used every 2 weeks at a cost of about US$500 (€450) each or about US$75,000 per year. The agency is not charged if the blood is rotated back into the hospital system. In contrast, Broward County Sheriff's Office Department of Fire Rescue pays for all of its blood products, used or unused, but in both cases, the cost has been deemed worthwhile especially with preliminary data indicating trends toward substantial lifesaving. Accordingly, both agencies plan on expanding their fleet of ground units carrying the blood.

29.5.3 Criteria and Triggers for EMS Infusing Whole Blood and Tranexamic Acid

The San Antonio Fire Department EMS crews will infuse blood into not only patients with blunt and/or penetrating trauma but also those with medical conditions associated with substantial blood loss such as severe gastrointestinal hemorrhage. To date, about 25% of the recipients of the whole blood had non-traumatic etiologies and the use included women of childbearing age and even pregnant patients [41].

Regardless of etiology, both San Antonio and Broward County EMS crews will use the blood product for patients with presumed large volume hemorrhage manifested by the following: systolic blood pressure <70 mmHg; systolic blood pressure <90 mmHg and a heart rate of ≥110 beats per minute; a witnessed post-traumatic or non-traumatic circulatory arrest <5 min prior to EMS arrival on-scene and continuous use of cardiopulmonary arrest (CPR) chest compressions throughout the resuscitation efforts; or a patient with likely bleeding who is ≥65 years of age and who has a systolic blood pressure ≤100 mmHg and heart rate ≥100 beats per minute.

In addition to the infusion of the 500 ml of blood over an approximate 3–4 min period, the patient simultaneously receives 1 g of tranexamic acid through another site of vascular access. Children <6 years of age are not treated according to the prescribed protocol, but they can still be given the blood after the medical director has been contacted for approval.

29.5.4 Infusing the Blood and Tranexamic Acid

Both the Broward County and San Antonio programs use a specialized infuser device called the Qinflow^R that immediately warms the blood from near freezing to 38 °C, reaching body temperature in a matter of seconds while delivering the blood at a rate of 200 ml/min through standard large bore peripheral intravenous catheters. In that respect, most patients receive the full benefit of the transfusion within minutes.

29.6 Conclusion

In addition to growing concerns about early resuscitation with crystalloids and other non-hematologic fluids, there is also a growing rationale and evolving evidence that bringing whole blood to the prehospital setting is not only feasible and superior to the component therapy approach but also lifesaving. Using low titer O+ whole blood avoids many of the prior concerns about using blood without blood type and crossmatching. Several strategic initiatives, as discussed in this chapter, may help to expedite and facilitate that lifesaving effect for other communities.

References

1. Pantridge JF, Geddes JS. A mobile intensive care unit in the management of myocardial infarction. Lancet. 1967;290:271–3.
2. Cobb LA, Alvarez H, Copass MK. A rapid response system for out-of-hospital cardiac emergencies. Med Clin North Am. 1976;60:283–93.
3. McManus WF, Tresch DD, Darin JC. An effective prehospital emergency system. J Trauma. 1977;17:304–10.
4. Page JO. The paramedics: an illustrated history of paramedics in their first decade in the U.S.A. Morristown, NJ: Backdraft Publications; 1979. p. 1–179.
5. Pepe PE, Copass MK, Fowler RL, Racht EM. Medical direction of emergency medical services systems. In: Cone DC, Fowler R, O'Connor RE, editors. Emergency medical services: clinical practice and systems oversight. Dubuque, IA: Textbook of the National Association of EMS Physicians, Kendall Hunt Publications; 2009. p. 22–52.
6. American College of Surgeons Committee on Trauma. Advanced trauma life support program for physicians. 6th ed. Chicago, IL: American College of Surgeons; 1997. p. 21–124.

7. Bickell WH, Pepe PE, Bailey ML, et al. Randomized trial of pneumatic anti-shock garments in the prehospital management of penetrating abdominal injury. Ann Emerg Med. 1987;16:653–8.
8. Bickell WH, Wall MJ, Pepe PE, et al. Immediate versus delayed fluid resuscitation for hypotensive patients with penetrating torso injury. N Engl J Med. 1994;331:1105–9.
9. Wiggers C. Physiology of shock. New York, NY: Commonwealth Fund; 1950. p. 121–46.
10. Shires T, Coln D, Carrico CJ, et al. Fluid therapy in hemorrhagic shock. Arch Surg. 1964;88:688–93.
11. Mattox KL, Maningas PA, Moore EE, et al. Prehospital hypertonic saline/dextran infusion for post-traumatic hypotension—the U.S.A. multi-center trial. Ann Surg. 1991;213:482–91.
12. Bickell WH, Bruttig SP, Millnamow GA, et al. The detrimental effects of intravenous crystalloid after aortotomy in swine. Surgery. 1991;110:529–36.
13. Capone A, Safar P, Stezoski W, et al. Improved outcome with fluid restriction in treatment of uncontrolled hemorrhagic shock. J Am Coll Surg. 1995;180:49–56.
14. Stern SA, Zink BJ, Mertz M, Wang Z, Dronen SC. Effect of initially limited resuscitation in a combined model of fluid-percussion brain injury and severe uncontrolled hemorrhagic shock. J Neurosurg. 2000;93:305–14.
15. Owens TM, Watson WC, Prough DS, et al. Limiting initial resuscitation of uncontrolled hemorrhage reduces internal bleeding and subsequent volume requirements. J Trauma. 1995;39:200–7.
16. Rafie AD, Rath PA, Michell MW, et al. Hypotensive resuscitation of multiple hemorrhages using crystalloid and colloids. Shock. 2004;22:262–9.
17. Shoemaker WC, Peitzman AB, Bellamy R, et al. Resuscitation from severe hemorrhage. Crit Care Med. 1996;24:S12–23.
18. Dutton RP, Mackenzie CF, Scalea T. Hypotensive resuscitation during active hemorrhage: impact on in-hospital mortality. J Trauma. 2002;52:1141–6.
19. Meuer WJ. Tranexamic acid reduced mortality in trauma patients who were bleeding or at risk for bleeding. Ann Intern Med. 2013;159:JC3.
20. Holcomb JB, Jenkins D, Rhee P, et al. Damage control resuscitation: directly addressing the early coagulopathy of trauma. J Trauma. 2007;62:307–10.
21. Holcomb JB, Tilley BC, Baraniuk S, et al. Transfusion of plasma, platelets, and red blood cells in a 1:1:1 vs a 1:1:2 ratio and mortality in patients with severe trauma: the PROPPR randomized clinical trial. JAMA. 2015;313:471–82.
22. Sperry JL, Guyette FX, Brown JB, et al. Prehospital plasma during air medical transport in trauma patients at risk for hemorrhagic shock (PAMPer Study Group). N Engl J Med. 2018;379:315–26.
23. Morte D, Lammers D, Bingham J, Kuckelman J, Eckert M, Martin M. Tranexamic acid administration following head trauma in a combat setting: does tranexamic acid result in improved neurological outcomes? J Trauma Acute Care Surg. 2019;87:125–9.
24. Roberts I, Shakur-Still H, Aeron-Thomas A, et al, writing group for the CRASH-2 Trial Collaborators. Effects of tranexamic acid on death, disability, vascular occlusive events and other morbidities in patients with acute traumatic brain injury (CRASH-3): a randomized, placebo-controlled trial. Lancet. 2019;394:1713–23.
25. Woolley T, Thompson P, Kirkman E, et al. Trauma hemostasis and oxygenation research network position paper on the role of hypotensive resuscitation as part of remote damage control resuscitation. J Trauma Acute Care Surg. 2018;84(suppl):S3–S13.
26. Holcomb JB, Pati S. Optimal trauma resuscitation with plasma as the primary resuscitative fluid: the surgeon's perspective. Hematology Am Soc Hematol Educ Program. 2013;1:656–9.
27. Zhu CS, Pokorny DM, Eastridge B, et al. Give the patient what they bleed, when and where they need it: establishing a comprehensive regional system of resuscitation based on patient need utilizing cold-stored, low titer O+ whole blood. Transfusion. 2019;59:1429–38.
28. Weymouth W, Long B, Koyfman A, Winckler CJ. Whole blood in trauma: a review for the emergency clinicians. J Emerg Med. 2019;56:491–8.

29. Schott U, Solomon C, Fries D, Bentzer P. The endothelial glycocalyx and its disruption, protection and regeneration: a narrative review. Scand J Trauma Resusc Emerg Med. 2016;24:48.
30. Guyette FX, Sperry JL, Peitzman AB, et al. Prehospital blood product and crystalloid resuscitation in the severely injured patient: a secondary analysis of the prehospital air medical plasma trial. Ann Surg. 2019 April 13. https://doi.org/10.1097/SLA.0000000000003324. [Epub ahead of print].
31. Moore HB, Moore EE, Chapman MP, et al. Plasma-first resuscitation to treat haemorrhagic shock during emergency ground transportation in an urban area: a randomised trial. Lancet. 2018;392:283–91.
32. Jones AR, Frazier SK. Increased mortality in adult patients with trauma transfused with blood components compared with whole blood. J Trauma Nurs. 2014;21:22–9.
33. Pidcoke HF, Aden JK, Mora AG, et al. Ten-year analysis of transfusion in operation Iraqi Freedom and operation Enduring Freedom: increased plasma and platelet use correlates with improved survival. J Trauma Acute Care Surg. 2012;73(6 Suppl 5):S445–52.
34. Spinella PC, Perkins JG, Grathwohl KW, Beekley AC, Holcomb JB. Warm fresh whole blood is independently associated with improved survival for patients with combat-related traumatic injuries. J Trauma. 2009;66(4 suppl):S69–76.
35. Spinella PC, Pidcoke HF, Strandenes G, et al. Whole blood for hemostatic resuscitation of major bleeding. Transfusion. 2016;56:S190–202.
36. Strandenes G, Berseus O, Cap AP, et al. Low titer group O whole blood in emergency situations. Shock. 2014;41(Suppl 1):70–5.
37. Berséus O, Boman K, Nessen SC, Westerberg LA. Risks of hemolysis due to anti-A and anti-B caused by the transfusion of blood or blood components containing ABO-incompatible plasma. Transfusion. 2013;53:114S–23S.
38. Porter TF, Silver RM, Jackson GM, Branch DW, Scott JR. Intravenous immune globulin in the management of severe Rh D hemolytic disease. Obstet Gynecol Surv. 1997;52:193–7.
39. Reed W, Lee T-H, Norris PJ, Utter GH, Busch MP. Transfusion associated microchimerism: a new complication of blood transfusions in severely injured patients. Semin Hematol. 2007;44:24–31.
40. McGinity AC, Zhu CS, Greebon L, et al. Prehospital low-titer cold stored whole blood: philosophy for ubiquitous utilization of O-positive product for emergency use in hemorrhage due to injury. J Trauma Acute Care Surg. 2018;84(6s Suppl):S115–9.
41. Newberry R, Winckler CJ, Luellwitz R, Greebon L, Xenakis E, Bullock W, Stringfellow M, Mapp J. Prehospital transfusion of low-titer O+ whole blood for severe maternal hemorrhage: a case report. Prehosp Emerg Care. 2019 Oct 14; https://doi.org/10.1080/10903127.2019.1671562. [Epub ahead of print].

Mobile Stroke Units: Taking the Emergency Room to the Patient

30

T. Bhalla, C. Zammit, and P. Leroux

30.1 Introduction

Stroke is a leading cause of death and disability: each year it is estimated that 5.5 million people die from a stroke worldwide. This accounts for 10% of total deaths. Current projections estimate the number of deaths from stroke worldwide will increase to >7 million in 2030. In the United States, 1 in 20 deaths are from stroke. Perhaps of greater significance, stroke is a leading cause of disability-adjusted loss of independent life-years, resulting in significant economic and societal costs.

The vast majority of strokes (80–90%) are ischemic in nature. Stroke management has historically been restricted to supportive measures with the majority of innovations, research, and treatment focused on prevention. Significant progress has occurred in ischemic stroke prevention, e.g., blood pressure control, use of antiplatelet agents, and carotid endarterectomy among other strategies. Despite this, the incidence of stroke is increasing globally, although a decrease has been observed in high-income countries. In 1995, the National Institute of Neurological Disorders and Stroke (NINDS) published a pivotal trial that described effective treatment for acute ischemic stroke, i.e., thrombolysis with intravenous tissue plasminogen activator (tPA) [1]. Since then, several subsequent trials have confirmed that intravenous tPA is an effective treatment [2]. More recent trials have demonstrated that endovascular clot retrieval is also beneficial [3].

Success of these therapies is time dependent. A pooled analysis of nine trials examining intravenous tPA for acute ischemic stroke showed that there are improved functional outcomes when treatment occurs within 4.5 h of stroke onset, and

---

T. Bhalla · C. Zammit · P. Leroux (✉)
Departments of Emergency Medicine, Neurology, and Neurosurgery,
University of Rochester Medical Center, Rochester, NY, USA

Division of Neurosurgery, Bassett HealthCare, Cooperstown, NY, USA
e-mail: peter.leroux@bassett.org

treatment benefits are greater with earlier initiation of treatment [2]. The time frame of benefit for endovascular clot retrieval is not as clearly defined, but there is decreasing benefit further from the ictus. Consequently there is now significant optimism about acute ischemic stroke management, and substantial efforts are being made to provide therapy as early as possible, ideally within the "golden hour." Despite the efficacy of thrombolysis, it remains underused. In addition, endovascular clot retrieval is only available at select hospitals and so available to only a small proportion of the acute ischemic stroke population.

Time to acute ischemic stroke treatment and organization of care remain priorities in stroke care and research [4]. Approaches to reduce time-to-treatment are constantly evolving and include public information campaigns, organization and streamlining of emergency medical services (EMS) and in-hospital logistics, and developing prehospital pre-alert systems. Imaging is essential in acute ischemic stroke. With this in mind, mobile stroke units or an ambulance equipped with a computed tomography (CT) scanner have evolved to take care to the patient and reduce time to treatment. This evolution is driven by several converging factors: (1) a realization that "time is brain"; (2) revascularization is underused; (3) organization of care; (4) advances in information technology and telemedicine; and (5) development of portable CT scanners. In this chapter, we will examine these factors and discuss the logistics of a mobile stroke unit, describe results of their use, explore alternatives and challenges to mobile stroke units, e.g., in remote or rural environments, and consider future use.

30.2 The Rationale Behind Mobile Stroke Units

30.2.1 Time Is Brain

In acute ischemic stroke, timely treatment with intravenous tPA or thrombectomy (endovascular clot retrieval) results in substantial clinical improvement. The treatment is time dependent [5–8]: for every 15-min reduction in "door-to-needle time," the odds of risk-adjusted in-hospital mortality are reduced by 5% [8]. The resulting axiom "time is brain" refers to the approximately two million neurons lost every minute in an acute ischemic stroke. As time passes from ictus, less neuronal tissue is salvageable with recanalization of the occluded vessel and more is risked, as hemorrhage-prone "dead brain" accumulates. Ideally, travel time to hospital should be 30 min or less but no more than 60 min, and the door-to-needle time should be within 60 min from hospital arrival [9].

30.2.2 Revascularization Is Underused

While there has been an increase in intravenous tPA administration in acute ischemic stroke [10], thrombolysis still remains underused; only 11.3% of patients receive intravenous tPA within 1.5 h of stroke onset [11]. There are many reasons for this which depend on patient, family and bystander recognition and action, prehospital care, and hospital care. In the United States, it is estimated that less than half the patients with acute ischemic stroke arrive at a stroke center within 3 h. In part this is associated with geography–less than one in four patients in the USA live where they could travel to a stroke center by land within 30 min [12] – and, in part, failure to recognize stroke symptoms. Although mobile stroke unit symptoms are well described, public knowledge of this remains poor worldwide [13]. The Get With The Guidelines Stroke registry found that only 26.2% of treatment-eligible patients with acute ischemic stroke (25,504 patients at 1082 U.S. sites) received intravenous tPA within 60 min of arriving at the hospital [8]. This hospital delay is associated with the time for an appropriate workup and treatment including calculation of a National Institute of Health Stroke Scale (NIHSS), assessment for contraindications, treatment of reversible contraindications (i.e., hypertension), and imaging to rule out intracerebral hemorrhage (ICH) among others.

Some studies suggest that if delays in patient and physician recognition and response to the signs and symptoms of acute ischemic stroke could be eliminated, the proportion of patients eligible for intravenous tPA could be doubled [14]. However, a community cluster-randomized controlled trial (RCT) that attempted to address this at multiple levels both in the community and in the hospital observed only a tendency to increased intravenous tPA use [15]. Rapid diagnostic assessment in the acute phase is crucial, hence taking care to the patient (a mobile stroke unit) makes sense. This shortened time-to-treatment can make a meaningful difference. The number needed to treat for a modified Rankin Scale (mRS) score of 0 or 1 is 4.5 for patients treated with intravenous tPA at <1.5 h from ictus, increases to 9 for those treated between 1.5 and 3 h, and is 14.1 for those treated between 3 and 4.5 h [16].

30.2.3 Organization of Care

Acute stroke care has evolved over time and, in particular, organization of care. A Cochrane analysis shows that this organization is associated with reduced mortality, institutionalized care, or dependency [17]. This organization extends beyond the hospital and also includes EMS systems and pre-planned, comprehensive, and coordinated statewide and local response networks. The value of this coordinated systems approach is well described in trauma. In acute ischemic stroke, effective communication between the stroke team and the EMS system, i.e., pre-notification of a patient's arrival, is associated with reduced time to physician evaluation and increased tPA use [18]. Streamlined and organized in-hospital logistics also makes a difference. For example, when 10 best practice guidelines are implemented, there is a 10-min decrease in the median door-to-needle time [19].

30.2.4 Portable CT Scanning

In patients with suspected stroke, immediate brain imaging is essential. CT scan, in large part to distinguish between an ischemic or hemorrhagic stroke, is used most frequently. Biomedical engineering advances have improved processing and acquisition speed, image quality, reduced radiation doses, and reduced weight and size, and with that portable CT scans have evolved. These devices initially were used at the bedside in the intensive care unit (ICU) for point-of-care testing. The efficacy, accuracy, and physiologic benefits of portable head CT scans and in particular similar image quality to conventional head CT scans are well described in intensive care and traumatic brain injury (TBI) [20, 21].

Portable CT scan devices are central to a mobile stroke unit, and several studies have demonstrated that prehospital head CT scans obtained in a mobile stroke unit are of adequate quality to detect radiological contraindications for thrombolysis [22]. In general, studies can be completed in <10 min [23]. According to American Heart Association Guidelines, head CT scans may be interpreted by any specialist if the physician acquires expertise in the field. This level of expertise is not fully defined, but agreement (kappa) levels >0.8 are recommended as the minimal accepted to use. In physicians other than radiologists, e.g., anesthesiologists who receive appropriate training, excellent inter-rater agreement using a portable CT scan is observed with in-hospital on-call radiologists to determine radiological selection for thrombolysis [23]. Furthermore with advances in information technology, an equivalent diagnostic accuracy is observed when using smartphone and laptops compared with medical monitors to interpret head CT images of acute stroke patients [24].

30.2.5 Information Technology and Telemedicine

Information technology and mobile devices have evolved exponentially in recent years and are now useful in many aspects of stroke care including education, prevention, acute care, imaging, and rehabilitation [24]. In acute stroke management, mobile telemedicine systems can deliver streaming video and audio and be used as supplementary tools for neurological examination and clinical decision-making. These systems permit similar accuracy and speed of use compared with face-to-face methods when assessing the NIHSS [25]. Interpretation of imaging studies is crucial in acute stroke care. Several studies have shown that in the emergency setting, a mobile device (e.g., smart phone, iPad) is just as effective in acute stroke management decisions, e.g., identification of intracranial hemorrhage, as a desktop using a Picture Archiving and Communications System [25, 26].

Telemedicine, defined as "the use of information and communication technology to provide healthcare services to individuals who are at a distance from the healthcare provider" [27], is central to a mobile stroke unit. Telemedicine for stroke was developed in the 1990s to improve access to acute stroke care and facilitate treatment decisions in remote or underserved areas. These "telestroke" consultations require high-speed, clear and reliable audio-video data transmission and traditionally involve an on-call stroke neurologist at a "hub" hospital interacting with physicians, e.g., emergency room doctors and the patient (or family members) at remote "spoke" sites through video teleconferencing. Several lines of evidence indicate that telestroke for stroke is safe and effective [28], and increases the number of CT scans read within 3 h, appropriate tPA use, and accuracy of treatment decisions and can be beneficial where immediate access to stroke expertise is not available [29–31].

Similarly, observational studies, both single and multicenter, have demonstrated the value of telemedicine, both at regional and at national levels for a variety of other neurologic conditions such as neurotrauma, intracranial hemorrhage, neurosurgical consults, and postoperative clinical care for patients undergoing elective neurosurgery [32–35]. In general, improvements have been observed in increased timeliness of diagnosis or triage, reduced unnecessary transfers, and expedited care at a receiving hospital with inter-facility transfers. This can translate into cost savings with adequate patient volume and patient travel distance [36].

30.2.6 Telemedicine in the Mobile Stroke Unit

A physician, e.g., a stroke neurologist or an appropriately trained intensivist or anesthesiologist, is part of the mobile stroke unit team onboard or remote through telemedicine. Several studies showed that acute stroke assessment and clinical decision-making in patients onboard a mobile stroke unit is feasible and can be accurately and reliably performed by a remote neurologist. This is associated with a decreased time to imaging and treatment [37, 38]. On average, time to initiation of a tPA bolus is 24 min for a telemedicine neurologist [39]. Technical failures (including failure of video connection) that limit a telemedicine assessment are infrequent (~5%). However, this may vary with local network structure and availability [38–41]. Not unexpectedly, 4G mobile communications provided higher quality of video-examination. In studies that have compared assessment between an onboard neurologist and a telemedicine neurologist, agreement is excellent (~90%) [42]. Furthermore, stroke severity quantification, e.g., the NIHSS or Unassisted TeleStroke Scale (UTSS), is reliable and can be completed in <5–10 min using a HIPAA-compliant mobile platform [43, 44]. The shortened NIHSS for EMS (sNIHSS-EMS) that consists of "level of consciousness," "facial palsy," "motor arm/leg," "sensory," "language," and "dysarthria" can further reduce assessment time and also permits parallel stroke recognition, severity grading, and large vessel occlusion prediction [45]. This in turn can help triage patients to specialized stroke centers with endovascular capability.

30.3 Mobile Stroke Unit Logistics and Organization

Setting, e.g., urban, metropolitan, or rural; high-income or low-income environment; traffic congestion and patterns; and existing EMS organization influence mobile stroke unit operation among other factors. There are several organizational models of mobile stroke units that describe location, distance, and availability. For example, the Berlin model operates the mobile stroke unit within a 16 min radius from a central location in a fire station [46]. A health economic analysis in Germany suggested that mobile stroke units could provide service up to 30 km radius from base [47]. Other models have not defined a clear distance from the base [48] or use a teaching hospital as a central base or have several units associated with multiple ambulance hubs. It is not clear if the distance/time threshold described in the Berlin model also applies to other locations, i.e., every mobile stroke unit program must adapt their processes and workflow to their own communities, and work closely with their local EMS and hospitals to ensure rapid patient management. This includes education of, and feedback from, first responders.

In part, the mobile stroke unit structure will depend on population, population density, and the number of emergency rooms and hospitals capable of tPA and endovascular therapy. In Australia, computational models based on Google maps that account for travel time (both for a mobile stroke unit and a conventional ambulance), time to process the patient at the scene, time to obtain a head CT, including advanced imaging, e.g., CT angiography or CT perfusion if used, telemedicine consult and proximity of a patient to a stroke center have helped define how best to deploy the mobile stroke unit across cities such as Melbourne and Sydney [49, 50] and is available as an app (https://gntem3.shinyapps.io/ambmc/). This geospatial optimization suggests that the mobile stroke unit can operate up to 76 min from its base, although this is city dependent [49, 50]. This form of analysis also permits identification of hospitals capable of endovascular clot retrieval that can serve as a mobile stroke unit hub. The model in Edmonton, Canada, which provides service in rural Alberta operates up to a radius of 250 km [51]. In this model, the mobile stroke unit will meet an incoming non-mobile stroke unit ambulance at a pre-designated site to reduce travel time. Much of the modeling is described for an ambulance that performs only non-contrast CT. Additional time needs to be considered when CT angiography or CT perfusion scans are used. These imaging studies can allow triage of patients with large vessel occlusion to endovascular clot retrieval-capable hospitals. However, the addition of further tests such as CT perfusion comes at the expense of reduced operating distance for a mobile stroke unit but can create go/no-go triage maps (salvageable tissue vs. large infarct core) for endovascular clot retrieval eligible patients [52].

Most mobile stroke units operate during business hours; few are operational 24/7. The initial 6-month experience from the group in Toledo, Ohio, who were the first 24/7 unit, demonstrated its value in a variety of emergencies including stroke, status epilepticus, and malignant hypertension. The mobile stroke unit covered a region of about 600 square miles that had an estimated population of 433,689. During the review period the mobile stroke unit was dispatched 248 times. Ten patients received intravenous tPA. Mobile stroke unit alarm to on-scene times and treatment times (tPA, anti-epileptics anti-hypertensive agents) were 35 and 50 min, respectively [53].

Scientific statements recommend the development of regional stroke care systems in which ambulances bring acute stroke patients directly to stroke center hospitals. Furthermore, these specialized centers should be organized according to the local and regional needs and classified in different levels of complexity according to available resources and treatments. Any mobile stroke unit should fit in with this organizational plan both at the regional and national levels. In England, the National Health Service (NHS) has sought to reconfigure nationwide stroke services based on the success of centralized stroke care in London which resulted in increased thrombolysis rates, reduced mortality, and reduced long-term costs. This organization is based on admission to a large (>600 stroke admissions a year) hyperacute stroke unit since increased institutional size is associated with reduced door-to-needle times [54] and travel time that ideally is <30 min but no more than 60 min [3, 5]. Modeling is associated with a "ceiling effect." For example, increasing the number of hyperacute stroke units reduces average and maximum road travel time but in so doing reduces the number of patients who reach a hospital with at least 600 admissions per year [55]. Furthermore, the models demonstrated that the maximum proportion of patients that would reach a hyperacute stroke unit with >600 admissions within 30 min travel was 82%. If travel time was increased to 45 min, then the maximum proportion of patients attending a hyperacute stroke unit of sufficient size is 95%. Modeling in other locations has shown that when the door to needle time is 45 min by usual ambulance route, a mobile stroke unit is superior in almost all cases [49]. This is geography dependent and care is needed when considering what appear to be mathematically "optimal" solutions.

30.4 Mobile Stroke Unit Components

The concept of a mobile stroke unit was first published by Fassbender et al. in 2003 as a way of "bringing treatment to the patient rather than the patient to the treatment" [56]. Once a patient arrives at a stroke center, care can be streamlined to expedite the delivery of personalized evidence-based stroke treatment. This however does nothing to accelerate prehospital care. Intuitively, a mobile stroke unit is a first step toward fast-tracking patients in this phase. Earlier CT scans, delivery of tPA, proper triage, and on-scene goal-directed care were the primary goals of early institution of mobile stroke units [56]. It was thought that these early benefits would shorten hospital length of stay and improve long-term outcomes in patients treated in mobile stroke units [57].

All mobile stroke units have the basic components to provide assessment and treatment of acute ischemic stroke, including standard ambulance equipment and medications, a CT scanner, point-of-care laboratory equipment, telemedicine capabilities, and, of course, tPA. In the first generation of mobile stroke units, standard ambulances could not house all the necessary components, but miniaturization of technology has now allowed all the necessary components to fit into a standard ambulance. In addition to the staff of a standard ambulance, the unit must also have a physician, either in person or via telemedicine, and a member trained, either primarily or cross-trained, as a CT technologist. These team members work to quickly and efficiently diagnose or rule out stroke and determine intravenous tPA eligibility. The entire team's sole focus is on the patient being evaluated with all the competing variables of in-hospital care removed from the equation. Instances where delays may arise due to triage of multiple patients, competing obligations of the hospitalist, availability of a CT scanner, or attention of emergency department nurses and technicians are effectively eliminated when the hospital is brought to the patient.

30.5 Do Mobile Stroke Units Make a Difference?

Multiple studies have shown both the benefits and limitations of mobile stroke unit care. In 2010, the University Hospital of the Saarland published their initial results of the first mobile stroke unit. They provided a proof of concept, with an average call to decision time of 35 min [58]. The second mobile stroke unit was created in Berlin and has been clinically used since February 2011 [59]. Since these pioneers developed the first mobile stroke units, many others have been created and deployed. The first mobile stroke unit in the United States was developed in Houston, Texas, and has been in clinical use since May 2014 [60]. Mobile stroke units are now operational in cities in Europe, Australia, Canada, and the USA. The concept continues to evolve and, while still being developed, are now available 24/7 [53], in metropolitan areas outside cities within health system networks or in rural regions [51].

The first RCT by the University of Saarland group found a decrease of 41 min from stroke alarm to therapeutic decision in the mobile stroke unit group (35 min total compared to the control group 76 min total) [57]. This occurred in the context of the mobile stroke unit operating only a short range from base. The trial was halted following the interim analysis of the first 100 patients, given the significant reduction in mobile stroke unit time to delivery of therapy. There was no increased risk of ICH, but given the small number of patients and short-term follow-up (mRS score at 7 days) a determination about clinical outcome could not be made. However, the study provided concrete "proof of concept" that mobile stroke units could be deployed effectively and safely to provide access to therapy in a shorter time period. Larger studies of patients with acute ischemic stroke treated in emergency departments show clearly that early treatment is associated with better outcomes suggesting that mobile stroke units will provide a clinical benefit.

The Saarland study was followed by the larger and more in-depth Phantom-S study from the Berlin group [61]. The initial pilot study found a decrease in time from stroke alarm to delivery of therapy when compared to registry times and no adverse outcomes associated with prehospital intravenous tPA treatment [62]. This was followed by the large-scale Phantom-S trial in 6182 patients, which found a significant decrease (25 min) in time-to-treatment when the mobile stroke unit was employed and a significantly increased thrombolysis rate from 21% in control weeks to 33% when the mobile stroke unit was used. There was no change in ICH risk or 7-day mortality [63]. Subsequent analysis showed that the rate of "golden hour" thrombolysis (treatment within 60 min of symptom onset) increased from 1.1% to 10.1% with mobile stroke units and that this was associated with increased discharge to home compared to nursing home [64]. In 2016, data on longer-term outcome were published: mobile stroke unit use significantly improved the 3-month 0–3 mRS (83% in mobile stroke unit patients, 74% in conventional care) and reduced 3-month mortality (6% in mobile stroke unit patients, 10% in conventional care) [65]. The study's primary endpoint, disability-free care, trended toward an improvement in mobile stroke unit patients but failed to reach statistical significance (53% mobile stroke unit patients, 47% conventional care).

From the Berlin registry, Nolte et al. [66] examined how mobile stroke units may influence care in patients with acute ischemic stroke who, pre-stroke, are dependent in activities of daily living (ADLs). This retrospective analysis included 264 patients, of whom 122 received mobile stroke unit-based care. Mobile stroke unit use was associated with a median reduction of 38 min from symptom onset to treatment compared with conventional care. Starting thrombolytic therapy in the mobile stroke unit was associated with a nearly twofold increased higher probability of a mRS score of 0–3 (39% vs. 25% with conventional care) but not improved 3-month survival rate. The risk of ICH was similar. Preliminary experience from Cleveland also shows that people experiencing stroke who are brought to the hospital in a mobile stroke unit are evaluated and treated nearly two times faster (or on average 40 min) than people taken in a regular ambulance. In addition, 44% received intravenous tPA within an hour-and-a-half, compared to 8% of other patients [37].

At the University of Rochester, we have observed mobile stroke unit door-to-needle times of <10 min by allowing the telestroke physician to participate in in-the-field evaluation of the possible stroke patient by the mobile stroke unit, and EMS providers via mobile-device, hands-free, Bluetooth-enabled teleconferencing on the telestroke platform. This also allows the CT technologist in the mobile stroke unit, who also has access to the telestroke platform, to listen to the evaluation, register the patient in the electronic health record (EHR), and prepare the mobile stroke unit for diagnostics and interventions decided by the telestroke physician before the patient is physically loaded in the mobile stroke unit (Fig. 30.1). In this workflow, the telestroke provider is able to learn pertinent exam findings, gather the historical information required to determine tPA eligibility, and enter orders for CT imaging, laboratory investigations, and tPA preparation before the patient enters the mobile stroke unit. Refinement and replication of this workflow may further enhance the potential efficacy of mobile stroke units.

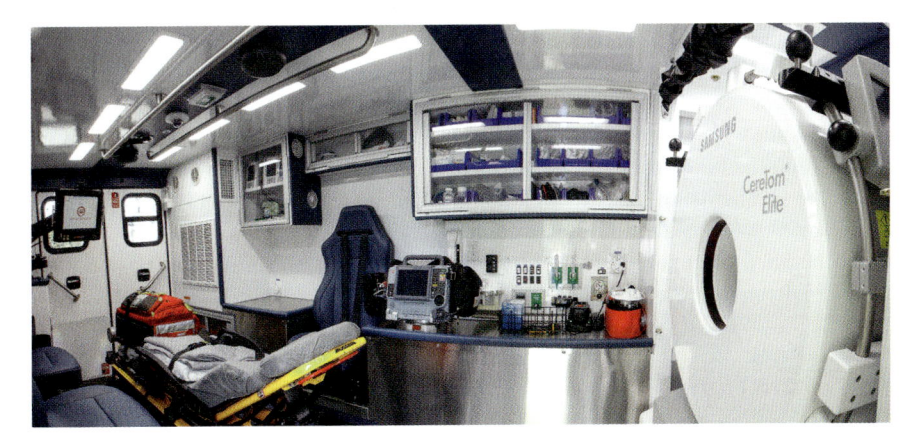

Fig. 30.1 Interior of the University of Rochester MSU showing the portable CT scanner (to the right)

Multiple "systems" benefits, with the potential to improve triage and delivery of care to stroke patients, have also been described. In a subset analysis of the Phantom-S trial, patients with acute ischemic stroke were more likely to be sent to hospitals without dedicated stroke units in the conventional care group (10.1%) than the mobile stroke unit group (3.9%) [67]. Similarly, patients with hemorrhagic stroke were delivered to a hospital without a neurosurgery department equipped to deal with hemorrhage in 43.0% of the conventional care group compared to 11.3% in the mobile stroke unit group. Mobile stroke units may also improve time to endovascular treatment, which, given the recent paradigm shifts in invasive stroke treatment, may enhance outcomes [68]. Consistent with this, data from the initial 6-month experience with a 24/7 mobile stroke unit showed that it was dispatched 248 times and transported 105 patients with alarm-to-treatment times of 50.6 min. Eight of these patients received intravenous tPA. Another 10 patients underwent endovascular clot retrieval based on mobile stroke unit diagnosis of large vessel obstruction [53].

30.6 Limitations of Mobile Stroke Units

While the studies above all show promising results, they were not without limitations. First, although none showed an increase in adverse events, such as hemorrhagic conversion or mortality, it is difficult to ascertain the degree of bias in these studies. Second, blinding of mobile stroke unit use is nearly impossible due to the obvious inherent differences in patient treatment. Third, with the exception of one subset of the Phantom-S study and a newer 2018 study out of Berlin, no other group has shown consistent differences in long-term outcomes with mobile stroke unit use [65, 66]. Consequently, effective cost–benefit analysis is limited. Fourth, these studies compare care delivered by a specialized mobile stroke unit team and one hospital to conventional care delivered by multiple hospitals. Fifth, the NIHSS is assessed in mobile stroke unit patients earlier than in patients who receive conventional care and subsequent worsening or improvement could result in a type of lead-time bias. Finally, the utility of mobile stroke units in an urban compared to suburban setting (or rural setting) where benefit might not be equivalent is still being elucidated. Future studies should target these limitations and ultimately may show mobile stroke units to be cost-effective and provide durable long-term outcome benefit [69]. The BEnefits of Stroke Treatment Delivered using a Mobile Stroke Unit (BEST-MSU) Study funded by the Patient-Centered Outcomes Research Institute and scheduled to conclude in 2022 (ClinicalTrials.gov Identifier: NCT02190500) should help answer the questions in the USA.

30.7 Are There Alternatives?

The value of a mobile stroke unit in large part is a reduction in time-to-treatment. Are there are organizational paradigms that may have the same effect not only for tPA but also for endovascular clot retrieval? In parts of Africa, comprehensive emergency obstetric care has been optimized through midwife obstetric units, staffed by midwifes and linked by telephone to a base hospital where an ambulance "flying squad" is on constant standby. Relevant to endovascular clot retrieval, cohort studies in patients with ST elevation myocardial infarction (STEMI) treated by primary percutaneous coronary intervention (PCI) show that by-passing the emergency room with direct admission to an angiography suite is associated with significantly shorter door-to-balloon times (e.g., 59 vs. 97 min) [70] and with an apparent survival benefit. Median door-to-balloon time is also reduced by 27 min with a correct diagnosis in 95% of patients when local emergency ambulance teams evaluate patients with STEMI eligible for direct PCI and transport them directly to the cardiac catheterization laboratory [71]. A variety of patient characteristics, hospital characteristics, physician characteristics, and care processes affect door-to-balloon times, these require identification to facilitate rapid initiation of treatment. For example, a prehospital electrocardiogram (EKG) that is telemetered through a mobile phone to a physician who with a single call activates the cardiac catheterization call team can bypass usual delays seen during emergency room triage. Similarly in TBI, prehospital activation of a full trauma alert has been shown to halve time to head CT scan [72].

In practical terms, these various methods to reduce time to treatment represent organization and a structured approach to care. An engineering and systems approach is required. This was first described in healthcare for handovers in pediatric cardiac surgery using a "pit crew" model adapted from Formula one racing [73]. In stroke, this same approach and a sigma-based quality-improvement process that clearly defines roles and even position of equipment has been demonstrated to improve efficiency. For example, Raj et al. [74] observed a 1-h reduction in emergency room arrival to groin puncture times, both during and outside of regular working hours when such a process was adopted. Similar organization and parallel processing of tasks is required for a successful mobile stroke unit particularly as a role for mobile stroke units in selecting patients for endovascular clot retrieval is evolving.

30.8 Low-Income Countries and Rural or Remote Settings

More than 80% of the annual deaths from stroke occur in low-income and middle-income countries. Many of these countries do not have widespread or dependable broadband internet access, but much of the population can access the internet using cell phones and this can facilitate mobile stroke units. However, thrombolysis is not frequent in low-income countries, e.g., in Africa, <5 countries have reported experiences with intravenous tPA. Furthermore in rural areas of low-income countries, specialist care is lacking. For example in India, >700 million people have to travel >75 km for specialist care. The number of neurologists ranges between 0.04 in low-income countries and 4.75 in high-income countries per 100,000 population [75]. Telemedicine and mobile stroke units can fill in these deficits but will need to be adapted to the social and geographic environment.

Many patients may suffer a stroke at a significant distance (or time) from a stroke center. For these patients, remoteness, i.e., accessibility, may be more important than distance [76]. The role of the mobile stroke unit in rural and remote environments is only beginning to be elucidated [51, 77, 78]. Early experience suggests it is feasible particularly when integrated into existing EMS services to enhance them [79]. For example, the Edmonton Stroke Program deploys a mobile stroke unit in a 250 km radius of the University of Alberta Hospital. Patients at a distance may already be in a non-mobile stroke unit ambulance or have presented to a remote hospital. The mobile stroke unit then travels toward the inbound ambulance to meet at a predetermined rendezvous location. A patient who does not require specialized care can then be triaged back to the referring hospital [51]. In remote and rural regions, the mobile stroke unit vehicle needs to be adapted to local conditions.

The limited access to specialists in remote or sparsely populated areas argues for a model run independently by the EMS rather than by in-hospital neurologists and neuroradiologists using a tele network service [80]. With advanced imaging capabilities, mobile stroke units can provide an additional resource for teleradiology and telestroke in these areas. However, cost and distance to travel may limit implementation of CT-carrying ground ambulances in dispersed rural areas. What about air transport? [81] The success of the Royal Flying Doctor Service in Australia providing medical care is well described [76, 82]. This includes air retrieval for mechanical thrombectomy of large vessel obstruction. For example, Crockett et al. [83] described air retrieval in 30 patients in Western Australia. The mean retrieval distance was 393 km and the longest 2600 km. Outcome was similar for these patients when compared to patients from urban regions treated during the same time period. An air mobile stroke unit is now being evaluated [81]. This can be a stand-alone air mobile stroke unit or integrate a ground mobile stroke unit and air retrieval.

Air mobile stroke units could use helicopter or fixed wing aircraft. Helicopters could also function in congested urban areas where time rather than distance may limit ground transport. In the United States, helicopter EMS (HEMS) are mainly for interhospital transfer. There are about 400,000 civilian HEMS missions a year in the United States. About 5% are for acute ischemic stroke; most of these flights are for interhospital transfer to a tertiary stroke center often while receiving tPA, i.e., drip and ship. The use of HEMS is associated with reduced time to treatment and in particular can facilitate thrombolytic therapy for patients who live far from primary stroke center facilities [84]. The benefit is more likely when distances exceed 50 km.

Helicopter-based mobile stroke units could be an alternative to ground mobile stroke units for rural areas. However, there are some intrinsic limitations. First, local regulations may determine the choice of HEMS or ground ambulances. These can generally be overcome. Second, helicopter (and fixed wing) flights are vulnerable to weather conditions. While the risk is low, crashes can still occur and these are more likely at night and during instrument-based flying (bad weather). Therefore, flight crews are blinded to patient age and diagnosis before making a go/no-go decision based on aeronautical factors, i.e., in bad weather they may not fly. Third, flights cannot be easily interrupted for unexpected events. Fourth, there are physical factors associated with flight, e.g., vibration, noise, changes in barometric pressure and oxygen levels that may affect clot constitution, the blood–brain barrier, blood pressure, and the ischemic penumbra. Finally, there are many barriers to installing a CT on a helicopter, e.g., radiation isolation in close quarters, electrical power consumption that may reduce drive train mechanical power, and electromagnetic interference with aircraft avionics. However, the main limitation is weight; excess weight will adversely affect performance. Larger helicopters could be used, but this would increase cost and limit access to smaller landing areas. Rather than a CT, the feasibility of other modalities to "image" the brain, e.g., Doppler, brain acoustic monitors, or the infrascanner, has been investigated but none has proved reliable in air transport.

30.9 Cost-effectiveness

Whether mobile stroke units are cost-effective is not well defined. The purchase cost of a mobile stroke unit, depending on its configuration, is estimated to be US$750,000–1,400,00 and most mobile stroke units in the USA have started with philanthropic gifts. Annual running costs during office hours are estimated to be about US$500,00–1,000,000. The cost of 24/7 mobile stroke units is still being elucidated. Cost-utility models that combine a decision tree with Markov modeling suggest that in-ambulance telemedicine is a cost-effective strategy compared to standard stroke care that starts after a time gain of 6 min and becomes dominant after 12 min [85]. Much of the running cost is associated with staffing; the use of telemedicine and elimination of an onboard neurologist reduces operational costs. It remains unclear whether mobile stroke units are financially sustainable or whether the money is better spent on improving the current EMS system, the availability of stroke centers, and earlier recognition of strokes due to large vessel obstruction.

30.10 The Future

Mobile stroke units will continue to proliferate and to evolve and rather than be used for acute ischemic stroke alone likely will become neurological emergency units. The feasibility of this has been shown in TBI, subarachnoid hemorrhage (SAH) and other neurologic emergencies, e.g., status epilepticus, blood pressure management, and reversal of anticoagulation in ICH [30, 53]. In addition, stroke treatment continues to evolve as does imaging equipment and in particular image acquisition and processing time. Portable CT scanners should therefore become more compact and weigh less and so be more suitable for helicopters. The introduction of CT angiography and CT perfusion into mobile stroke units now allows detection of major arterial occlusions. These patients can then be diverted to specialized hospitals that offer endovascular clot retrieval [86]. The role of mobile stroke units in access to endovascular clot retrieval and intra-arterial thrombectomy is a pre-specified BEST-MSU substudy. Initial analysis shows that door-to-puncture-time is shorter in mobile stroke unit patients [87].

30.11 Conclusion

In conclusion, mobile stroke units, i.e., specially equipped ambulances that bring a diagnostic CT scanner and therapeutic thrombolysis directly to patients in the field, are proliferating. Mobile stroke units are setting dependent, but accumulating evidence demonstrates that time to treatment in acute ischemic stroke is reduced and that more patients eligible for treatment receive intravenous tPA. In addition, patients can be triaged rapidly to centers capable of endovascular clot retrieval. The success of a mobile stroke unit depends on integration into and organization of stoke systems and the involvement of major stakeholders in the stroke field. However, mobile stroke units remain investigational and there is at present a lack of robust evidence for clinical benefit or cost-effectiveness.

References

1. National Institute of Neurological Disorders and Stroke rt-PA Stroke Study Group. Tissue plasminogen activator for acute ischemic stroke. N Engl J Med. 1995;333:1581–7.
2. Lees KR, Emberson J, Blackwell L, et al. Effects of alteplase for acute stroke on the distribution of functional outcomes: a pooled analysis of 9 trials. Stroke. 2016;47:2373–9.
3. Goyal M, Menon BK, van Zwam WH, et al. Endovascular thrombectomy after large-vessel ischaemic stroke: a meta-analysis of individual patient data from five randomised trials. Lancet. 2016;387:1723–31.
4. Hachinski V, Donnan GA, Gorelick PB, et al. Stroke: working toward a prioritized world agenda. Stroke. 2010 Jun;41:1084–99.
5. Emberson J, Lees KR, Lyden P, et al. Effect of treatment delay, age, and stroke severity on the effects of intravenous thrombolysis with alteplase for acute ischaemic stroke: a meta-analysis of individual patient data from randomised trials. Lancet. 2014;384:1929–35.
6. Saver JL. Time is brain—quantified. Stroke. 2006;37:263–6.
7. Saver JL, Goyal M, van der Lugt A, et al. HERMES Collaborators. Time to treatment with endovascular thrombectomy and outcomes from ischemic stroke: a meta-analysis. JAMA. 2016;316:1279–88.
8. Fonarow GC, Smith EE, Saver JL, et al. Timeliness of tissue-type plasminogen activator therapy in acute ischemic stroke: patient characteristics, hospital factors, and outcomes associated with door-to-needle times within 60 minutes. Circulation. 2011;123:750–8.
9. Jauch EC, Saver JL, Adams HP Jr, et al. Guidelines for the early management of patients with acute ischemic stroke: a guideline for healthcare professionals from the American Heart Association/American Stroke Association. Stroke. 2013;44:870–947.
10. Quain DA, Parsons MW, Loudfoot AR, et al. Improving access to acute stroke therapies: a controlled trial of organized pre-hospital and emergency care. Med J Aust. 2008;189:429–33.
11. Kim JT, Fonarow GC, Smith EE, et al. Treatment with tissue plasminogen activator in the golden hour and the shape of the 4.5-hour time-benefit curve in the national United States Get With The Guidelines-Stroke population. Circulation. 2017;135:128–39.
12. Albright KC, Branas CC, Meyer BC, et al. ACCESS: acute cerebrovascular care in emergency stroke systems. Arch Neurol. 2010;67:1210–8.
13. Anderson BE, Rafferty AP, Lyon-Callo S, Fussman C, Reeves MJ. Knowledge of tissue plasminogen activator for acute stroke among Michigan adults. Stroke. 2009;40:2564–7.
14. Boode B, Welzen V, Franke C, van Oostenbrugge R. Estimating the number of stroke patients eligible for thrombolytic treatment if delay could be avoided. Cerebrovasc Dis. 2007;23:294–8.

15. Scott PA, Meurer WJ, Frederiksen SM, Kalbfleisch JD, Xu Z, et al. INSTINCT Investigators. A multilevel intervention to increase community hospital use of alteplase for acute stroke (INSTINCT): a cluster-randomised controlled trial. Lancet Neurol. 2013;12:139–48.
16. Lees KR, Bluhmki E, von Kummer R, et al. Time to treatment with intravenous alteplase and outcome in stroke: an updated pooled analysis of ECASS, ATLANTIS, NINDS, and EPITHET trials. Lancet. 2010;375:1695–703.
17. Stroke Unit Trialists' Collaboration. Organised inpatient (stroke unit) care for stroke. Cochrane Database Syst Rev. 2013;9:CD000197.
18. Kim SK, Lee SY, Bae HJ, et al. Pre-hospital notification reduced the door-to-needle time for iv t-PA in acute ischaemic stroke. Eur J Neurol. 2009;16:1331–5.
19. Fonarow GC, Smith EE, Saver JL, et al. Improving door-to-needle times in acute ischemic stroke: the design and rationale for the American Heart Association/American Stroke Association's Target: Stroke initiative. Stroke. 2011;42:2983–9.
20. Peace K, Maloney E, Frangos S, et al. The use of a portable head CT scanner in the ICU. J Neurosci Nurs. 2010;42:109–16.
21. Agrawal D, Saini R, Singh PK, et al. Bedside computed tomography in traumatic brain injury: experience of 10,000 consecutive cases in neurosurgery at a level 1 trauma center in India. Neurol India. 2016;64:62–5.
22. John S, Stock S, Cerejo R, et al. Brain imaging using mobile CT: current status and future prospects. J Neuroimaging. 2015;26:5–15.
23. Hov MR, Zakariassen E, Lindner T, et al. Interpretation of brain CT scans in the field by critical care physicians in a mobile stroke unit. J Neuroimaging. 2018;28:106–11.
24. Salazar AJ, Useche N, Bermúdez S, et al. Evaluation of the accuracy equivalence of head CT interpretations in acute stroke patients using a smartphone, a laptop, or a medical workstation. J Am Coll Radiol. 2019;16:1561–71.
25. Demaerschalk BM, Vegunta S, Vargas BB, Wu Q, Channer DD, Hentz JG. Reliability of real-time video smartphone for assessing National Institutes of Health Stroke Scale scores in acute stroke patients. Stroke. 2012;43:3271–7.
26. Panughpath SG, Kumar S, Kalyanpur A. Utility of mobile devices in the computerized tomography evaluation of intracranial hemorrhage. Indian J Radiol Imaging. 2013;23:4–7.
27. Roine R, Ohinmaa A, Hailey D. Assessing telemedicine: a systematic review of the literature. CMAJ. 2001;165:765–71.
28. Kazley AS, Wilkerson RC, Jauch E, et al. Access to expert stroke care with telemedicine: reach MUSC. Front Neurol. 2012;3:44.
29. Meyer BC, Raman R, Hemmen T, et al. Efficacy of site-independent telemedicine in the STRokE DOC trial: a randomised, blinded, prospective study. Lancet Neurol. 2008;7:787–95.
30. Schwindling L, Ragoschke-Schumm A, Kettner M, et al. Prehospital imaging based triage of head trauma with a mobile stroke unit; first evidence and literature review. J Neuroimaging. 2016;26:489–93.
31. Whetten J, van der Goes DN, Tran H, Moffett M, Semper C, Yonas H. Cost-effectiveness of Access to Critical Cerebral Emergency Support Services (ACCESS): a neuro-emergent telemedicine consultation program. J Med Econ. 2018;21:398–405.
32. Ashkenazi I, Zeina AR, Kessel B, et al. Effect of teleradiology upon pattern of transfer of head injured patients from a rural general hospital to a neurosurgical referral centre: follow-up study. Emerg Med J. 2015;32:946–50.
33. Kahn EN, La Marca F, Mazzola CA. Neurosurgery and telemedicine in the United States: assessment of the risks and opportunities. World Neurosurg. 2016;89:133–8.
34. Migliaretti G, Ciaramitaro P, Berchialla P, et al. Teleconsulting for minor head injury: the Piedmont experience. J Telemed Telecare. 2013;19:33–5.
35. Reider-Demer M, Raja P, Martin N, Schwinger M, Babayan D. Prospective and retrospective study of videoconference telemedicine follow-up after elective neurosurgery: results of a pilot program. Neurosurg Rev. 2018;41:497–501.

36. Thakar S, Rajagopal N, Mani S, et al. Comparison of telemedicine with in-person care for follow-up after elective neurosurgery: results of a cost-effectiveness analysis of 1200 patients using patient-perceived utility scores. Neurosurg Focus. 2018;44:E17.
37. Taqui A, Cerejo R, Itrat A, et al. Reduction in time to treatment in prehospital telemedicine evaluation and thrombolysis. Neurology. 2017;88:1305–12.
38. Itrat A, Taqui A, Cerejo R, et al. Telemedicine in prehospital stroke evaluation and thrombolysis: taking stroke treatment to the doorstep. JAMA Neurol. 2016;73:162–8.
39. Bowry R, Parker SA, Yamal JM, et al. Time to decision and treatment with tPA (tissue-type plasminogen activator) using telemedicine versus an onboard neurologist on a mobile stroke unit. Stroke. 2018;49:1528–30.
40. Geisler F, Kunz A, Winter B, et al. Telemedicine in prehospital acute stroke care. J Am Heart Assoc. 2019;e011729:8.
41. Winter B, Wendt M, Waldschmidt C, et al. 4G versus 3G-enabled telemedicine in prehospital acute stroke care. Int J Stroke. 2019;14:620–9.
42. Wu TC, Parker SA, Jagolino A, et al. Telemedicine can replace the neurologist on a mobile stroke unit. Stroke. 2017;48:493–6.
43. Van Hooff RJ, Cambron M, Van Dyck R, et al. Prehospital unassisted assessment of stroke severity using telemedicine: a feasibility study. Stroke. 2013;44:2907–9.
44. Barrett KM, Pizzi MA, Kesari V, et al. Ambulance-based assessment of NIH Stroke Scale with telemedicine: a feasibility pilot study. J Telemed Telecare. 2017;23:476–83.
45. Purrucker JC, Härtig F, Richter H, et al. Design and validation of a clinical scale for prehospital stroke recognition, severity grading and prediction of large vessel occlusion: the shortened NIH Stroke Scale for emergency medical services. BMJ Open. 2017;e016893:7.
46. Koch PM, Kunz A, Ebinger M, et al. Influence of distance to scene on time to thrombolysis in a specialized stroke ambulance. Stroke. 2016;47:2136–40.
47. Dietrich M, Walter S, Ragoschke-Schumm A, et al. Is pre-hospital treatment of acute stroke too expensive? An economic evaluation based on the first trial. Cerebrovasc Dis. 2014;38:457–63.
48. Audebert HJ, Clarmann von Clarenau S, Schenkel J, et al. Problems of emergency transfers of patients after a stroke. Results of a telemedicine pilot project for integrated stroke accommodation in southeast Bavaria (Tempis). Dtsch Med Wochenschr. 2005;130:2495–500.
49. Phan TG, Beare R, Parsons M, et al. Googling boundaries for operating mobile stroke unit for stroke codes. Front Neurol. 2019;10:331.
50. Phan TG, Beare R, Srikanth V, Ma H. Googling location for operating base of mobile stroke unit in metropolitan Sydney. Front Neurol. 2019;10:810.
51. Shuaib A, Jeerakathil T, Alberta Mobile Stroke Unit Investigators. The mobile stroke unit and management of acute stroke in rural settings. CMAJ. 2018;190:E855–8.
52. Nogueira RG, Jadhav AP, Haussen DC, et al. Thrombectomy 6 to 24 hours after stroke with a mismatch between deficit and infarct. N Engl J Med. 2018;378:11–21.
53. Lin E, Calderon V, Goins-Whitmore J, Bansal V, Zaidat O. World's first 24/7 mobile stroke unit: initial 6-month experience at mercy health in Toledo, Ohio. Front Neurol. 2018;9:283.
54. Bray BD, Campbell J, Cloud GC, et al. Bigger, faster? Associations between hospital thrombolysis volume and speed of thrombolysis administration in acute ischemic stroke. Stroke. 2013;44:3129–35.
55. Allen M, Pearn K, Villeneuve E, Monks T, Stein K, James M. Feasibility of a hyper-acute stroke unit model of care across England: a modeling analysis. BMJ Open. 2017;7:e018143.
56. Fassbender K, Walter S, Liu Y, et al. "Mobile stroke unit" for hyperacute stroke treatment. Stroke. 2003;e44:34.
57. Walter S, Kostopoulos P, Haass A, et al. Diagnosis and treatment of patients with stroke in a mobile stroke unit versus in hospital: a randomised controlled trial. Lancet Neurol. 2012;11:397–404.
58. Walter S, Kostpopoulos P, Haass A, et al. Bringing the hospital to the patient: first treatment of stroke patients at the emergency site. PLoS One. 2010;e13758:5.
59. Ebinger M, Lindenlaub S, Kunz A, et al. Prehospital thrombolysis: a manual from Berlin. J Vis Exp. 2013;18:e50534.

60. Parker SA, Bowry R, Wu TC, et al. Establishing the first mobile stroke unit in the United States. Stroke. 2015;46:1384–91.
61. Ebinger M, Rozanski M, Waldschmidt C, et al. PHANTOM-S: the prehospital acute neurological therapy and optimization of medical care in stroke patients—study. Int J Stroke. 2012;7:348–53.
62. Weber JE, Ebinger M, Rozanski M, et al. Prehospital thrombolysis in acute stroke: results of the PHANTOM-S pilot study. Neurology. 2013;80:163–8.
63. Ebinger M, Winter B, Wendt M, et al. Effect of the use of ambulance-based thrombolysis on time to thrombolysis in acute ischemic stroke: a randomized clinical trial. JAMA. 2014;311:1622–31.
64. Ebinger M, Kunz A, Wendt M, et al. Effects of golden hour thrombolysis: a Prehospital Acute Neurological Treatment and Optimization of Medical Care in Stroke (PHANTOM-S) substudy. JAMA Neurol. 2015;72:25–30.
65. Kunz A, Ebinger M, Geisler F, et al. Functional outcomes of pre-hospital thrombolysis in a mobile stroke treatment unit compared with conventional care: an observational registry study. Lancet Neurol. 2016;15:1035–43.
66. Nolte CH, Ebinger M, Scheitz JF, et al. Effects of prehospital thrombolysis in stroke patients with prestroke dependency. Stroke. 2018;49:646–51.
67. Wendt M, Ebinger M, Kunz A, et al. Improved prehospital triage of patients with stroke in a specialized stroke ambulance: results of the pre-hospital acute neurological therapy and optimization of medical care in stroke study. Stroke. 2015;46:740–5.
68. Bowry R, Parker S, Rajan SS, et al. Benefits of stroke treatment using a mobile stroke unit compared with standard management: the BEST-MSU Study run-in phase. Stroke. 2015;46:3370–4.
69. Yamal JM, Rajan SS, Parker SA, et al. Benefits of stroke treatment delivered using a mobile stroke unit trial. Int J Stroke. 2017;13:321–7.
70. Lubovich A, Dobrecky-Mery I, Radzishevski E, et al. Bypassing the emergency room to reduce door-to-balloontime and improve outcomes of ST elevation myocardial infarction patients: analysis of data from 2004-2010 ACSIS registry. J Interv Cardiol. 2015;28:141–6.
71. Van de Loo A, Saurbier B, Kalbhenn J, Koberne F, Zehender M. Primary percutaneous coronary intervention in acute myocardial infarction: direct transportation to catheterization laboratory by emergency teams reduces door-to-balloon time. Clin Cardiol. 2006;29:112–6.
72. Rados A, Tiruta C, Xiao Z, et al. Does trauma team activation associate with the time to CT scan for those suspected of serious head injuries? World J Emerg Surg. 2013;8:4.
73. Catchpole K, De Leval M, McEwan A, et al. Patient handover from surgery to intensive care: using formula 1 pit-stop and aviation models to improve safety and quality. Pediatr Anesth. 2007;17:470–8.
74. Rai AT, Smith MS, Boo S, Tarabishy AR, Hobbs GR, Carpenter JS. The 'pit-crew' model for improving door-to-needle times in endovascular stroke therapy: a Six-Sigma project. J Neurointerv Surg. 2016;8:447–52.
75. World Federation of Neurology, World Health Organization. ATLAS. Country Resources for Neurological Disorders. 2nd ed. Geneva: Department of Mental Health and Substance Abuse; 2017.
76. Fatovich DM, Phillips M, Jacobs IG, Langford SA. Major trauma patients transferred from rural and remote Western Australia by the Royal Flying Doctor Service. J Trauma. 2011;71:1816–20.
77. Lippman JM, Smith SN, McMurry TL, et al. Mobile telestroke during ambulance transport is feasible in a rural EMS setting: the iTREAT study. Telemed J E Health. 2015;22:507–13.
78. Mathur S, Walter S, Grunwald IQ, Helwig SA, Lesmeister M, Fassbender K. Improving prehospital stroke services in rural and underserved settings with mobile stroke units. Front Neurol. 2019;10:159.
79. Hov MR, Nome T, Zakariassen E, et al. Assessment of acute stroke cerebral CT examinations by anaesthesiologists. Acta Anaesthesiol Scand. 2015;59:1179–86.

80. Bradford NK, Caffery LJ, Smith AC. Telehealth services in rural and remote Australia: a systematic review of models of care and factors influencing success and sustainability. Rural Remote Health. 2016;16:3808.
81. Walter S, Zhao H, Easton D, et al. Air-Mobile Stroke Unit for access to stroke treatment in rural regions. Int J Stroke. 2018;13:568–75.
82. Margolis SA, Ypinazar VA. Aeromedical retrieval for critical clinical conditions: 12 years of experience with the Royal Flying Doctor Service, Queensland, Australia. J Emerg Med. 2009;36:363–8.
83. Crockett MT, Jha N, Hooper AJ, et al. Air retrieval for clot retrieval; time-metrics and outcomes of stroke patients from rural and remote regions air-transported for mechanical thrombectomy at a state stroke unit. J Clin Neurosci. 2019;70:151–56.
84. Hutton CF, Fleming J, Youngquist S, et al. Stroke and helicopter emergency medical service transports: an analysis of 25,332 patients. Air Med J. 2015;34:348–56.
85. Valenzuela Espinoza A, Devos S, van Hooff RJ, et al. Time gain needed for in-ambulance telemedicine: cost-utility model. JMIR Mhealth Uhealth. 2017;5:e175.
86. John S, Stock S, Masaryk T, et al. Performance of CT angiography on a mobile stroke treatment unit: implications for triage. J Neuroimaging. 2016;26:391–4.
87. Czap AL, Grotta JC, Parker SA, et al. Emergency department door-to-puncture time since 2014. Stroke. 2019;50:1774–80.

Part X

Trauma

Evaluating Quality in Trauma Systems

31

A. J. Mahoney and M. C. Reade

31.1 Introduction

Do you work in a high-quality trauma system? For many of us, trauma is a familiar clinical entity, which comprises a substantial proportion of our caseload. Trauma is the cause of 25% of presentations to emergency departments [1], and 50% of hospitalized trauma patients require intensive care unit (ICU) admission [2]. But does our familiarity translate into the best outcomes for our patients? On face value, this question seems simple; we each have an impression of how care in our own institution "measures up." But quality is not a monolithic concept, either present or absent. Nor, from the patient's perspective, can it be equated with the performance of one clinical team or hospital unit. Rather, appraising the quality of a trauma system requires consideration of the entire patient journey, from injury to rehabilitation, using carefully selected measures of structure, process, and outcome. Here, we consider an innovative system-based approach to trauma quality assurance and improvement that is likely to guide the work of intensivists and emergency physicians in the near future.

A. J. Mahoney (✉)
Royal Hobart Hospital, Hobart, TAS, Australia

2nd General Health Battalion, Australian Regular Army, Brisbane, QLD, Australia
e-mail: adam.mahoney@ths.tas.gov.au

M. C. Reade
Faculty of Medicine & Jamieson Trauma Institute, The University of Queensland, Brisbane, QLD, Australia

Joint Health Command, Australian Defence Force, Canberra, ACT, Australia

31.2 Context

Trauma remains a major cause of mortality in developed and developing countries, responsible for around 9% of global mortality. The most recent Global Burden of Disease (GBD) study estimated that in 2013 at least 4.5 million people died as a result of injury. In the GBD analysis, the most common causes of trauma death, together accounting for nearly 50% of fatalities, were road injury, falls, and interpersonal violence [3].

Acknowledging the ongoing burden of disease from trauma, it is important to recognize that much progress has already been made. In the 23 years between the first and most recent GBD study, there has been a 30% reduction in disability-adjusted life years (DALYs) lost to trauma. However, this trend is not universal, and improvements have been achieved predominately in developed nations [4]. Since the 1990s, developed health systems have invested in quality improvement and quality assurance processes that have enabled identification of modifiable risk factors for trauma death and allowed implementation of strategies for both primary prevention and injury management [5, 6]. However, improvements have not been uniform even in these high-performing systems, suggesting scope for the further innovation outlined in this chapter.

31.3 What Is a Trauma System?

"Trauma systems are an integrated and systematic structure designed to facilitate and coordinate a multidisciplinary system response to provide optimal care to injured patients from onset of injury through rehabilitation and return of ideal functioning" [7].

Arguably, trauma services represent a "system of systems" in that they pool the resources and capabilities of a collection of task-oriented organizations. Many of the components of a trauma system, from the prehospital retrieval service to pathology, surgery to rehabilitation, are operationally and managerially independent. They may also be geographically dispersed. Each of these stakeholders will undergo independent evolutionary development and, in delivering the clinical effect of "trauma care," they demonstrate emergent behavior. Emergent behaviors or qualities are those that arise as a result of interactions between the components of a complex system and which cannot be predicted from scrutiny of the components in isolation. A common rendering of this concept is the notion that "the whole is greater than the sum of the parts." Comprehensive management of trauma casualties cannot be delivered by an emergency department, radiology service, blood bank, or hospital switchboard alone; but through their relationships they can produce the "health effect" of trauma care. This point is of great importance because, where systems demonstrate emergent behavior, it is not possible to reliably predict their performance solely through analysis of their constituent parts.

31.4 What Are the Goals of a Trauma System?

Earlier, we said that trauma systems aim to provide "optimal care to injured patients," but such nebulous yardsticks are difficult to use in practice. Each clinician will have their own view of "optimal" care within their domain. It is more helpful to map the goals of a trauma system against the World Health Organization (WHO) dimensions of healthcare quality [8]. Healthcare should be as follows:

- Effective, in that it adheres to an evidence base and results in improved outcomes for individuals and communities
- Efficient, in that it maximizes the use of available resources, avoiding waste
- Acceptable (patient centered), accounting for the preferences and aspirations of individuals and communities
- Accessible, in that care is timely, geographically proximate and resourced sufficiently for the community's needs
- Equitable, without variation in quality based on personal characteristics or geographical location
- Safe, in that it minimizes the risks and harms to patients

Using the dimensions of healthcare quality as a lens during quality assurance and quality improvement activities can help to avoid missing opportunities to enhance service provision, as might occur if the focus is too narrowly upon metrics of effectiveness and efficiency.

31.5 What Is Meant By "Quality Assurance" and "Quality Improvement"?

One definition of quality assurance is "an organized process designed to ensure the maintenance of a desired level of safety and quality in a service or product" [9]. Quality improvement on the other hand represents an "iterative process to continuously improve the safety and quality of care provided to patients" [9]. It might be said that quality assurance aims to bring care up to an established standard, while quality improvement aims to lift the standard itself. In practice, quality assurance and quality improvement overlap substantially, and it is important for a trauma system to seek opportunities both to enhance performance and to monitor for deterioration in areas of service that are already highly effective. For both quality improvement and quality assurance, it is crucial that analysis employs the best available measures of quality, as outlined below.

31.6 Selecting Measures of Quality

It is clear that monitoring trauma system quality is complex. Unsurprisingly, one systematic review from 2010 identified over 1500 quality indices in fewer than 200 articles [10]. Given the financial and personnel constraints within most trauma services, it is not possible for all relevant quality indicators to be measured [11]. How then are we to choose?

Historically, trauma systems have benchmarked themselves primarily according to risk-adjusted mortality and case fatality rates, and preventable deaths [12], in much the same way as might be done in some ICUs. However, it is important to consider all the abovementioned dimensions of quality, and limiting analysis to "hard" endpoints such as death, ventilator days, or hospital length of stay results in an incomplete picture of performance.

One way of classifying quality indices is to divide them into measures of structure, process, and outcome, as proposed by Donabedian [13]: structure reflects the environment in which healthcare is provided, including organization of clinical services and materiel; process reflects the manner in which healthcare is delivered; and outcome reflects the consequences of healthcare delivery, both positive and negative, for individuals and the community. There is some evidence that trauma systems that perform well against structural metrics are more likely to perform well against process metrics, and that higher performance against both structure and process metrics correlates with improved patient outcomes [14].

Within these categories, indicators may be judged according to their importance, usability, scientific soundness, and feasibility [15]. Importance relates to impact upon patient outcomes and perceived scope for improvement. Usability reflects the ease with which data can be analyzed, communicated, and used in decision-making. Scientific soundness relates to the existence of an established process-outcome relationship, akin to biological plausibility, and the validity and reliability of measurement [16]. Feasibility denotes the extent to which the benefit of collecting data outweighs the administrative burden of its collection [17]. Ultimately, each measure can be mapped to one or more dimensions of quality, allowing appreciation of the extent to which a quality management process is delivering a holistic appraisal of performance [18]. There are numerous examples of intuitively attractive indicators that fail these criteria. For example, while trauma patients with Glasgow Coma Scale (GCS) scores <13 who did not have a computed tomography (CT) head scan had a significantly increased risk of death (suggesting this might be a good indicator), patients with an epidural or subdural hematoma who had surgery delayed >4 h (a similarly intuitively negative process measure) actually had a *lower* risk of death, presumably because these were the least unwell patients [19].

Quality evaluation in intensive care is often focused upon "benchmarking" one unit against a qualitatively similar unit using standardized mortality ratios (SMR). In doing so, quality is largely viewed through the lens of efficacy, efficiency, and safety. Less consideration is usually given to dimensions of quality such as accessibility, equity, and acceptability. This is not necessarily unreasonable: in most developed countries, nearly all hospital patients at risk of preventable death can be admitted to an ICU. Therefore in-unit deaths, both preventable and unpreventable, are of sufficient frequency to make SMR a useful comparator between institutions. If we wished to assess the other dimensions of quality, theoretically it would be possible to incorporate measures of the social and cultural acceptability of care, or the extent to which hospital bed-flow limited accessibility, by retaining focus at the hospital level. But would this be an adequate measure of quality, for trauma in particular?

A trauma system must serve a population and its component parts cannot be validly assessed in isolation. Indeed, to do so may lead us to draw specious conclusions. For example, in the recent conflicts in Afghanistan, improvements in the prehospital trauma system were associated with *increasing* in-hospital mortality [20]. Rather than being considered a cause for concern, this observation was thought by many to reflect the success of a system that enabled critically injured patients to reach hospital who in previous conflicts would have died at the scene or en route. In this setting, comparison of one military hospital with another would not be without value, but such comparisons must necessarily give us an incomplete picture. From the perspective of the individual patient, it is not emergency department or ICU mortality that is of greatest importance, but their overall chance of survival from the point of injury to the time of discharge. Trauma is almost unique in the extent to which outcomes depend upon time-sensitive integration of prehospital and critical care services, as well as comprehensive inpatient care and rehabilitation. Therefore, unlike in general intensive care or in virtually any other area of medicine, we cannot approach trauma system quality evaluation armed only with the same tools we employ to judge the overall performance of individual clinical services. It is this requirement for an "injury-to-community" approach that differentiates the evaluation of trauma systems from quality assurance and improvement approaches commonly applied in ICUs, emergency departments, and surgical services.

In the following sections, we review some widely employed quality indices, outlining their strengths and limitations, before exploring emerging system-level evaluation opportunities offered by data linkage and temporospatial analysis techniques that are likely to guide the work of clinicians worldwide in the near future.

31.7 Structure and Process Measures

We do not propose to deal with structure and process measures in detail, save to flag their significance and to provide resources for further consideration. Most structure and process measures are intuitive, and many will be familiar to clinicians working within established trauma systems; a selection is presented in Table 31.1, alongside a number of common outcome measures. Structure and process measures carry great weight in trauma verification processes, such as that undertaken by the American College of Surgeons [21] and the Royal Australasian College of Surgeons [22]. As indirect evidence of the importance of evaluating these indices, trauma verification has been identified as an independent predictor of survival, at least in smaller trauma centers [23].

Notwithstanding this, structure and process indicators must still be carefully selected. Even "intuitive" measures, where high compliance might be expected to produce measurably better patient outcomes, often lack substantial published evidence to support their use. Partly this is due to the dilution of research effort by the plethora of reported indicators. Additionally, well performing trauma systems may exhibit high compliance with a large cluster of structure and process indicators, making it difficult to identify which individual metrics are most important. Where evidence is scarce, standardization is an appropriate goal and we highly

Table 31.1 Quality indicators by category and phase of care

	Structure	Process	Outcome
Prehospital	Sufficient number of trained clinicians Adequate communication systems Dispatch protocols Retrieval triage protocol Facility bypass protocol Procedural skill training program	On-scene time Retrieval time Completeness of prehospital documentation	Preventable death rate
Intrahospital	Sufficient number of trained clinicians Trauma team activation protocol Massive transfusion protocol Direct transfer to theater protocol Trauma death review committee Existence of trauma registry	Time to trauma team activation Time to antibiotics for open fracture Time to first blood product transfusion Time to CT trauma series Tertiary survey completeness	Preventable death rate Standardized mortality ratio Unplanned returns to theatre Unplanned admissions to ICU Procedural complication rate Deep vein thrombosis rate
Posthospital	Protocol for follow-up of traumatic brain injury Protocol for follow-up of substance abuse or dependence Standardized rehabilitation protocols	Time to review by rehabilitation service Time to rehabilitation admission following acceptance of care. Substance abuse screening rate	Evaluation of functional status Return to work Return to independent living Welfare dependence Proportion of patients returning with new substance-use-related injuries

commend the work of Stelfox and colleagues, who have endeavored to narrow the field of potential quality indicators based upon published evidence and expert consensus [10, 18].

31.8 Outcome Measures

31.8.1 Death

Inpatient mortality, adjusted to injury severity, is one of the most commonly reported quality indices [10]. It has been used both for internal quality assurance and for benchmarking of institutions. It rates highly in terms of usability and feasibility. However, its importance has decreased over time for several reasons: first, preventable inpatient deaths have decreased to the point where further gains are likely to be much smaller in magnitude; second, 80–90% of trauma deaths occur in the prehospital environment and therefore presumably it is in this phase of care that most preventable deaths will be identified; and third, reduction in trauma deaths is not necessarily mirrored by reduction in trauma-related burden of disease. Consequently, inpatient mortality or case fatality rates alone are inadequate measures of quality [12] and should not be the primary means of determining the efficacy of structure or process changes within a developed trauma system. It does not follow that we should expunge death-related indices; spikes in fatality rates may sound a warning within an established system and sharp reductions in mortality may accompany introduction of a trauma system where none previously existed. Yet we should look beyond simple statistical methods when examining patterns of trauma death, exploring the possibilities offered by large linked datasets and temporospatial analysis as outlined later in this chapter.

31.8.2 Functional Outcomes

Given the inherent limitations of death rate quality indices, it is unsurprising that many authors have sought indicators that more closely reflect trauma's burden of disease for individuals and communities. Putative measures have included quality of life (QoL) measures, return to work, welfare dependence, need for assistance with activities of daily living (ADL), and physical function at discharge, among many others.

Unfortunately, functional outcome indices are much less feasible to measure than death outcome measures. The administrative burden of data gathering is much greater, resulting in inconsistent collection, and the lack of commonly accepted QoL and other function-based instruments also significantly hampers benchmarking. Further, if measurement occurs solely at the time of discharge, rather than following a fixed post-injury interval, functional indices may reflect variation in discharge practices more than patients' independence or lack thereof. Indeed, if we wished to approximate a patient's ultimate functional status, we would need to collect data around 1 year after injury [24]; this is beyond the capability of many trauma registries. However, linkage of patient records with non-clinical administrative databases, as explored later in this chapter, may afford the ability to evaluate long-term outcomes such as return to work, welfare dependence, and the requirement for residential care.

Presently, it is true to say that no ideal functional outcome measure has yet been identified in the literature. Nevertheless, it is also true that the importance of assessing function is widely accepted by academics in the field of quality improvement and by clinicians in major trauma centers [18]. Trauma system leaders should select one or more functional indicators appropriate to their context using the general markers of a good indicator as outlined above.

31.9 Limitations of "Traditional" Epidemiology

Descriptive epidemiology theoretically considers three main factors: person, place, and time. Traditionally, however, "place" has been given less prominence. For those who work in hospitals rather than public health units, this is unsurprising;

patients present to the emergency department, are managed in various hospital units and are discharged to "the community." For some illnesses, it would not be unreasonable for a clinician to give little thought to the location from which a patient was collected by an ambulance. In this person- and time-centric approach to epidemiology, outcome measures may be reported for an entire patient cohort or for various subgroups defined by age, sex, comorbidities, or reported demographic characteristics.

Overall and subgroup mortality rates remain valuable outcome indicators for components of a trauma system. Nonetheless, they have several key limitations. First, in-hospital mortality alone cannot account for variation in patients' prehospital clinical journeys. Patients with identical injuries cannot be assumed to have an equal chance of survival if they vary in their time to retrieval and prehospital management. Second, tabulated statistics do not facilitate the detection of "clustering," where there is a non-random pattern in disease incidence or outcome (adjusted for incidence) with respect to geography. Third, if we return to the WHO dimensions of quality, mortality rates do not significantly aid us in making a determination as to the accessibility or equity of healthcare within a trauma system.

31.10 Why "Place" Matters

Thus far, we have established that trauma is a global public health concern and that substantial improvement in trauma outcomes can be achieved through implementation of trauma systems. We have identified that best-practice trauma management requires the time-sensitive integration of many different teams, making it nearly unique among the clinical conditions encountered by intensive care and emergency physicians. Further, we have concluded that outcome measures that focus on a single institution or its component parts rather than the system as a whole are of limited value. In short, the evaluation of trauma care is very different to the evaluation of systems for managing other critical illnesses. We are compelled therefore to seek a different form of analysis, one in which the integrated effects of time, place, and person may be explored—spatial analysis.

31.11 Spatial Analysis

As applied to trauma systems, spatial analysis refers to the description and analysis of geographically indexed outcome data with respect to patient, environmental, and social risk factors [25]. Research has traditionally been focused in two domains: identification of risk factors for trauma and analysis of the spatial organization of trauma care [26]. Several forms of spatial analysis have been used within these fields of enquiry, including disease mapping, geographic correlation studies, and cluster detection. In this chapter, we will explore disease mapping and its applications, touching upon geographical correlation techniques in some of the case studies [27].

31.11.1 Disease Maps

Disease mapping has been used for well over a century. Perhaps the most common form of disease map is called a "choropleth," from "*choro-*"(area) and "*pleth*" (value). These maps aggregate a given parameter, be it deaths or another desired indicator, within a defined boundary, representing the calculated value according to a change in color or intensity of shading of the area. Choropleth maps can afford the viewer a synoptic view of complex epidemiological data, and many clinicians find identification of visual patterns easier on a map than in a table. Maps of trauma incidence or mortality, including separate figures for different subgroups or time periods, can be employed purely for descriptive purposes or to help hypothesis generation within a quality improvement cycle [25].

In trauma, the most basic form of choropleth mapping would involve aggregating trauma deaths within existing population divisions, such as statistical or local government areas. Simple death counts are misleading because areas with higher populations will have more deaths. One way to overcome this problem is to use mortality rates, in order to account for population inequality between areas. However, where areas are of unequal size, larger polygons tend to have greater "visual weight" than smaller polygons of the same color; this tends to produce an exaggerated impression of mortality in larger areas and minimize perceived mortality in smaller areas.

The limitations of using raw mortality rates have led many trauma researchers to employ an alternative statistic in their map, the SMR. The SMR for area i is calculated by dividing the number of deaths observed in a particular area (O_i) by the number of deaths expected in that area (E_i). There are many ways of determining E_i; commonly, this term is derived by applying global age- and sex-adjusted mortality rates to the population of the region in question. Mapping the SMR allows identification of "hotspots" where observed trauma deaths greatly exceed expected deaths. These areas can then be subjected to detailed scrutiny in order to identify whether there are modifiable risk factors or aspects of management that can be manipulated in order to improve trauma system performance.

The fundamental advantage of identifying trauma SMR outlier hotspots by population area rather than by hospital is that this is what matters more to patients. Knowing that a particular hospital has a higher than expected mortality would no doubt be of some interest, but few severe trauma patients are able to choose their treating hospital and indeed (as we have seen was true in the military Afghanistan example) this might lead to a misleading conclusion. Rather, knowing they live in an area at particularly high risk should prompt community agitation to identify and fix the root problems wherever they are in the system—be they road infrastructure, availability of prehospital services, or "quality" of hospital care.

31.11.2 The "Small Numbers" Problem

Without additional efforts by the researcher, all rate-based measures are vulnerable to the effects of the "small numbers problem." The small numbers problem refers to the observation that rates calculated for areas with low population counts exhibit high variance. One death in an area with a population of 50 people has more influence on the mortality rate than one death in a much more populated area. Hence, the rates calculated for sparsely populated areas are inherently unstable. The implication of unstable rates is that it becomes more difficult for the researcher to determine whether an observed increase in mortality or SMR reflects a meaningful finding or an artifact of small mortality denominators.

31.11.3 Addressing the Small Numbers Problem

There are many approaches to "stabilizing" the values of unstable ratios. Two of the most common are the spatial empirical Bayes method and kernel density estimation. In the spatial empirical Bayes method, rates are adjusted toward a global or local mean using an *a priori* determination of risk distribution. The *a priori* estimate can be based either on a global mean (global empirical Bayes estimate) or on the mean of adjacent areas (local empirical Bayes estimate). Rates are only adjusted for areas where margins of error exceed a predetermined threshold; hence empirical Bayesian smoothing tends to "shrink" the estimate rates of low population areas toward the local or global mean, leaving highly populated areas unchanged.

31.11.4 Kernel Density Estimation and "Heat Maps"

An alternative approach, if individual case data are available, employs kernel density estimation. In this method, a series of overlapping spatial filters, kernels, are placed over the study area, and a kernel function is employed to fit a smoothly curved surface over each point. Basic kernel density analysis, in which kernel radius is specified empirically, still suffers from the small numbers problem. If kernel radius is too small, then in some areas the population covered will be insufficient to generate a stable rate. Conversely, if the radius is too large, the rates will be stable, but there will be a loss of geographic detail (Fig. 31.1). However, the problem of over- and under-"smoothing" can be addressed using adaptive spatial filters, which use kernels of varying radii that expand or contract to include data from adjacent grid points until a stable rate is achieved. Interpolation of the area between the grid points results in a "heat map" of disease burden. Adaptive spatial filters therefore afford a compromise between stable rates and preservation of the geographical detail needed to identify areas of higher than expected trauma morbidity or mortality.

31.11.5 Examples of Using Spatial Analysis to Evaluate Trauma System Quality

Spatial analysis techniques are particularly useful in evaluating the accessibility and equity dimensions of trauma system quality. One example is the work by Brown and

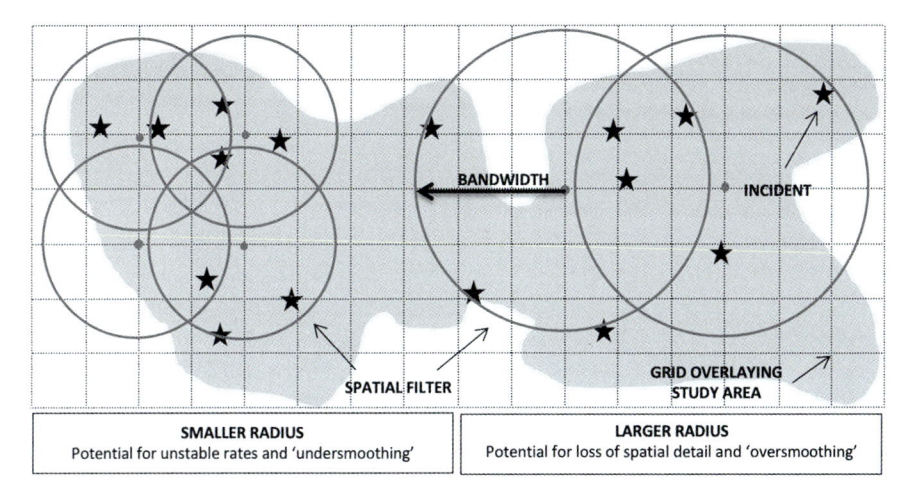

Fig. 31.1 Kernel density estimation with fixed radius spatial filters. Choice of kernel radius size affects the degree to which the reported rates represent the data for a broader or more constrained area. Individualizing the kernel radii to the data such that a stable and representative rate is achieved in each area (adaptive spatial filtering) achieves an optimal balance between detail and smoothing

colleagues in Pennsylvania [28]. In their study of fatal motor vehicle collisions, each injury location was mapped, as were the locations of major trauma centers and aeromedical retrieval bases. An empiric Bayes method of interpolation was used to create a map of fatality rates within the trauma system boundary. This facilitated a "hotspot" analysis that identified a surfeit of trauma deaths in the geographical areas most distant from major trauma centers. The importance of trauma center proximity was reinforced by the observation of "cold spots" around trauma centers, representing fewer deaths, even in regions exhibiting high overall fatality rates (Fig. 31.2). Regression analysis confirmed a relationship between the mean distance between point of injury and the closest trauma system resource, and mortality. The authors then modeled a number of scenarios in which trauma system resources, such as aeromedical retrieval bases, were reallocated to improve accessibility of trauma care.

An even more sophisticated analysis of the impact of retrieval distance on outcome was performed by Tansley and colleagues [29]. They employed a method called cost distance analysis, in which the time cost in minutes of patient retrieval is calculated using a road network map, taking into account local speed limits. The authors were then able to map predicted ground-based patient transport times for the entire area covered by their trauma system (Fig. 31.3). Bivariate analysis demonstrated that patients suffering injury as a result of motor vehicle collision or penetrating trauma in a location with a predicted travel time of >30 min to a trauma center had both higher on-scene and overall mortality. Interestingly, patients with higher predicted travel times were also more likely to have been ejected from their vehicle, hinting at lower rates of seatbelt use in remote areas. In this study therefore, spatial analysis has been used both to evaluate trauma system accessibility and to

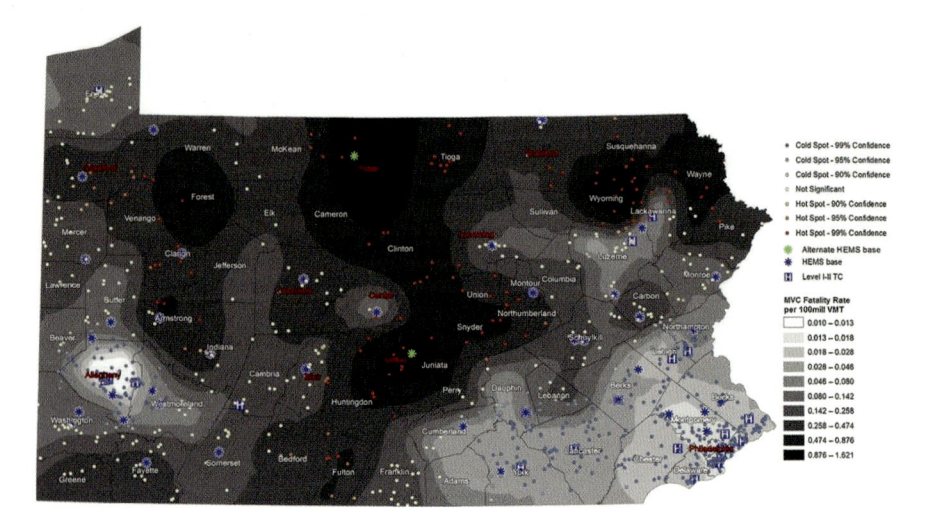

Fig. 31.2 Heat map of fatal motor vehicle collisions per 100 million vehicle miles traveled. "Cold spots" around trauma centers, representing fewer deaths, even in regions exhibiting high overall fatality rates, highlight the importance of proximity to trauma care (From [28] with permission)

generate a hypothesis as to risk factors for worse trauma outcomes in some parts of a trauma system dependency.

The abovementioned case studies demonstrate the pivotal importance of the geographic organization of trauma systems and the utility of spatial analysis of incident-level data in identifying regions or communities with outcomes that are better or worse than expected. Variation alone does not allow us to comment on which of several similar communities has the "appropriate" rate of trauma mortality; however, where all patient characteristics are similar, the highest and lowest rates are likely to differ according to system-level risk factors [30]. For example, spatial analysis allows comparison of regions with similar distances to major trauma centers, and apparently similar trauma system structures and process indices, which might have quite different SMRs. Targeted examination of outliers in spatial analysis can therefore form part of the trauma system quality improvement cycle.

Evidently, spatial analysis has potential as a means of investigating system-wide quality. However, in order to make the most use of both spatial analysis and other epidemiological techniques, we must possess data reflecting the entire patient journey, from the point of injury to rehabilitation.

31.12 Trauma Registries and Linked Data

For many years, trauma centers have kept hospital or departmental records of trauma patients, containing abundant clinical details for the period from triage to discharge. Often though, these repositories contain only sparse information about potential quality indicators such as the location of injury or the time from injury to ambulance arrival.

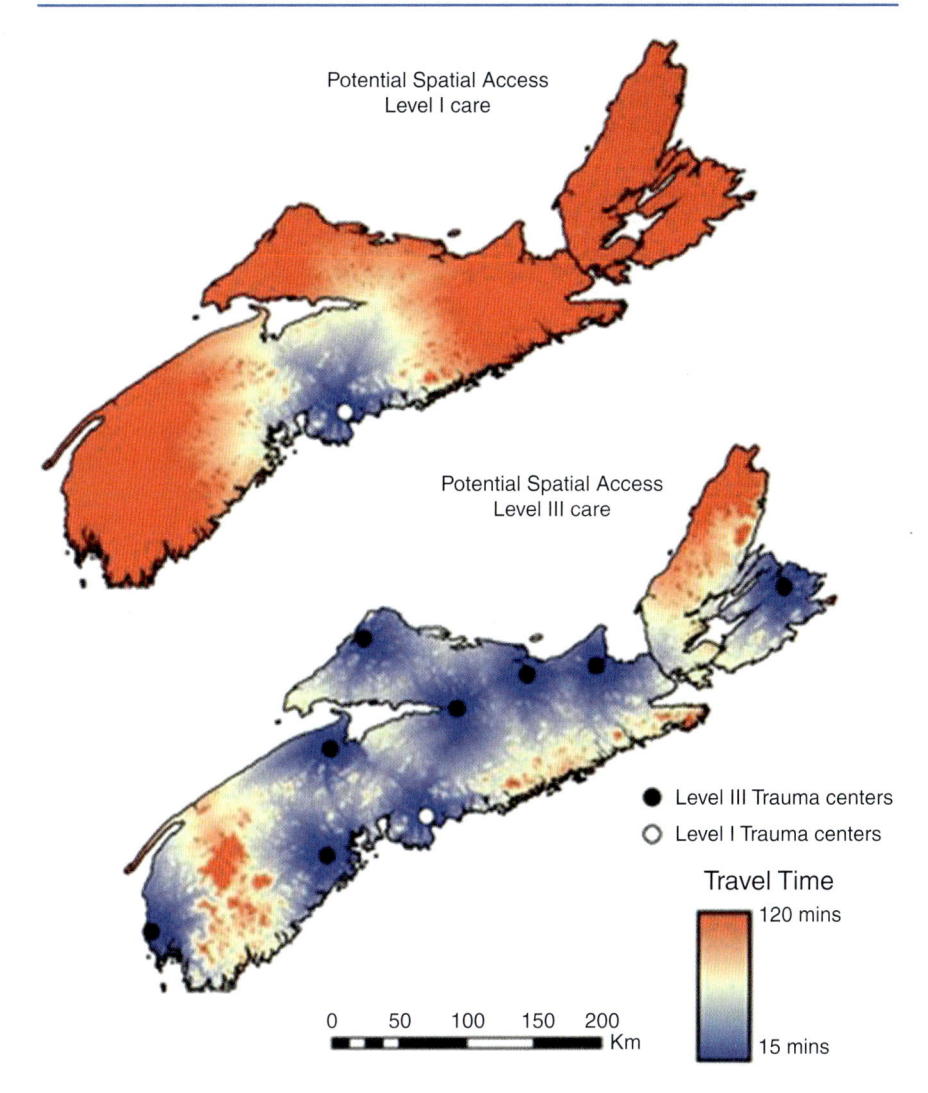

Fig. 31.3 Predicted ground retrieval times to Level I and Level III Trauma Centers. Patients injured more than 30 min from a trauma center had both higher on-scene and overall mortality (From [29] with permission)

One approach to addressing the need for comprehensive data is a geographically based trauma registry. A common model for trauma registries is to identify patients meeting predetermined major trauma criteria at the point of admission to emergency departments or intensive care units. The records of patients who meet or who are likely to meet inclusion criteria are then reviewed by professional data coders, who extract information relating to each patient's injury, transport, and admission. Frequently, a mechanism will exist to allow retrospective checking of case capture, for example comparing registry entries against an International Classification of Diseases (ICD)-10 report for all hospital discharges [31].

In a system where there is only one major trauma center, an established trauma registry with high capture and completeness is an excellent foundation for trauma system quality assurance and improvement. However, in more complex trauma systems with multiple major trauma centers, or where historically separate trauma networks have been amalgamated, we can be faced with the problem of multiple institutional registries, each with different inclusion criteria and coding processes. Where such fragmentation of data occurs, there can be great value in adopting streamlined geographically based registry processes [31, 32].

Even in systems that have achieved standardization of terms and data collection processes, geographically based trauma registries tend not to produce a complete picture of system performance. One of the main reasons for this is that information relating to prehospital deaths tends to be systematically excluded from trauma registries that recruit patients at their first point of hospital contact. A further potential gap is the failure to include patients transferred from other hospitals, if the discharge ICD-10 code for the second admission does not reflect the patient's initial injury [32]. Thus, even with adequate resources and robust data collection methodology, trauma registries cannot be regarded as a panacea.

Data linkage techniques represent one method of enhancing the capture of meaningful quality indicators. Linkage refers to the process of uniting records from two or more files, aiming to combine records belonging to the same patient [33]. In evaluating trauma systems, linkage can be used to match ambulance, police, and other emergency service records with emergency department, inpatient and rehabilitation records in order to complete the injury continuum [34]. Often, linkage makes use of data that is already being captured by these individual services for reasons other than trauma system analysis; hence once a linkage process is established, there may be little additional requirement for resources to facilitate data collection. Further, linking records from predominately administrative databases can afford rich data relating to employment, race, religion, and other social determinants of health, which may not be included as trauma registry variables; this again facilitates appraising the equity and accessibility dimensions of trauma system quality.

Unfortunately, like trauma registries, data linkage processes are imperfect. Linkage can be impeded by cumbersome processes for obtaining approval to access records, the records themselves may be incomplete, and the quality of data obtained from administrative sources can be highly variable [34]. In some countries, such as the United States, there are legal barriers to retention of identifying information, which means that researchers need to employ probabilistic techniques that use variables such as age, sex, injury date, and location to calculate the likelihood of two records belonging to the same person [32]. Notwithstanding these limitations, data linkage remains a powerful tool for achieving holistic evaluation of trauma systems.

31.13 Conclusion

We return now to the original question—do you work in a high-quality trauma system? For each of us, this is a complex question, and one that is difficult to answer without having a framework against which to evaluate quality. In this chapter, we have advocated a holistic approach that considers all dimensions of quality across the entire continuum of injury, not only the measures of efficacy and efficiency that can dominate consideration of in-hospital trauma outcomes.

A purposive approach to setting quality goals will allow selection of the best structure, process, and outcome indicators with regard to their importance, usability, scientific soundness, and feasibility within the local context. We encourage those interested in trauma system evaluation to consider the opportunities afforded by spatial analysis, particularly in that spatial analysis introduces new ways of presenting data to both clinical and lay audiences, allowing us to advocate more effectively for the resources require to investigate and remedy potential shortfalls in system capability. We also look forward to the opportunities that may be offered in future by streamlined, near real-time data linkage, with its potential to accelerate the quality improvement cycle for the entire continuum of trauma care.

Finally, we emphasize that the data needed to drive quality improvement are already being collected for routine administrative purposes in many healthcare systems. In order to realize the benefits we have outlined in this chapter, clinicians need to move beyond their direct responsibilities for patient care and engage with quality evaluation at a system level. Only in doing so can we continue to approach the trauma system ideal of providing care to the right patient, at the right place, at the right time.

References

1. Australian Institute of Health and Welfare. Emergency Department Care 2017-2018: Australian Hospital Statistics. Canberra: AIHW; 2018.
2. Prin M, Li G. Complications and in-hospital mortality in trauma patients treated in intensive care units in the United States, 2013. Inj Epidemiol. 2016;3:18.
3. Haagsma JA, Graetz N, Bolliger I, et al. The global burden of injury: incidence, mortality, disability-adjusted life years and time trends from the Global Burden of Disease study 2013. Inj Prev. 2016;22:3–18.
4. World Health Organization. Injuries and violence: the facts. Geneva: WHO; 2014.
5. Lendru R, Locke D. Trauma system development. Anaesthesia. 2013;68:30–9.
6. Mora C, Lecky FE, Bouamr O, et al. Changing the system—major trauma patients and their outcomes in the NHS (England) 2008-17. EClinicalMedicine. 2018;2:13–21.
7. Mullin R, Man C. Introduction to the academic symposium to evaluate evidence regarding the efficiency and efficacy of trauma systems. J Trauma. 1999;47:S3–7.
8. World Health Organization. Quality of care: a process for making strategic choices in health systems. Paris: WHO; 2006.
9. Australian and New Zealand College of Anaesthetists. Guidelines on quality assurance and quality improvement in anaesthesia. Melbourne: ANZCA; 2018.
10. Stelfo H, Bobranska-Artiuc B, Nathen A, Strau S. Quality indicators for evaluating trauma care: a scoping review. JAMA Surg. 2010;145:286–95.
11. Merr AF, Shuke C, Hambli R. Patient safety and the Triple Aim. Intern Med J. 2017;47:1103–6.
12. Grue R, Gabb B, Stelfo H, Cameron P. Indicators of the quality of trauma care and the performance of trauma systems. Br J Surg. 2012;99:97–104.
13. Donabedia A. Evaluating the quality of medical care. Milbank Q. 2005;83:691–7.
14. Moor L, Lavoi A, Bourgeoi G, Lapoint J. Donabedian's structure-process-outcome quality of care model: validation in an integrated trauma system. J Trauma Acute Care Surg. 2015;78:1168–75.

15. Husse P, Mattke S, Mors L, Ridgele M. Evaluation of the use of AHRQ and other quality indicators. Rockville: Agency for Health Research and Quality; 2007.
16. McGlyn E, Adam J. What makes a good quality measure? JAMA. 2015;312:1517–8.
17. McGlyn E. Selecting common measures of quality and system performance. Med Care. 2003;41:I39–47.
18. Santan MJ, Stelfox HT, on behalf of the Trauma Quality Indicator Consensus Panel. Development and evaluation of evidence-informed quality indicators for adult injury care. Ann Surg. 2014;259:186–92.
19. Glance LG, Dick AW, Mukamel DB, Osler TM. Association between trauma quality indicators and outcomes for injured patients. Arch Surg. 2012;147:308–15.
20. Holcomb JB, Stansbury LG, Champion HR, Wade C, Bellamy RF. Understanding combat casualty care statistics. J Trauma. 2006;60:397–401.
21. American College of Surgeons. About the Verification, Review and Consultation Program: ACS; 2019. Available from: https://www.facs.org/quality-programs/trauma/tqp/center-programs/vrc. Accessed 5 Nov 2019.
22. Royal Australasian College of Surgeons. Trauma Verification: RACS; 2019. Available from: https://www.surgeons.org/research-audit/trauma-verification. Accessed 5 Nov 2019.
23. Brown J, Watson G, Forsythe R, et al. American college of surgeons trauma center verification vs state designation: are level II centers slipping through the cracks? J Trauma Acute Care Surg. 2013;75:44–9.
24. Holbrook TL, Anderson JP, Sieber WJ, Browner D, Hoyt DB. Outcome after major trauma: 12-month and 18-month follow-up results from the Trauma Recovery Project. J Trauma. 1999;46:765–71.
25. Elliott P, Wartenberg D. Spatial epidemiology: current approaches and future challenges. Environ Health Perspect. 2004;112:998–1006.
26. Schuurman N, Hameed SM, Fiedler R, Bell N, Simons RK. The spatial epidemiology of trauma: the potential of geographic information science to organize data and reveal patterns of injury and services. Can J Surg. 2008;51:389–95.
27. Kirby R, Delmelle E, Eberth J. Advances in spatial epidemiology and geographic information systems. Ann Epidemiol. 2017;27:1–9.
28. Brown JB, Rosengart MR, Billiar TR, Peitzman AB, Sperry JL. Distance matters: effect of geographic trauma system resource organization on fatal motor vehicle collisions. J Trauma Acute Care Surg. 2017;83:111–8.
29. Tansley G, Schuurman N, Erdogan M, et al. Development of a model to quantify the accessibility of a Canadian trauma system. Can J Emerg Med. 2017;19:285–92.
30. Merry AF. An overview of quality and safety in health care. Can J Anesth. 2013;60:101–10.
31. Cameron P, Gabbe B, McNeill J, et al. The Trauma Registry as a Statewide quality improvement tool. J T. 2005;59:1469–76.
32. Zehtabchi S, Nishijima DK, McKay MP, Clay MN. Trauma registries: history, logistics, limitations, and contributions to emergency medicine research. Acad Emerg Med. 2011;18:637–43.
33. Bohensky MA, Jolley D, Sundararajan V, et al. Data linkage: a powerful research tool with potential problems. BMC Health Serv Res. 2010;10:346.
34. Mitchell RJ, Cameron CM, Bambach MR. Data linkage for injury surveillance and research in Australia: perils, pitfalls and potential. Aust N Z J Public Health. 2014;38:275–80.

Vasopressors for Post-traumatic Hemorrhagic Shock: Friends or Foe?

32

J. Richards, T. Gauss, and P. Bouzat

32.1 Introduction

Management of shock after trauma remains a clinical challenge, in particular if associated with active hemorrhage [1]. Prevailing dogma precludes the use of vasopressors in shock after trauma until hemorrhage is excluded or controlled and advocates a hypotensive strategy [2]. The use of vasopressors is considered deleterious and associated with a risk of increased bleeding and organ damage due to excessive vasoconstriction. Despite the controversy and discouraged use in hemorrhagic shock, particularly in trauma centers in the United States and the United Kingdom [3], vasopressors are part of the recommended therapeutic arsenal and routinely used by clinicians in Europe to manage trauma patients in shock [4].

Mounting evidence suggests that the effect of vasopressors in shock and hemorrhage after trauma justifies a more nuanced position. A differentiated approach appears indicated, because not all cardio- and vasoactive agents are the same when it comes to their inotropic and vasoconstrictive capacities. Among all agents, norepinephrine and vasopressin have emerged as the molecules of choice if any cardio/vasoactive effect is to be achieved. In this chapter, we attempt to provide a balanced perspective on the use of norepinephrine and vasopressin in traumatic shock and hemorrhage, based on recent physiological, epidemiological, and clinical data.

J. Richards
Department of Anesthesiology, Divisions of Trauma Anesthesiology and Critical Care Medicine, R Adams Cowley Shock Trauma Center, Baltimore, MD, USA

T. Gauss
Department of Anesthesia and Critical Care, Hôpital Beaujon, HUPNVS, AP-HP, Clichy, France

P. Bouzat (✉)
Department of Anesthesia and Critical Care, Grenoble Alps Trauma Centre, Grenoble University Hospital, Grenoble, France
e-mail: PBouzat@chu-grenoble.fr

32.2 Pharmacology

32.2.1 Cardiovascular Effects of Norepinephrine

Norepinephrine is a neurohormone, released from sympathetic, postganglionic nerve fibers. Norepinephrine is a product of the decarboxylation of dopamine, stored in presynaptic granules that release their content into the synaptic space upon depolarization. In the adrenal gland, a methylene group is added, modifying norepinephrine to epinephrine.

After release, norepinephrine acts on postsynaptic alpha- and, to a lesser extent, beta-receptors [5, 6]. The effects on both receptors are dose dependent and with increasing doses the alpha effect dominates. The intracellular signal transmission is G-protein coupled and activates a cAMP-kinase cycle. This results in (1) contraction of smooth muscle fibers in arterial and venous vessels inducing vasoconstriction and (2) myocardial inotropic and chronotropic stimulation [5, 6].

32.2.2 Cardiovascular Effects of Vasopressin

The physiology of vasopressin is complex and beyond the scope of this review; readers are referred to the excellent work by Holmes et al. [7, 8]. Vasopressin is a neuroendocrine nonapeptide, produced in the neurons of the paraventricular and supraoptic nuclei in the posterior hypothalamus. Vasopressin acts on multiple G-protein-coupled receptors and uses the phosphatidylinositol pathway [7] to increase Ca^{2+} influx. Vasopressin 1R (V1R) receptors are densely situated on vascular smooth muscles of the systemic, splanchnic, renal, and coronary circulations; their stimulation leads to potent vasoconstriction [7] and concomitant increase in cardiac output and centralization of blood volume [9]. They are also found on cardiac myocytes and in many other organs, such as liver, brain, and renal medulla. In renal efferent arterioles, this vasoconstriction increases glomerular filtration rate (GFR). In the pulmonary vasculature, vasopressin induces less vasoconstriction than norepinephrine. V1R receptor stimulation on platelets facilitates their aggregation. V2R receptors located in the renal collecting system induce antidiuresis by shuttling aquaporin-2-containing vesicles to the cell surface and stimulation of synthesis of aquaporin-2 mRNA. There is also a complex physiologic interaction of vasopressin on oxytocin and purinergic receptors. Purinergic receptors on cardiac endothelium seem to exert positive inotropic stimulation without concomitant positive chronotropy and increase in oxygen demand [10].

32.2.3 Metabolic and Immunomodulatory Effects of Norepinephrine and Vasopressin

Apart from the hemodynamic manifestations, norepinephrine and vasopressin exert a number of endocrine, metabolic, and immunomodulatory effects. For example, norepinephrine alters the function of most immune cells, reducing the activity of macrophage, T-helper, and natural killer (NK) cells, and up- or downregulates certain cytokines (e.g., interleukin [IL]-6 and -10, tumor necrosis factor [TNF]-α) [11]. A wealth of research indicates that vasopressin appears to have a beneficial effect on the immune system, such as reduction of mRNA of TNF-α, nuclear factor-kappa B (NF-κB), and IL-1β [12]. Norepinephrine increases glycogenolysis and glucose production and modifies lipid metabolism [13]. Via V3R receptors in the pituitary, vasopressin seems to increase adrenocorticotropic secretion and ultimately influences cortisol secretion. The effects of norepinephrine and vasopressin are part of the highly complex immunologic, endocrine, and metabolic response to trauma, shock, and hemorrhage triggering a systemic inflammatory (SIRS) and compensatory anti-inflammatory (CARS) response described as persistent inflammatory and catabolic syndrome (PICS) [14].

32.3 The Physiologic Response to Traumatic Shock and Hemorrhage

The complex physiology of the response to hemorrhage and shock cannot be reduced to a simple loss of blood volume. An intricate and coordinated series of adaptive mechanisms and interactions has emerged in our understanding of the pathophysiology of hemorrhagic shock [15]. On a macrovascular level, the organism responds to shock and hemorrhage with an intense sympathetic stimulation propelled by the peripheral and central nervous systems [16]. This neurohormonal response induces intense vasoconstriction, an increase in heart rate, respiratory drive and venous return, improved coronary perfusion, and cardiac contractility [16, 17]. Combined, these augment, or at least maintain, stroke volume, cardiac output, arterial pressure, and oxygen delivery. Norepinephrine and vasopressin play crucial roles in this response at the peripheral and central levels.

If the initial source of hemorrhage is not quickly controlled, this phase of compensated hypovolemic shock may evolve to a state of vasodilatory shock. Ultimately all shock forms are considered to decompensate to a form of distributive shock [18, 19]. This vasodilatory phase is caused by numerous mechanisms such as xanthine oxidase [20], prostanoids (PG-1, thromboxane), reactive oxygen species (ROS), hydrogen sulfide, and, probably the most important, nitric oxide (NO) and potassium channels [21]. NO is increased by augmented activation of inducible NO synthase (iNOS) acting via cyclic guanosine monophosphate (cGMP) to reduce intracellular calcium and activate calcium-sensitive (Kca) and ATP-dependent K-channels. The subsequent hyperpolarization and decreased influx of calcium [8, 22] demonstrate that the synergy between K-channels and reduced Ca^{2+} influx further exacerbates the hyporesponsiveness to catecholamines and results in profound hypotension. Furthermore, adrenoceptors are desensitized and downregulated [23, 24]. The vasopressin response is also subject to desensitization, receptor internalization, and store depletion [7, 19]. In the decompensation phase, even blood transfusion cannot restore normal intravascular pressures [25].

To understand the process at the microvascular level, it is helpful to consider the endothelium as a whole organ system, with a weight of 1 kg and a surface of 5000 m^2 [26]; the role of the endothelium in health and disease has probably been underestimated and it is the target of a number of pathophysiologic alterations. At the microvascular level, the onset of hemorrhagic shock reflects a myriad of physical, chemical, cellular, and genomic interactions [15]. Some interactions are triggered by the macrovascular response and many prompt the measurable and clinically apparent macrovascular and hemodynamic response. In addition to the above-described neurohormonal response, vascular injuries expose the endothelial surface and cells to lower oxygen concentration and acidosis. Profound rheological changes accompany a modified vascular reactivity depending on the affected regional perfusion. A variety of cytokines and messengers alter endothelial surface reactivity and permeability, including leukocyte and platelet adhesion and activation. Leukocyte activation triggers synthesis of ROS. Activated protein-C initiates coagulopathy that is induced by cleavage of plasminogen activator inhibitor and increases tissue plasminogen activator. Thrombomodulin is released and platelets become dysfunctional. Numerous cytokines circulate and initiate transcription of adhesion molecules and other pro- and anti-inflammatory mediators, modifying further vascular permeability and vessel reactivity and reducing functional capillary density; the endothelial surface swells, increasing O_2 diffusion distance [15].

A body of experimental and clinical evidence points towards the concept of shock-induced endotheliopathy [27] as the central element to the above-described process. The endothelium is covered with a layer of glycosylated proteins (proteoglycans), called the glycocalyx. The interaction between this layer and albumin is now considered as a surrogate for oncotic pressure. In shock, hypoxia, hypotension, acidosis, cytokines, and neurohormones (epinephrine) contribute to the destruction of the glycocalyx, leading to increased vessel permeability and endothelial and end-organ dysfunction. Glycocalyx degradation at the onset of shock/hemorrhage can be quantified by syndecan-1 levels [28, 29]. In trauma patients, syndecan-1 plasma concentration is correlated to the level of injury, mortality, and epinephrine concentration [30].

32.4 Vasopressors in Shock and Hemorrhage in Trauma: Experimental Evidence

Considering experimental and animal data about the effects of norepinephrine and vasopressin in the physiopathology of hemorrhagic shock it seems important to acknowledge two aspects. First, the mechanisms in septic shock are far better investigated and understood and some observations about norepinephrine and vasopressin have been extrapolated from studies on septic shock to hemorrhagic shock [21]. Second, it is crucial to consider the type of animal model used and which aspect of the shock response is studied [31].

It is usually considered that vasopressors increase afterload and oxygen consumption and decrease organ perfusion [32]. It is noteworthy that some of these experimental studies used vasopressors without concomitant fluid expansion. When applied to achieve a systolic blood pressure of 80–90 mmHg, a critical rise in afterload cannot be documented with norepinephrine administration in patients with vasoplegic shock [5]. In fact, both norepinephrine and vasopressin seem to improve coronary perfusion pressure, venous return, and cardiac output and subsequently organ perfusion in shock [8]. Norepinephrine and vasopressin are part of the physiological response to hemorrhage and the mechanisms responsible for the vasodilatory phase of prolonged shock when physiological compensation is exhausted (see above) may require exogenous vasopressor administration as neurohormonal augmentation therapy [33].

Another important argument against norepinephrine and vasopressin use in hemorrhagic shock is the danger of intensifying bleeding from noncontrolled sources by increasing hydrostatic pressure ("pop the clot"), the rationale behind permissive hypotension. However, recent evidence indicates that even with fluid-only resuscitation, profound and prolonged hypotension is associated with increased end-organ damage. In a model of controlled hemorrhage and shock of 30% blood loss after blast injury, pigs were randomized to two systolic blood pressure levels, 110 mmHg and 80 mmHg, resuscitated with fluids only [34]. Survival was shorter in the 80 mmHg group associated with important metabolic derangement. This finding was confirmed in another pig model of uncontrolled hemorrhagic shock comparing three mean arterial pressure (MAP) levels of 60, 80, and 100 mmHg obtained with fluid resuscitation alone [35]. Both the 60 and 100 mmHg groups demonstrated more organ dysfunction and histopathological damage.

Several studies have explored the effect of norepinephrine or vasopressin use in animal shock models. In a model of hemorrhagic shock in rodents, the use of norepinephrine with fluid expansion was associated with higher survival [36]. In a rat model of shock, Poloujadoff et al. demonstrated that MAP-targeted resuscitation associating norepinephrine and fluids proved beneficial in terms of survival [37]. Liu et al. successfully tested a combination of norepinephrine and vasopressin and fluids in rats to maintain perfusion pressure until definitive hemorrhage control [38]. These studies have in common that the investigating groups used both vasopressor therapy and fluid expansion. Furthermore, administration of norepinephrine or vasopressin does not necessarily induce end-organ damage in shock models; the effects are organ-, dose-, and time-dependent [7, 34, 35]. In fact, Harrois et al. demonstrated protection of intestinal villi in hemorrhage in mice [39]. Dunberry-Poissant et al. revealed no difference comparing various parameters of organ damage after fluid resuscitation versus fluid and norepinephrine in a controlled rat shock model during resuscitation to MAP levels of 55–60 mmHg and after reperfusion [20]. The administration of norepinephrine in this model was associated with a considerably reduced volume of fluid administration.

Of note, different resuscitation strategies (fluid only versus norepinephrine/vasopressin plus fluid) and varying pressure levels at different times affect organs differently [7, 20, 34, 35]. For example, a MAP of 100 mmHg caused more organ damage in the lungs than in the liver and kidney compared to a pressure level of 60 mmHg [7, 20, 34, 35].

The topic becomes more complicated with regard to vasopressor effects on the endothelial surface and glycocalyx. There seems to be an undeniable association between circulating endogenous epinephrine, endothelial damage, and mortality in animals and patients [27]. Sympathectomy appears to protect against this phenomenon in an animal model [40]. In fact, recently, in a controlled hemorrhagic shock model in rats, there was raised capillary permeability in the lung and higher lactate and base excess in the group resuscitated with fluids and vasopressin compared to groups resuscitated with fluids only and those resuscitated with fluids and blood.

In summary, this wealth of experimental knowledge and observations can be interpreted in favor of or against the use of norepinephrine (Table 32.1) and vasopressin (Table 32.2) in shock and hemorrhage after trauma. The complexity of the adaptive physiological and pathophysiologic patterns demonstrates that the potential beneficial or detrimental effects of both agents are not reduced to macrohemodynamic effects and are part of the physiological response to injury.

Table 32.1 Risks and benefits of norepinephrine

	Risk	Benefit
Physiologic	• Increased oxygen consumption • Increased right ventricular and left ventricular afterload, when mean arterial pressure in excess • Decreased regional perfusion due to excessive vasoconstrictive effects • Immunosuppression	• Augments venous return and increases central systemic vascular compartment volume • Increases coronary artery perfusion • Supports cardiac contractility
Clinical	• Retrospective studies, conflicting data for in-hospital mortality [45–47]	• No prospective evidence available to support clinical use compared to standard care

Table 32.2 Risks and benefits of vasopressin

	Risk	Benefit
Physiologic	• Increased visceral ischemia due to splanchnic vasoconstriction and translocation of intestinal bacteria • Exacerbates cerebral edema • Coronary ischemia due to vasoconstriction	• Activates V1 receptors and counteracts nitric oxide synthesis, thereby increasing vascular tone • Augments renal perfusion by vasoconstriction of renal efferent arterioles • Promotes von Willebrand factor release from endothelium, platelet activation, and thrombin generation • Regulates intravascular volume resorption via V2 receptors in collecting tubules • Immunostimulation
Clinical	• Expensive • Lack of significant mortality benefit in prospective studies [48]	• Decreased transfusion requirements (blood product and overall volume) [48] • No excess mortality in prospective study

32.5 Clinical Evidence of Permissive Hypotension and Vasopressor Use

One of the hallmark pathophysiologic signs of advanced hemorrhagic shock is hypotension. Hypotension is a time-sensitive and dose-dependent event such that the following questions remain: "How much hypotension is acceptable in a trauma patient?" "And for how long?" Unfortunately, the answers to these questions remain elusive. Despite traumatic mechanisms of injury typically occurring in younger patients with few medical comorbidities, hypotension is significantly associated with increased mortality. In addition, there is a growing population of older patients with comorbidities, such as hypertension and peripheral vascular disease, who are sustaining traumatic injuries. Does all traumatic hemorrhagic shock require the same approach to hemodynamic resuscitation? And do the same hypotensive thresholds apply across all trauma patients? The seemingly obvious answer would be no. However, while few data are available on the duration of hypotension in critically injured trauma patients, there is substantial evidence in the perioperative and critical care literature to support that longer periods, and even single episodes, of hypotension are associated with organ dysfunction and increased mortality [41]. Yet, as previously discussed, there is a pervasive opinion especially among certain trauma providers that hypotension is potentially beneficial in trauma patients and should be acceptable, especially early in the resuscitation phase following hemorrhage.

The topic of hypotensive resuscitation and permissive hypotension in resuscitation from traumatic hemorrhagic shock has been formulated over the last three decades. While early resuscitation strategies emphasized volume replacement with isotonic crystalloid formulations, Bickell et al. [42] demonstrated in a swine model of vascular injury that initial large volumes of crystalloid administration led to decreased animal survival. In a subsequent prospective, randomized trial of immediate versus delayed fluid resuscitation in hypotensive patients who sustained penetrating traumatic injuries, those who received less prehospital crystalloid (mean volume of 92 ml compared to 870 ml) had greater rates of survival [43]. However, the difference in systolic blood pressure upon arrival to the trauma center was clinically negligible (72 mmHg vs. 79 mmHg, respectively), albeit statistically significant. In recent years, attempts to replicate such findings and support tolerating a lower blood pressure during initial trauma resuscitation have failed to demonstrate an improvement in mortality [44]. Unfortunately, the enthusiasm and support for hypotensive resuscitation, and admonishment for the use of vasopressors, are extrapolated primarily from a clinical study in which a blood pressure target was not the primary outcome nor was the systolic blood pressure clinically different among treatment groups. Therefore, it should be clarified that minimizing excessive volumes of crystalloid, or overall excessive volume in general, does not equate to accepting a lower blood pressure in a bleeding patient.

Blood volume replacement remains the initial primary method of resuscitation from hemorrhagic shock. Recent publications in blood component administration and reinvigoration of whole blood therapy have advanced the science of hemorrhagic shock resuscitation towards a cell-based approach that minimizes excess crystalloid administration and emphasizes restoration of the endothelial glycocalyx [27]. As previously discussed, disruption and damage to the endothelium lining the inner vasculature lumen result in release of anticoagulant molecules that contribute to the trauma-induced coagulopathy and exacerbate acute blood loss. In addition, endothelial dysfunction is characterized by a release of iNO with subsequent vascular hyporesponsiveness, vasoplegia, and loss of vascular tone [21]. Patients with severe and profound hemorrhagic shock may continue to demonstrate hypotension despite replacement of adequate blood volume. In a cyclical fashion, this very hypotension and continued hypoperfusion lead to further endothelial dysfunction and further hypotension unresponsive to volume resuscitation. It would therefore seem logical that administration of vasopressor therapy and restoration of vascular tone would serve a valuable function in such patients.

While there is no level 1 clinical evidence to suggest that early administration of vasopressors or vasopressor use in the initial resuscitation of traumatic hemorrhagic shock results in worse outcomes, evidence from some retrospective studies is conflicting. Some studies suggest that vasopressors are associated with increased in-hospital mortality. Sperry et al. reported that early vasopressor use (i.e., phenylephrine, norepinephrine, or vasopressin), within 12 h of injury, was associated with mortality even after adjusting for volume of crystalloid resuscitation [45]. Of note, patients who survived <48 h were excluded, when in fact it is this very population of patients with early mortality as a result of hemorrhage that are of significant interest with regard to vasopressor therapy (i.e., patients who failed to respond to initial resuscitation efforts as a result of profound shock with subsequent vasoplegia may have been salvageable with vasopressor therapy). Dose and duration of vasopressor use were also not reported and the study excluded patients with traumatic brain injury (TBI) or a spinal cord injury, which represents a population that may also be well served by augmented systemic blood pressure and vasopressor therapy. More recent work by Aoki et al. from the Japan Trauma Databank demonstrated that in a propensity-matched cohort, vasopressor use within 24 h of hospital admission was associated with in-hospital mortality [46]. However, there was no difference in emergency department mortality among patients who received early vasopressor treatment. A limitation of this large investigation was that the type of vasopressor, dose, and duration of treatment were unavailable from the trauma databank.

In contrast, there is emerging evidence to suggest that specific vasopressors (i.e., norepinephrine or vasopressin) are not associated with increased mortality in hemorrhagic shock. Gauss et al. performed a retrospective analysis of patients in hemorrhagic shock (defined as patients receiving 4 units of red blood cells [RBCs] within the first 6 h of hospital admission) and after propensity score matching observed that early norepinephrine administration was not associated with in-hospital mortality [47]. A recently published prospective, randomized trial from a single center in the United States has also provided valuable evidence in support of early vasopressor treatment in patients with hemorrhagic shock. The Arginine Vasopressin During the Early Resuscitation of Traumatic Shock (AVERT Shock) [48] trial randomized patients receiving at least 6 units of blood products (packed RBCs, fresh frozen plasma [FFP], and platelets) within 12 h of injury to an intervention that consisted of a bolus of 4 units of vasopressin and then continuous infusion up to 0.04 units/min to achieve a MAP of 65 mmHg versus standard component-based resuscitation. Efforts to achieve hemostatic resuscitation were performed in each study arm and the intervention was continued for 48 h. Patients in the vasopressin group required less total volume of blood products and crystalloid with no overall difference in complication rates, such as acute kidney injury (AKI), acute respiratory distress syndrome (ARDS), prolonged mechanical ventilation, or mortality. These results provide some of the most encouraging clinical evidences that specific vasopressor therapy may potentially be considered as part of the initial resuscitation of trauma patients in hemorrhagic shock (Fig. 32.1).

Possible explanations for the utility of vasopressors in hemorrhagic shock resuscitation are the restoration of an adequate perfusing blood pressure in order to maintain vital organ function. Our current understanding of aggressive volume administration, even in the form of blood products, is known to be associated with increased complications such as dilutional coagulopathy, lung injury, and cardiac overload. Therefore, it may be hypothesized that early initiation of vasopressors, in conjunction with appropriate volume administration and correction of coagulation derangements, will reduce overall total resuscitation volumes (both blood products and crystalloid) and minimize post-resuscitation

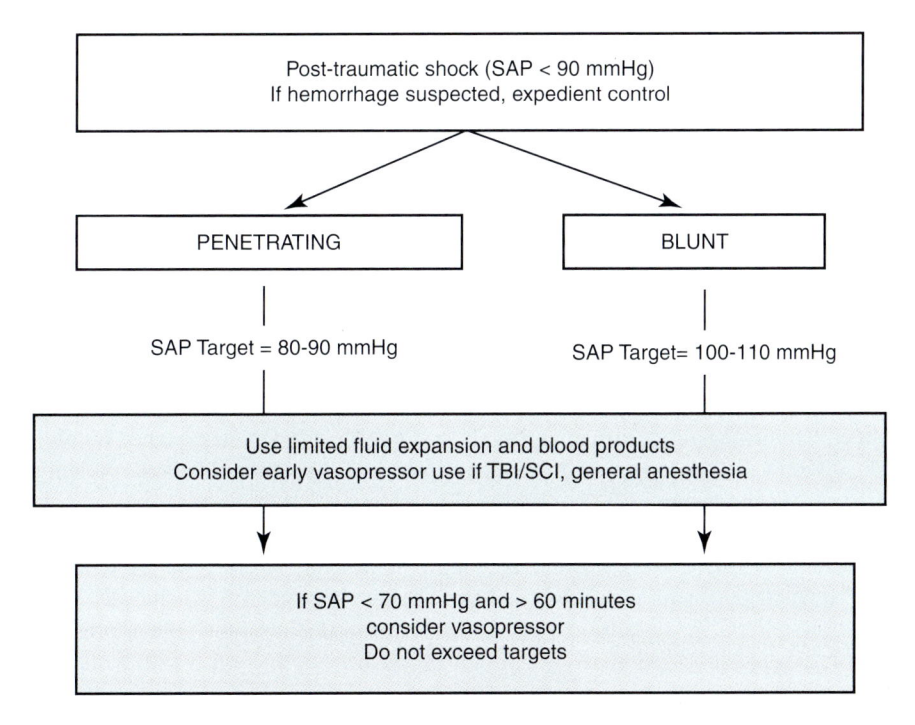

Fig. 32.1 Suggested practical algorithm for vasopressor use after severe trauma. *SAP* systolic arterial blood pressure, *TBI* traumatic brain injury, *SCI* spinal cord injury

complications. Intrinsic pharmacologic properties of specific vasopressors may target pathophysiologic processes involved in hemorrhagic shock. For example, as previously described, norepinephrine exerts alpha-1 sympathomimetic activity that would be of benefit to a severely injured trauma patient in profound hemorrhagic shock with vasoplegia [37]. Intrinsic beta-1 activity would also augment cardiac contractility and improve oxygen delivery to hypoperfused organs [5, 6]. It is also well described that severely injured and critically ill trauma patients present with endocrine insufficiency, to which vasopressin deficiency may significantly contribute [48]. Administration of exogenous vasopressin may therefore restore components of endothelial integrity, intravascular volume, and platelet function. However, it cannot be overstated that inappropriate use of vasopressors in hemorrhagic shock can result in severe deleterious consequences.

32.6 A Practical Approach to Vasopressor Use for an Updated Resuscitation Strategy

From the prehospital environment to the intensive care unit (ICU), hemorrhaging trauma patients progress through different phases of shock, defined by the complex physiologic response and the therapeutic strategy. Prohibiting vasopressor use within the first 24 h in patients with shock and hemorrhage may considerably limit the therapeutic arsenal to adapt and shift the response as needed. As exposed in the preceding sections, the available experimental and clinical evidence is insufficient to preclude in principle the use of norepinephrine or vasopressin in the initial 24-h management.

Based on these data, it seems obvious that vasopressor use can only be considered after a fluid challenge, probably between 500 and 1000 ml, fails to achieve hemodynamic stabilization, as recommended. If fluid fails, it is likely that the patient is decompensating into the distributive phase of shock and fluid and blood alone will not be able to prevent further clinical deterioration; vasopressors may be required to prevent prolonged hypotension, associated with an increase in organ damage. Many mature trauma systems manage to increase survival of very critically sick and severely bleeding patients, but even the most efficient systems struggle to obtain hemorrhage control within 1 h [1] and transport times may exceed 60 min. Yet, it seems that the longer the hypotensive phase lasts, the more likely the patient's risks of organ damage [34]. As much as it is obvious that permissive hypotension should remain a central element of the damage control strategy to limit blood loss, in particular in penetrating trauma, there is an increasingly strong rationale to maintain adequate perfusion pressure even before hemorrhage control is achieved. If the duration of hypotension is too long (>60) or too profound (systolic arterial pressure <60 mmHg), hemodynamic resuscitation may be difficult to control with fluids and blood products only. This constellation is frequently observed in the distributive, decompensated phase of shock and more so in blunt trauma and often associated with a sympatholytic component, such as the required use of induction agents, sedation/anesthesia, brain, or medullary injury. Shock in trauma patients cannot be reduced to bleeding, with bleeding being the main rationale behind the strategy of permissive hypotension. Yet all forms of shock require the restoration of adequate perfusion.

It is true that the definition of adequate perfusion remains a challenge. However, an increase in global trauma mortality has been described for arterial systolic blood pressure lower than 110 mmHg after severe trauma [49]. Recent guidelines from the Trauma Hemostasis and Oxygenation Research Network also highlight this point, raising the systolic arterial blood pressure target from 80–90 to 100 mmHg [49]. These pressure levels cannot be obtained with fluid expansion and blood products only in patients with profound and prolonged traumatic shock. Large volumes of fluid resuscitation are in fact quite harmful. The use of vasopressors becomes mandatory to reach these hemodynamic goals. Higher targets seem crucial, particularly in patients with associate traumatic brain or medullary injury and multisystem trauma [50], to control cerebral and medullary perfusion pressure.

For these reasons, the authors share the assumption that norepinephrine and vasopressin have a place in the therapeutic arsenal to treat trauma patients in shock, including those with active hemorrhage (Fig. 32.1). Both agents should be part of a bridging strategy to maintain tissue perfusion if hypotension is too long or too profound. In no case however should this strategy become a substitute for expedient hemorrhage control. Furthermore, the pressure levels targeted with norepinephrine/vasopressin use require a reasonable trade-off between tissue perfusion and overcorrection, which may increase bleeding by increasing the hydrostatic pressure.

32.7 Conclusion

Traumatic hemorrhagic shock is a complex disease process that incorporates a dynamic physiologic response to blood loss and tissue injury. While restoration of circulating blood volume is the mainstay of initial treatment of hemorrhagic shock, maintenance of adequate perfusion pressure is essential in order to minimize organ dysfunction. While historically it has been advocated to treat hemorrhagic shock with aggressive blood product transfusion and the use of vasopressors is discouraged, severe injury with profound shock and prolonged hypotension will decompensate to a distributive form of vasoplegia that is unresponsive to further volume administration. Therefore, it appears intuitive that appropriate and targeted use of specific vasopressors has a beneficial contribution to the management of early hemorrhagic shock. We advocate that specific, targeted vasopressor therapy has an integral and necessary role in the early resuscitation of traumatic hemorrhagic shock and that further large-scale scientific and clinical research will more clearly define vasopressor administration in patients with hemorrhagic shock.

References

1. Alarhayem AQ, Myers JG, Dent D, et al. Time is the enemy: mortality in trauma patients with hemorrhage from torso injury occurs long before the "golden hour". Am J Surg. 2016;212:1101–5.
2. Nevin DG, Brohi K. Permissive hypotension for active haemorrhage in trauma. Anaesthesia. 2017;72:1443–8.
3. Gupta B, Garg N, Ramachandran R. Vasopressors: do they have any role in hemorrhagic shock? J Anaesthesiol Clin Pharmacol. 2017;33:3–8.
4. Rossaint R, Bouillon B, Cerny V, et al. The European guideline on management of major bleeding and coagulopathy following trauma: fourth edition. Crit Care. 2016;20:100.
5. Hamzaoui O, Jozwiak M, Geffriaud T, et al. Norepinephrine exerts an inotropic effect during the early phase of human septic shock. Br J Anaesth. 2018;120:517–24.
6. De Backer D, Pinsky M. Norepinephrine improves cardiac function during septic shock, but why? Br J Anaesth. 2018;120:421–4.
7. Holmes CL, Landry DW, Granton JT. Science review: vasopressin and the cardiovascular system part 1 – receptor physiology. Crit Care. 2003;7:427–34.
8. Holmes CL, Landry DW, Granton JT. Science review: vasopressin and the cardiovascular system part 2 - clinical physiology. Crit Care. 2004;8:15–23.
9. Bown LS, Ricksten SE, Houltz E, et al. Vasopressin-induced changes in splanchnic blood flow and hepatic and portal venous pressures in liver resection. Acta Anaesthesiol Scand. 2016;60:607–15.
10. Mei Q, Liang BT. P2 purinergic receptor activation enhances cardiac contractility in isolated rat and mouse hearts. Am J Physiol Heart Circ Physiol. 2001;281:H334–41.
11. Stolk RF, van der Poll T, Angus DC, et al. Potentially inadvertent immunomodulation: norepinephrine use in sepsis. Am J Respir Crit Care Med. 2016;194:550–8.
12. Russell JA, Walley KR. Vasopressin and its immune effects in septic shock. J Innate Immun. 2010;2:446–60.
13. Ensinger H, Geisser W, Brinkmann A, et al. Metabolic effects of norepinephrine and dobutamine in healthy volunteers. Shock. 2002;18:495–500.
14. Lord JM, Midwinter MJ, Chen YF, et al. The systemic immune response to trauma: an overview of pathophysiology and treatment. Lancet. 2014;384:1455–65.
15. Torres Filho IP, Torres LN, Salgado C, Dubick MA. Novel adjunct drugs reverse endothelial glycocalyx damage after hemorrhagic shock in rats. Shock. 2017;48:583–9.
16. Schadt JC, Ludbrook J. Hemodynamic and neurohumoral responses to acute hypovolemia in conscious mammals. Am J Phys. 1991;260(2 Pt 2):H305–18.
17. Hamzaoui O, Georger JF, Monnet X, et al. Early administration of norepinephrine increases cardiac preload and cardiac output in septic patients with life-threatening hypotension. Crit Care. 2010;14:R142.
18. Barrett LK, Singer M, Clapp LH. Vasopressin: mechanisms of action on the vasculature in health and in septic shock. Crit Care Med. 2007;35:33–40.
19. Landry DW, Oliver JA. The pathogenesis of vasodilatory shock. N Engl J Med. 2001;345:588–95.
20. Dunberry-Poissant S, Gilbert K, Bouchard C, et al. Fluid sparing and norepinephrine use in a rat model of resuscitated haemorrhagic shock: end-organ impact. Intensive Care Med Exp. 2018;6:47.
21. Lambden S, Creagh-Brown BC, Hunt J, Summers C, Forni LG. Definitions and pathophysiology of vasoplegic shock. Crit Care. 2018;22:174.
22. Quayle JM, Nelson MT, Standen NB. ATP-sensitive and inwardly rectifying potassium channels in smooth muscle. Physiol Rev. 1997;77:1165–232.
23. Hotchkiss RS, Karl IE. The pathophysiology and treatment of sepsis. N Engl J Med. 2003;348:138–50.

24. Saito T, Takanashi M, Gallagher E, et al. Corticosteroid effect on early beta-adrenergic down-regulation during circulatory shock: hemodynamic study and beta-adrenergic receptor assay. Intensive Care Med. 1995;21:204–10.
25. Dalibon N, Schlumberger S, Saada M, Fischler M, Riou B. Haemodynamic assessment of hypovolaemia under general anaesthesia in pigs submitted to graded haemorrhage and retransfusion. Br J Anaesth. 1999;82:97–103.
26. Aird WC. Endothelium in health and disease. Pharmacol Rep. 2008;60:139–43.
27. Johansson PI, Stensballe J, Ostrowski SR. Shock induced endotheliopathy (SHINE) in acute critical illness - a unifying pathophysiologic mechanism. Crit Care. 2017;21:25.
28. Haywood-Watson RJ, Holcomb JB, Gonzalez EA, et al. Modulation of syndecan-1 shedding after hemorrhagic shock and resuscitation. PLoS One. 2011;e23530:6.
29. Ostrowski SR, Henriksen HH, Stensballe J, et al. Sympathoadrenal activation and endotheliopathy are drivers of hypocoagulability and hyperfibrinolysis in trauma: a prospective observational study of 404 severely injured patients. J Trauma Acute Care Surg. 2017;82:293–301.
30. Johansson PI, Henriksen HH, Stensballe J, et al. Traumatic endotheliopathy: a prospective observational study of 424 severely injured patients. Ann Surg. 2017;265:597–603.
31. Tremoleda JL, Watts SA, Reynolds PS, Thiemermann C, Brohi K. Modeling acute traumatic hemorrhagic shock injury: challenges and guidelines for preclinical studies. Shock. 2017;48:610–23.
32. Beloncle F, Meziani F, Lerolle N, Radermacher P, Asfar P. Does vasopressor therapy have an indication in hemorrhagic shock? Ann Intensive Care. 2013;3:13.
33. Myburgh J. Norepinephrine: more of a neurohormone than a vasopressor. Crit Care. 2010;14:196.
34. Garner J, Watts S, Parry C, Bird J, Cooper G, Kirkman E. Prolonged permissive hypotensive resuscitation is associated with poor outcome in primary blast injury with controlled hemorrhage. Ann Surg. 2010;251:1131–9.
35. Bai X, Yu W, Ji W, Duan K, Tan S, Lin Z, et al. Resuscitation strategies with different arterial pressure targets after surgical management of traumatic shock. Crit Care. 2015;19:170.
36. Lee JH, Kim K, Jo YH, Kim KS, et al. Early norepinephrine infusion delays cardiac arrest after hemorrhagic shock in rats. J Emerg Med. 2009;37:376–82.
37. Poloujadoff MP, Borron SW, Amathieu R, et al. Improved survival after resuscitation with norepinephrine in a murine model of uncontrolled hemorrhagic shock. Anesthesiology. 2007;107:591–6.
38. Liu L, Tian K, Xue M, et al. Small doses of arginine vasopressin in combination with norepinephrine "buy" time for definitive treatment for uncontrolled hemorrhagic shock in rats. Shock. 2013;40:398–406.
39. Harrois A, Baudry N, Huet O, et al. Norepinephrine decreases fluid requirements and blood loss while preserving intestinal villi microcirculation during fluid resuscitation of uncontrolled hemorrhagic shock in mice. Anesthesiology. 2015;122:1093–102.
40. Xu L, Yu WK, Lin ZL, et al. Chemical sympathectomy attenuates inflammation, glycocalyx shedding and coagulation disorders in rats with acute traumatic coagulopathy. Blood Coagul Fibrinolysis. 2015;26:152–60.
41. Wesselink EM, Kappen TH, Torn HM, Slooter AJC, van Klei WA. Intraoperative hypotension and the risk of postoperative adverse outcomes: a systematic review. Br J Anaesth. 2018;121:706–21.
42. Bickell WH, Bruttig SP, Millnamow GA, O'Benar J, Wade CE. The detrimental effects of intravenous crystalloid after aortotomy in swine. Surgery. 1991;110:529–36.
43. Bickell WH, Wall MJ Jr, Pepe PE, et al. Immediate versus delayed fluid resuscitation for hypotensive patients with penetrating torso injuries. N Engl J Med. 1994;331:1105–9.
44. Carrick MM, Morrison CA, Tapia NM, et al. Intraoperative hypotensive resuscitation for patients undergoing laparotomy or thoracotomy for trauma: early termination of a randomized prospective clinical trial. J Trauma Acute Care Surg. 2016;80:886–96.

45. Sperry JL, Minei JP, Frankel HL, et al. Early use of vasopressors after injury: caution before constriction. J Trauma. 2008;64:9–14.
46. Aoki M, Abe T, Saitoh D, Hagiwara S, Oshima K. Use of vasopressor increases the risk of mortality in traumatic hemorrhagic shock: a nationwide cohort study in Japan. Crit Care Med. 2018;46:e1145–e51.
47. Gauss T, Gayat E, Harrois A, et al. Effect of early use of noradrenaline on in-hospital mortality in haemorrhagic shock after major trauma: a propensity-score analysis. Br J Anaesth. 2018;120:1237–44.
48. Sims CA, Holena D, Kim P, et al. Effect of low-dose supplementation of arginine vasopressin on need for blood product transfusions in patients with trauma and hemorrhagic shock: a randomized clinical trial. JAMA Surg. 2019. Aug 28. https://doi.org/10.1001/jamasurg.2019.2884. [Epub ahead of print].
49. Woolley T, Thompson P, Kirkman E, et al. Trauma Hemostasis and Oxygenation Research Network position paper on the role of hypotensive resuscitation as part of remote damage control resuscitation. J Trauma Acute Care Surg. 2018;84:S3–S13.
50. Spaite DW, Hu C, Bobrow BJ, et al. Association of out-of-hospital hypotension depth and duration with traumatic brain injury mortality. Ann Emerg Med. 2017;70:522–30.

Extracranial Tsunami After Traumatic Brain Injury

G. Bonatti, C. Robba, and G. Citerio

33.1 Introduction

Traumatic brain injury (TBI) is a leading cause of death and disability, with an incidence of more than 50 million people each year [1]. However, TBI is often accompanied by extracranial lesions and, later, by extracranial complications that might influence the outcome.

The presence of major extracranial injuries in a large cohort of TBI from the CRASH trial was associated with increased early mortality (odds ratio 1.53–1.15, respectively, in high/low-middle-income countries) and death or severe disability (odds ratio 1.62–1.73) at 6 months [2]. In a meta-analysis including more than 39,000 patients, extracranial injuries with an Abbreviated Injury Score (AIS) ≥3 adjusted for age, Glasgow Coma Score (GCS) motor, and pupillary reactivity were related to increased mortality [3]. The strength of the effect was greater in less severe TBI (2.14 in mild, 1.46 in moderate, and 1.18 in severe TBI). In high-income countries, we are currently facing a decrease in severe, traffic-related TBI and an increase in fall-related TBI [1]. Older patients might initially be less severe but,

---

G. Bonatti
Department of Surgical Sciences and Integrated Diagnostics, University of Genoa, Genoa, Italy

Anaesthesia and Intensive Care, Policlinico San Martino Hospital, IRCCS for Oncology and Neuroscience, Genoa, Italy

C. Robba
Anaesthesia and Intensive Care, Policlinico San Martino Hospital, IRCCS for Oncology and Neuroscience, Genoa, Italy

G. Citerio (✉)
School of Medicine and Surgery, University Milano Bicocca, Milan, Italy

Neurointensive Care Unit, San Gerardo Hospital, ASST-Monza, Monza, Italy
e-mail: giuseppe.citerio@unimib.it

during the intensive care unit (ICU) stay, are more prone to extracranial complications, such as pneumonia, sepsis, or multiple organ dysfunction syndromes. These complications have been described as the leading causes of late morbidity and mortality in TBI [4].

In this chapter, we review the prevalence, pathophysiological basis, and features of extracranial complications after TBI.

33.2 Respiratory Complications

Respiratory failure is the most common non-neurological complication after TBI [4, 5]. ICU stay is significantly increased in these patients, but mortality seems not to be affected [5] (Table. 33.1).

33.2.1 Brain-Lung Interaction

Brain-lung interaction has been widely investigated in the experimental setting. In a pig model, Heuer et al. proved that extreme acute intracranial hypertension induced lung injury in healthy lungs [6]. The mechanism of lung damage after acute brain injury is described through a "double-hit model": the systemic spread of inflammatory mediators and catecholamine release—first hit—creates a systemic inflammatory environment responsible for the activation of biological mechanisms that make the lung more vulnerable to insults, such as the increase in vascular hydrostatic pressures—second hit [7]. Several respiratory complications have been described after TBI including neurogenic pulmonary edema, respiratory tract infections, acute respiratory distress syndrome (ARDS), ventilator-induced lung injury (VILI), and aspiration pneumonia.

33.2.2 Neurogenic Pulmonary Edema

Up to 20% of patients with TBI develop neurogenic pulmonary edema [8]. Neurogenic pulmonary edema is described as an intra-alveolar accumulation of proteinaceous fluid and hemorrhage, along with perivascular interstitial fluid, not explained by cardiovascular or pulmonary causes.

The exact mechanisms involved in the development of neurogenic pulmonary edema are not clear [8]. Some authors have described a neurocardiac model: TBI and raised intracranial pressure (ICP) can increase sympathetic outflow and catecholamine excess causing subendocardial ischemia, myocyte death, and cardiac dysfunction. These mechanisms could lead to elevated pulmonary artery occlusion pressures and true cardiogenic pulmonary edema. The neuro-hemodynamic model describes hydrostatic pulmonary edema with a rapid fall in aortic compliance and subsequent increase in sympathetic outflow and left ventricular failure.

The "blast theory" proposes that the hydrostatic forces occur synergistically with a direct pulmonary endothelial injury mediated by dramatic and transient surges in

Table 33.1 Overview of extracranial complications

	Incidence	Clinical features	Management	Outcome
	23–67% [33–35]	NPE Hypoxia and ARDS Infections VAP Aspiration pneumonia	Fluid balance Protective ventilation (V_T 7 ml/kg, PEEP 6–8 mmHg) $PaCO_2$ target: 36–40 mmHg (with normal ICP) Antibiotics	↓ Neurological function ↑ ICU LOS [5, 33, 36]
	0–50% [33, 37–39]	Hemodynamic instability EKG changes Stress cardiomyopathy Conduction abnormalities Dysautonomia	Early cardiac assessment (e.g., EKG, echocardiography) Advanced cardiac monitoring (e.g., CO, GEDI, SVV, PPV, SVRI) Fluids Vasopressors Blood transfusions β-Blockers	↑ Secondary brain injury ↑ Mortality [18–20, 23]
	0–2% [25, 26]	Acute kidney injury Chronic kidney disease Electrolyte disturbances (i.e., ↓ and ↑ NA^+)	Avoid/correct hemodynamic instability Fluid balance ↓ Nephrotoxic agents (i.e., colloids, antibiotics, contrast media, NSAIDs) RRT in selected cases	↓ Good outcome ↑ ICU LOS ↑ Mortality [25, 29]
	49% (↑ ALT) [30]	Liver failure Peptic ulceration Hypermetabolic status	Avoid hypotension ↓ Hepatotoxic drugs (i.e., acetaminophen, antiepileptics, antibiotics) Prefer propofol for sedation and fentanyl or hydromorphone for analgesia N-acetylcysteine	Impaired immunological function [30]
	10–97% [33]	Trauma-induced coagulopathy Thromboembolic disease	Frequent coagulation monitoring (routine lab or viscoelastic test) Fresh frozen plasma/platelets Tranexamic acid Thromboembolic prophylaxis	↑ ICU LOS ↑ Mortality [31, 33]

ALT alanine aminotransferase, *ARDS* acute respiratory distress syndrome, *CO* cardiac output, *GEDI* global end-diastolic volume index, *ICU* intensive care unit, *LOS* length of stay, *NPE* neurogenic pulmonary edema, *NSAID* nonsteroidal anti-inflammatory drugs, *PEEP* positive end-expiratory pressure, *PPV* pulse pressure variation, *RRT* renal replacement therapy, *SIRS* systemic inflammatory response syndrome, *SVRI* systemic vascular resistance index, *SVV* stroke volume variation, *VAP* ventilator-associated pneumonia, V_T tidal volume pulmonary arterial pressures related to the sympathetic storm experienced at the time of significant TBI or raised ICP. Other authors explain neurogenic pulmonary edema through a mechanism of pulmonary venule adrenergic hypersensitivity: it has been hypothesized that the excess catecholamines directly stimulate α- and β-adrenergic receptors in the pulmonary circulation causing vascular injury.

Patients with neurogenic pulmonary edema manifest clinical signs of oxygenation failure, crackles and rales on auscultation, and pulmonary edema with bilateral diffuse alveolar infiltrates on chest radiograph. The treatment of neurogenic pulmonary edema, along with hemodynamic optimization, includes the application of positive end-expiratory pressure (PEEP) to guarantee adequate oxygenation [8].

33.2.3 Hypoxia and Hypercapnia

Hypoxia is known to cause adverse outcomes in patients with TBI. Early hypoxia is strongly associated with a poorer outcome (odds ratios of 2.1) and the addition of hypotension induces poorer outcomes than either insult alone [9]. Volpi et al. observed in 967 patients with TBI that hypoxia was associated with an unfavorable outcome when it was manifest in both pre- and in-hospital phases, but also when it was resolved at hospital admission [10].

After an acute brain injury, patients are at high risk of developing ARDS. In addition to major ARDS risk factors (aspiration, pneumonia, and lung contusion), therapeutic approach, including positive fluid balance, blood products and vasopressors, may also contribute to the development of ARDS in patients with acute brain injury [7]. The CENTER-TBI researchers, in a pre-study survey, declared that they aimed for a supernormal PaO_2, with an initial arterial oxygen saturation goal of >95% [11]. However, caution is needed in exposing patients to hyperoxia even though all the studies did not demonstrate a link between hyperoxia and negative long-term outcomes [12].

Carbon dioxide levels directly control cerebral blood vessels and have immediate effects on ICP. Ventilator management is challenging in patients with TBI and the literature is not clear regarding the best strategy to adopt in this group of patients. The fear of hypercapnia in TBI patients led clinicians in a dated study to set high tidal volumes [13], which might cause VILI. Appropriate use of lung-protective ventilation (tidal volume 7 ml/kg), optimal PEEP (6–8 mmHg), oxygen titration, and neuromuscular blocking agents reduced days of mechanical ventilation and mortality in patients with acute brain injury [14]. Clinicians, in the absence of raised ICP, target a $PaCO_2$ of 36–40 mmHg and move to lower $PaCO_2$ values (30–35 mmHg) only when ICP is increased [11].

33.2.4 Ventilator-Associated Pneumonia

Ventilator-associated pneumonia (VAP) is a frequent nosocomial infection in ICU patients admitted for TBI, with an incidence of up to 61% [15]. A recent meta-analysis indicated a VAP incidence of 36%, identifying smoking, blood transfusion on admission, barbiturate infusion, and injury severity score as risk factors. VAP prolonged mechanical ventilation time and ICU/hospital length of stay without increasing the risk of mortality [16].

A preliminary analysis of the CENTER-TBI cohort, a large, prospective, observational, multicenter, longitudinal cohort study on TBI [17], evaluated the incidence of VAP. In 962 patients mechanically ventilated for >48 h and with an ICU length of stay >72 h, 20.4% developed VAP at a median time of 5 days from intubation. Patients developing VAP were younger, with a higher incidence of alcohol and drug abuse and thoracic trauma and less prophylactic antibiotic use. This new evidence confirms that patients developing VAP had no increased mortality or worse neurological outcome but only an increased hospital length of stay.

33.3 Cardiac Dysfunction

Cardiac dysfunction consequent to TBI contributes to increased morbidity and mortality [18, 19]. Indeed, cardiac dysfunction can contribute to cerebral hypoperfusion and secondary injury after TBI [20].

The catecholamine surge following TBI causes peripheral vessel vasoconstriction and, subsequently, increase in systemic arterial pressure (neurogenic hypertension). Therefore, early hemodynamic instability, including hypotension and hypertension, is common in patients after severe TBI. Recent studies have suggested that this hemodynamic profile is related to myocardial dysfunction. Although early treatment of hypotension in TBI patients has been suggested by international TBI guidelines [21], no studies have assessed cardiac status before using hemodynamic-controlling drugs following TBI.

33.3.1 Electrocardiogram Changes

In TBI, up to 73% of patients have electrocardiogram (EKG) changes. Studies have demonstrated that EKG alterations correlate with the severity of TBI and are related to worse outcomes. The EKG changes can appear without known atherosclerotic coronary artery disease and could be associated with elevated cardiac biomarkers. As with echocardiographic changes, EKG modifications post-TBI seem to reflect a hemodynamic issue or an intracranial injury effect rather than a direct or primary cardiac insult.

33.3.2 Myocardial Dysfunction

Several studies have evaluated changes in myocardial function after TBI. However, most of these studies showed a selection bias and lack of statistical power. Thus, there are not enough data to design evidence-based guidelines concerning early diagnosis, acute treatment, and preventive management [22].

Elevated systolic blood pressure multiplied by heart rate could be protective by supporting cerebral blood flow when cerebral autoregulation is impaired. However, Krishnamoorthy et al., in a retrospective cohort study designed to evaluate the early myocardial workload profile following isolated severe TBI, noticed that both depressed and elevated myocardial workload profiles are common, and that the admission myocardial workload profile is associated with ischemic cardiac events and with in-hospital mortality in a "U-shaped" fashion [23].

Stress cardiomyopathy related to a primary neurologic condition (such as TBI) is identified as neurogenic stunned myocardium. This condition is characterized by a classic triad: transient left ventricular wall motion abnormality, EKG alterations, and a modest rise in cardiac biomarkers, without coronary artery disease. The mechanism of catecholamine-mediated myocardial stunning could be described by direct myocyte damage, sympathetically mediated microcirculatory dysfunction, or epicardial coronary arterial spasm. Neurogenic stunned myocardium can impair the outcome of TBI patients: heart failure, pulmonary edema, and cardiac arrhythmias can occur. Systolic dysfunction usually improves over the first week of hospitalization. Thus, after neurologic injury, optimal cardiac performance is central to maintaining cardiac output and, consequently, cerebral blood flow. The administration of vasopressors, fluids or blood transfusions should be guided by the cardiac function, assessed through continuous EKG, cardiac biomarkers, echocardiography [24], and, in more severe cases, continuous advanced cardiac monitoring.

33.4 Kidney Complications

The incidence of renal failure in TBI has been reported as 0.45–1.9% [25, 26]. A mechanism of brain-kidney crosstalk has been recently proposed [27]: acute cerebral injuries can produce cerebral salt wasting and excess secretion of antidiuretic hormone, resulting in hyponatremia, and the excess of sympathetic nervous activity with the increase of plasma catecholamine levels can lead to hemodynamic instability and reduced renal perfusion.

Moreover, the injured brain is subject to post-traumatic neuroinflammation, including complement activation and release of pro-inflammatory chemokines and cytokines that can leak, through the dysfunctional blood-brain barrier, into the systemic circulation. Furthermore, blood loss from trauma, aggressive fluid resuscitation, use of hypertonic solutions, vasopressor support, exposure to contrast media, nephrotoxic sepsis, and administration of antibiotics and nonsteroidal anti-inflammatory drugs may exacerbate renal dysfunction.

On the other hand, in acute kidney injury (AKI) patients, urea and other solutes are increased and these substances can pass into the brain because of the damage to the blood-brain barrier in patients with TBI. This inflow is initially compensated by astrocytes taking up additional ions and water. However, this compensation mechanism is unsettled in TBI, and cerebral edema can worsen. Moreover, AKI can alter the concentration of neurotransmitters or circulating cytokines, acid-base balance, hemostasis, and drug metabolism that can lead to disruption of the brain-blood barrier.

33.4.1 AKI After TBI

There is limited information on the incidence of AKI in patients with TBI. A recent large, retrospective, multicenter study by Harrois and colleagues [28], including 3111 patients, showed that AKI generally has an early onset after trauma (within 5 days from admission in 96% of patients) and occurs in 13% of cases, increasing up to 42.5% in patients presenting with hemorrhagic shock; prehospital hemodynamic variables including mean arterial pressure (MAP), heart rate, and hemorrhagic shock as well as severity of trauma (as for injury severity score), presence of renal trauma, blood lactate levels, and rhabdomyolysis severity were independent risk factors for AKI. However, this study presents several limitations including missing data on comorbidities and blood tests as well as on the administration of nephrotoxic agents, such as colloids and antibiotics. A preliminary analysis of the CENTER-TBI cohort, using the KDIGO criteria, found that 17.6% of TBI patients had risk/injury AKI and 6.2% acute kidney failure AKI, occurring, respectively, 2 and 3 days after TBI. Both categories are strongly associated with worse long-term outcome. The mortality rate is higher and outcome worse in patients with AKI than in patients with normal renal function, even if the dysfunction is mild [25]. This finding was confirmed by a recent systematic review and meta-analysis of AKI in trauma patients showing an association between AKI and increased hospital length of stay and mortality [29].

33.5 Liver Dysfunction

There is a paucity of literature addressing liver complications in patients after head injury. Increased alanine aminotransferase (ALT) values were common (49%) in patients admitted to the rehabilitation unit following TBI. For the majority of these patients, enzymes returned to normal with conservative management. In most cases, no specific etiology was ever identified [30].

Regardless of the cause, liver injury is directly related to impaired immunological function. Interestingly, neuroinflammatory responses triggered by TBI have been demonstrated to change the expression of nearly a thousand genes in the liver. Studies have demonstrated that TBI leads to an increase in acute-phase effector proteins (such as tumor necrosis factor [TNF]-α, interleukin [IL]-1β, interleukin IL-6, and interferon [IFN]γ) in the brain and serum. Elevated serum levels, binding to hepatocytes, stimulate the hepatic acute-phase response, which is a major component of the systemic response to tissue damage, infection, inflammation, and trauma.

Previous studies disagree regarding whether TBI activates the acute-phase response. These discrepancies can be justified by differential sensitivity of the markers or lack of temporal specificity. Furthermore, it could be that not all brain injuries induce the acute-phase response.

33.5.1 Effect of Drugs on Liver Function

In the general population, the four main classes of drugs responsible for acute liver failure necessitating transplantation are acetaminophen, antituberculosis, antiepileptic, and antibiotic drugs. Three out of four of these drugs are widely used in patients with TBI; thus, this population could be at high risk of toxic hepatopathy. Concerning antiepileptics, phenytoin and carbamazepine can cause an idiosyncratic reaction (dose independent, and unpredictable), while valproic acid and phenobarbital may lead to anticonvulsant hypersensitivity syndrome.

Analgesia and sedation are often required in patients following TBI. The γ-aminobutyric acid theory in the pathogenesis of hepatic encephalopathy hypothesizes that increased drug-binding sites enhance sensitivity to benzodiazepines and barbiturates in patients with acute liver dysfunction. Thus, propofol is preferred for use because of its rapid onset, short duration of action, and antiepileptogenic properties. Hourly doses should be set based on the Richmond Agitation-Sedation Scale and not exceed 5 mg/kg of body weight to avoid the risk of propofol infusion syndrome.

Concerning analgesic agents, those with inactive metabolites, such as fentanyl and hydromorphone, are favored. Similarly, pain score-directed titration of bolus administration rather than continuous infusion is recommended to avoid brain and liver dysfunction worsening.

33.6 Hematologic Complications

The incidence of TBI-associated coagulopathy is highly variable ranging from 7% to 63%, reflecting the wide difference in definitions of coagulopathy [31]. The ICU mortality risk of TBI is multiplied 4.2 times by cardiovascular complications and 3.13 times by the presence of coagulopathy [31].

The origin of TBI-associated coagulopathy is multifactorial, involving tissue factor, fibrinolysis, platelets, von Willebrand factor, anionic phospholipids, and brain-derived microparticles. Tissue factor plays a key role in the initiation of hemostasis and thrombin production. The resulting microvascular thrombosis and depletion of clotting factors can cause a functionally hypocoagulable state, which can initiate disseminated intravascular coagulation (DIC). Endothelial activation with related thrombomodulin expression and increased activated protein C also contribute to endogenous fibrinolysis and anticoagulation. Due to the dynamic coagulation changes, routine coagulation tests should be performed frequently in all patients with TBI using routine laboratory or viscoelastic tests. In the CENTER-TBI collaboration, trauma-related hemostatic abnormalities were most frequently treated with fresh frozen plasma (73%) or platelets (52%), followed by the supplementation of vitamin K (39%) [32].

As TBI may alter coagulation along with immobilization, this can increase the risk of venous thromboembolism. Therefore, the benefits of thromboembolism prevention should be balanced with the risk of intracranial bleeding extension. Some reports suggest that early prophylaxis with enoxaparin within the first 3 days did not increase intracranial hemorrhage progression. Most CENTER-TBI researchers reported using deep venous thrombosis prophylaxis with anticoagulants frequently or always (94%). In the absence of hemorrhagic brain lesions, 21% delayed deep venous thrombosis prophylaxis until 72 h after trauma. If hemorrhagic brain lesions were present, the number of centers delaying deep venous thrombosis prophylaxis for 72 h increased to 46% [32].

33.7 Conclusion

Patients with TBI commonly manifest clinically significant extracranial organ impairment. ICU physicians should have a clear knowledge of all these complications to ensure prompt and proper management because some of them have an impact on long-term outcome. Data from the large CENTER-TBI cohort will help us to better understand these complications and use comparative effective analysis to identify better treatment strategies.

References

1. Maas AIR, Menon DK, Adelson PD, et al. Traumatic brain injury: integrated approaches to improve prevention, clinical care, and research. Lancet Neurol. 2017;16:987–1048.
2. MRC CRASH Trial Collaborators, Perel P, Arango M, et al. Predicting outcome after traumatic brain injury: practical prognostic models based on large cohort of international patients. BMJ. 2008;336:425–9.
3. van Leeuwen N, Lingsma HF, Perel P, et al. Prognostic value of major extracranial injury in traumatic brain injury: an individual patient data meta-analysis in 39,274 patients. Neurosurgery. 2012;70:811–8.
4. Piek J, Chesnut RM, Marshall LF, et al. Extracranial complications of severe head injury. J Neurosurg. 1992;77:901–7.
5. Corral L, Javierre CF, Ventura JL, Marcos P, Herrero JI, Mañez R. Impact of non-neurological complications in severe traumatic brain injury outcome. Crit Care. 2012;16:R44–7.
6. Heuer JF, Pelosi P, Hermann P, et al. Acute effects of intracranial hypertension and ARDS on pulmonary and neuronal damage: a randomized experimental study in pigs. Intensive Care Med. 2011;37:1182–91.
7. Mascia L. Acute lung injury in patients with severe brain injury: a double hit model. Neurocrit Care. 2009;11:417–26.
8. Busl KM, Bleck TP. Neurogenic pulmonary edema. Crit Care Med. 2015;43:1710–5.
9. McHugh GS, Engel DC, Butcher I, et al. Prognostic value of secondary insults in traumatic brain injury: results from the IMPACT study. J Neurotrauma. 2007;24:287–93.
10. Volpi PC, Robba C, Rota M, Vargiolu A, Citerio G. Trajectories of early secondary insults correlate to outcomes of traumatic brain injury: results from a large, single centre, observational study. BMC Emerg Med. 2018;18:52–9.
11. Huijben JA, Volovici V, Cnossen MC, et al. Variation in general supportive and preventive intensive care management of traumatic brain injury: a survey in 66 neurotrauma centers participating in the Collaborative European NeuroTrauma Effectiveness Research in Traumatic Brain Injury (CENTER-TBI) study. Crit Care. 2018;22:90.
12. Briain DÓ, Nickson C, Pilcher DV, Udy AA. Early hyperoxia in patients with traumatic brain injury admitted to intensive care in Australia and New Zealand: a retrospective multicenter cohort study. Neurocrit Care. 2018;29:443–51.

13. Pelosi P, Ferguson ND, Frutos-Vivar F, et al. Management and outcome of mechanically ventilated neurologic patients. Crit Care Med. 2011;39:1482–92.
14. Asehnoune K, Roquilly A, Cinotti R. Respiratory management in patients with severe brain injury. Crit Care. 2018;22:76.
15. Esnault P, Nguyen C, Bordes J, et al. Early-onset ventilator-associated pneumonia in patients with severe traumatic brain injury: incidence, risk factors, and consequences in cerebral oxygenation and outcome. Neurocrit Care. 2017;7:728–12.
16. Li Y, Liu C, Xiao W, Song T, Wang S. Incidence, risk factors, and outcomes of ventilator-associated pneumonia in traumatic brain injury: a meta-analysis. Neurocrit Care. 2019;128:579.
17. Maas AIR, Menon DK, Steyerberg EW, et al. Collaborative European NeuroTrauma Effectiveness Research in Traumatic Brain Injury (CENTER-TBI): a prospective longitudinal observational study. Neurosurgery. 2015;76:67–80.
18. Wijayatilake DS, Sherren PB, Jigajinni SV. Systemic complications of traumatic brain injury. Curr Opin Anaesthesiol. 2015;28:525–31.
19. Morris NA, Chatterjee A, Adejumo OL, et al. The risk of Takotsubo cardiomyopathy in acute neurological disease. Neurocrit Care. 2018;30:171–6.
20. Mazzeo AT, Micalizzi A, Mascia L, Scicolone A, Siracusano L. Brain-heart crosstalk: the many faces of stress-related cardiomyopathy syndromes in anaesthesia and intensive care. Br J Anaesth. 2014;112:803–15.
21. Carney N, Totten AM, O'Reilly C, et al. Guidelines for the Management of Severe Traumatic Brain Injury, Fourth Edition. Neurosurgery. 2017;80:6–15.
22. Ibrahim MS, Samuel B, Mohamed W, Suchdev K. Cardiac dysfunction in neurocritical care: an autonomic perspective. Neurocrit Care. 2018;30:508–21.
23. Krishnamoorthy V, Vavilala MS, Chaikittisilpa N, et al. Association of early myocardial workload and mortality following severe traumatic brain injury. Crit Care Med. 2018;46:965–71.
24. Patel HC, Bouamra O, Woodford M, et al. Trends in head injury outcome from 1989 to 2003 and the effect of neurosurgical care: an observational study. Lancet. 2005;366:1538–44.
25. Li N, Zhao W-G, Zhang W-F. Acute kidney injury in patients with severe traumatic brain injury: implementation of the acute kidney injury network stage system. Neurocrit Care. 2011;14:377–81.
26. Berthiaume L, Zygun D. Non-neurologic organ dysfunction in acute brain injury. Crit Care Clin. 2006;22:753–66.
27. Lu R, Kiernan MC, Murray A, Rosner MH, Ronco C. Kidney–brain crosstalk in the acute and chronic setting. Nat Rev Nephrol. 2015;11:707–19.
28. Harrois A, Soyer B, Gauss T, et al. Prevalence and risk factors for acute kidney injury among trauma patients: a multicenter cohort study. Crit Care. 2018;22:344.
29. Søvik S, Isachsen MS, Nordhuus KM, et al. Acute kidney injury in trauma patients admitted to the ICU: a systematic review and meta-analysis. Intensive Care Med. 2019;45:407–19.
30. Fox A, Sanderlin JB, McNamee S, Bajaj JS, Carne W, Cifu DX. Elevated liver enzymes following polytraumatic injury. J Rehabil Res Dev. 2014;51:869–74.
31. Maegele M, Schöchl H, Menovsky T, et al. Coagulopathy and haemorrhagic progression in traumatic brain injury: advances in mechanisms, diagnosis, and management. Lancet Neurol. 2017;16:630–47.
32. Huijben JA, van der Jagt M, Cnossen MC, et al. Variation in blood transfusion and coagulation management in traumatic brain injury at the intensive care unit: a survey in 66 neurotrauma centers participating in the Collaborative European Neurotrauma Effectiveness Research in Traumatic Brain Injury Study. J Neurotrauma. 2017;35:323–32.
33. Goyal K, Bindra A, Kumar N, et al. Non-neurological complications after traumatic brain injury: a prospective observational study. Indian J Crit Care Med. 2018;22:632–8.
34. Ramtinfar S, Chabok S, Chari A, Reihanian Z, Leili E, Alizadeh A. Early detection of nonneurologic organ failure in patients with severe traumatic brain injury: multiple organ dysfunction score or sequential organ failure assessment? Indian J Crit Care Med. 2016;20:575–80.

35. Aiolfi A, Benjamin E, Khor D, Inaba K, Lam L, Demetriades D. Brain trauma foundation guidelines for intracranial pressure monitoring: compliance and effect on outcome. World J Surg. 2017;41:1543–9.
36. Mascia L, Zavala E, Bosma K, et al. High tidal volume is associated with the development of acute lung injury after severe brain injury: an international observational study. Crit Care Med. 2007;35:1815–20.
37. Prathep S, Sharma D, Hallman M, et al. Preliminary report on cardiac dysfunction after isolated traumatic brain injury. Crit Care Med. 2014;42:142–7.
38. Krishnamoorthy V, Rowhani-Rahbar A, Chaikittisilpa N, et al. Association of early hemodynamic profile and the development of systolic dysfunction following traumatic brain injury. Neurocrit Care. 2017;26:379–87.
39. Cuisinier A, Maufrais C, Payen JF, Nottin S, Walther G, Bouzat P. Myocardial function at the early phase of traumatic brain injury: a prospective controlled study. Scand J Trauma Resusc Emerg Med. 2016;24:129.

Part XI
Neurological Aspects

Ten False Beliefs About Mechanical Ventilation in Patients with Brain Injury

34

D. Battaglini, P. Pelosi, and C. Robba

34.1 Introduction

Patients with brain injury often require mechanical ventilation in order to protect the airways, optimize carbon dioxide and oxygen levels, and minimize secondary brain damage [1]. Unfortunately, respiratory targets and ideal ventilator settings in this group of patients are unclear; currently accepted lung-protective ventilation principles are not generally applied in the brain-injured population, as they can be detrimental for cerebral hemodynamics [2]. Traditionally, high tidal volumes are used in brain-injured patients to avoid hypercapnia and consequent cerebrovascular vasodilation, and positive end-expiratory pressure (PEEP), recruitment maneuvers, and prone position are avoided as they can negatively affect intracranial pressure (ICP). Furthermore, respiratory weaning is challenging, extubation is often delayed, and optimal timing of tracheostomy is unclear [3]. However, recent evidence is progressively modifying these traditional concepts, thus paving the way for the application of protective ventilator settings and rescue therapies even in this group of patients [4].

The aim of this chapter is to review the current knowledge concerning mechanical ventilation management, rescue therapies, weaning, and tracheostomy in patients with brain injury, by discussing and debulking ten traditional "false beliefs."

D. Battaglini · P. Pelosi
Department of Surgical Sciences and Integrated Diagnostics, University of Genoa, Genoa, Italy

Anesthesia and Intensive Care, San Martino Policlinico Hospital, IRCCS for Oncology and Neuroscience, Genoa, Italy

C. Robba (✉)
Anesthesia and Intensive Care, San Martino Policlinico Hospital, IRCCS for Oncology and Neuroscience, Genoa, Italy

34.2 Brain-Lung Crosstalk Does Not Exist

Brain-lung interaction—"brain-lung crosstalk"—has been studied by several authors over the last decades [5]. Traditionally, the brain and the lung have always been considered as two separate organs with no connection to each other [4, 6]. Even so, recent literature suggests a bidirectional interaction in neurocritically ill patients receiving mechanical ventilation, strongly supporting the theory of the existence of a strict interaction between the brain and the lung [5].

According to this theory, Samary et al. described the role of an immunogenic response after stroke [7]: the blood-brain barrier increases its permeability and immune cells, such as macrophages, neutrophils, and lymphocytes, enter the damaged tissue, having both neuroprotectant and neurodegenerative effects. Not only is there a local immune response during brain damage, but systemic innate and adaptive immune responses are both heightened, leading to the release of interleukin-10 (IL-10), which is capable of enhancing pro-inflammatory responses in peripheral organs, such as the lung [7]. Thereby, primary brain injury triggers increased sympathetic activity, which leads to high capillary permeability and pulmonary venoconstriction, causing increased endothelial dysfunction, neutrophil infiltrates, and a systemic inflammatory response [6]. Therefore, pulmonary complications, such as bronchitis, pneumonia [6], and acute respiratory distress syndrome (ARDS) [8], are common after brain injury, and are associated with a high risk of death [6, 8]. On the other hand, mechanical ventilation itself, via a mechano-transduction mechanism [8] caused by repeated opening and closing of atelectatic lung regions, may contribute to enhance the inflammatory cascade affecting distal organs, thus promoting or worsening existing pulmonary damage [5]. This mechanism is one of the key causes of ventilator-induced lung injury (VILI), which along with ARDS may promote brain injury through the release of systemic inflammatory mediators [5]. This theory involves specific pathways. Mechanical ventilation may *per se* have a dangerous impact on lung function and structure, and could promote early gene *c-fos* expression in some brain areas. This gene is a marker of neuronal activation expressed in response to proliferation, transcription, and apoptosis [5]. In addition, the inflammatory response was mostly mediated by tumor necrosis factor-α (TNF-α), especially in mice ventilated with higher tidal volumes [8]. Accordingly, in another experimental study, authors suggested that lung epithelial cells, when stimulated by pro-inflammatory mediators, increased the release of cytokines and exerted apoptosis and necrosis on brain cells [6]. In addition, brain damage is responsible for intra-alveolar edema and reduction of the phagocytic capability of macrophages, demonstrating that the brain and the lung strongly affect each other [6].

In summary, most authors agree that the brain and the lung are highly connected and minimal changes in brain or lung pathophysiology can promote deep changes in inflammatory systemic response, causing secondary brain and lung injuries, which could be nicknamed as "dangerous crosstalk" [5].

34.3 The More Oxygen We Give, the Better It Is

Reduced cerebral oxygenation after brain injury could lead to secondary brain damage and, therefore, maintaining adequate oxygen concentration is fundamental in brain-injured patients [9]. In particular, hypoxia is linked to a higher risk of mortality and higher intensive care unit (ICU) length of stay and should be avoided [9]. However, recent evidence suggests that *hyper*oxia is also independently associated with higher mortality risk and poor outcome in patients with acute brain injury [9]. Supplemental oxygen level is associated with the production of reactive oxygen species (ROS) that overcome physiological antioxidant defenses [9, 10]. Damaged cells release endogenous damage-associated molecular pattern molecules (DAMPs), stimulating the inflammatory response and inducing cell apoptosis [9]. Thus, although oxygen therapy might be essential for patient management, high oxygen concentration in blood and tissues may be harmful [9, 10]. Hyperbaric hyperoxia is well known for its effects on vasoreactivity, cerebral metabolism, and cerebral blood flow. Hyperbaric hyperoxia (250/250 kPa) and normobaric normoxia (101/21 kPa) were tested in healthy subjects, and single-photon emission computed tomography (CT) was used to observe the changes in cerebral regional blood flow. During hyperbaric hyperoxia, cerebral blood flow increased in the sensor-motor, visual, and cingulate cortices and cognition area, suggesting a possible positive effect in brain trauma and stroke patients [10]. However, more recent evidence highlights the risks associated with hyperbaric hyperoxia and in brain-injured patients oxygen supplementation is recommended only when oxygen saturation (SpO_2) is <95% [9]. Similarly, in traumatic brain injury (TBI) patients, the target arterial partial oxygen pressure (PaO_2) is >60 mmHg, titrating the fraction of inspired oxygen (FiO_2) to this value [9]. In this context, bedside multimodal monitoring systems, such as jugular venous oxygen saturation, can be helpful to avoid cerebral hypoxemia [11]. In a randomized clinical trial on mechanically ventilated TBI patients, two different FiO_2 levels administered within the first 6 h after traumatic accident were compared. No differences in Barthel index (a scale used to measure performance in activities of daily living) and length of stay were observed, but the normobaric oxygen group had a better neurological outcome as assessed using the modified Rankin Scale (mRS) [12]. Taken together, recent data suggest avoiding high FiO_2 values during mechanical ventilation, and that oxygen administration should be individualized: FiO_2 should be titrated to achieve an SpO_2 of 95% or PaO_2 >60 mmHg [9]; both hypoxia and hyperoxia should be avoided, and multimodal neuromonitoring could be of help in the early detection of brain ischemia.

34.4 Brain-Injured Patients Must Be Hyperventilated

Hyperventilation has been suggested as a treatment to decrease the ICP in the neurocritical care setting, especially in TBI patients [11, 13]. Hypocapnia leads to a reduction in arterial extracerebral $PaCO_2$ with brain tissue alkalosis and cerebral arteriolar vasoconstriction. These changes are responsible for decreased cerebral blood flow, cerebral blood volume, and ICP [11]. Despite the efficacy of hyperventilation in reducing ICP, cerebral vasoconstriction can lead to cerebral ischemia and tissue hypoxia [11]. In a randomized controlled trial, patients were assigned to receive normal ventilation ($PaCO_2$ 35 mmHg ± 2 standard deviation [SD]), hyperventilation ($PaCO_2$ 25 mmHg ± 2 SD) or hyperventilation ($PaCO_2$ 25 mmHg ± 2 SD) with addition of the buffer tromethamine. The authors found that at 3 and 6 months, patients in the hyperventilation only group had a worst Glasgow Outcome Scale compared to the other two groups, suggesting that sustained hyperventilation was deleterious in this cohort of patients [13]. Recently, Brandi et al. observed the effects of hyperventilation in the acute phase of TBI through transcranial color-coded sonography of the middle cerebral artery. Cerebral perfusion pressure and microdialysis, ICP, $SatO_2$, end-tidal carbon dioxide ($ET-CO_2$), and brain tissue oxygen tension ($PbrO_2$) were continuously monitored. Cerebral mean flow velocity in the middle cerebral artery and ICP decreased during moderate short-term hyperventilation, without significant alteration of oxygenation and brain metabolites, suggesting that moderate hyperventilation ($PaCO_2$ 30–35 mmHg) could be safely used in patients with TBI [11]. Despite this evidence, it is common knowledge that preventive hyperventilation ($PaCO_2$ ≤25 mmHg) should be avoided; hyperventilation should be considered only as rescue therapy in emergency cases of cerebral herniation [13].

34.5 Tidal Volume Must Be High and PEEP Must Be ZEEP

In observational data, a low tidal volume ventilation setting (4.6 ml/kg predicted body weight [PBW]) has been validated in patients with ARDS [14], although its application in patients without ARDS and specifically in neurocritically ill patients requiring mechanical ventilation is still controversial [15]. Low tidal volume and consequent permissive hypercapnia can cause cerebrovascular vasodilation, thus posing the risk of intracranial hypertension [9]. Because of this concern, brain-injured patients have always been excluded from the major trials exploring the effects of lung-protective ventilation [16] and, traditionally, a high tidal volume (9 ml/kg PBW) is the most common strategy applied in clinical practice in neurocritically ill patients [16]. Moreover, recent evidence suggests that the use of high tidal volumes might be associated with the development of acute lung injury even in the severely brain-injured population [15]. A recent experimental study using an open lung approach with low tidal volume mechanical ventilation in a rat model with massive brain damage demonstrated that this ventilatory strategy attenuated lung injury [17]. Tejerina and colleagues, in a large cohort of brain-injured patients, did not find any positive association between tidal volume and increased risk of ARDS development [4]. This may be explained by the fact that most of the patients were ventilated with a range of tidal volumes within 10 ml/kg PBW [4]. In a recent large, randomized controlled trial in patients without ARDS, use of low (4–6 ml/kg PBW) and intermediate

(8–10 ml/kg PBW) tidal volumes, while maintaining a plateau pressure (P_{plat}) <25 cmH$_2$O, resulted in similar primary outcome (ventilator-free days at day 28) [18]. Further, as secondary non-planned outcomes, low tidal volume was more frequently associated with hypercapnia and lower pH, with a trend toward a higher frequency of delirium [18]. Thus, current evidence in patients without ARDS suggests that low tidal volume should be initially applied in these patients, but if increased sedation is required to maintain strict low tidal volume, assisted ventilation might be implemented and higher tidal volume levels tolerated up to 10 ml/kg PBW with a P_{plat} <25 cmH$_2$O [18]. However, in case of progressive deterioration of lung function, yielding ARDS criteria (from mild to severe), low tidal volumes between 4 and 6 ml/kg PBW should be immediately applied [18]. For this reason, when intermediate tidal volume is used in patients without ARDS, careful and daily monitoring of respiratory function is necessary to avoid delay in the application of a low tidal volume strategy. Moreover, only 5% of the PReVENT trial population was neurologic patients, making it impossible to generalize the results of the trial to this specific population of patients [18]. Among ventilator parameters, driving pressure, i.e., the difference between respiratory system plateau pressure and PEEP, is the only ventilator parameter that has been associated with an increased risk of developing ARDS [4]. Thus, driving pressure could be considered to optimize tidal volume in this group of patients, since it has to be maintained at <15 cmH$_2$O [4]. Further, no studies have unequivocally shown that mechanical ventilation with high tidal volumes *per se* increases ICP [15]. Consequently, the concept of tidal volume sizing in acute brain-injured patients is not evidence based, and further studies are necessary to overcome this issue. However, we suggest keeping low tidal volumes and P_{plat} <25 cmH$_2$O in mechanically ventilated patients with head trauma or brain injury, unless clinically contraindicated.

PEEP is considered as another key component of lung-protective ventilation, able to keep the alveoli open and guarantee oxygenation [19]. A recent trial showed that in non-ARDS patients the use of a PEEP value >5 cmH$_2$O was not associated with better outcome. However, the number of neurologic patients included in the analysis was limited [20]. Results from two systematic reviews and meta-analyses showed a beneficial effect on mortality using the "open lung strategy" with the application of high PEEP only in those affected by severe ARDS [21]. Nevertheless, recent experimental evidence regarding safe application of the "open lung concept" is limited [19]. Indeed, some authors demonstrated that pro-inflammatory cytokines were especially released during alveolar static overdistention, leading to the innovative concept of "close the lungs and keep them rested" [19]. Therefore, experts recently made a conditional recommendation for high PEEP ($\geq$15 cmH$_2$O) to be used only in patients with moderate-to-severe ARDS [22]. Results from the LUNG-SAFE study showed that, in patients with mild ARDS who worsened over the first week after inclusion, PEEP was significantly higher as compared with those in whom ARDS improved or remained at a mild stage [23]. However, PEEP application remains doubtful in neuro-damaged patients because it has been linked to cerebral hemodynamic impairment, due to the rise in intrathoracic pressure and the decrease in venous drainage and cardiac output [24]. Although the use of zero PEEP (ZEEP) has been proposed by some authors to overcome the problem in neurocritically ill patients [25], the use of ZEEP (when compared with an 8 cmH$_2$O PEEP strategy) was shown to increase the risk for ARDS development and VILI within 5 days even in neurocritical care patients [25]. The effect of PEEP on cerebral dynamics seems to be primarily related to the respiratory system compliance [24]. In patients with low respiratory system compliance, such as in ARDS patients, PEEP is not associated with significant cerebral impairment, whereas ICP can be affected by PEEP when lung compliance is high [24]. In a recent pilot study, the application of different levels of PEEP (from 5 to 10 and from 10 to 15 cmH$_2$O) in TBI and lung-injured patients resulted in an increased brain tissue oxygen pressure and oxygen saturation without affecting ICP or cerebral perfusion [26]. These results suggest that PEEP levels able to optimize alveolar recruitment can be safely applied in brain-injured patients, providing that PEEP does not cause alveolar hyperinflation or hemodynamic instability [27]. An ongoing randomized controlled study, the REstricted versus Liberal positive end-expiratory pressure in patients without ARDS (RELAx) trial, is investigating low (less than 5 cmH$_2$O) and down-titrated versus high (8 cmH$_2$O) PEEP, in non-ARDS patients. This trial could be essential to clarify some open points, even in the subgroup of brain-injured patients [2].

In summary, in the general population of patients without ARDS, evidence suggests that a protective ventilatory strategy with "enough" PEEP to assure adequate gas exchange (basically a PEEP value ≤5 cmH$_2$O), associated with a low tidal volume, can be safely applied also in brain-damaged patients to prevent VILI [19] and to reduce the risk of developing secondary brain damage [5]. However, higher PEEP levels obtained by individual titration can be used in patients who need to improve oxygenation.

34.6 Recruitment Maneuvers Are Forbidden

The "open lung approach" also includes recruitment maneuvers to open up the collapsed lung by a transient elevation in airway pressure, followed by a high PEEP application to maintain the alveoli open [21]. Many authors have investigated the role of recruitment maneuvers as rescue therapy for respiratory failure to improve systemic oxygenation in ARDS patients [28]. A recent meta-analysis investigated the role of recruitment maneuvers in ICU mortality and ventilator-free days, demonstrating that a protective ventilation strategy that includes recruitment maneuvers reduces ICU mortality, but does not affect ventilator-free days and in-hospital mortality [28]. Another meta-analysis showed that recruitment maneuvers in ARDS patients could improve oxygenation without harmful effects, albeit not reducing mortality [29].

Although recruitment maneuvers have been very promising in experimental ARDS models [21], in patients without ARDS their use is still controversial and limited to sudden alveolar derecruitment as rescue therapy to temporarily increase the lung area available for gas exchange and oxygenation improvement [19]. Thus, recruitment maneuvers have been advocated as part of a lung-protective ventilation strategy notwithstanding that their role in the general ICU population is still unclear [19].

In the specific subpopulation of brain-injured patients, because recruitment maneuvers increase intrathoracic pressure they can have a detrimental effect on cerebral physiology [30]. Bein et al. showed that the application of volume recruitment maneuvers with 30-s progressive increase in peak pressure (P_{peak}) up to 60 cmH$_2$O and maintained for 30 s increased ICP and reduced mean arterial pressure (MAP) and cerebral perfusion pressure, with only marginal improvement in systemic oxygenation [30]. Similarly, a recent randomized crossover study suggested that during application of a P_{peak} of 30 cmH$_2$O for 30 s, subdural pressure increased and cerebral perfusion pressure significantly reduced [31]. However, in a cohort of subarachnoid hemorrhage patients with ARDS, the application of recruitment maneuvers with continuous positive airway pressure (CPAP) of 35 cmH$_2$O for 40 s resulted in increased ICP and decreased cerebral perfusion pressure, whereas for recruitment maneuvers during pressure support ventilation with 35 cmH$_2$O of pressure control above 15 cmH$_2$O of PEEP for 2 min, arterial oxygenation improved without significant changes in ICP and cerebral perfusion pressure [32]. Moreover, other authors found that stepwise recruitment maneuvers with 3 cmH$_2$O applied during pressure control ventilation seemed not to cause significant changes in systemic or cerebral hemodynamics [33].

In summary, although having a potentially dangerous effect on ICP, recruitment maneuvers can improve oxygenation. Nevertheless, even if recruitment maneuvers can be safely adopted in brain-injured patients with careful neuromonitoring, evidence that this maneuver can improve clinical outcomes in neurologic patients is absent. Therefore, it should only be considered in selected cases.

34.7 Assisted Ventilation Is Contraindicated

Cerebral masses, hemorrhage, and brain stem lesions are frequently associated with respiratory drive impairment and specific breathing patterns [34]. Although the use of controlled ventilation has been associated with good PaCO$_2$ control, controlled ventilation needs deep sedation resulting—when compared with assisted ventilation—in worse outcomes and longer ICU lengths of stay [35]. Moreover, to maintain patient-ventilator synchrony, neuromuscular paralysis is often used, which can cause muscular atrophy, reduced compliance, and atelectasis [35]. Assisted ventilation allows spontaneous breathing, use of diaphragm musculature, and avoidance of deep sedation with neuromuscular blockade agents [36]. Its main benefit is the ability to provide ventilator support at the patient's demand, improving synchrony and comfort. However, the use of assisted ventilation requires a stable respiratory condition with sufficient drive, and the ability to initiate the breath [36]. Over the past years, assisted ventilation has been proposed in non-brain-damaged patients as the first step through the weaning phase to reduce the level of sedation and synchronize respiratory triggers [37]. Nevertheless, the role of assisted ventilation in acute brain-injured patients is still controversial. In a retrospective study, comatose patients admitted to the ICU who were ventilated with pressure support ventilation plus sigh presented lower values of ICP compared to patients with continuous positive pressure ventilation [37]. In a retrospective study of TBI patients, ICP values together with neurological examination were found to be the main factors influencing the decision for selection of ventilatory assistance; worse neurologic condition and more elevated ICP were associated with the use of controlled ventilation [37]. However, the use of assisted ventilation was found to be a feasible and safe alternative to controlled ventilation even in the acute phase of trauma [37], but only if patient-ventilator asynchrony, diaphragmatic myo-trauma, respiratory effort, and respiratory drive were properly monitored [34]. Unfortunately, no large randomized controlled studies have been conducted to evaluate assisted ventilation in brain-damaged patients. Nevertheless, in front of new evidence, the use of early assisted ventilation is gaining popularity and should be taken into consideration also in the neurocritical care population.

34.8 Extubation Should Be Delayed

When possible, an early weaning process followed by extubation is preferred to continuation of mechanical ventilation, to avoid possible mechanical ventilation-related complications and high ventilation-related costs [38]. Unnecessary prolonged mechanical ventilation is associated with a greater risk of developing pneumonia and pulmonary or airway trauma. On the other hand, premature removal of mechanical ventilation is linked to difficulty in re-establishing artificial airways and impaired gas exchange with consequent respiratory failure [38]. Many studies have investigated the criteria for successful extubation in non-brain-injured critically ill patients [39]. However, in brain-injured patients this issue is even more relevant. The brain stem is the generator of spontaneous breaths; thus structural or functional damage to the breath generator nuclei or the involved pathways could result in weaning and extubation failure [38]. In fact, neurocritically ill patients are particularly prone to extubation failure or late extubation, due to the loss of ventilator control or the need for strict $PaCO_2$ control [38]. Thus, the weaning process and optimal tracheostomy timing in this population are challenging. The latest available guidelines concerning weaning were developed more than 10 years ago, without any specific recommendation for neuropatients [39]. A before-after study was performed to investigate ventilatory management and extubation phase in brain-injured patients. During the pre-intervention phase, ventilatory management and weaning were initiated according to the physician's decision. In the interphase, a tidal volume of 7 ml/kg PBW, PEEP of 6–8 cmH$_2$O, and respiratory rate adjusted to reach normocapnia were applied. Results showed that these protective ventilatory and early extubation strategies did not alter outcomes in brain-injured patients. In patients managed with greater compliance to the protective interventional phase, there were more invasive ventilation-free days and the mortality rate at day 90 was lower [40]. Because of the lack of specific guidelines, in daily clinical practice, the weaning process is usually started at the discretion of the intensivist. To help in the daily decision-making, a systematic approach for weaning and extubation in neurosurgical and neurological patients was suggested many years ago, demonstrating a reduction in the re-intubation rate, duration of mechanical ventilation, ICU stay, rate of tracheostomy, and mortality when applied [41]. More recently, Asehnoune et al. developed the VISAGE score for the prediction of extubation success in severe brain-damaged patients. This score assigns 1 point for each of these variables, age <40 years old, visual pursuit, swallowing attempts, and Glasgow Coma Scale >10, and rates extubation success at 23% for 0 point, 56% for 1 point, 70% for 2 points, and 90% for 3 points. The VISAGE score has been demonstrated to be quite sensitive (62%) and specific (79%) to detect patients at risk of extubation failure [1]. Hopefully, new randomized controlled trials will help solve the open issue concerning the preferable weaning timing and the criteria for extubation failure in the neurocritically ill population.

34.9 Tracheostomy Should Be Performed Late

Tracheostomy is a common procedure in the ICU, which is performed in about 10–15% of critically ill patients with the aim of facilitating the weaning process in long-term ventilated patients [42]. The procedure helps to prevent long-term intubation-related complications, such as ventilator-associated pneumonia (VAP), tracheal stenosis, and sinusitis [43]. An estimated timing for extubation within 7–15 days of mechanical ventilation is quite customary, followed by tracheostomy if extubation is not deemed feasible within a few days [43]. Neurocritically ill patients are particularly prone to require tracheostomy. Results from a cohort of 546 critically ill patients demonstrated that tracheostomy was performed more frequently in brain-injured patients compared to the general population (55% versus 10.7%, respectively) [3]. The decision and timing of tracheostomy in brain-injured patients present peculiar features, as extubation failure and difficult weaning may be related not only to respiratory failure, but also to poor neurological outcome [1]. Evidence on the advantages of early (within 1 week) versus late tracheostomy (after 1 week) is somewhat conflicting and no real differences in mortality have been identified in the general population [42]. Gessler et al., in a cohort of subarachnoid hemorrhage patients, noted that the majority of the patients underwent late tracheostomy (between 8 and 20 days), and that late tracheostomy was associated with an increased occurrence of pneumonia and pulmonary complications [44]. A recent meta-analysis including ten trials investigating early versus late tracheostomy timing in brain-injured patients found that early tracheostomy was associated with reduced long-term mortality, ICU length of stay, and duration of mechanical ventilation, while it did not reduce short-term mortality [43]. In the SETPOINT randomized controlled trial, including patients with stroke and comparing a strategy based on very early tracheostomy (within 1–3 days from intubation) versus standard-late tracheostomy (from 7 to 14 days), no differences were found in the length of stay, but sedation needed, ICU mortality, and 6-month mortality were lower in the early tracheostomy group [45]. Likewise, in a recent study including brain-injured patients undergoing decompressive craniectomy, early tracheostomy (within 10 days from mechanical ventilation) was associated with increased ventilator-free days, and reduced mortality, VAP, and hospital length of stay [46]. By contrast, evidence confirms that early tracheostomy within the first 4 days of ICU admission is not associated with an improvement in 30-day mortality in the general ICU population [42]. Since no randomized controlled trials have elucidated the open question concerning early versus late tracheostomy, future trials are needed to clarify this point. A new multicenter observational trial may be the first step toward this.

34.10 Prone Position Is Contraindicated

ARDS is common in brain-injured patients, especially those with TBI, impacting the morbidity and mortality of neurocritical care patients [6], and *per se* is associated with increased mortality, longer length of stay, and poor outcomes [6]. High PEEP, recruitment maneuvers, and prone position are useful mechanical ventilation strategies commonly used in ARDS patients, as they have been shown to improve gas exchange, respiratory mechanics, intrapulmonary shunt, and ventilation/perfusion mismatch [22]. Although these strategies have shown a beneficial effect on mortality in ARDS patients [22], the increase in intrathoracic pressure is associated with impaired jugular venous flow by reduced venous return to the right atrium, possibly causing intracranial hypertension [28]. Therefore, brain-injured patients have always been excluded from the major trials exploring the role of protective ventilation strategies and in particular prone position [22], and there is a lack of literature on the use of prone position in patients with both TBI and ARDS [47]. In a small study on severe brain-damaged patients with intracranial aneurysm rupture who developed ARDS, prone position increased brain tissue oxygen partial pressure, ICP, and decreased cerebral perfusion pressure [47]. In a retrospective study on brain-injured patients receiving prone positioning for ARDS, Roth et al. demonstrated that arterial oxygenation increased significantly in the prone position when compared to supine, but at the expense of an increase in ICP [48]. However, in a retrospective study on subarachnoid hemorrhage patients undergoing prone positioning [47], ICP increased from 9.3 ± 5.2 mmHg to 14.8 ± 6.7 mmHg and cerebral perfusion pressure decreased from 73 ± 10.5 mmHg to 67.7 ± 10.7 mmHg, suggesting that the beneficial effect of prone position on cerebral tissue oxygenation outweighed the expected adverse effect on ICP and cerebral perfusion pressure. Therefore, prone positioning in brain-injured patients should be considered when refractory hypoxia occurs, under strict neuromonitoring to avoid secondary brain injury [11].

34.11 No Role for ECMO

Extracorporeal oxygenation techniques, such as veno-venous extracorporeal membrane oxygenation (VV-ECMO), are useful temporary lifesaving strategies applied in severe ARDS patients when conventional strategies have failed [49]. However, use of ECMO in trauma patients is limited by serious concerns regarding the risk of hemorrhage during and after cannulation, in particular in the presence of severe coagulopathy and risk of intracranial hemorrhage [49]. Anticoagulation is always required during ECMO. Usually, a bolus of 50–100 U/kg heparin is administered, followed by a continuous infusion that aims to maintain an activated clotting time between 180 and 200 s or a prothrombin time between 40 and 50 s [50]. Although the need for anticoagulation has always been traditionally considered a relative contraindication for the use of ECMO in brain-injured patients, recent evidence suggests that VV-ECMO can be feasible and safe even in this group of patients [50]. A case series and literature review with a cumulative number of 31 patients undergoing VV-ECMO for hypoxemic respiratory failure secondary to ARDS in trauma found a survival rate of 85% with none of these patients dying because of ECMO-related complications [50]. Moreover, improvement in ECMO techniques, including the introduction of centrifugal pumps and heparin-coated circuits, is progressively reducing the amount of heparin required; indeed, the application of heparin-free ECMO showed good outcomes and minimal complications [50]. In summary, ECMO can be considered as a safe and feasible rescue therapy even in trauma patients, including neurological injury. The decision to start VV-ECMO in neurocritically ill patients is challenging and patient selection and timing, as well as a multidisciplinary approach including cardio-anesthesiologists, neuro-intensivists, and perfusionists, are crucial for achieving success [50].

34.12 Conclusion

Although the literature concerning ventilatory management in neurocritically ill patients is still limited, current evidence suggests that the principles of protective ventilation strategies can potentially be applied even in brain-injured mechanically ventilated patients (Fig. 34.1). Whether or not ARDS is present, ventilator settings and rescue therapies should be individualized, balancing the risks and benefits of each and performing them under strict systemic and neuromonitoring surveillance.

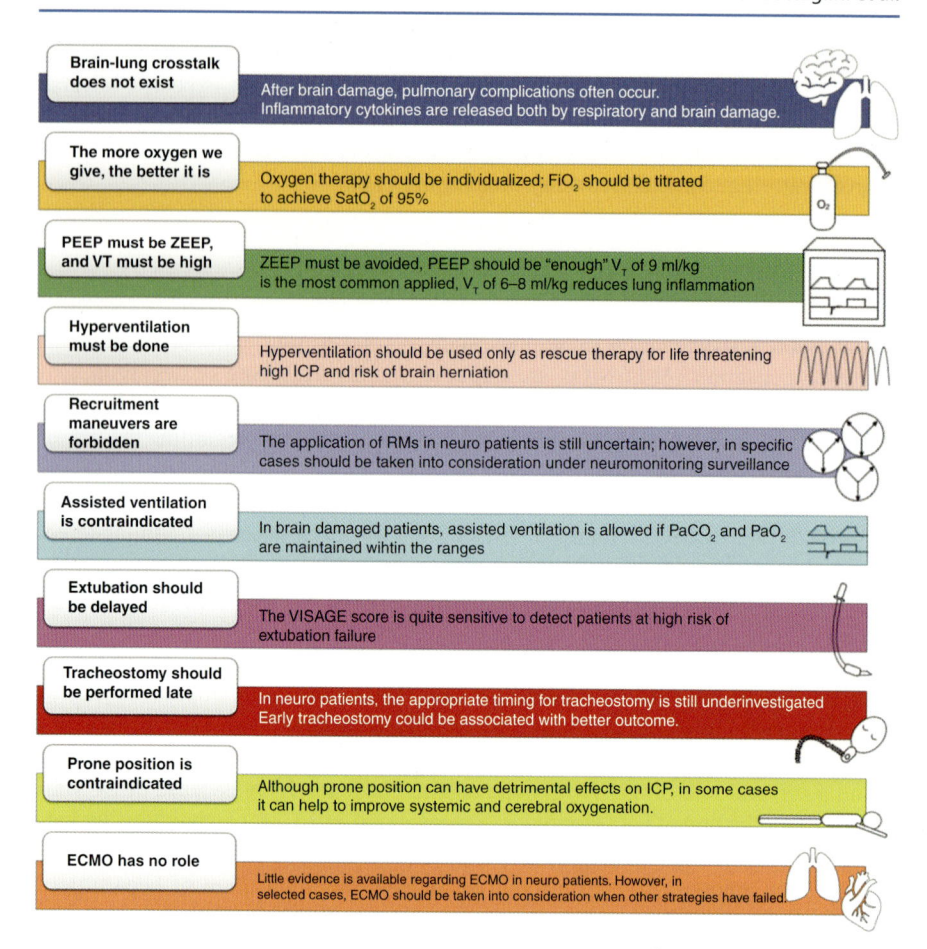

Brain-lung crosstalk does not exist	After brain damage, pulmonary complications often occur. Inflammatory cytokines are released both by respiratory and brain damage.
The more oxygen we give, the better it is	Oxygen therapy should be individualized; FiO_2 should be titrated to achieve $SatO_2$ of 95%
PEEP must be ZEEP, and VT must be high	ZEEP must be avoided, PEEP should be "enough" V_T of 9 ml/kg is the most common applied, V_T of 6–8 ml/kg reduces lung inflammation
Hyperventilation must be done	Hyperventilation should be used only as rescue therapy for life threatening high ICP and risk of brain herniation
Recruitment maneuvers are forbidden	The application of RMs in neuro patients is still uncertain; however, in specific cases should be taken into consideration under neuromonitoring surveillance
Assisted ventilation is contraindicated	In brain damaged patients, assisted ventilation is allowed if $PaCO_2$ and PaO_2 are maintained wihtin the ranges
Extubation should be delayed	The VISAGE score is quite sensitive to detect patients at high risk of extubation failure
Tracheostomy should be performed late	In neuro patients, the appropriate timing for tracheostomy is still underinvestigated Early tracheostomy could be associated with better outcome.
Prone position is contraindicated	Although prone position can have detrimental effects on ICP, in some cases it can help to improve systemic and cerebral oxygenation.
ECMO has no role	Little evidence is available regarding ECMO in neuro patients. However, in selected cases, ECMO should be taken into consideration when other strategies have failed.

Fig. 34.1 Ten false beliefs on mechanical ventilation in brain-injured patients. FiO_2 fraction of inspired oxygen, $SatO_2$ oxygen saturation, *PEEP* positive end-expiratory pressure, V_T tidal volume, *ZEEP* zero PEEP, *RM* recruitment maneuvers, PaO_2 arterial oxygen pressure, $PaCO_2$ carbon dioxide partial pressure, *ECMO* extracorporeal membrane oxygenation

References

1. Asehnoune K, Seguin P, Lasocki S, et al. Extubation success prediction in a multicentric cohort of patients with severe brain injury. Anesthesiology. 2017;127:338–46.
2. Algera AG, Pisani L, Bergmans DCJ, et al. RELAx - REstricted versus liberal positive end-expiratory pressure in patients without ARDS: protocol for a randomized controlled trial. Trials. 2018;19:272.
3. Frutos-Vivar F, Esteban A, Apezteguía C, et al. Outcome of mechanically ventilated patients who require a tracheostomy. Crit Care Med. 2005;33:290–8.
4. Tejerina E, Pelosi P, Muriel A, et al. Association between ventilatory settings and development of acute respiratory distress syndrome in mechanically ventilated patients due to brain injury. J Crit Care. 2017;38:341–5.
5. Pelosi P, Rocco PRM. The lung and the brain: a dangerous cross-talk. Crit Care. 2011;15:168.

6. Samary CS, Ramos AB, Maia LA, et al. Focal ischemic stroke leads to lung injury and reduces alveolar macrophage phagocytic capability in rats. Crit Care. 2018;22:249.
7. Samary CS, Pelosi P, Leme Silva P, Rocco PRM. Immunomodulation after ischemic stroke: potential mechanisms and implications for therapy. Crit Care. 2016;20:391.
8. Quilez ME, Fuster G, Villar J, et al. Injurious mechanical ventilation affects neuronal activation in ventilated rats. Crit Care. 2011;15:R124.
9. Vincent JL, Taccone FS, He X. Harmful effects of hyperoxia in postcardiac arrest, sepsis, traumatic brain injury, or stroke: the importance of individualized oxygen therapy in critically ill patients. Can Respir J. 2017;2017:2834956.
10. Micarelli A, Jacobsson H, Larsson SA, Jonsson C, Pagani M. Neurobiological insight into hyperbaric hyperoxia. Acta Physiol. 2013;209:69–76.
11. Brandi G, Stocchetti N, Pagnamenta A, Stretti F, Steiger P, Klinzing S. Cerebral metabolism is not affected by moderate hyperventilation in patients with traumatic brain injury. Crit Care. 2019;23:45.
12. Taher A, Pilehvari Z, Poorolajal J, Aghajanloo M. Effects of normobaric hyperoxia in traumatic brain injury: a randomized controlled clinical trial. Trauma Mon. 2016;21:e26772.
13. Muizelaar JP, Marmarou A, Ward JD, et al. Adverse effects of prolonged hyperventilation in patients with severe head injury: a randomized clinical trial. J Neurosurg. 1991;75:731–9.
14. Putensen C, Theuerkauf N, Zinserling J, Wrigge H, Pelosi P. Meta-analysis: ventilation strategies and outcomes of the acute respiratory distress syndrome and acute lung injury. Ann Intern Med. 2009;151:566–76.
15. Mascia L, Zavala E, Bosma K, et al. High tidal volume is associated with the development of acute lung injury after severe brain injury: an international observational study. Crit Care Med. 2007;35:1815–20.
16. Pelosi P, Ferguson ND, Frutos-Vivar F, et al. Management and outcome of mechanically ventilated neurologic patients. Crit Care Med. 2011;39:1482–92.
17. Krebs J, Tsagogiorgas C, Pelosi P, et al. Open lung approach with low tidal volume mechanical ventilation attenuates lung injury in rats with massive brain damage. Crit Care. 2014;18:R59.
18. Simonis FD, Serpa Neto A, Binnekade JM, et al. Effect of a low vs. intermediate tidal volume strategy on ventilator-free days in intensive care unit patients without ARDS. JAMA. 2018;320:1872.
19. Pelosi P, Rocco PRM, Gama de Abreu M. Close down the lungs and keep them resting to minimize ventilator-induced lung injury. Crit Care. 2018;22:72.
20. Serpa Neto A, Filho RR, Cherpanath T, et al. Associations between positive end-expiratory pressure and outcome of patients without ARDS at onset of ventilation: a systematic review and meta-analysis of randomized controlled trials. Ann Intensive Care. 2016;6:109.
21. Lu J, Wang X, Chen M, et al. An open lung strategy in the management of acute respiratory distress syndrome: a systematic review and meta-analysis. Shock. 2017;48:43–53.
22. Fan E, Del Sorbo L, Goligher EC, et al. An official American Thoracic Society/European Society of intensive care medicine/society of critical care medicine clinical practice guideline: mechanical ventilation in adult patients with acute respiratory distress syndrome. Am J Respir Crit Care Med. 2017;195:1253–63.
23. Pham T, Serpa Neto A, Pelosi P, et al. Outcomes of patients presenting with mild acute respiratory distress syndrome: insights from the LUNG SAFE study. Anesthesiology. 2019;130:263–83.
24. Caricato A, Conti G, Della Corte F, et al. Effects of PEEP on the intracranial system of patients with head injury and subarachnoid hemorrhage: the role of respiratory system compliance. J Trauma. 2005;58:571–6.
25. Korovesi I, Papadomichelakis E, Orfanos S, et al. Exhaled breath condensate in mechanically ventilated brain-injured patients with no lung injury or sepsis. Anesthesiology. 2011;114:1118–29.
26. Nemer SN, Caldeira JB, Santos RG, et al. Effects of positive end-expiratory pressure on brain tissue oxygen pressure of severe traumatic brain injury patients with acute respiratory distress syndrome: a pilot study. J Crit Care. 2015;30:1263–6.

27. Mascia L, Grasso S, Fiore T, Bruno F, Berardino M, Ducati A. Cerebro-pulmonary interactions during the application of low levels of positive end-expiratory pressure. Intensive Care Med. 2005;31:373–9.
28. Hodgson C, Goligher E, Young M, et al. Recruitment manoeuvres for adults with acute respiratory distress syndrome. Cochrane Database Syst Rev. 2016;17:CD006667.
29. Kang H, Yang H, Tong Z. Recruitment manoeuvres for adults with acute respiratory distress syndrome receiving mechanical ventilation: a systematic review and meta-analysis. J Crit Care. 2019;50:1–10.
30. Bein T, Kuhr L-P, Bele S, Ploner F, Keyl C, Taeger K. Lung recruitment maneuver in patients with cerebral injury: effects on intracranial pressure and cerebral metabolism. Intensive Care Med. 2002;28:554–8.
31. Flexman AM, Gooderham PA, Griesdale DE, Argue R, Toyota B. Effects of an alveolar recruitment maneuver on subdural pressure, brain swelling, and mean arterial pressure in patients undergoing supratentorial tumour resection: a randomized crossover study. Can J Anesth. 2017;64:626–33.
32. Nemer SN, Caldeira JB, Azeredo LM, et al. Alveolar recruitment maneuver in patients with subarachnoid hemorrhage and acute respiratory distress syndrome: a comparison of 2 approaches. J Crit Care. 2011;26:22–7.
33. Zhang X, Yang Z, Wang Q, Fan H. Impact of positive end-expiratory pressure on cerebral injury patients with hypoxemia. Am J Emerg Med. 2011;29:699–703.
34. Vaporidi K, Akoumianaki E, Telias I, Goligher EC, Brochard L, Georgopoulos D. Respiratory drive in critically ill patients: pathophysiology and clinical implications. Am J Respir Crit Care Med. 2020;201:20–32.
35. Aragón RE, Proaño A, Mongilardi N, et al. Sedation practices and clinical outcomes in mechanically ventilated patients in a prospective multicenter cohort. Crit Care. 2019;23:130.
36. Chiumello D, Pelosi P, Calvi E, Bigatello LM, Gattinoni L. Different modes of assisted ventilation in patients with acute respiratory failure. Eur Respir J. 2002;20:925–33.
37. Cormio M, Portella G, Spreafico E, Mazza L, Pesenti A, Citerio G. [Role of assisted breathing in severe traumatic brain injury]. Minerva Anestesiol. 2002;68:278–284.
38. MacIntyre NR, Cook D, Ely EWJ, et al. Evidence-based guidelines for weaning and discontinuing ventilatory support. Chest. 2003;120:375S–95S.
39. Boles J-M, Bion J, Connors A, et al. Weaning from mechanical ventilation. Eur Respir J. 2007;29:1033–56.
40. Asehnoune K, Mrozek S, Perrigault PF, et al. A multi-faceted strategy to reduce ventilation-associated mortality in brain-injured patients. The BI-VILI project: a nationwide quality improvement project. Intensive Care Med. 2017;43:957–70.
41. Navalesi P, Frigerio P, Moretti MP, et al. Rate of reintubation in mechanically ventilated neurosurgical and neurologic patients: evaluation of a systematic approach to weaning and extubation. Crit Care Med. 2008;36:2986–92.
42. Esperanza JA, Pelosi P, Blanch L. What's new in intensive care: tracheostomy-what is known and what remains to be determined. Intensive Care Med. 2019;45:1619–21.
43. McCredie VA, Alali AS, Scales DC, et al. Effect of early versus late tracheostomy or prolonged intubation in critically ill patients with acute brain injury: a systematic review and meta-analysis. Neurocrit Care. 2017;26:14–25.
44. Gessler F, Mutlak H, Lamb S, et al. The impact of tracheostomy timing on clinical outcome and adverse events in poor-grade subarachnoid hemorrhage. Crit Care Med. 2015;43:2429–38.
45. Bösel J, Schiller P, Hook Y, et al. Stroke-related early tracheostomy versus prolonged orotracheal intubation in neurocritical care trial (SETPOINT): a randomized pilot trial. Stroke. 2013;44:21–8.
46. Qureshi MSS, Shad ZS, Shoaib F, et al. Early versus late tracheostomy after decompressive craniectomy. Cureus. 2018;10:e3699.

47. Reinprecht A, Greher M, Wolfsberger S, Dietrich W, Illievich UM, Gruber A. Prone position in subarachnoid hemorrhage patients with acute respiratory distress syndrome: effects on cerebral tissue oxygenation and intracranial pressure. Crit Care Med. 2003;31:1831–8.
48. Roth C, Ferbert A, Deinsberger W, et al. Does prone positioning increase intracranial pressure? A retrospective analysis of patients with acute brain injury and acute respiratory failure. Neurocrit Care. 2014;21:186–91.
49. Combes A, Hajage D, Capellier G, et al. Extracorporeal membrane oxygenation for severe acute respiratory distress syndrome. N Engl J Med. 2018;378:1965–75.
50. Robba C, Ortu A, Bilotta F, et al. Extracorporeal membrane oxygenation for adult respiratory distress syndrome in trauma patients: a case series and systematic literature review. J Trauma Acute Care Surg. 2017;82:165–73.

Manifestations of Critical Illness Brain Injury

35

S. Williams Roberson, E. W. Ely, and J. E. Wilson

35.1 Introduction

Critical illness brain injury is an acute disorder of consciousness and/or one or more cognitive or psychomotor domains (e.g., attention, perceptual awareness, or volition) and is common among intensive care unit patients [1]. Such injury is associated with increased intensive care unit (ICU)-related morbidity and mortality as well as long-term cognitive impairment. Commonly recognized manifestations of critical illness brain injury include delirium and coma, but recent work has shed light on a third form of brain dysfunction that may be seen in the ICU: catatonia. This chapter describes these three manifestations of critical illness brain injury and provides a conceptual framework for their distinct but potentially overlapping presentations in ICU patients. Underlying pathophysiology, assessment, and management recommendations are provided, and areas of future research are discussed.

35.2 Delirium

Delirium is the most common form of acute brain dysfunction in the ICU and is manifested by inattention, disorientation, altered arousal, changes in cognition, and at times abnormalities in thought and perception [2]. Around 70% of patients on mechanical ventilation will experience delirium during their critical illness and almost a third of days in the ICU are days spent with delirium [3]. Delirium is characterized by motor abnormalities, including hypoactive (decreased movement and decreased arousal), hyperactive (increased movement and agitation), and mixed (exhibiting features of both motor subtypes that may fluctuate) presentations [4]. The hypoactive form predominates (perhaps due to prompt treatment of hyperactive patients with sedation, etc.); however it is underdiagnosed and is associated with worse outcomes [5].

35.2.1 Pathophysiology and Etiologic Considerations

Risk factors for the development of delirium include, but are not limited to, older age, preexisting dementia, hypertension, pre-ICU emergency surgery or trauma, elevated Acute Physiology and Chronic Health Evaluation (APACHE)-II score, mechanical ventilation, metabolic acidosis, delirium on the prior day, coma, and use of certain medications, including benzodiazepines and anticholinergic medications among others [6, 7]. Distinct etiologic mechanisms leading to the development of delirium remain unknown; however preliminary evidence suggests neural disconnectivity of the dorsolateral prefrontal cortex and the posterior cingulate cortex as well as reversible reduction of functional connectivity of subcortical regions [8]. Neuroinflammation leading to hippocampal and extra-hippocampal dysfunction may also contribute to the development of delirium [8]; however, given the heterogeneous phenotype, there may be several neurobiological mechanisms contributing to its development instead of one distinct causal pathway.

35.2.2 Assessment of Delirium During Critical Illness

The gold standard for assessment of delirium is a full psychiatric interview according to Diagnostic and Statistical Manual of Mental Disorders (DSM)-5 criteria [2]. This is impractical, however, as a screening tool in the ICU due to the high prevalence of this disorder, the length of time and expertise required to conduct a thorough DSM-5 evaluation and the acute nature of medical care making an exhaustive evaluation over-burdensome for the critically ill patient. In the critical care setting, the most widely used instrument to screen for delirium is the Confusion Assessment Method for the ICU (CAM-ICU). In a recent meta-analysis, the CAM-ICU (969 patients from nine studies) had a pooled sensitivity of 80.0% (95% confidence interval [CI] 77.1–82.6%), and the pooled specificity was 95.9% (95% CI 94.8–96.8%) [9].

35.2.3 Management

Antipsychotic medications have historically been the treatment of choice for delirium; however recent findings suggest that haloperidol (a typical antipsychotic) and ziprasidone (an atypical antipsychotic) have no effect on the duration of delirium in the ICU [10]. Despite these findings, these medications may still have an indication for psychotic symptoms (delusions, hallucinations, and agitation) secondary to critical illness delirium, although further research is needed. Delirium is characterized by alterations in the sleep/wake cycle; therefore melatonin (hormone released by the pineal gland with a key role in circadian rhythm regulation) or ramelteon (melatonin receptor agonist) may have a role in the treatment or prevention of delirium [11, 12]. Non-pharmacological interventions such as adherence to the ABCDEF (*A*ssess, prevent, and manage pain; *B*oth spontaneous awakening and breathing trials; *C*hoice of analgesia and sedation; *D*elirium assess, prevent, and manage; *E*arly mobility and exercise; *F*amily engagement/empowerment) bundle have shown the greatest effectiveness in reducing delirium occurrence in the ICU [3].

35.2.4 Prognosis

Delirium is known to be independently predictive of increased in-hospital and post-discharge mortality, new-onset dementia akin to an Alzheimer's-type dementia, depression, post-traumatic stress disorder (PTSD), longer length of stay in the hospital, new institutionalization at discharge, inability to return to work, and increased cost of care, amongst others [13–17]. Profound brain volume loss and white matter disruptions in survivors of critical illness may help to explain newfound dementia [18] although the exact neuropathologic insults underlying these cognitive and functional changes remain a mystery.

35.2.5 Summary

Delirium is the most commonly identified form of critical illness brain dysfunction, characterized by inattention, disorientation, altered arousal, and cognitive changes. The wide variety of risk factors and motoric subtypes suggest that there may be several neurobiological mechanisms. The CAM-ICU is the most widely used and best-validated screening method in the ICU. Management relies heavily on avoidance of risk factors and implementation of established protocols based on the

ABCDEF bundle. More work is needed to understand this disorder, its association with long-term cognitive decline, and its pathophysiologic relationship with other forms of critical illness brain injury.

35.3 Coma

From the Greek κῶμα, meaning "deep sleep" or "trance," coma is characterized by closed eyes and unresponsiveness, with absence of any appropriate response to even the most vigorous stimulation [19]. Patients in coma do not localize stimuli or make any defensive movements in response to painful stimuli, although they may grimace or demonstrate stereotyped posturing. Interestingly, grimacing and stereotyped posturing are also features of catatonia, although the stereotypical posturing in canonical forms of coma is characterized by dystonic flexion or extension of the extremities in response to noxious stimuli. Sudden coma is a neurologic emergency—it indicates acute onset of one or more potentially fatal but possibly reversible conditions resulting in severe impairment of brain activity.

35.3.1 Pathophysiology and Etiologic Considerations

Coma is a disorder of profoundly impaired arousal and, possibly as a by-product, awareness. The presence of coma in a patient indicates dysfunction of one or more components of brain networks mediating the intrinsic ability to maintain and regulate a state of alertness. These networks include several brainstem nuclei, most notably the reticular activating system of the pons and ventral medulla [20] as well as their projections to the midbrain reticular formation, thalamic intralaminar nucleus, dorsal hypothalamus, and basal forebrain [21, 22]. These subcortical and brainstem structures interact with each other and with the cortex in a complex interplay of activation and inhibition, mediated by several neurotransmitters including acetylcholine, gamma-aminobutyric acid (GABA), glutamate, dopamine, and serotonin [23]. Coma in the critical care setting may thus result from focal disruption of brainstem or subcortical arousal networks or from widespread disruption of cortical activity.

35.3.2 Assessment of Coma During Critical Illness

One of the oldest measures of the level of consciousness in common clinical use today is the Glasgow Coma Scale (GCS). The GCS grades quality of eye opening (4 points), verbal responses (5 points), and motor responses (6 points) to auditory and tactile stimuli. It was initially validated for assessment and prognostication after traumatic brain injury (TBI) [24]. The Full Outline of UnResponsiveness (FOUR) Score is another well-validated scale that is based on eye responses, motor responses, brainstem reflexes, and respiratory patterns [25]. Compared to the GCS, the FOUR Score has the advantage of avoiding dependence on verbal responses, and thus is not confounded by the inability to speak (e.g., due to intubation). The Richmond Agitation–Sedation Scale (RASS) is a 10-point scale ranging from −5 (coma) to +4 (severely agitated) with 0 being normal. The RASS differs from the GCS and FOUR Score in two aspects: (1) the RASS focuses on arousal and does not require intact comprehension or command following to obtain a normal score; and (2) the RASS also includes values indicating hyperarousal or agitation. This scale is well validated as a monitoring tool to guide sedative titration and to evaluate agitation in the adult ICU.

There are several other scales published for monitoring the level of sedation in the ICU or intraoperatively, e.g., the Ramsay Sedation Scale, the Riker Sedation-Agitation Scale, the Motor Activity Assessment Scale, and the University of Michigan Sedation Scale. These can be used to assess the level of consciousness but do not include multiple levels indicating deeper stages of coma.

Electroencephalography (EEG) is a useful and easily accessible technology to assess for potential etiologies of coma and rule out locked-in syndrome, an infrequent but important mimic of coma that is characterized by profound motor impairment with preserved sensory awareness. EEG patterns most commonly seen in coma include burst suppression, very low voltage or discontinuous activity, generalized periodic discharges (with or without triphasic morphology), and absence of reactivity. Electrographic seizures or status epilepticus can also be recorded in patients unresponsive to external stimuli and suggest a potential epileptic etiology for the coma.

35.3.3 Management

Initial management of the comatose patient involves stabilization. Airway protection, assurance of hemodynamic stability, and respiratory support are potentially lifesaving measures in the minutes to hours after onset of coma. Physical examination should screen for signs of trauma and focal neurologic deficits. Early laboratory studies should include blood glucose measurement, electrocardiogram, complete blood count, comprehensive metabolic panel, and brain computerized tomography (CT) scan. Additional evaluations, such as cerebrospinal fluid (CSF) studies, EEG, and/or brain magnetic resonance imaging (MRI), should be guided by the clinical history and examination. Treatment in the acute phase largely consists of addressing the underlying etiology and minimizing risks of adverse neurologic sequelae, e.g., resuscitation and targeted temperature management (TTM) in the case of cardiac arrest.

Subsequent management is guided by the differential diagnosis and risk of complications. In general it is important to avoid medications that may confound the coma assessment such as sedatives or other central nervous system (CNS) suppressants. Some advocate for standard pain management during procedures, given that 15–40% of patients deemed comatose may yet be aware of their surroundings but may be unable to mount a motor response sufficient to express suffering. Nevertheless, global sedatives and anxiolytics may augment coma and worsen outcome; thus local or regional anesthetics is preferred where possible.

Patients in prolonged unresponsive states are at high risk for skin breakdown, musculoskeletal injury, and neuromuscular dysfunction due to disuse and inability to spontaneously adjust their position. Nursing and respiratory care with frequent turning and attention to positioning are crucial to limit such injury. Finally, in the patient with prolonged coma, no spontaneous sleep/wake cycles, and absence of brainstem reflexes in the context of a known devastating intracerebral insult, brain death evaluation may be considered.

35.3.4 Prognosis

In general, coma portends worse prognosis in the critically ill population. Depth and duration of TBI-induced coma are predictors of functional status at 3 months post-injury. Lower GCS score at presentation is associated with increased in-hospital mortality in non-trauma patients as well [26]. Clinical signs of coma after cardiac arrest strongly predict death or poor neurologic outcome [27]. Mechanically ventilated patients with burst suppression (an EEG-based measure consistent with coma) are twice as likely to die by 6 months post-discharge as those without burst suppression [28]. The trajectory of level of arousal and interaction with the environment also informs prognosis. Serial assessment is important, as is an exhaustive search for and remediation of reversible contributing factors.

35.3.5 Summary

Coma is a condition of profoundly impaired arousal and unresponsiveness to even the most vigorous stimuli. Diverse etiologies can lead to disruption of the ascending reticular activating system and subcortical arousal networks, or diffuse cortical dysfunction, or both. Regular assessment using a standardized scale is a key component of monitoring. EEG can assist with assessment and help rule out locked-in syndrome, a rare but important mimic. Coma is generally associated with poorer ICU outcomes. Its acute presentation requires emergent stabilization, identification and management of potential etiologies, and mitigation of risk factors.

35.4 Catatonia

Catatonia is a syndrome of psychomotor abnormalities (decreased, increased, and abnormal motor behaviors such as waxy flexibility and echo phenomenon) and volition (or will). Catatonia has historically been linked with schizophrenia; however more recently it has been described in patients with severe mood and general medical disorders.

35.4.1 Pathophysiology and Etiologic Considerations

The prevalence of catatonia, in acute inpatient psychiatric settings, has ranged from 9% to 18% [29, 30]. Work by Abrams and Taylor has suggested a higher prevalence in patients with primary mood disorders, with up to 20% of patients with bipolar disorder exhibiting catatonic signs [31, 32]. Up to 10% of the general medical population may exhibit catatonic signs during their acute hospitalization [33] with catatonia manifesting as a feature of many general medical conditions [33–35]. Studies into the prevalence of catatonia on a psychiatric liaison service showed that it was 1.6–8.9% across all medical services, varying across age groups and associated medical conditions [36]. Recent literature has suggested neurobiological and neuroinflammatory hypotheses for the development of catatonia, such as increased neural activity in premotor areas in patients with hypokinetic catatonia [37] and downstream autoimmunity effects of specific actions on extracellular antigens (e.g., as seen in N-methyl-D-aspartate receptor [NMDAR] encephalitis) [38] as potential etiologic theories for catatonia.

35.4.2 Assessment of Catatonia During Critical Illness

Catatonia has increasingly become recognized as a manifestation of acute brain dysfunction in the ICU, although universally it remains underreported, and in critical illness it is generally not a part of routine screening programs [39, 40]. Although classical descriptions of catatonia include depictions of mental status abnormalities consistent with delirium [4], and classical descriptions of delirium include depictions of catatonia [41], modern diagnostic criteria (such as the DSM-5) do not recognize the co-occurrence of delirium and catatonia. In fact, DSM-5 criterion C for catatonia states that "the disturbance (e.g., catatonia) [should] not occur exclusively during the course of a delirium" [2]. Perhaps in part due to this, catatonia has not routinely been screened for or diagnosed in medically ill populations, especially in the critically ill, where the prevalence of delirium is high, thus limiting further research in this area.

The most widely used assessment tool for catatonia is the Bush Francis Catatonia Rating Scale (BFCRS), a 23-item rating scale, which relies on observation, physical exam, and interview of the patient (if possible) [42]. The BFCRS score is calculated from the totaling of individual items (rated 0–3, with higher scores indicating increased severity of that sign). In recent years, some researchers have begun to explore the association between delirium and catatonia, with estimates up to one-third of critically ill patients screening positively for catatonia in the ICU [39, 40,

43]. Among patients with DSM-5 catatonia (≥3 of 12 criterion A signs present) ($n = 46$), 91.3% also screened positive for delirium with the CAM-ICU [44]. Revised cutoff points on the BFCRS have been suggested for use in the critically ill given the phenotypic overlap between delirium and catatonia [44]. Despite our increased appreciation of catatonic signs in critical illness the clinical relevance of the occurrence of catatonia is unknown [39, 40, 43].

35.4.3 Management

Fortunately, for most patients, prompt recognition of catatonia and treatment with anticonvulsant medications (benzodiazepines or barbiturates) or electroconvulsive therapy can be lifesaving, regardless of underling etiology [45–47]; however, there remains general ambiguity as to whether sedative hypnotics can be safety used in a delirious or comatose individual with catatonia, as these medications are associated with the development of delirium [6]. Studies in this area are urgently needed. Additionally, antipsychotics are generally avoided in catatonic individuals especially those with excited or agitated catatonia, given the concern for conversion to neuroleptic malignant syndrome, although data supporting this clinical assumption are lacking.

35.4.4 Prognosis

Catatonia is a potentially lethal condition if left untreated. Its presence puts patients at risk for a variety of medical complications including aspiration, dehydration, malnutrition, contractures, pulmonary embolism, and rhabdomyolysis leading to renal failure [48]. Despite effective treatments, some evidence suggests that patients with catatonia have increased morbidity compared to their counterparts [49, 50]; however, additional studies are needed.

35.4.5 Summary

Catatonia is a common but under-recognized neuropsychiatric manifestation of acute brain dysfunction in the ICU. Catatonia is frequently comorbid with delirium; however the optimal treatment and clinical relevance in this context remain understudied.

35.5 A Conceptual Framework for Manifestations of Critical Illness Brain Injury

Figure 35.1 provides a schematic overview for understanding the interrelations among manifestations of critical illness brain injury. Catatonia, a poorly recognized disorder of psychomotor function, has overlapping features with both delirium

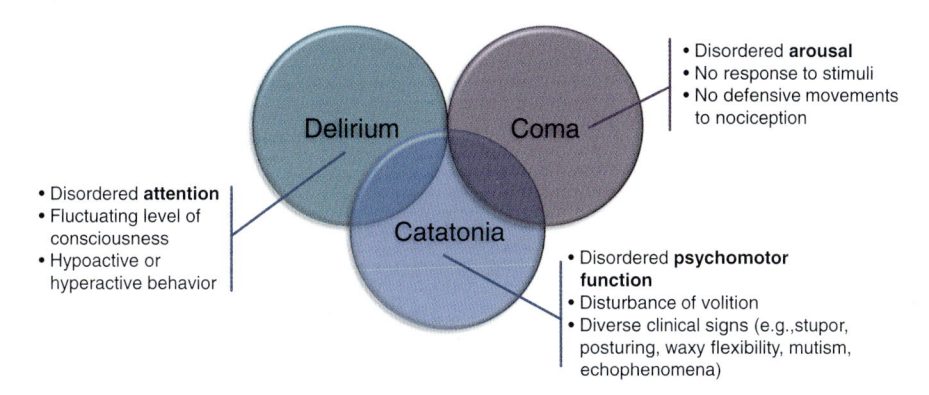

Fig. 35.1 Conceptual schematic of manifestations of critical illness brain injury

(characterized by fluctuating level of arousal and inattention) and coma (characterized by profound hypoarousal and unresponsiveness).

35.6 Conclusion

We present a conceptual framework for understanding critical illness brain injury. Delirium manifests with fluctuating levels of arousal and inability to maintain attention. Coma is characterized by profoundly impaired arousal and absent responses to external stimuli. Catatonia, a recently recognized manifestation of critical illness brain injury, has a variable presentation including diverse psychomotor, behavioral, and emotional disturbances that may overlap with delirium or coma. The key distinctions that help separate the three conditions are abnormal attention and cognition (delirium), depressed consciousness (coma), and profoundly abnormal motor behavior which relies on a physical examination (catatonia). The pathophysiologic mechanisms underlying these syndromes are incompletely understood, but likely include shared components and these three conditions may exist on a spectrum of acute brain dysfunction in the ICU. Given that management approaches differ depending on the clinical presentation (A-F bundle for delirium, reducing risk factors for coma and possibly lorazepam challenge for catatonia with avoidance of antipsychotics), recognition and disambiguation of these syndromes are crucially important. Future studies exploring the natural history and optimal management, especially in cases of ICU-related catatonia, are warranted.

References

1. Girard TD, Dittus RS, Ely EW. Critical illness brain injury. Annu Rev Med. 2016;67:497–513.
2. American Psychiatric Association. Diagnostic and statistical manual of mental disorders. 5th ed. Arlington: American Psychiatric Association Publishing; 2013.
3. Pun BT, Balas MC, Barnes-Daly MA, et al. Caring for critically ill patients with the ABCDEF bundle: results of the ICU Liberation Collaborative in over 15,000 adults. Crit Care Med. 2019;47:3–14.

4. Lipowski ZJ. Transient cognitive disorders (delirium, acute confusional states) in the elderly. Am J Psychiatry. 1983;140:1426–36.
5. Han JH, Wilber ST. Altered mental status in older patients in the emergency department. Clin Geriatr Med. 2013;29:101–36.
6. Pandharipande P, Shintani A, Peterson J, et al. Lorazepam is an independent risk factor for transitioning to delirium in intensive care unit patients. Anesthesiology. 2006;104:21–6.
7. Inouye SK. Predisposing and precipitating factors for delirium in hospitalized older patients. Dement Geriatr Cogn Disord. 1999;10:393–400.
8. Cascella M, Bimonte S. The role of general anesthetics and the mechanisms of hippocampal and extra-hippocampal dysfunctions in the genesis of postoperative cognitive dysfunction. Neural Regen Res. 2017;12:1780–5.
9. Gusmao-Flores D, Salluh JI, Chalhub RA, Quarantini LC. The confusion assessment method for the intensive care unit (CAM-ICU) and intensive care delirium screening checklist (ICDSC) for the diagnosis of delirium: a systematic review and meta-analysis of clinical studies. Crit Care. 2012;16:R115.
10. Girard TD, Exline MC, Carson SS, et al. Haloperidol and ziprasidone for treatment of delirium in critical illness. N Engl J Med. 2018;379:2506–16.
11. Baumgartner L, Lam K, Lai J, et al. Effectiveness of melatonin for the prevention of intensive care unit delirium. Pharmacotherapy. 2019;39:280–7.
12. Hatta K, Kishi Y, Wada K, et al. Preventive effects of ramelteon on delirium: a randomized placebo-controlled trial. JAMA Psychiat. 2014;71:397–403.
13. Milbrandt EB, Deppen S, Harrison PL, et al. Costs associated with delirium in mechanically ventilated patients. Crit Care Med. 2004;32:955–62.
14. Ely EW, Shintani A, Truman B, et al. Delirium as a predictor of mortality in mechanically ventilated patients in the intensive care unit. JAMA. 2004;291:1753–62.
15. Ely EW, Gautam S, Margolin R, et al. The impact of delirium in the intensive care unit on hospital length of stay. Intensive Care Med. 2001;27:1892–900.
16. Pandharipande PP, Girard TD, Jackson JC, et al. Long-term cognitive impairment after critical illness. N Engl J Med. 2013;369:1306–16.
17. Girard TD, Jackson JC, Pandharipande PP, et al. Delirium as a predictor of long-term cognitive impairment in survivors of critical illness. Crit Care Med. 2010;38:1513–20.
18. Morandi A, Rogers BP, Gunther ML, et al. The relationship between delirium duration, white matter integrity, and cognitive impairment in intensive care unit survivors as determined by diffusion tensor imaging: the VISIONS prospective cohort magnetic resonance imaging study. Crit Care Med. 2012;40:2182–9.
19. Posner JB, Saper CB, Schiff ND, Plum F. Plum and Posner's diagnosis of stupor and coma. 4th ed. Oxford: Oxford University Press; 2007.
20. Moruzzi G, Magoun HW. Brain stem reticular formation and activation of the EEG. Electroencephalogr Clin Neurophysiol. 1949;1:455–73.
21. Parvizi J, Damasio AR. Neuroanatomical correlates of brainstem coma. Brain. 2003;126(Pt 7):1524–36.
22. Fuller PM, Sherman D, Pedersen NP, Saper CB, Lu J. Reassessment of the structural basis of the ascending arousal system. J Comp Neurol. 2011;519:933–56.
23. McClenathan BM, Thakor NV, Hoesch RE. Pathophysiology of acute coma and disorders of consciousness: considerations for diagnosis and management. Semin Neurol. 2013;33:91–109.
24. Teasdale G, Jennett B. Assessment and prognosis of coma after head injury. Acta Neurochir. 1976;34:45–55.
25. Iyer VN, Mandrekar JN, Danielson RD, Zubkov AY, Elmer JL, Wijdicks EF. Validity of the FOUR score coma scale in the medical intensive care unit. Mayo Clin Proc. 2009;84:694–701.
26. Bastos PG, Sun X, Wagner DP, Wu AW, Knaus WA. Glasgow Coma Scale score in the evaluation of outcome in the intensive care unit: findings from the Acute Physiology and Chronic Health Evaluation III study. Crit Care Med. 1993;21:1459–65.
27. Booth CM, Boone RH, Tomlinson G, Detsky AS. Is this patient dead, vegetative, or severely neurologically impaired? Assessing outcome for comatose survivors of cardiac arrest. JAMA. 2004;291:870–9.

28. Watson PL, Shintani AK, Tyson R, Pandharipande PP, Pun BT, Ely EW. Presence of electroencephalogram burst suppression in sedated, critically ill patients is associated with increased mortality. Crit Care Med. 2008;36:3171–7.
29. Rosebush PI, Hildebrand AM, Furlong BG, Mazurek MF. Catatonic syndrome in a general psychiatric inpatient population: frequency, clinical presentation, and response to lorazepam. J Clin Psychiatry. 1990;51:357–62.
30. Lee JW, Schwartz DL, Hallmayer J. Catatonia in a psychiatric intensive care facility: incidence and response to benzodiazepines. Ann Clin Psychiatry. 2000;12:89–96.
31. Abrams R, Taylor MA. Catatonia. A prospective clinical study. Arch Gen Psychiatry. 1976;33:579–81.
32. Taylor MA, Abrams R. Catatonia. Prevalence and importance in the manic phase of manic-depressive illness. Arch Gen Psychiatry. 1977;34:1223–5.
33. Morrison JR. Catatonia: diagnosis and management. Hosp Community Psychiatry. 1975;26:91–4.
34. Fink M, Taylor MA. Catatonia: A clinician's guide to diagnosis and treatment. 1st ed. Cambridge: Cambridge University Press; 2003.
35. Gelenberg AJ. The catatonic syndrome. Lancet. 1976;1:1339–41.
36. Jaimes-Albornoz W, Serra-Mestres J. Prevalence and clinical correlations of catatonia in older adults referred to a liaison psychiatry service in a general hospital. Gen Hosp Psychiatry. 2013;35:512–6.
37. Walther S, Stegmayer K, Wilson JE, Heckers S. Structure and neural mechanisms of catatonia. Lancet Psychiatry. 2019;6:610–9.
38. Rogers JP, Pollak TA, Blackman G, David AS. Catatonia and the immune system: a review. Lancet Psychiatry. 2019;6:620–30.
39. Saddawi-Konefka D, Berg SM, Nejad SH, Bittner EA. Catatonia in the ICU: an important and underdiagnosed cause of altered mental status. A case series and review of the literature∗. Crit Care Med. 2014;42:e234–41.
40. Grover S, Ghosh A, Ghormode D. Do patients of delirium have catatonic features? An exploratory study. Psychiatry Clin Neurosci. 2014;68:644–51.
41. Aurelianus C. On Acute Diseases and on Chronic Diseases. Edited and translated by IE Drabkin. Chicago, University of Chicago Press, 1950.
42. Bush G, Fink M, Petrides G, Dowling F, Francis A. Catatonia. I. Rating scale and standardized examination. Acta Psychiatr Scand. 1996;93:129–36.
43. Quinn DK. "Burn catatonia": a case report and literature review. J Burn Care Res. 2014;35:e135–42.
44. Wilson JE, Carlson R, Duggan MC, et al. Delirium and catatonia in critically ill patients: The Delirium and Catatonia Prospective Cohort Investigation. Crit Care Med. 2017;45:1837–44.
45. Bush G, Fink M, Petrides G, Dowling F, Francis A. Catatonia. II. Treatment with lorazepam and electroconvulsive therapy. Acta Psychiatr Scand. 1996;93:137–43.
46. Schmider J, Standhart H, Deuschle M, Drancoli J, Heuser I. A double-blind comparison of lorazepam and oxazepam in psychomotor retardation and mutism. Biol Psychiatry. 1999;46:437–41.
47. England ML, Ongur D, Konopaske GT, Karmacharya R. Catatonia in psychotic patients: clinical features and treatment response. J Neuropsychiatry Clin Neurosci. 2011;23:223–6.
48. Levenson J. Medical aspects of catatonia. Prime Psychiatry. 2009;16:23–6.
49. Cornic F, Consoli A, Tanguy ML, et al. Association of adolescent catatonia with increased mortality and morbidity: evidence from a prospective follow-up study. Schizophr Res. 2009;113:233–40.
50. McCall WV, Mann SC, Shelp FE, Caroff SN. Fatal pulmonary embolism in the catatonic syndrome: two case reports and a literature review. J Clin Psychiatry. 1995;56:21–5.

has become easily applicable also by neurointensivists, in part due to the development of more user-friendly devices. These three components represent the concept of essential noninvasive multimodality neuromonitoring, which we describe in this chapter.

36.2 Automated Pupillometry

One of the most important parameters to evaluate when performing a clinical neurological examination of the brain stem reflexes is the pupillary light reflex. The pupil constricts when the light signal is carried to the tectal plate in the midbrain, then to the Edinger-Westphal nucleus, and then to the eye where it causes the motor fibers to contract, visualized clinically by pupil constriction. The pupillary light reflex, along with size and size differences between pupils (anisocoria), provides information regarding the functional status of both the optic and the oculomotor nerves.

Until recently, evaluation of the pupils was performed through simple observation of the pupil's reaction to light evoked by flashlights. Similarly, the pupil's diameter and anisocoria were assessed by an approximate estimation. However, manual examination of the pupillary light reflex is subject to large inter-examiner discrepancies, as high as 40%, particularly when miosis is present. The discrepancy may be further increased in the presence of other confounding factors such as alcohol, drugs, or hypothermia [1]. Couret et al. observed an error rate of 20% and a 50% failure rate in the detection of anisocoria even for pupils of an intermediate size (2–4 mm) [2]. Larson et al. demonstrated that there was a complete failure in detecting the pupillary light reflex when manual examination was performed when the reflex amplitude was <0.3 mm [3]. The examiner would score the initial diameter of the pupil, followed by light stimulation. Reactivity was described as present or absent, or briskly reactive versus sluggishly reactive.

Recently, automated infrared pupillometry has been introduced into clinical practice, quickly gaining popularity due to its quantitative precision, low cost, noninvasiveness, bedside applicability, and easy-to-use technology, contributing to a modern precision-oriented approach to medicine. With the event of this new technology, it is now possible to add important prognostic and diagnostic information to clinical practice when dealing with the patient with brain injury of various origins.

A few devices are available on the market and are composed of an infrared light-emitting diode, a digital camera that captures the outer border of the iris and senses the reflected infrared light, a data processor, and a screen display showing measured variables in response to the light stimulation, in both a numerical and a graphical format (Fig. 36.1). The measured variables are size, asymmetry, constriction change to light stimulation, latency, and constriction and dilation velocity. The average reported values are shown in Table 36.1.

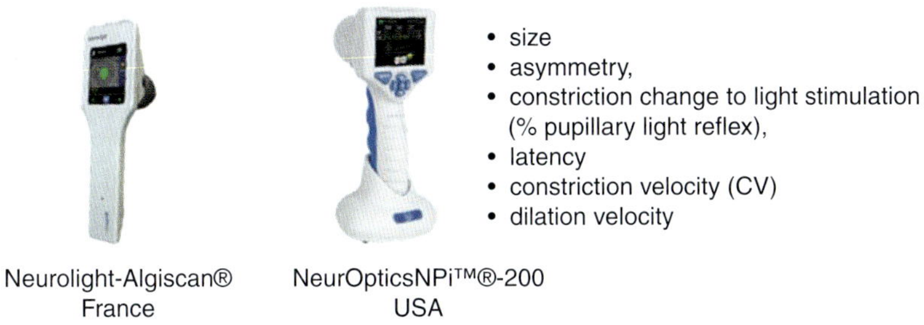

- size
- asymmetry,
- constriction change to light stimulation (% pupillary light reflex),
- latency
- constriction velocity (CV)
- dilation velocity

Neurolight-Algiscan® France

NeurOpticsNPi™®-200 USA

Fig. 36.1 Examples of the automated infrared pupillometry devices available on the market

Table 36.1 Parameters provided by manufacturers of two automated infrared pupillometry devices: *Neuroptics NPi-200 and **NeuroLight-Algiscan

Type of stimulation	Parameters	Normal values
Pupil constriction to light	Diameter (mm)	<0.5 mm
	Asymmetry (mm)	<0.5 mm
	% Pupillary constriction to light (%PLR)	35–40%
	Latency (s)	
	Constriction velocity (mm/s)	1.5 mm/s (<1 mm/s: pathological)
	Dilation velocity (mm/s)	2.83
	Neurological pupillary index (NPi)*	≥3
Pupil dilation to pain	Pupillary dilation reflex (%)**	33
	Pupillary pain index**	Depends on intensity of stimulation [16–19]

PLR pupillary light reflex

36.2.1 Prognosis Following Cardiac Arrest

Clinicians have been checking the pupils of patients with suspected or known brain injury or impaired consciousness for over 100 years. The use of the automated pupillary light reflex has been applied in various forms of brain injury for both prognostic and diagnostic reasons. Its use as a prognostic tool has been mostly studied in the comatose post-cardiac arrest patient. Rossetti et al. showed that bilateral absence of the standard manual pupillary light reflex at day 3 following cardiac arrest was a strong predictor of poor outcome [4]. However, these patients may be under opioid sedation and the pupillary light reflex may be subject to confounding effects, therefore reducing the prognostic accuracy.

Behrends et al. [5] were the first to show that quantitative pupillometry had strong prognostic predictive value during cardiopulmonary resuscitation (CPR) in in-hospital cardiac arrest patients and strong correlations between return to spontaneous circulation and quantitative pupillary were also demonstrated by Yokobori et al. [6]. Pupillometry has been shown to be equally accurate in predicting poor 1-year outcome compared to absent reactivity on the EEG and bilaterally absent N20 waves on SSEPs [5, 6].

One multicenter study recently compared quantitative automated pupillary light reflex and neurological pupillary index (NPi; using the NeurOptics NPi-200, NeurOptics, Laguna Hills, CA) to manual pupillary light reflex in comatose cardiac arrest patients and found that an NPi ≤2, performed between days 1 and 3 following cardiac arrest, was 100% specific for an unfavorable 3-month neurological outcome when compared to manual pupillary light reflex [7].

36.2.2 Traumatic Brain Injury

Pupillary light reactivity is a well-described prognostic variable in the setting of severe head injury. The literature is full of evidence demonstrating that alterations of the pupillary light reflex, pupil size, and/or anisocoria are correlated with outcome following traumatic brain injury (TBI) [8]. In fact, neurosurgeons triage patients to surgical evacuation of mass lesions or conservative therapy according to the pupillary status [9]. It has also been shown that patients who undergo prompt treatment after a new pupil abnormality, whether it be medical or surgical, have a better outcome [3].

In patients with acute traumatic epidural hematoma and Glasgow Coma Scale (GCS) score <8, anisocoria was present in 67% of patients and reducing the surgery interval to <90 min was associated with a better outcome [10]. TBI patients with a GCS = 3 and fixed, dilated pupils had no chance of survival, whereas patients with a GCS = 3 with pupils that were not fixed or dilated had an excellent survival rate [11]. Intracranial hypertension is associated with decreased NPi, and patients with elevated ICP had an improvement in NPi values after treatment with osmotic therapy. Therefore, pupillometry has the potential as a noninvasive tool to assess the efficacy of osmotic therapy [12].

Stevens et al. performed a prospective observational study on 40 patients with TBI requiring invasive ICP monitoring and showed a weak relationship between ICP events and a preceding NPi event. The strength of this trend appeared to diminish post-decompressive surgery [13]. Jahns et al. assessed 54 patients with severe TBI with abnormal lesions on head computed tomography (CT) imaging who underwent parenchymal ICP monitoring and repeated NPi assessment through four consecutive measurements over intervals of 6 h prior to sustained elevated ICP >20 mmHg and found that episodes of elevated ICP correlated with a concomitant decrease in NPi. Sustained abnormal NPi was in turn associated with a more complicated ICP course and worse outcome [14].

Vassilieva et al. assessed the feasibility of automated pupillometry for the detection of command following in patients with altered consciousness. They enrolled 20 healthy volunteers and 48 patients with a wide range of neurological disorders who were asked to engage in mental arithmetic [15]. Fourteen of 20 (70%) healthy volunteers and 17 of 43 (39.5%) neurological patients fulfilled pre-specified criteria for command following by showing pupillary dilations during 4 or 5 arithmetic tasks.

None of the five sedated and unconscious ICU patients passed this threshold. Therefore, automated infrared pupillometry combined with mental arithmetic appears to be a promising paradigm for the detection of covert consciousness in unresponsive patients with brain injury and may have potential in the future of providing a tool that can reveal covert consciousness in patients in whom standard investigations have failed to detect signs of consciousness (Fig. 36.2).

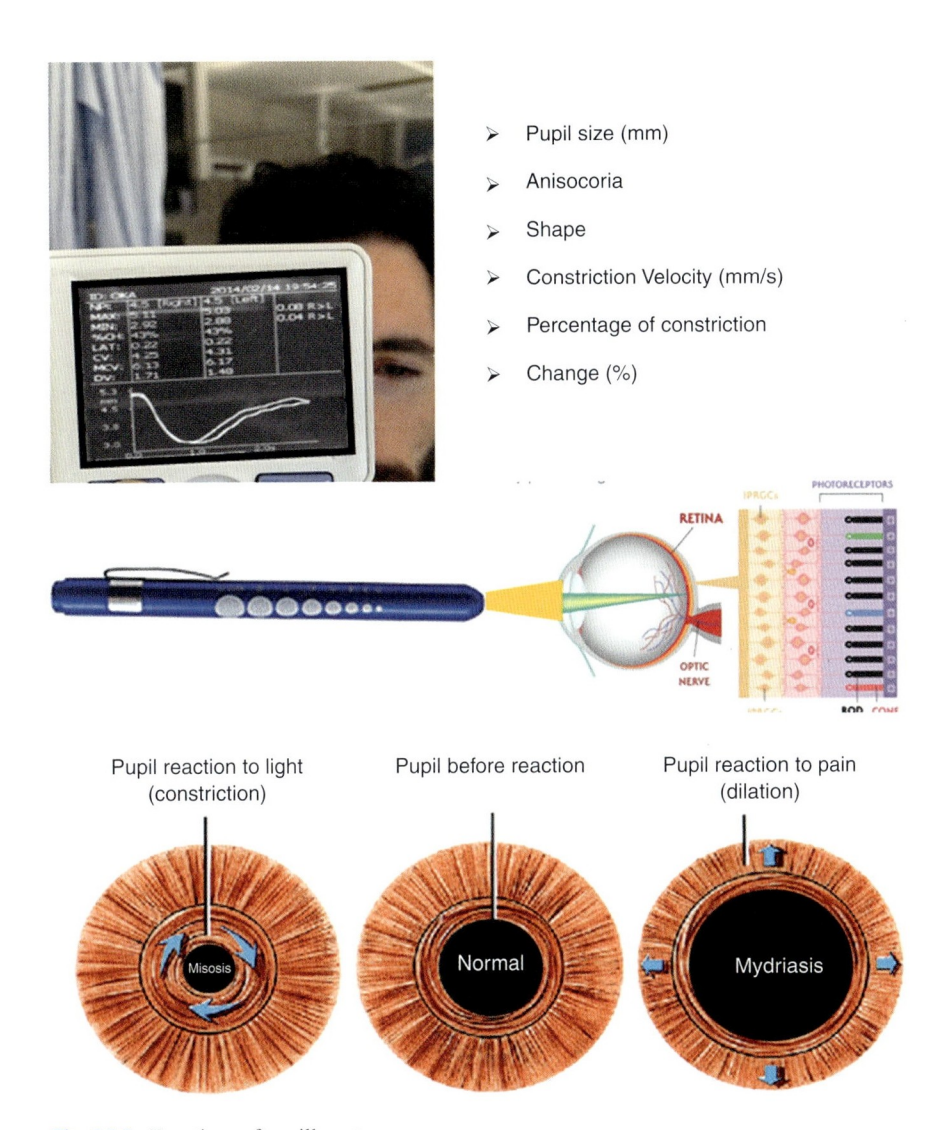

➢ Pupil size (mm)
➢ Anisocoria
➢ Shape
➢ Constriction Velocity (mm/s)
➢ Percentage of constriction
➢ Change (%)

Fig. 36.2 Functions of pupillometry

36.2.3 Pain Assessment in Unconscious Patients

Objective nociceptive assessment and optimal pain management have gained increasing attention and adequate nociceptive monitoring remains challenging in noncommunicative, critically ill adults. In the intensive care unit (ICU), routine nociceptive evaluation in mechanically ventilated patients is usually carried out through scales such as the Behavior Pain Scale (BPS). However, this assessment is limited by medication use (e.g., neuromuscular blocking agents) and the inherent subjective character of nociceptive evaluation by third parties.

Since pupillary reflexes are submitted to controlled regulation by the autonomic nervous system, pupillometry allows the assessment of pain in patients subjected to painful stimulation. In fact, pupillary constriction is mediated by the parasympathetic system, whereas dilation is mediated by the noradrenergic sympathetic fibers that are under the influence of stimuli, including stress and pain. A painful stimulus would typically evoke a pupillary dilation reflex. The potential for application of pupillometry for pain evaluation becomes even greater when dealing with the unconscious patient, during general anesthesia for example, where pain assessment scores have no value. Several studies have suggested the use of pupillometry in noncommunicative ICU adults. Paulus et al. demonstrated that pupillary dilation reflex evaluation may predict analgesia requirements during endotracheal aspiration [16]. Moreover, this method may be able to reveal different levels of analgesia and could have discriminatory properties regarding different types of noxious procedures [17]. Recently, scientific interest has been directed toward the use of specific protocols for pupillary dilation reflex assessment because of their low stimulation currents. The pupillary pain index protocol suggested in our approach has been previously investigated in anesthetized adults, revealing a significant correlation between pupillary dilation reflex and opioid administration [18]. Furthermore, Sabourdin et al. demonstrated that pupillary dilation reflex can be used to guide individual intraoperative remifentanil administration and therefore reduce intraoperative opioid consumption and postoperative rescue analgesia requirements [19].

36.3 Brain Ultrasound

Bedside ultrasonography is becoming increasingly widespread in modern medicine, especially in the intensive care setting where this kind of resource is easily accessible and always available to physicians. Brain ultrasonography is a safe, noninvasive way to assess brain anatomy, pathology, and intracranial blood flow. Transcranial Doppler was first introduced in 1982 by Aaslid et al. to record flow velocity in basal cerebral arteries [20]. Advances in technology introduced transcranial color-coded duplex ultrasonography which allows us to assess anatomical features of the brain, rather than just identify brain vessels blindly.

Brain ultrasonography can be applied in different settings, even outside of neurosurgical ICUs: stroke units, enabling physicians to assess the effectiveness of a fibrinolytic therapy, and operating rooms for monitoring CBF during carotid vascular surgery are just some examples of its potential.

Despite being less reliable compared to CT scans and magnetic resonance imaging (MRI), transcranial color-coded duplex ultrasonography is a useful tool to monitor intracranial lesions, such as hematomas, which might cause a midline shift. It might even enable the clinician to assess the ventricles and parenchyma in selected patients with a good acoustic window [21].

36.3.1 Different Approaches

There are four main acoustic windows accessible for brain ultrasonography, usually performed with a 2–2.5 MHz probe (Fig. 36.3):

1. Transtemporal approach: between the tragus and the lateral orbit wall, with the probe marker facing toward the eye. The first landmark is the contralateral skull, which is normally around 15 cm deep. The midbrain (Fig. 36.4 left panel) appears as a hypoechoic shaped heart in the middle of the scan. Once found, the power Doppler can be selected to explore the circle of Willis. This approach is generally used to identify midline shifts (when scanning the third ventricle, which appears as a hypoechoic band between two hyperechoic lines, as shown in Fig. 36.5) and assess blood flow (Fig. 36.6).

Fig. 36.3 Main approaches to transcranial ultrasonography

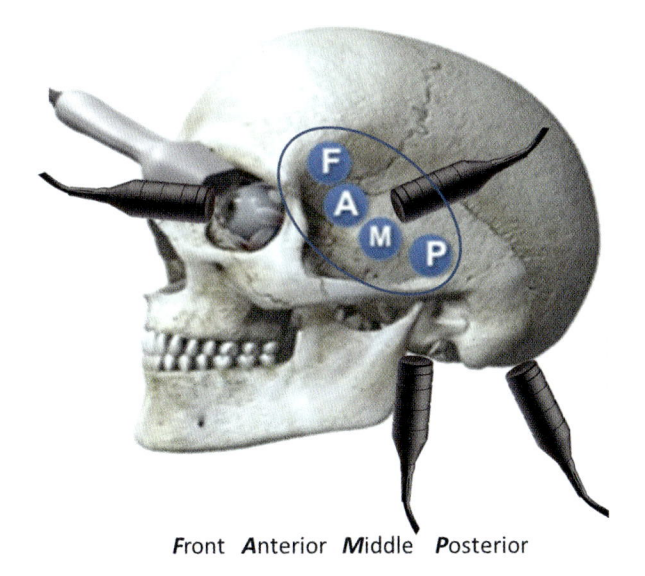

Front Anterior Middle Posterior

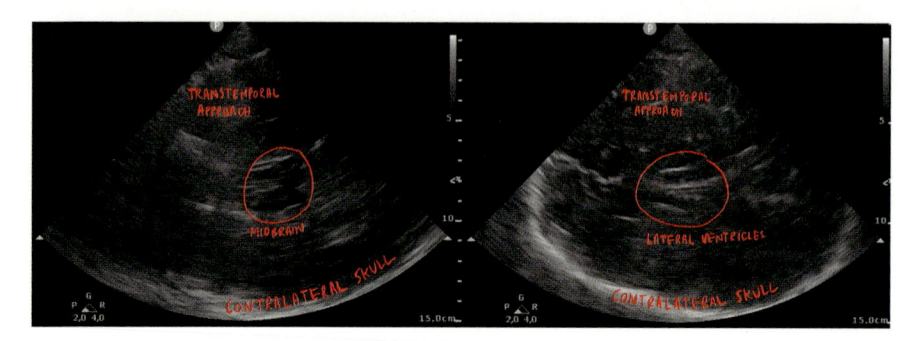

Fig. 36.4 Left panel: Midbrain as the main landmark to explore the circle of Willis; once that is found, the power Doppler can be started to scan for intracranial arteries. Right panel: Lateral ventricles in a severe TBI patient with pronounced midline shift and trans-tentorial herniation

Fig. 36.5 Midline shift in a patient with severe traumatic brain injury. The third ventricle appears as a hypoechoic band between two hyperechoic lines

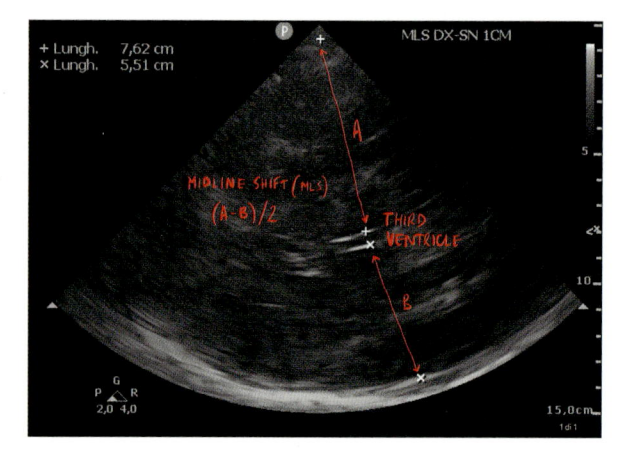

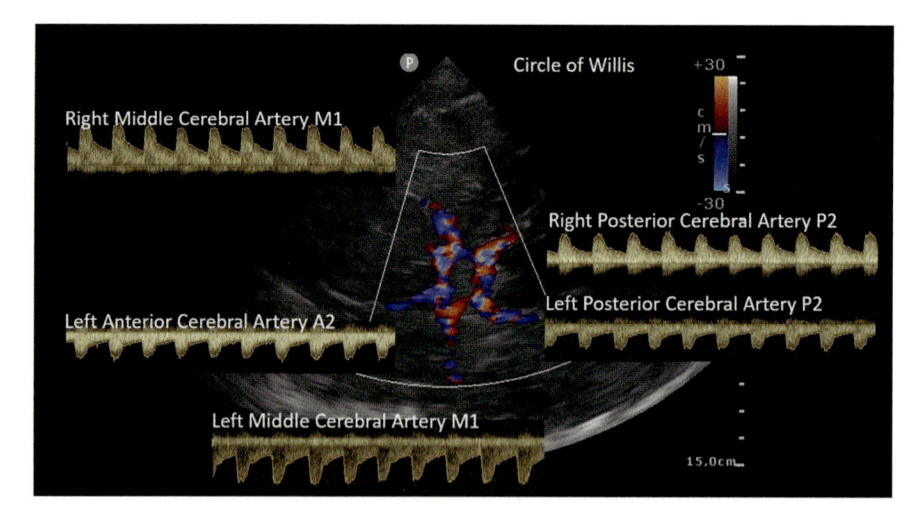

Fig. 36.6 The circle of Willis, as scanned from a transtemporal approach in a patient who underwent a decompressive craniectomy. The different shapes of the arterial flows are shown in the picture

Fig. 36.7 The optic nerve sheath diameter can be measured using a transorbital approach

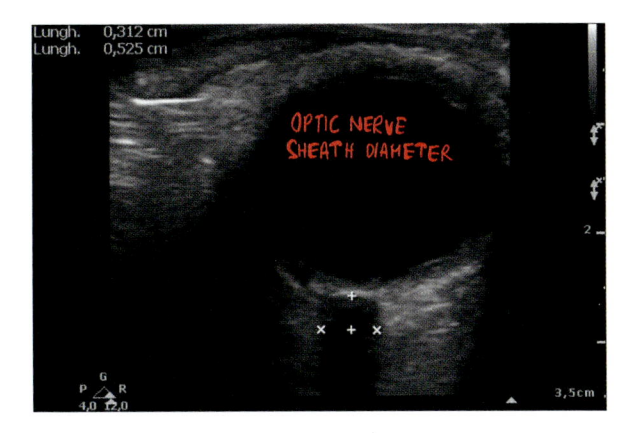

Fig. 36.8 An occipital approach to assess vertebral and basilar blood flow. Landmarks are the hyperechoic clivus and hypoechoic foramen magnum

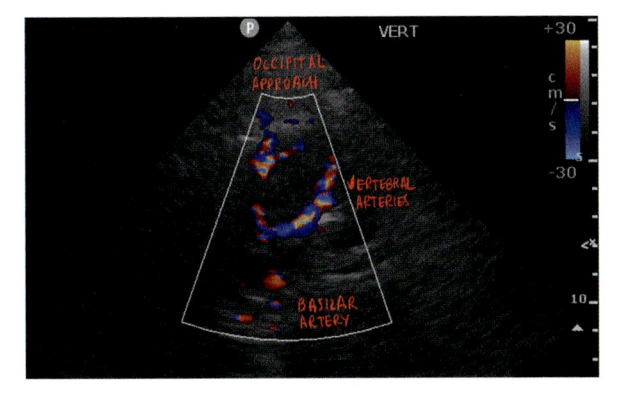

2. Transorbital approach: Through transorbital ultrasonography it is possible to assess the optic nerve sheath diameter (Fig. 36.7), as well as blood flow in the ophthalmic artery.
3. Occipital approach: The landmark for this approach is 1 cm below the external occipital protuberance, aiming forward and superiorly (toward the eyes), starting with a large scale (11–13 cm); the anatomic landmarks which can be seen with ultrasound are the clivus (hyperechoic structure) and the foramen magnum (hypoechoic). Using the power Doppler function, it is possible to scan for both vertebral arteries ending the basilar artery (Fig. 36.8).
4. Submandibular approach: The submandibular window allows assessment of the extracranial and intracranial or extradural segment of the internal carotid artery. The probe should be placed at the angle of the mandible, directed slightly medially and posteriorly. The internal carotid artery can usually be identified at a depth of 40–60 mm.

36.3.2 The Optic Nerve Sheath Diameter

The optic nerve sheath diameter is a good surrogate measurement for ICP [22]; cutoffs >0.5 cm correlate well with an ICP >20 mmHg. This noninvasive, quick, repeatable way to assess ICP carries a sensitivity of 0.90 and therefore a good level of diagnostic accuracy to quickly detect increased ICP [23]. Using a linear probe placed transversally over the closed eyelid of the patient, the clinician can scan the optic nerve behind the eye, as a hypoechoic structure extending posteriorly from the retina. Measurements of its diameter should be taken 3 mm from the globe perpendicularly (as shown in Fig. 36.7), using an electronic caliper. The rationale behind this technique is related to the anatomy of the optic nerve, which originates directly from the central nervous system (CNS) and is surrounded by the meningeal sheaths and cerebrospinal fluid (CSF): increases in ICP shift CSF into this space, which increases in diameter. This easy and repeatable technique carries one important pitfall, which is the artifact created by the retinal artery. This vessel runs close to the nerve and might appear as a hypoechoic bump that is particularly difficult to distinguish from the optic nerve. When any suspicion arises, color Doppler mode should be used to evaluate the presence of blood flow.

36.3.3 Noninvasive ICP Measurement

ICP can be estimated using brain ultrasonography, through a transtemporal approach, assessing blood flow in the middle cerebral artery. The formula used was first introduced by Czosnyka et al. in 1998 [24], originally to estimate CPP noninvasively:

$$CPP = MAP \times FVd / FVm + 14$$

where MAP is the mean arterial pressure, FVd the diastolic flow velocity, and FVm the mean flow velocity. However, given that MAP-ICP=CPP, the formula can be written as

$$ICP = MAP - [MAP \times FVd / FVm + 14].$$

Evidence shows that this method can accurately exclude intracranial hypertension in patients with acute brain injury. The best ICP threshold estimated was 24.8 mmHg, which carried a sensitivity of 100% and a specificity of 91.2% [25]. Another useful tool to consider while estimating ICP using this technique is the pulsatility index. This is calculated as the difference between systolic and diastolic flow velocities, divided by the mean velocity. Many studies have supported the interpretation of the pulsatility index as a tool to reflect distal cerebrovascular resistances, attributing a higher pulsatility index to higher cerebrovascular resistances [26]. However, the pulsatility index is not dependent solely on cerebrovascular resistances, but its value is the result of an interplay between cerebrovascular resistances, CPP, and compliance of the arterial bed. Some authors consider this parameter as less reliable for estimation of ICP [27], and it should therefore be used together with other noninvasive methods for estimation of ICP (transcranial color-coded duplex ultrasonography—optic nerve sheath diameter, as already described).

36.3.4 Aneurysmal Subarachnoid Hemorrhage and Vasospasm

Vasospasm after aneurysmal subarachnoid hemorrhage (SAH) is the main cause of delayed cerebral ischemia and is associated with severe mortality and morbidity. Guidelines agree on the importance of monitoring blood flow velocities noninvasively [28]. Transcranial Doppler and transcranial color-coded duplex ultrasonography play a pivotal role in the detection of this complication after aneurysmal SAH. Monitoring mean flow velocities is not enough, as an increase in flow velocity does not necessarily imply arterial narrowing. To differentiate this from cerebral hyperemia, Lindegaard et al. [29] introduced a ratio between either the middle cerebral artery or the anterior cerebral artery and the internal carotid artery, using a threshold of 3 as a diagnostic criterion. A Lindegaard ratio of 3 or above was diagnostic for vasospasm, a Lindegaard ratio of less than 3 indicated hyperemia, and a Lindegaard ratio of 6 was highly predictive of severe vasospasm. A blunt increase in flow velocities of 50 cm/s or more within 24 h is also predictive of vasospasm. In 2002, a modified Lindegaard ratio was published for the assessment of basilar vasospasm as a ratio between basilar artery and extracranial vertebral artery, using a cutoff of 2 to differentiate between vasospasm and hyperemia [30].

36.3.5 Midline Shift

Midline shift can be effectively determined using the transtemporal window, axial plane on ultrasound. The main landmarks are the contralateral skull bone and the mesencephalon, and once those are found and centered in the image, the probe can be tilted cranially 10° until the third ventricle appears in the middle of the scan (diencephalic plane), as two parallel hyperechoic lines in the middle of the field, according to the technique described by Seidel et al. in 1996 [19]. Having identified the third ventricle, the clinician should use an electronic caliper to measure the distance between the ventricle and the inner part of the skull bone, bilaterally. The difference between the two measurements divided by two is the estimation of the midline shift. This relates well with the midline shift measured on CT scan (compared with the Bland-Altman method), regardless of the cause of the shift (space-occupying lesion, hematoma) [31] (Fig. 36.5).

36.3.6 Cerebral Circulatory Arrest

Digital subtraction angiography is considered the gold standard for the confirmation of cerebral circulatory arrest and brain death. However, it requires transport of a hemodynamically unstable patient to the radiology suite to perform an invasive procedure. CBF can be assessed using transcranial Doppler. Increased ICP blunts diastolic flow velocities and, when ICP equals the diastolic arterial blood pressure, flow velocity becomes zero. When ICP increases even further, there is a backflow of

Fig. 36.9 Reverberating flow in a patient with severe brain injury who developed an isoelectric encephalogram trace minutes after this recording and was confirmed brain dead a few hours later

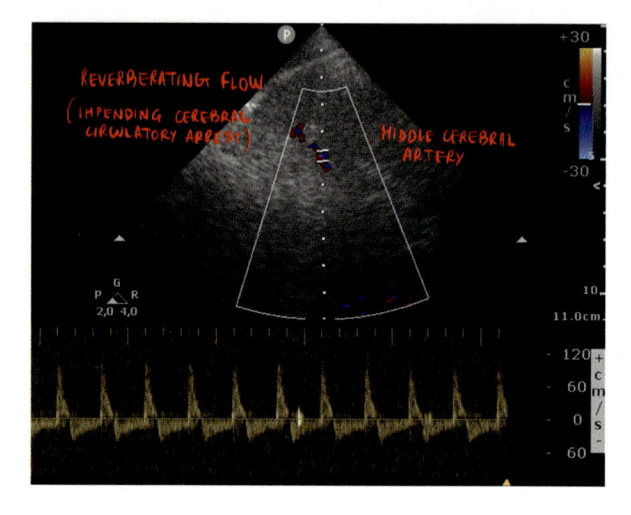

blood during the diastolic phase. This phenomenon is called reverberating flow, after diastolic peak blood flows in the opposite direction, and can be assessed with transcranial Doppler. Brunser et al. reported that power mode transcranial Doppler had high sensitivity and specificity for diagnosis of brain death, respectively 100% and 98% (flow velocity was assessed in the middle cerebral artery using a transtemporal approach) [32] (Fig. 36.9).

36.4 Processed Electroencephalography

Precision medicine represents "a new era of medicine through research, technology, and policies that empower patients, researchers, and providers to work together toward development of individualized care." With these words, Barack Obama, former president of the United States, launched the Precision Medicine Initiative on January 20, 2015. Funds were dedicated to creating treatments tailored to individual patients' biologic (genetic and molecular) profiles. Interestingly, current attempts toward standardization of care—protocols, checklists, algorithms, evidence-based medicine, guidelines, consensus papers, and enhanced recovery after surgery programs—challenge precision medicine. While protocols provide guidelines derived from strong evidence that decreases standard variability of care, eventual personalization discovered through clinical algorithms may provide better outcomes [33].

Drug response to sedatives and hypnotics is just one example of interindividual variability related to pharmacogenomics. In this light, identification of the correct dose of sedatives for optimal sedation in the ICU, through proper monitoring and within specific institutional protocols, matches well with the concept of precision and personalized medicine.

Intensivists continuously monitor their patients' organs and systems during the ICU stay: of the cardiovascular system using invasive and noninvasive methods; the respiratory system using blood gas and ventilator curve analysis; and renal function using urine output, creatinine, and biomarker levels. The brain is the main target of the sedatives frequently administered to critically ill patients, but no monitor is usually applied to monitor their effect on brain electrical activity, at least outside the neuro-ICU. The main reason for this reality is that electroencephalography (EEG) [34] is a complex investigation system that few intensivists can interpret. Technological evolution has developed a variety of (simplified) EEG-derived indices that can be used to make this information more available. Use of processed EEG indices has been shown to improve intraoperative anesthetic titration during anesthesia but also sedation in the ICU: bispectral index [BIS, Medtronic, Boulder, CO), E-Entropy (GE Healthcare, Helsinki, Finland), Narcotrend (Narcotrend Gruppe, Hannover, Germany), Masimo SEDLine (SEDline, Masimo Corp, Irvine, CA), and NeuroSENSE (NeuroWave Systems, Inc., Cleveland Heights, OH) are a few examples of the tools now available on the market (Fig. 36.10). There is as yet no evidence for superiority of one device over the others and differences in trace visualization, shape and characteristics of the sensor, institutional habits, and budgets are the main reasons for operator choice [35].

A detailed description of the EEG signal recording and processing is beyond the aim of this chapter, and the reader is referred to dedicated articles [36]. Briefly, subcortical regions (e.g., the thalamus) produce small potentials that cannot be identified from electrodes placed on the scalp because an electric field decreases in

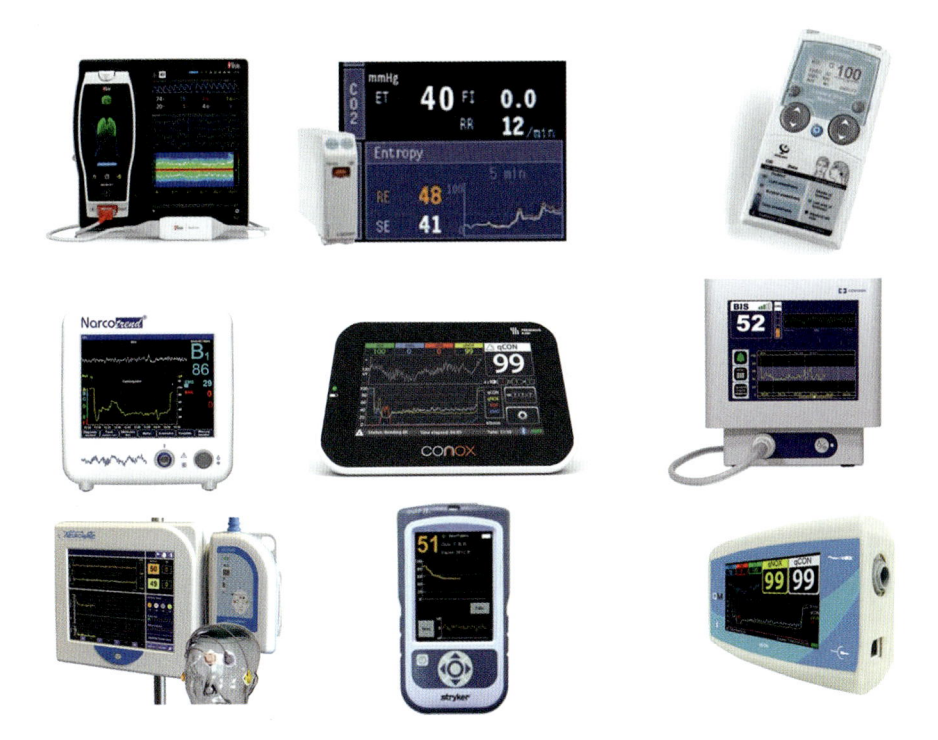

Fig. 36.10 Devices commercially available for processed EEG monitoring

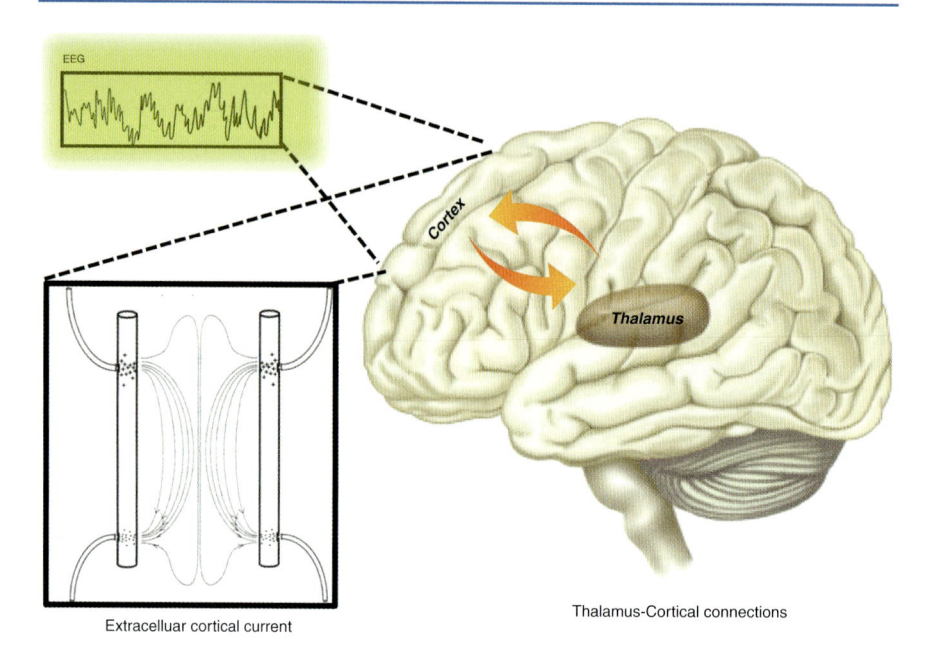

Fig. 36.11 Subcortical-cortical interactions

strength by the square of the distance from its source (Fig. 36.11). However, because of the close and continuous interconnection between superficial and deep brain structures, surface EEG reflects the states of both cortical and subcortical areas. Dedicated monitors that automatically elaborate the frontal EEG trace are needed because a full-montage EEG during sedation requires cumbersome equipment and specialized training, not available to all intensivists. Moreover, a frontal processed EEG trace is considered reliable for the purposes of anesthesia/sedation monitoring even if some clinical conditions (see later) eventually require some knowledge of basic EEG principles. Processed EEG monitors deliver three main pieces of information: (1) the raw trace, (2) the numerical index of anesthesia/sedation depth, and (3) the 2D spectrogram (Fig. 36.12). The reader is referred to dedicated articles for details about the specific parameters [37].

Processed EEG was originally intended for the management of the anesthetic state during surgery to avoid accidental awareness and to titrate sedation in critically ill patients where clinical scales represent the gold standard. The inclusion of processed EEG into many multiparametric ICU monitors reflects the perceived need for ICU caregivers to use a comprehensive approach in the management of sedated patients. Deep sedation is clearly associated with poor short- and long-term outcomes in critically ill patients: prolonged mechanical ventilation and cognitive and psychological complications all increase hospital and ICU length of stay and mortality [38]. Although light sedation, with patients being able to communicate and cooperate at any time, represents a modern target of sedation and a standard of care in ICUs, moderate-to-deep sedation (e.g., a Richmond Agitation–Sedation Scale

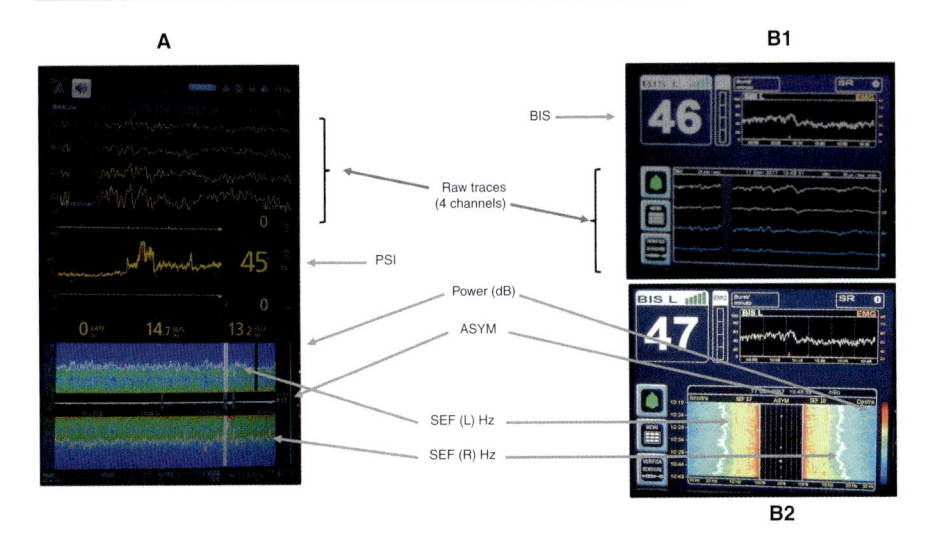

Fig. 36.12 Data delivered by processed EEG devices. A: SEDLine, Masimo Corp, Irvine, CA; B1 and B2: BIS, Medtronic, Boulder, CO. *ASYM* asymmetry, *SEF* spectral edge frequency, *L* left, *R* right

[RASS] ≤3) may be needed in a non-negligible number of patients, including those with alcohol weaning syndromes complicated by uncontrolled agitation; complex ventilator–patient desynchrony; refractory status epilepticus; intracranial hypertension; patients receiving neuromuscular blocking agents; postsurgical patients requiring hemodynamic, temperature, or bleeding stabilization; post-cardiac arrest therapy (post-resuscitation care); or TBI. In these categories of patients, clinical scales (e.g., RASS, Riker Sedation-Agitation Scale [SAS]), unless they represent standardized assessment of sedation levels, cannot be applied. Moreover, they are commonly evaluated every 4–6 h, and may not detect periods of inadequate sedation occurring between assessments, whereas processed EEG is a continuous method of analysis. In addition, clinical scale assessment is performed by disturbing sedated or sleeping patients (processed EEG does not require modification of the sedation state) and can never identify phases of burst suppression or isoelectric traces (total suppression) [39], which are associated with negative outcomes (e.g., delirium occurrence, prolonged mechanical ventilation, mortality). In this context, in a *post hoc* analysis of a prospective observational study performed in 125 ICU patients under mechanical ventilation, burst suppression occurred in 39% of the cases and was an independent predictor of increased risk of death at 6 months [40]. Processed EEG values can vary greatly in patients sedated in the ICU because, unlike those undergoing painful surgery, patients in the ICU may not experience strong stimulation and therefore require relatively low levels of sedation, appearing calm with BIS values of around 60–80. Clinical procedures, spontaneous patient arousal, physiological sleep cycles, noise, and nursing activities may cause sedation levels to fluctuate. What is important to consider is that muscle activity (mainly) and electric devices (less frequently) may interfere with the ability of the system to process the raw trace, leading to falsely increased sedation indexes [41]. In order to limit this sort of artifact the companies are improving their devices keeping them more "resistant" to EMG interference.

36.4.1 Recommendations from International Guidelines

In a change from the previous version published in 2013, the recent international guidelines on sedation practice in the ICU [42] (Clinical Practice Guidelines for the Prevention and Management of Pain, Agitation/Sedation, Delirium, Immobility, and Sleep Disruption in Adult Patients in the ICU) report that processed EEG monitoring systems, although best suited for sedative titration during deep sedation or for patients who receive neuromuscular blockade, may also have potential benefits in lighter sedation states and that processed EEG monitoring, compared with the standard clinical scales, may improve sedative titration [43]. Using processed EEG systems as an objective guide for sedative dosing in critically ill patients can decrease the medical complications of oversedation, such as depressed cardiac contractility and hypotension. There are few studies on processed EEG monitoring in the ICU. The first was a prospective trial that randomized patient sedation to be assessed using the Ramsay Scale or BIS monitoring during propofol sedation that was stopped every 2 h [44]. A nurse-guided Ramsey score of 4 was the target in controls, and a BIS value of 70–80 was the target for the study group. A reduction in propofol of 50% was obtained in the BIS group versus controls. The second study [45] was a prospective randomized trial in which patients sedated with morphine and midazolam were randomized to sedation titration based on a BIS >0 versus clinical assessment. No difference was found in the total amount of administered sedative drugs, length of mechanical ventilation, or ICU length of stay. In a recent study on 110 trauma patients, use of BIS resulted in a decrease in sedation and analgesia use, decrease in agitation, less failure to extubate, and fewer tracheostomies, with an approximate 4-day decreased length of stay [46].

Beyond its use for sedative titration purposes, processed EEG may have some additional applications in ICU patients, including identification of subclinical/unrecognized seizures or seizures occurring when neuromuscular blocking agents are administered. Nevertheless, depending on the frequencies of the ictal waveforms, processed EEG may have variable values that only skilled intensivists are able to read on the raw EEG trace to successfully understand this clinical condition. Processed EEG monitors can also be used to guide therapy aimed at minimizing cerebral metabolism rate to reach predefined levels of burst suppression [47]. A significant proportion of critically ill patients with altered mental status have nonconvulsive subclinical seizures and nonconvulsive status epilepticus [48]. Continuous EEG assessment for nonconvulsive subclinical seizures and nonconvulsive status epilepticus in patients with altered mental status can be indicated in patients with a history of epilepsy, fluctuating level of consciousness, acute brain injury, recent convulsive status epilepticus, stereotyped activity such as paroxysmal movements, nystagmus, twitching, jerking, hippus, and autonomic variability [49]. Nonconvulsive subclinical seizures, seizures with little or no overt clinical manifestations, can be detected with EEG monitoring.

36.5 Conclusion

Noninvasive neuro-multimodality monitoring is now possible. We present an essential bundle of noninvasive neuromonitoring composed of pupillometry, brain ultrasound, and processed EEG. Although some of these noninvasive tools are not yet reliable enough to completely substitute invasive monitoring, they do represent an important adjunct for the clinician in both neuroanesthesia and neurocritical care environments.

We have only described the basic features and the potential that transcranial color-coded duplex Doppler and brain ultrasonography have to offer to the clinician. Bedside ultrasounds are becoming increasingly popular with clinicians because they are quick, reliable, and repeatable. While not yet being a substitute for invasive ICP monitoring, ultrasound can give the clinician useful information when indications for such invasive devices are blurred or contraindicated (liver failure, anticoagulation). Moreover, it has become a mainstay for the early detection of vasospasm in patients with aneurysmal SAH. In the emergency department, expanding focused assessment with sonography in trauma (FAST) assessment to brain ultrasound may enable the physician to become aware of increased ICP even before the patient is transported for a CT scan, and prompt early neuroprotective medical intervention.

EEG is a fundamental tool for monitoring human brain electrical activity during changing states of consciousness like sleep, sedation, or general anesthesia. Processed EEG may contribute to help anesthesiologists and intensivists optimize drug doses in individuals with different pharmacogenomics and clearance of sedatives. Processed EEG devices are not simple plug-and-play units providing a well-interpretable dimensionless number. They require a global knowledge of technology and of EEG tracings to avoid misinterpretation, especially when muscle activity interferes with the processing algorithm. The use of processed EEG in the ICU could be much more complex than during anesthesia in the operating rooms. Nevertheless, processed EEG monitors offer advantages in the management of patients under moderate and deep sedation and in patients receiving neuromuscular blocking agents to avoid both awareness and burst suppression. Some pathological states, such as seizures or altered EEG states (iatrogenic burst suppression or areflexic coma), may be revealed by processed EEG and trigger a complete EEG examination.

References

1. Meeker M, Du R, Bacchetti P, et al. Pupil examination: validity and clinical utility of an automated pupillometer. J Neurosci Nurs. 2005;37:34–40.
2. Couret D, Boumaza D, Grisotto C, et al. Reliability of standard pupillometry practice in neurocritical care: An observational, double-blinded study. Crit Care. 2016;20:99.
3. Larson MD, Muhiudeen I. Pupillometric analysis of the 'absent light reflex'. Arch Neurol. 1995;52:369–72.
4. Rossetti AO, Rabinstein AA, Oddo M. Neurological prognostication of outcome in patients in coma after cardiac arrest. Lancet Neurol. 2016;15:597–609.
5. Behrends M, Niemann CU, Larson MD. Infrared pupillometry to detect the light reflex during cardiopulmonary resuscitation: a case series. Resuscitation. 2012;83:1223–8.
6. Yokobori S, Wang KKK, Yang Z, et al. Quantitative pupillometry and neuron-specific enolase independently predict return of spontaneous circulation following cardiogenic out-of-hospital cardiac arrest: a prospective pilot study. Sci Rep. 2018;8:15964.
7. Oddo M, Sandroni C, Citerio G, et al. Quantitative versus standard pupillary light reflex for early prognostication in comatose cardiac arrest patients: an international prospective multicentre double-blinded study. Intensive Care Med. 2018;44:2102–11.
8. Cnossen MC, Huijben JA, van der Jagt M, et al. Variation in monitoring and treatment policies for intracranial hypertension in traumatic brain injury: a survey in 66 neurotrauma centers participating in the CENTER-TBI study. Crit Care. 2017;21:233.
9. Manley G, Larson M. Infrared pupillometry during uncal herniation. J Neurosurg Anesthesiol. 2002;14:223–8.
10. Cohen JE, Montero A, Israel ZH. Prognosis and clinical relevance of anisocoria-craniotomy latency for epidural hematoma in comatose patients. J Trauma. 1996;41:120–2.
11. Lieberman JD, Pasquale MD, Garcia R, Cipolle MD, Mark Li P, Wasser TE. Use of admission Glasgow Coma Score, pupil size, and pupil reactivity to determine outcome for trauma patients. J Trauma. 2003;55:437–42.
12. Ong C, Hutch M, Barra M, Kim A, Zafar S, Smirnakis S. Effects of osmotic therapy on pupil reactivity: quantification using pupillometry in critically ill neurologic patients. Neurocrit Care. 2019;30:307–15.
13. Stevens AR, Su Z, Toman E, Belli A, Davies D. Optical pupillometry in traumatic brain injury: neurological pupil index and its relationship with intracranial pressure through significant event analysis. Brain Inj. 2019;33:1032–8.
14. Jahns FP, Miroz JP, Messerer M, et al. Quantitative pupillometry for the monitoring of intracranial hypertension in patients with severe traumatic brain injury. Crit Care. 2019;23:155.
15. Vassilieva A, Olsen MH, Peinkhofer C, Knudsen GM, Kondziella D. Automated pupillometry to detect command following in neurological patients: a proof-of-concept study. PeerJ. 2019;7:e6929.
16. Paulus J, Roquilly A, Beloeil H, Théraud J, Asehnoune K, Lejus C. Pupillary reflex measurement predicts insufficient analgesia before endotracheal suctioning in critically ill patients. Crit Care. 2013;17:R161.
17. Constant I, Nghe MC, Boudet L, et al. Reflex pupillary dilatation in response to skin incision and alfentanil in children anaesthetized with sevoflurane: a more sensitive measure of noxious stimulation than the commonly used variables. Br J Anaesth. 2006;96:614–9.
18. Wildemeersch D, Baeten M, Peeters N, Saldien V, Vercauteren M, Hans G. Pupillary dilation reflex and pupillary pain index evaluation during general anaesthesia: a pilot study. Rom J Anaesth Intensive Care. 2018;25:19–23.
19. Sabourdin N, Barrois J, Louvet N, Rigouzzo A. Pupillometry-guided intraoperative remifentanil administration versus standard practice influences opioid use: a randomized study. Anesthesiology. 2017;127:284–92.
20. Aaslid R, Markwalder TM, Nornes H. Noninvasive transcranial Doppler ultrasound recording of flow velocity in basal cerebral arteries. J Neurosurg. 1982;57:769–74.

21. Robba C, Simonassi F, Ball L, Pelosi P. Transcranial color-coded duplex sonography fir bedside monitoring of central nervous system infection as a consequence of decompressive craniectomy after traumatic brain injury. Intensive Care Med. 2019;45:1143–4.
22. Robba C, Cardim D, Tajsic T, et al. Non-invasive intracranial pressure assessment in brain injured patients using ultrasound-based methods. Acta Neurochir Suppl. 2018;126:69–7.
23. Sekhon MS, Griesdale DE, Robba C, et al. Optic nerve sheath diameter on computed tomography is correlated with simultaneously measured intracranial pressure in patients with severe traumatic brain injury. Intensive Care Med. 2014;40:1267–74.
24. Czosnyka M, Matta BF, Smielewski P, Kirkpatrick PJ, Pickard JD. Cerebral perfusion pressure in head-injured patients: a noninvasive assessment using transcranial Doppler ultrasonography. J Neurosurg. 1998;88:802–8.
25. Rasulo FA, Bertuetti R, Robba C, et al. The accuracy of transcranial Doppler in excluding intracranial hypertension following acute brain injury: a multicenter prospective pilot study. Crit Care. 2017;21:44.
26. Giller CA, Hodges K, Batjer HH. Transcranial Doppler Pulsatility in vasodilation and stenosis. J Neurosurg. 1990;72:901–6.
27. De Riva N, Budohoski KP, Smielewski P, et al. Transcranial Doppler Pulsatility Index: what it is and what it isn't. Neurocrit Care. 2012;17:58–66.
28. Le Roux P, Menon DK, Citerio G, et al. Consensus summary statement of the international multidisciplinary consensus conference on multimodality monitoring in neurocritical care. Neurocrit Care. 2014;17:58–66.
29. Lindegaard KF, Nornes H, Bakke SJ, Sorteberg W, Nakstad P. Cerebral vasospasm after subarachnoid hemorrhage investigated by means of transcranial Doppler ultrasound. Acta Neurochir Suppl (Wein). 1988;42:81–4.
30. Soustiel JF, Shik V, Shreiber R, Tavor Y, Goldsher D. Basilar vasospasm diagnosis: investigation of a modified "Lindegaard Index" based on imaging studies and blood velocity measurements of the basilar artery. Stroke. 2002;33:72–7.
31. Cattalani A, Grasso VM, Vitali M, Gallesio I, Magrassi L, Barbanera A. Transcranial color-coded duplex sonography for evaluation of midline-shift after chronic-subdural hematoma evacuation (TEMASE): A prospective study. Clin Neurol Neurosurg. 2017;162:101–7.
32. Brunser AM, Lavados PM, Cárcamo DA, et al. Accuracy of Power mode transcranial Doppler in the diagnosis of brain death. J Med Ultrasound. 2015;23:29–33.
33. Iravani M, Lee LK, Cannesson M. Standardized care versus precision medicine in the perioperative setting: Can point-of-care testing help bridge the gap? Anesth Analg. 2017;124:1347–53.
34. Rampil I. A primer for EEG signal processing in anesthesia. Anesthesiology. 1998;89:980–1002.
35. Scheeren TWL, Kuizenga MH, Maurer H, Struys MMRF, Heringlake M. Electroencephalography and brain oxygenation monitoring in the perioperative period. Anesth Analg. 2019;128:265–77.
36. Fahy BG, Chau DF. The technology of processed electroencephalogram monitoring devices for assessment of depth of anesthesia. Anesth Analg. 2018;126:111–7.
37. Purdon P, Pierce E, Mukamel E, et al. Electroencephalogram signatures of loss and recovery of consciousness from propofol. Proc Natl Acad Sci U S A. 2013;110:E1142–51.
38. Shehabi Y, Chan L, Kadiman S, et al. Sedation depth and long-term mortality in mechanically ventilated critically ill adults: a prospective longitudinal multicentre cohort study. Intensive Care Med. 2013;39:910–8.
39. Wang ZH, Chen H, Yang YL, et al. Bispectral index can reliably detect deep sedation in mechanically ventilated patients: a prospective multicenter validation study. Anesth Analg. 2017;125:176–83.
40. Watson P, Shintani A, Tyson R, Pandharipande P, Pun B, Ely E. Presence of electroencephalogram burst suppression in sedated, critically ill patients is associated with increased mortality. Crit Care Med. 2008;36:3171–7.
41. Dahaba A. Different conditions that could result in the bispectral index indicating an incorrect hypnotic state. Anesth Analg. 2005;101:765–73.
42. Barr J, Fraser GL, Puntillo K, et al. Clinical practice guidelines for the management of pain, agitation, and delirium in adult patients in the intensive care unit. Crit Care Med. 2013;41:263–306.

43. Devlin JW, Skrobik Y, Gélinas C, et al. Clinical Practice Guidelines for the Prevention and Management of Pain, Agitation/Sedation, Delirium, Immobility, and Sleep Disruption in Adult Patients in the ICU. Crit Care Med. 2018;46:e825–73.
44. Olson DM, Thoyre SM, Peterson ED, Graffagnino C. A randomized evaluation of bispectral index-augmented sedation assessment in neurological patients. Neurocrit Care. 2009;11:20–7.
45. Weatherburn C, Endacott R, Tynan P, Bailey M. The impact of Bispectral Index monitoring on sedation administration in mechanically ventilated patients. Anaesth Intensive Care. 2007;35:204–8.
46. Mahmood S, Parchani A, El-Menyar A, Zarour A, Al-Thani H, Latifi R. Utility of bispectral index in the management of multiple trauma patients. Surg Neurol Int. 2014;5:141.
47. Musialowicz T, Mervaala E, Kälviäinen R, Uusaro A, Ruokonen E, Parviainen I. Can BIS monitoring be used to assess the depth of propofol anesthesia in the treatment of refractory status epilepticus? Epilepsia. 2010;51:1580–6.
48. Towne A, Waterhouse E, Boggs J, et al. Prevalence of nonconvulsive status epilepticus in comatose patients. Neurology. 2000;54:340–5.
49. Friedman D, Claassen J, Hirsch LJ. Continuous electroencephalogram monitoring in the intensive care unit. Anesth Analg. 2009;109:506–23.

Part XII
Organ Donation

Brain Death After Cardiac Arrest: Pathophysiology, Prevalence, and Potential for Organ Donation

C. Sandroni, M. Scarpino, and M. Antonelli

37.1 Introduction

Sudden cardiac arrest is a major cause of death in developed countries [1]. Each year, over 350,000 people in the United States [2] and over 270,000 in Europe [3] have an out-of-hospital cardiac arrest (OHCA) attended by the emergency medical system. Unfortunately, most of these patients will die despite provision of cardiopulmonary resuscitation (CPR). Data reported in the North American CARES Registry in 2018 [4] show that among 23,069 patients resuscitated from nontraumatic OHCA who achieved a sustained return of spontaneous circulation and were admitted to hospital, only 8489 (36.8%) survived to hospital discharge. The majority of in-hospital deaths in patients who are comatose after resuscitation from cardiac arrest are due to hypoxic-ischemic brain injury [5, 6]. Most of these deaths result from active withdrawal of life-sustaining treatment in patients where the severity of hypoxic-ischemic brain injury indicates that survival with a poor neurological outcome is very likely [7, 8]. However, in the remaining cases these deaths occur as a direct consequence of hypoxic-ischemic brain injury, which causes an irreversible loss of all brain functions, i.e., brain death [9]. In these patients, a timely diagnosis of brain death opens an important opportunity to save other patients' lives through organ donation [10].

C. Sandroni (✉) · M. Antonelli
Istituto Anestesiologia e Rianimazione Università Cattolica del Sacro Cuore, Fondazione Policlinico Universitario "Agostino Gemelli" IRCCS, Rome, Italy
e-mail: claudio.sandroni@policlinicogemelli.it

M. Scarpino
SODc Neurofisiopatologia, Dipartimento Neuromuscolo-Scheletrico e degli Organi di Senso, AOU Careggi, Florence, Italy

IRCCS Fondazione Don Carlo Gnocchi, Florence, Italy

© Springer Nature Switzerland AG 2020
J.-L. Vincent (ed.), *Annual Update in Intensive Care and Emergency Medicine 2020*, Annual Update in Intensive Care and Emergency Medicine,
https://doi.org/10.1007/978-3-030-37323-8_37

37.2 Pathophysiology of Brain Death After Cardiac Arrest

Cardiac arrest results in ischemia-reperfusion injury to vital organs, namely the heart and the brain. However, the brain is more sensitive than the heart to tissue ischemia as it has no myoglobin oxygen stores [11]. As a result, severe brain injury from cardiac arrest may be observed even when spontaneous circulation is restarted achieving a relative hemodynamic stability.

The diagnosis of brain death presumes an irreversible loss of both cortical and brainstem functions [12]. Although hypoxic-ischemic brain injury is known to affect mainly supratentorial structures such as the cortex, hippocampus, and basal ganglia, while relatively sparing the brainstem [13, 14], the occurrence of brain death after cardiac arrest demonstrates that hypoxic-ischemic brain injury can be sufficiently diffuse and severe to cause extensive neuronal death to the entire encephalon. Neuronal death after global cerebral ischemia and reperfusion results from both a primary and a secondary injury (Fig. 37.1), the first being due to direct neuronal ischemia during cardiac arrest, and the second being activated by subsequent reperfusion [15].

37.2.1 Cerebral Edema

One possible mechanism for brain death after cardiac arrest is the occurrence of cerebral edema leading to intracranial hypertension compromising cerebral perfusion. Increased intracranial pressure (ICP) can occur in comatose patients with hypoxic-ischemic brain injury [16] and it is associated with unfavorable outcome [17]. Massive cerebral edema after cardiac arrest leading to brain death has been described [18].

Cerebral edema from hypoxic-ischemic brain injury may be both cytotoxic and vasogenic. During cardiac arrest, lack of oxygen delivery to neurons causes cessation of adenosine triphosphate (ATP) production and a consequent stop of the membrane-bound Na-K-ATPase pump. This leads to intracellular accumulation of sodium ions (Na^+) resulting in cytotoxic edema [15, 19]. After reperfusion, vasogenic edema results from increased vascular permeability, leading to fluid shift from the intravascular to the extracellular space. Aquaporin-4, a bidirectional water-channel protein located at the astrocyte perivascular endfeet (Fig. 37.1), may play a role in this process [20].

On brain computed tomography (CT), brain edema after cardiac arrest appears as sulcal effacement and a reduction in the density ratio between the gray matter and the white matter (GM/WM ratio). In prognostication studies conducted on comatose resuscitated patients, a GM/WM ratio <1.2 within 24 h from return of spontaneous circulation was consistently associated with death or poor neurological outcome [21]. In a single-center study on 160 comatose resuscitated patients, a GM/WM ratio <1.07 predicted the occurrence of brain death with 95% specificity [22].

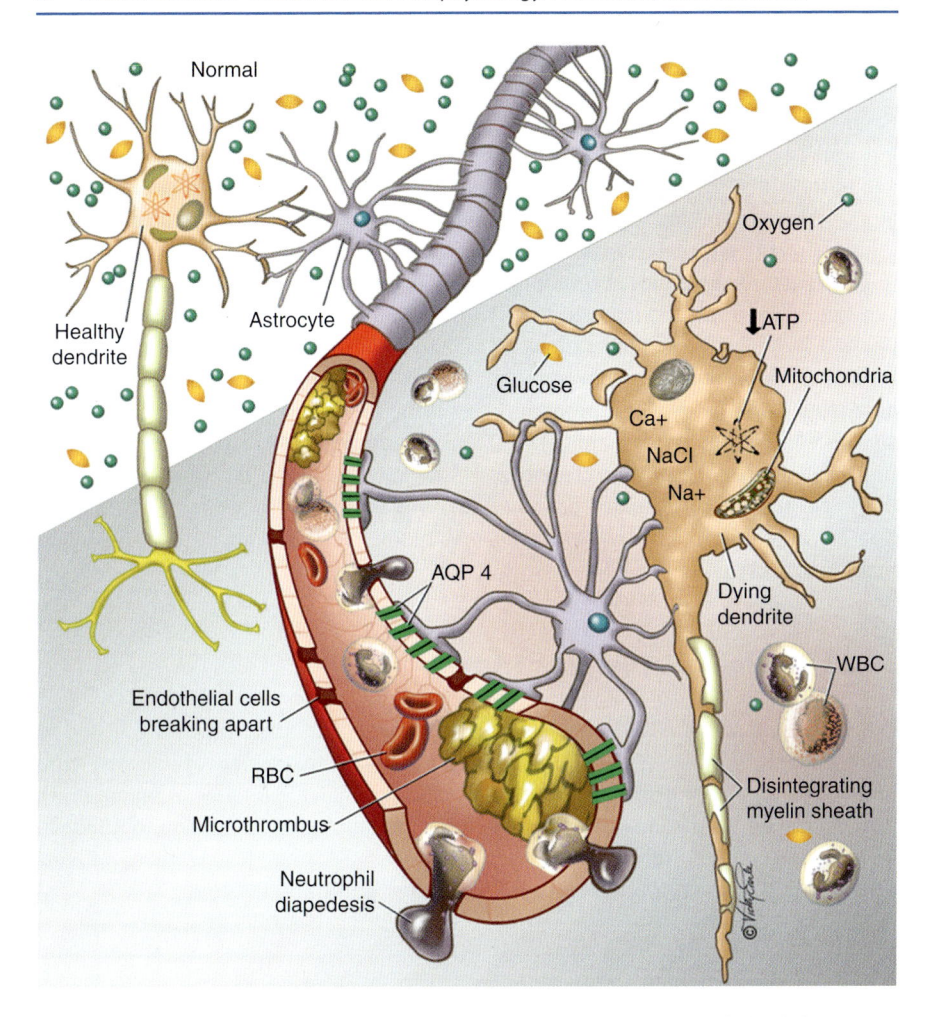

Fig. 37.1 Pathophysiology of hypoxic-ischemic brain injury. Ischemia-reperfusion injury causes direct neuronal damage by reducing the availability of adenosine triphosphate (ATP). Energy-dependent ion channel failure leads to intracellular increase in calcium, and to sodium and water retention. In addition, microvascular changes lead to vasogenic edema and microthrombosis, aggravating neuronal injury via reduced perfusion. *AQP 4* aquaporin-4, *RBC* red blood cell, *WBC* white blood cell (From [15], distributed under the terms of the Creative Commons Attribution 4.0 International License (http://creativecommons.org/licenses/by/4.0/))

In patients with hypoxic-ischemic brain injury, cytotoxic edema results in restricted intracellular water motion, which is detected on magnetic resonance imaging (MRI) as hyperintensity on diffusion-weighted imaging of various areas of the brain, including the brainstem [23]. Reduced diffusion measured with apparent diffusion coefficient on brain MRI is associated with severe neurological injury and death after cardiac arrest [21, 23].

37.2.2 Neuronal Apoptosis and Cerebral Hypoperfusion

Brain death after cardiac arrest can occur even in the absence of intracranial hypertension [24]. As a result of neuronal ischemia, Ca^{++} influx from cellular membranes and intracellular Ca^{++} release lead to mitochondrial dysfunction and release of excitatory neurotransmitters triggering neuronal apoptosis. Further neuronal injury after reperfusion occurs as a result of increased free radical production [15].

Experimental evidence showed that following return of spontaneous circulation, cerebral blood flow is characterized by an initial phase of hyperemia followed by marked hypoperfusion ("no reflow") [25]. In addition to increased intravascular resistance from extravascular edema, suggested mechanisms for this include decreased nitric oxide (NO) production resulting in vasoconstriction and thrombosis of cerebral microvasculature [15]. This phenomenon may be exacerbated by impaired autoregulation. Cerebral blood flow autoregulation is lost in about one-third of comatose resuscitated patients [26], while in others the zone of autoregulation is right-shifted [27] so that a normal blood pressure can be insufficient to maintain cerebral perfusion.

37.2.3 Neurological Causes of Arrest

When cardiac arrest is due to a neurological cause, the same process that led to cardiac arrest may also cause brain death. In a retrospective review of intensive care unit (ICU) databases from three regional referral centers in France, Arnaout et al. [28] described 86 patients resuscitated from nontraumatic OHCA due to a neurological cause, mainly subarachnoid hemorrhage ($n = 74/86$; 85%). All these patients died within 3 days after arrest, most of them (56%) from brain death.

37.3 Prevalence

The prevalence of brain death after cardiac arrest has been investigated only recently. In 2016, a systematic review from our group [9] searched for studies reporting the rate of brain death in adult patients resuscitated from either OHCA or in-hospital cardiac arrest. The review identified 26 studies published between 2002 and 2016, enrolling a total of 23,388 patients. Of these, 22,744 were resuscitated using conventional CPR (16 studies), while the remaining 644 patients were resuscitated using extracorporeal CPR (ECPR; 10 studies). A total of 17,779 (76.0%) patients died before hospital discharge, of whom 1830 developed brain death at a mean duration of 3 days after return of spontaneous circulation. The overall prevalence of brain death was 12.6 [10.2–15.2]% among patients who died and 8.9 [7.0–11.0]% among the total population of resuscitated patients.

In that systematic review, patients resuscitated with ECPR were three times more likely to develop brain death than those resuscitated with conventional CPR (27.9 [19.7–36.6]% vs. 8.3 [6.5–10.4]%; $p < 0.0001$). The most likely reason for a higher severity of hypoxic-ischemic brain injury in ECPR patients is that they had significantly longer arrest times than those resuscitated with conventional CPR (mean 94.7 ± 2.9 vs. 24.0 ± 1.7 min; $p = 0.0001$), because ECPR is generally used when conventional CPR fails to restore spontaneous circulation and it requires longer to initiate. Another possible explanation is that in some patients resuscitated using ECPR, brain death could have been due to cerebral hemorrhage induced by anticoagulation needed to maintain the extracorporeal circulation. This is supported by the fact that brain death is relatively common even in patients not in cardiac arrest undergoing veno-venous extracorporeal membrane oxygenation (VV-ECMO) for respiratory failure. In a report including 4988 adult patients supported with VV-ECMO included in the Extracorporeal Life Support Organization (ELSO) Registry [29], 356 (7%) had a neurological complication, the most common of which (181/356; 43%) was intracranial hemorrhage. Of these patients, 100 (28%) had brain death.

Limited evidence suggests that the prevalence of brain death after cardiac arrest in children is particularly high. In a retrospective study [30] performed at the Children's Hospital of Philadelphia, Du Pont-Thibodeau et al. investigated the timing and mode of death in patients admitted to the pediatric ICUs from 2005 to 2013 after resuscitation from OHCA. Among 86 children who died before hospital discharge, brain death was the commonest cause (40/86; 47%), followed by withdrawal of life-sustaining treatment due to unfavorable neurological prognosis. Brain death occurred at a median of 4 [2–5] days from cardiac arrest. All brain-dead patients had severe signs of hypoxic-ischemic brain injury on brain CT.

37.4 Potential for Organ Donation

The success of programs for organ donation after circulatory death in patients with OHCA [31] demonstrates that extracerebral organs can still be viable despite prolonged whole-body ischemia-reperfusion injury in patients that cannot be resuscitated. Therefore, we can expect that the same should be true for patients who evolve towards brain death after successful restoration of spontaneous circulation. In their seminal study published in 2008 [32], Adrie et al. included 246 adult patients resuscitated from OHCA, 40 (16%) of whom evolved towards brain death at a median of 2.5 (2–4) days after cardiac arrest. Of these 40 patients, 19 donated 52 solid organs (29 kidneys, 14 livers, 7 hearts, and 2 lungs). Both 1-year and 5-year survival of kidneys and livers donated from these patients did not differ from those of organs donated from a reference population of patients with brain death not due to cardiac arrest extracted from the French Organ Transplant Agency. Similar results were demonstrated in a systematic review on 858 organs transplanted from 741 donors, 91 of whom had brain death after cardiac arrest [33].

In the systematic review from our group mentioned above [9], organ donation was reported in 9/26 studies, of which 4 were conducted on conventional CPR patients (total 1224 donors) and 5 on ECPR patients (total 40 donors). The estimated pooled rate of donors among brain-dead patients was 41.8 [20.2–51.0]%.

Little information is available about donation after post-cardiac arrest brain death in children. In the retrospective study from Du Pont-Thibodeau et al. [30], 20 (50%) brain-dead patients donated organs. No information was available on survival rates of these organs after transplant.

The potential of organ donation from patients brain dead after resuscitation from cardiac arrest is remarkable. According to recent statistics [2], each year about 174,000 adults are resuscitated from nontraumatic OHCA by the emergency medical services in the United States. Of these, 49,000 (29%) are successfully resuscitated and admitted to an ICU. Based on the 5.4 [3.9–7.1]% overall prevalence of brain death among conventional CPR patients in our review, an estimated 2648 patients [95% CI 1962–3433] will evolve to brain death, 40% of whom could donate organs.

Despite the absence of detailed statistics, there are data suggesting that the number of cardiac arrest patients as organ donors has been increasing in the last years. In a retrospective review of the UK Intensive Care National Audit & Research Centre database on 63,417 patients admitted to ICU after resuscitation from cardiac arrest [34], the proportion of those who became organ donors increased by more than 300%, from 34/1582 (3.1%) in 2004 to 278/4147 (10.1%) in 2014. In a Canadian study [35] comparing the characteristics of 1040 brain-dead donors included in a transplant database between two consecutive study periods (2000–2005 vs. 2006–2012), hypoxic-ischemic brain injury as a cause of death increased from 8.1% to 17.3%, while traumatic injury decreased from 27% to 19.7%.

37.5 Detecting Brain Death After Cardiac Arrest

The occurrence of brain death in comatose resuscitated patients should be identified early and systematically, in order to avoid missing potential donors on the one side, and continuing ineffective intensive treatment in patients with no chance of recovery on the other side. This last aspect is particularly important in those countries or communities [36, 37] where brain death is the only universally accepted reason for suspending all life-support measures, and withdrawal of life-sustaining treatment in alive patients based on the presence of severe hypoxic-ischemic brain injury is not common practice.

Neuronal death after hypoxic-ischemic brain injury is typically delayed [38] and it is not complete until 3–4 days after return of spontaneous circulation. According to current guidelines [8], clinical prognostic assessment should be performed at 72 h after return of spontaneous circulation or later. However, several studies [39–42] have shown that in up to 40% of resuscitated comatose patients, withdrawal of life-sustaining treatment occurs earlier. This carries the risk of missing patients with potential chances of recovery [39, 43], and those who might evolve towards brain death and potentially become donors. Both in adult and in pediatric studies, brain death is detected on average 3–4 days after return of spontaneous circulation but in some studies this occurred up to 6 days or more [9, 16, 30, 32] after return of spontaneous circulation.

Figure 37.2 shows a suggested algorithm for brain death screening in patients with severe hypoxic-ischemic brain injury after cardiac arrest. An early brain death occurrence can be expected when the cause of arrest is neurological [28]. During targeted temperature management (TTM), even when sedation and/or paralysis precludes a full clinical examination, clinical signs such as loss of pupillary reactivity, hemodynamic instability, or diabetes insipidus suggest impending brain death. The diagnosis of brain death is confirmed once all potential confounders, like sedative agents or artificially induced hypothermia, have been excluded.

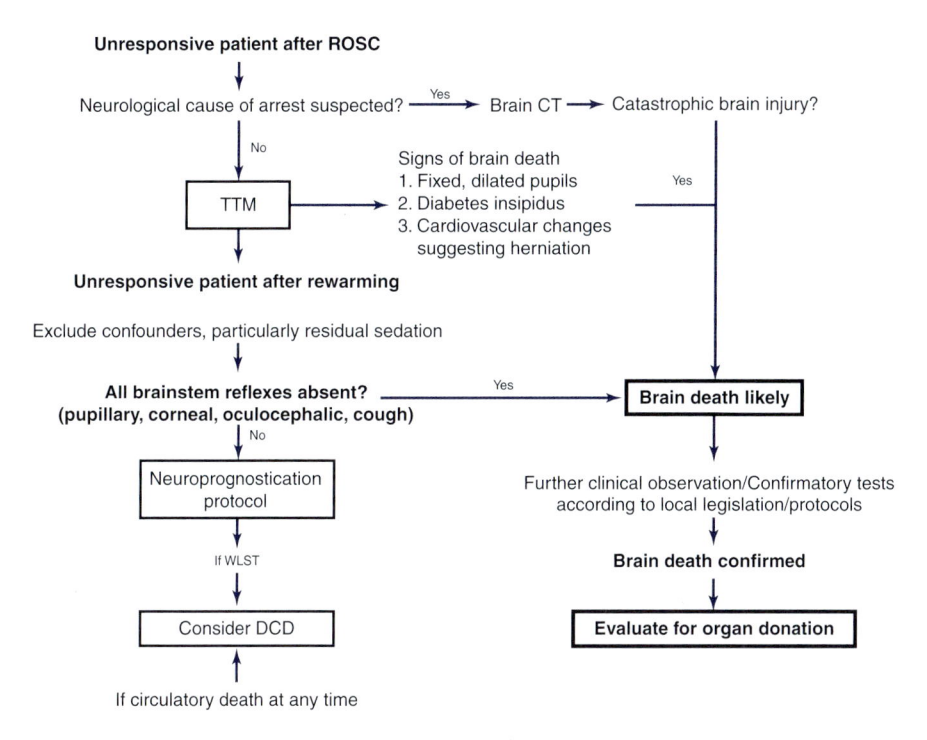

Fig. 37.2 Suggested algorithm for brain death screening after cardiac arrest. In a resuscitated comatose patient, brain death is suspected shortly after return of spontaneous circulation (ROSC) if a catastrophic brain injury is demonstrated on computed tomography (CT) or if the patient shows signs like fixed, dilated pupils, diabetes insipidus, or cardiovascular changes suggesting herniation. After rewarming from targeted temperature management (TTM), and after having excluded confounders, brain death is suspected if brainstem reflexes are all absent. The diagnosis of brain death is confirmed by clinical observation and/or by confirmatory tests according to local legislation or protocols. Organ donation should be considered after brain death ascertainment. When circulatory death occurs, either spontaneously or after withdrawal of life-sustaining treatment (WLST), donation after circulatory death (DCD) can be considered (From [9], distributed under the terms of the Creative Commons Attribution l 4.0 International License (http://creativecommons.org/licenses/by-nc/4.0/))

37.6 Future Developments

Identifying the risk factors for brain death in patients resuscitated from cardiac arrest is important, both to prevent progression towards brain death and to be ready to detect brain death when it occurs. Although these factors have not been systematically reviewed yet, evidence from the literature suggests that progression towards brain death is more likely in pediatric patients [30], in those resuscitated with ECPR [9], and when arrest is due to a neurological cause [28]. In a recent retrospective study [44] enrolling 42/214 adults who developed brain death in a French ICU after resuscitation from OHCA, the most important independent risk factor for brain death was a neurological cause of arrest (odds ratio [OR] 14.72, 95% CI 3.03–71.37), followed by hemodynamic instability (OR 6.20 [2.41–15.93]) and a low-flow period longer than 16 min (OR 2.94 [1.21–7.16]). Female sex was associated with an increased risk (OR 2.34; 95% CI [1.02–5.35]), while older age was associated with a lower risk of developing brain death (OR per year 0.95 [0.92–0.98]).

One of the possible mechanisms for brain death occurrence after cardiac arrest is development of brain edema with consequent impaired cerebral perfusion. Performing brain CT within 24 h from return of spontaneous circulation to assess cerebral edema from hypoxic-ischemic brain injury, as recommended by current prognostication guidelines [21], can predict progression towards brain death with high specificity [22]. New noninvasive techniques for monitoring ICP [45] and measuring cerebral perfusion pressure [46] after cardiac arrest are now available. Automated pupillometry provides a precise and quantitative assessment of pupillary reflex that can be used not only to assess the severity of hypoxic-ischemic brain injury [47], but also to detect the occurrence of elevated ICP leading to brainstem compression [48].

The occurrence of brain death after cardiac arrest is still insufficiently documented in the medical literature. In 2016, only 10% of studies considered for inclusion in our systematic review reported it [9]. The main reason for this is that neither of the two recommended measures of neurological outcome after cardiac arrest—cerebral performance categories (CPC) and modified Rankin Score (mRS)—includes brain death as a separate outcome. The term "death" in both scores (corresponding to a CPC = 5 or mRS = 6) implicitly refers to death from neurological cause, but without actually distinguishing between brain death directly caused from hypoxic-ischemic brain injury and death from withdrawal of life-sustaining treatment based on prognostication of severe neurological disability. Furthermore, the vast majority of studies make no distinction between death from a neurological and death from a circulatory cause when reporting the outcome of cardiac arrest [49].

Due to underreporting and interference from early withdrawal of life-sustaining treatment in patients with severe hypoxic-ischemic brain injury, the 5.4% overall prevalence of brain death after cardiac arrest reported in the current literature [9] is probably underestimated. In a recent Italian prognostication study [37] conducted in a cohort of resuscitated comatose patients where withdrawal of life-sustaining treatment was not performed, brain death occurred in 34/183 (19%) patients. The 2019

Standards for Studies on Neurological Prognostication after Cardiac Arrest issued by the American Heart Association [50] suggested that every study investigating prognosis after cardiac arrest should report the cause of death (brain vs. cardiac), along with the rates of and reasons for withdrawal of life-sustaining treatment.

Finally, despite the increased number of organ donations from patients resuscitated from cardiac arrest [34], there are few data from recent studies regarding the outcomes of organs donated from these patients and what donor characteristics affect transplant success. Future studies are needed to evaluate this important outcome.

37.7 Conclusion

Brain death due to severe hypoxic-ischemic brain injury after cardiac arrest is an underestimated event that needs to be prevented and detected timely. Due to the high incidence of cardiac arrest in developed countries, and due to the high rates of unfavorable outcome in patients resuscitated from cardiac arrest, there is great potential of organ donation from patients whose death is ascertained using neurological criteria. These criteria allow organ donation after cardiac arrest even in those countries or communities where donation after withdrawal of life-sustaining treatment based on neurological prognostication is not common practice. The general principle of providing "CPR to save lives" is not limited to the life of the patients who are resuscitated but it extends also to the potential recipients of organs retrieved from resuscitated patients who evolve towards brain death. Future studies on neurological prognosis after cardiac arrest should comply with recent recommendations indicating that the cause of death and the reasons for and rates of withdrawal of life-sustaining treatment should be reported.

References

1. Stecker EC, Reinier K, Marijon E, et al. Public health burden of sudden cardiac death in the United States. Circ Arrhythm Electrophysiol. 2014;7:212–7.
2. Benjamin EJ, Muntner P, Alonso A, et al. Heart disease and stroke statistics-2019 update: a report from the American Heart Association. Circulation. 2019;139:e56–e528.
3. Grasner JT, Lefering R, Koster RW, et al. EuReCa ONE-27 Nations, ONE Europe, ONE Registry: a prospective one month analysis of out-of-hospital cardiac arrest outcomes in 27 countries in Europe. Resuscitation. 2016;105:188–95.
4. CARES Cardiac Arrest Registry to Enhance Survival CARES Summary Report 2018. Demographic and Survival Characteristics of OHCA. https://mycares.net/sitepages/uploads/2019/2018%20Non-Traumatic%20National%20Summary%20Report.pdf. Accessed 3 Aug 2019.
5. Laver S, Farrow C, Turner D, Nolan J. Mode of death after admission to an intensive care unit following cardiac arrest. Intensive Care Med. 2004;30:2126–8.
6. Lemiale V, Dumas F, Mongardon N, et al. Intensive care unit mortality after cardiac arrest: the relative contribution of shock and brain injury in a large cohort. Intensive Care Med. 2013;39:1972–80.

7. Dragancea I, Rundgren M, Englund E, Friberg H, Cronberg T. The influence of induced hypothermia and delayed prognostication on the mode of death after cardiac arrest. Resuscitation. 2013;84:337–42.
8. Sandroni C, Cariou A, Cavallaro F, et al. Prognostication in comatose survivors of cardiac arrest: an advisory statement from the European Resuscitation Council and the European Society of Intensive Care Medicine. Intensive Care Med. 2014;40:1816–31.
9. Sandroni C, D'Arrigo S, Callaway CW, et al. The rate of brain death and organ donation in patients resuscitated from cardiac arrest: a systematic review and meta-analysis. Intensive Care Med. 2016;42:1661–71.
10. Orioles A, Morrison WE, Rossano JW, et al. An under-recognized benefit of cardiopulmonary resuscitation: organ transplantation. Crit Care Med. 2013;41:2794–9.
11. Casas AI, Geuss E, Kleikers PWM, et al. NOX4-dependent neuronal autotoxicity and BBB breakdown explain the superior sensitivity of the brain to ischemic damage. Proc Natl Acad Sci U S A. 2017;114:12315–20.
12. Citerio G, Cypel M, Dobb GJ, et al. Organ donation in adults: a critical care perspective. Intensive Care Med. 2016;42:305–15.
13. Barelli A, Della Corte F, Calimici R, Sandroni C, Proietti R, Magalini SI. Do brainstem auditory evoked potentials detect the actual cessation of cerebral functions in brain dead patients? Crit Care Med. 1990;18:322–3.
14. Bjorklund E, Lindberg E, Rundgren M, Cronberg T, Friberg H, Englund E. Ischaemic brain damage after cardiac arrest and induced hypothermia—a systematic description of selective eosinophilic neuronal death. A neuropathologic study of 23 patients. Resuscitation. 2014;85:527–32.
15. Sekhon MS, Ainslie PN, Griesdale DE. Clinical pathophysiology of hypoxic ischemic brain injury after cardiac arrest: a "two-hit" model. Crit Care. 2017;21:90.
16. Sakabe T, Tateishi A, Miyauchi Y, et al. Intracranial pressure following cardiopulmonary resuscitation. Intensive Care Med. 1987;13:256–9.
17. Naito H, Isotani E, Callaway CW, Hagioka S, Morimoto N. Intracranial pressure increases during rewarming period after mild therapeutic hypothermia in postcardiac arrest patients. Ther Hypothermia Temp Manag. 2016;6:189–93.
18. Bergman R, Tjan DH, Adriaanse MW, van Vugt R, van Zanten AR. Unexpected fatal neurological deterioration after successful cardio-pulmonary resuscitation and therapeutic hypothermia. Resuscitation. 2008;76:142–5.
19. Rungta RL, Choi HB, Tyson JR, et al. The cellular mechanisms of neuronal swelling underlying cytotoxic edema. Cell. 2015;161:610–21.
20. Hubbard JA, Szu JI, Binder DK. The role of aquaporin-4 in synaptic plasticity, memory and disease. Brain Res Bull. 2018;136:118–29.
21. Sandroni C, D'Arrigo S, Nolan JP. Prognostication after cardiac arrest. Crit Care. 2018;22:150.
22. Scarpino M, Lanzo G, Lolli F, et al. Is brain computed tomography combined with somatosensory evoked potentials useful in the prediction of brain death after cardiac arrest? Neurophysiol Clin. 2017;47:327–35.
23. Choi SP, Park KN, Park HK, et al. Diffusion-weighted magnetic resonance imaging for predicting the clinical outcome of comatose survivors after cardiac arrest: a cohort study. Crit Care. 2010;14:R17.
24. Nguyen M, Bievre T, Nadji A, Bouhemad B. Rapid brain death following cardiac arrest without intracranial pressure rise and cerebral circulation arrest. Case Rep Crit Care. 2018;2018:2709174.
25. Bottiger BW, Krumnikl JJ, Gass P, Schmitz B, Motsch J, Martin E. The cerebral 'no-reflow' phenomenon after cardiac arrest in rats—influence of low-flow reperfusion. Resuscitation. 1997;34:79–87.
26. Sekhon MS, Griesdale DE. Individualized perfusion targets in hypoxic ischemic brain injury after cardiac arrest. Crit Care. 2017;21:259.

27. Ameloot K, Genbrugge C, Meex I, et al. An observational near-infrared spectroscopy study on cerebral autoregulation in post-cardiac arrest patients: time to drop 'one-size-fits-all' hemodynamic targets? Resuscitation. 2015;90:121–6.
28. Arnaout M, Mongardon N, Deye N, et al. Out-of-hospital cardiac arrest from brain cause: epidemiology, clinical features, and outcome in a multicenter cohort. Crit Care Med. 2015;43:453–60.
29. Lorusso R, Gelsomino S, Parise O, et al. Neurologic injury in adults supported with veno-venous extracorporeal membrane oxygenation for respiratory failure: findings from the Extracorporeal Life Support Organization Database. Crit Care Med. 2017;45:1389–97.
30. Du Pont-Thibodeau G, Fry M, Kirschen M, et al. Timing and modes of death after pediatric out-of-hospital cardiac arrest resuscitation. Resuscitation. 2018;133:160–6.
31. Minambres E, Rubio JJ, Coll E, Dominguez-Gil B. Donation after circulatory death and its expansion in Spain. Curr Opin Organ Transplant. 2018;23:120–9.
32. Adrie C, Haouache H, Saleh M, et al. An underrecognized source of organ donors: patients with brain death after successfully resuscitated cardiac arrest. Intensive Care Med. 2008;34:132–7.
33. Sandroni C, Adrie C, Cavallaro F, et al. Are patients brain-dead after successful resuscitation from cardiac arrest suitable as organ donors? A systematic review. Resuscitation. 2010;81:1609–14.
34. Nolan JP, Ferrando P, Soar J, et al. Increasing survival after admission to UK critical care units following cardiopulmonary resuscitation. Crit Care. 2016;20:219.
35. Hassanain M, Simoneau E, Doi SA, et al. Trends in brain-dead organ donor characteristics: a 13-year analysis. Can J Surg. 2016;59:154–60.
36. Heo DS. Life-sustaining medical treatment for terminal patients in Korea. J Korean Med Sci. 2013;28:1–3.
37. Scarpino M, Lanzo G, Lolli F, et al. Neurophysiological and neuroradiological multimodal approach for early poor outcome prediction after cardiac arrest. Resuscitation. 2018;129:114–20.
38. Horn M, Schlote W. Delayed neuronal death and delayed neuronal recovery in the human brain following global ischemia. Acta Neuropathol. 1992;85:79–87.
39. Elmer J, Torres C, Aufderheide TP, et al. Association of early withdrawal of life-sustaining therapy for perceived neurological prognosis with mortality after cardiac arrest. Resuscitation. 2016;102:127–35.
40. Grossestreuer AV, Abella BS, Leary M, et al. Time to awakening and neurologic outcome in therapeutic hypothermia-treated cardiac arrest patients. Resuscitation. 2013;84:1741–6.
41. Cristia C, Ho ML, Levy S, et al. The association between a quantitative computed tomography (CT) measurement of cerebral edema and outcomes in post-cardiac arrest-a validation study. Resuscitation. 2014;85:1348–53.
42. Albaeni A, Chandra-Strobos N, Vaidya D, Eid SM. Predictors of early care withdrawal following out-of-hospital cardiac arrest. Resuscitation. 2014;85:1455–61.
43. Sandroni C, Taccone FS. Does early withdrawal of life-sustaining treatment increase mortality after cardiac arrest? Resuscitation. 2016;102:A3–4.
44. Cour M, Turc J, Madelaine T, Argaud L. Risk factors for progression toward brain death after out-of-hospital cardiac arrest. Ann Intensive Care. 2019;9:45.
45. Cardim D, Griesdale DE, Ainslie PN, et al. A comparison of non-invasive versus invasive measures of intracranial pressure in hypoxic ischaemic brain injury after cardiac arrest. Resuscitation. 2019;137:221–8.
46. Taccone FS, Crippa IA, Creteur J, Rasulo F. Estimated cerebral perfusion pressure among post-cardiac arrest survivors. Intensive Care Med. 2018;44:966–7.
47. Oddo M, Sandroni C, Citerio G, et al. Quantitative versus standard pupillary light reflex for early prognostication in comatose cardiac arrest patients: an international prospective multicenter double-blinded study. Intensive Care Med. 2018;44:2102–11.

48. Solari D, Miroz J-P, Oddo M. Opening a window to the injured brain: non-invasive neuromonitoring with quantitative pupillometry. In: Vincent JL, editor. Annual Update in Intensive Care and Emergency Medicine 2018. Heidelberg: Springer; 2018. p. 503–18.
49. Taccone FS, Horn J, Storm C, et al. Death after awakening from post-anoxic coma: the "Best CPC" project. Crit Care. 2019;23:107.
50. Geocadin RG, Callaway CW, Fink EL, et al. Standards for studies of neurological prognostication in comatose survivors of cardiac arrest: a scientific statement from the American Heart Association. Circulation. 2019;140:e517–42.

Organ Recovery Procedure in Donation After Controlled Circulatory Death with Normothermic Regional Perfusion: State of the Art

R. Badenes, B. Monleón, and I. Martín-Loeches

38.1 Introduction

Organ transplantation has become a consolidated therapy extending or improving the quality of life of 139,024 patients around the world in 2018, but this barely covers 10% of the global organ transplant needs [1, 2]. The majority of transplants from deceased organ donors use organs recovered from patients whose death has been declared on the basis of the irreversible cessation of neurological function, i.e., donation after brain death or more recently called death by neurological criteria [3]. However, the shortage of organs for transplantation, along with technical developments leading to improved posttransplant outcomes, has resulted in renewed interest in donation from persons whose death has been determined by circulatory criteria, i.e., donation after circulatory death or, also called, donation after the circulatory determination of death.

The first attempt to classify donors after circulatory death dates back to 1995, when the first International Workshop on what was then called "non-heart-beating donation" took place in Maastricht (the Netherlands) [4]. Donors were classified

R. Badenes
Department of Anesthesiology and Surgical-Trauma Intensive Care, Hospital Clínic Universitari de Valencia, Valencia, Spain

Faculty of Medicine, Department of Surgery, University of Valencia, Valencia, Spain

INCLIVA Health Research Institute, Valencia, Spain

B. Monleón
Department of Anesthesiology and Surgical-Trauma Intensive Care, Hospital Clínic Universitari de Valencia, Valencia, Spain

I. Martín-Loeches (✉)
Multidisciplinary Intensive Care Research Organization (MICRO), St. James's Hospital, Dublin, Ireland

Hospital Clinic, Universidad de Barcelona, CIBERes, Barcelona, Spain
e-mail: Imartinl@tcd.ie

Table 38.1 Updated Maastricht classification for donation after circulatory death (DCD)

Category	Type of DCD	Description	
I	N/A	Found dead – IA: out-of-hospital – IB: in-hospital	Unexpected cardiac arrest with no attempt at resuscitation. Can donate tissues (not suitable as organ donor)
II	Uncontrolled	Witnessed cardiac arrest – IIA: out-of-hospital – IIB: in-hospital	Unexpected cardiac arrest with unsuccessful resuscitation
III	Controlled	Withdrawal of life-sustaining therapy	Primary mode of DCD (only in some countries)
IV	Uncontrolled/controlled	Cardiac arrest after brain death determination	Unexpected cardiac arrest in a brain-dead patient scheduled for donation

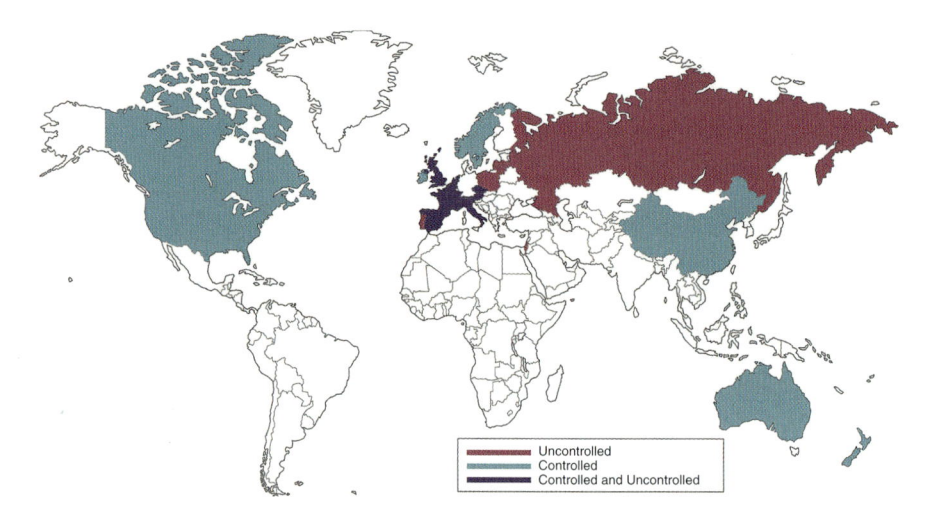

Fig. 38.1 Current donation after circulatory death practices in countries around the world

into four categories, depending on the circumstances of the cardiac arrest preceding death. The Maastricht classification was updated at a dedicated conference held in Paris (France) in February 2013 (Table 38.1) [5] to more accurately represent current donation after circulatory death practices in countries which have this form of donation (Fig. 38.1).

There are two broad categories of donation after circulatory death—controlled and uncontrolled. Donation after controlled circulatory death refers to organ donation after death following the planned withdrawal of life-sustaining therapies because these are no longer determined to be in the best interests of the patient (primarily Maastricht category III).

The potential for donation after controlled circulatory death can be considered in any hospital location after failed cardiopulmonary resuscitation (CPR) or whenever withdrawal of life-sustaining therapies is being considered. However, given the patients' morbidities and concomitant disease states contributing to the decision to withdraw life-sustaining therapies, donation after controlled circulatory death is most often considered in the intensive care unit (ICU) and emergency department (ED) [6].

The aim of this narrative review is to provide the state-of-the-art of the process of donation after controlled circulatory death, highlighting factors for success at each step provided that this activity is possible within a given jurisdiction.

38.2 Donation After Controlled Circulatory Death Pathway

38.2.1 Withdrawal of Life-Sustaining Therapies

The decision to withdraw life-sustaining treatment should always be made in accordance with national guidance on end-of-life care [7]. The majority of published documents acknowledge the fundamental principle that a decision to withdraw treatment must always be made in the best interests of the patient and independent of any subsequent consideration of organ donation [8]. National end-of-life care guidance that recognizes organ donation as a routine part of end-of-life care is helpful in reducing the perception of any conflict of interest, even though none may exist [7].

Individual hospitals should be encouraged to develop practical guidelines for treatment withdrawal in accordance with national regulations. Although the need to develop and comply with such protocols applies to all end-of-life care decisions, it is particularly important that units practicing donation after controlled circulatory death make the process consistent and transparent. These protocols should not only address the principles of the decision-making process but also give practical guidance on how to manage treatment withdrawal, particularly with regard to airway management and use of sedation and analgesia provided during the hospital stay. If the personal representative, that is usually the next of kin, agrees, withdrawal of life-sustaining therapies must be delayed until the clinical transplant coordinators and transplant physicians are ready and prepared in the operating room. Those responsible for organ allocation and recovery should do everything to minimize delays, recognizing the needs of the donor and their relatives at this time. The site and timing of subsequent withdrawal of life-sustaining therapies should facilitate organ procurement as rapidly as possible after death to minimize the warm ischemia time after cardiac arrest. The operating room presents considerable logistical advantages for withdrawal of life-sustaining therapies, but challenges privacy for the patient and relatives, and may lack appropriate staffing and range of resources. There are no clear data on the most appropriate location for withdrawal of life-sustaining therapies, only evidence of variability [9].

38.2.2 Consent and Authorization

Potential donors after controlled circulatory death usually lack the capacity for decision-making while being cared for in an ICU or ED. A prior decision for withdrawal of life-sustaining therapies is a prerequisite for an approach to a patient or their relative(s) to discuss donation after death. The approach should not be made until the clinical team is satisfied that the patient's relatives understand and accept the reasons for treatment withdrawal and the inevitability of death thereafter. To ensure this, the conversation on withdrawing treatment should be dissociated from the approach for organ donation. This also helps to reduce any perception that a decision on withdrawal of life-sustaining therapies is linked to a need for donor organs. The approach should be planned between the medical and nursing staff caring for the patients and the clinical lead for organ donation to clarify the clinical situation, identify key relatives, define key social circumstances, seek evidence of prior consent (e.g., checking donor registries), agree the timing and setting of the approach, and agree who will be involved [9]. Subsequent approaches for organ donation should be undertaken by trained requestors as this improves authorization rates, usually the clinical lead for organ donation [10]. The clinical lead for organ donation will also collect all the information required to assess whether the patient is suitable for undergoing organ donation and may discuss whether certain interventions are acceptable to the relatives before the patient dies.

38.2.3 Antemortem Procedures

Some procedures before cardiac arrest occurs can be justified ethically, on the basis of organ donation optimization, if they facilitate the wishes of the patient to promote and optimize the process of organ donation, and if they do not cause harm or distress to that patient or the relatives and/or can be reasonably controlled [11]. Where legal framework allows, a variety of procedures before the event of cardiac arrest arrives are actually possible to minimize ischemic injury and improve organ outcomes, including femoral cannulation for regional organ perfusion, anticoagulation, vasodilatation, or intravascular balloons [12, 13].

38.2.4 Determination of Death

The diagnosis of death must be made by experienced clinicians not involved in the process of organ donation or transplantation. Death should be diagnosed expeditiously while meeting appropriate legal standards [14]. Declaration of death is made on the absence of circulatory activity (e.g., no pulse, blood pressure, heart-beating sounds, neurologic response, or breathing) [15], confirmed by the absence of pulsatile flow on an arterial line or by absence of ventricular contraction on transesophageal echocardiography, on rare occasions as ancillary tests [16].

The permanence of death is confirmed by a mandatory but internationally variable "no-touch" period of observation (usually 5 min, but varying across countries) of cardiorespiratory arrest before organ procurement can begin [14].

38.2.5 Timeline

The surgical team should arrive at the donor hospital prior to withdrawal of life-sustaining therapies. A team briefing is mandatory, particularly when both thoracic and abdominal teams are present, and allows a common strategy to be agreed to ensure safe organ recovery. The outcome of transplantation with organs from donation after controlled circulatory death is significantly influenced by the duration of warm ischemia. Following withdrawal of life-sustaining therapies, several time periods have been defined [17] (Fig. 38.2):

1. Withdrawal time (agonal phase): the time from operating room to circulatory arrest.
2. First/primary warm ischemia time: the time from circulatory arrest to the start of normothermic regional perfusion.
3. Functional warm ischemia time: the time between the first episode of significant hypoperfusion (the start of which depends on national guidelines) and the start of normothermic regional perfusion.
4. Donor warm ischemia time: withdrawal time (agonal phase) + first warm ischemia time, also referred to as total warm ischemia time.

The definition for the start of functional warm ischemia time (significant hypoperfusion) is yet to be universally agreed upon, but in general a sustained fall in mean arterial blood pressure (MAP) ≤50 or 60 mmHg is accepted in Europe, while a fall in systolic blood pressure (SBP) <80 mmHg and/or O_2 saturation <80% is accepted in the United States [15–18].

One of the most significant factors in organ viability is likelihood of death occurring within a window period for each individual organ (liver and heart 20–30 min, lungs and pancreas 60 min, kidneys 90–120 min), with the duration of functional and warm ischemia times impacting transplant outcomes. The acceptable functional

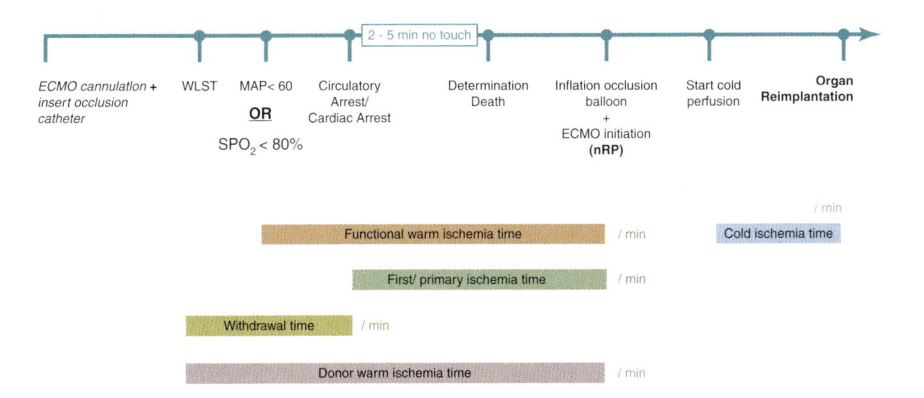

Fig. 38.2 Controlled donation after circulatory death timeline. *ECMO* extracorporeal life support, *WLST* withdrawal of life-sustaining therapies, *MAP* mean arterial blood pressure, *nRP* normothermic regional perfusion

warm ischemia time varies for different organs and ranges from 30 min (liver and heart) and 60 min (pancreas and lungs) to 90–120 min (kidneys). These times are likely to change with the use of normothermic regional perfusion [19–21].

Following withdrawal of life-sustaining therapies, the clinical lead for organ donation must communicate the vital signs (saturation, pulse, and blood pressure) and inform the procurement team when certain values or time points are met. During the process of determination of death, preservation, and organ recovery, respect for the dying donor must be ensured. At each step, their privacy and dignity must be maintained, and the end-of-life wishes of the donor and relatives must be honored as far as possible. All personnel involved should make an effort to personalize care within the given time constraints (Fig. 38.3).

38.2.6 Normothermic Regional Perfusion

The use of extracorporeal membrane oxygenation (ECMO) devices for the preservation of abdominal organs with oxygenated blood was first proposed by Spanish teams as the ideal approach for the practice of donation after uncontrolled circulatory death [22]. Normothermic regional perfusion enables cellular energy substrates to be restored and potentially improves the quality of ischemically damaged organs. Normothermic regional perfusion can turn an urgent into an elective organ recovery procedure and reduce organ damage and organ losses due to surgical events [23]. It also provides the opportunity to evaluate the macroscopic appearance of the liver and monitor alanine aminotransferase/aspartate aminotransferase (ALT) levels, and hence to assess the viability of the liver prior to transplantation [22]. Normothermic regional perfusion also seems to allow a safe extension of donor age, a factor which has classically been a major determinant of recipient outcomes [24].

The optimal duration of abdominal normothermic regional perfusion in donation after controlled circulatory death is to be determined. Most groups maintain abdominal normothermic regional perfusion for at least 90–120 min [25–27].

38.2.6.1 Specific Procedure

If antemortem cannulation is allowed for normothermic regional perfusion, femoral vessels are cannulated percutaneously (preferably) or surgically with adequate sedation, analgesia, and anticoagulation. An aortic occlusion balloon is placed at the contralateral groin to restrict preservation measures to the abdominal cavity during normothermic regional perfusion [28]. The position of the balloon must be radiologically confirmed prior to withdrawal of life-sustaining therapies. Two arterial lines, one from the femoral arterial cannula and the other from the left radial artery, are used for monitoring purposes. After the determination of death, the balloon is inflated and normothermic regional perfusion initiated. During normothermic

CRITICAL ILLNESS

- Yes
  - End of life decision
- Yes
  - Donation request → No → END OF LIFE CARE
- Yes
  - DCD potential → No → END OF LIFE CARE
- Yes
  - Screening   Matching   Organ allocation
- Yes
  - **Insert** *ECMO Catheters and* **Insert** *Aortic occlusion catheters*
- Yes
  - Initiation of end of life care
- Yes
  - WLST
- Yes
  - Cardiorespiratory arrest → No → END OF LIFE CARE
- Yes
  - No touch period
- Yes
  - Declaration of death
- Yes
  - Fill in occlusion aortic catheter and start ECMO

ORGAN PROCUREMENT

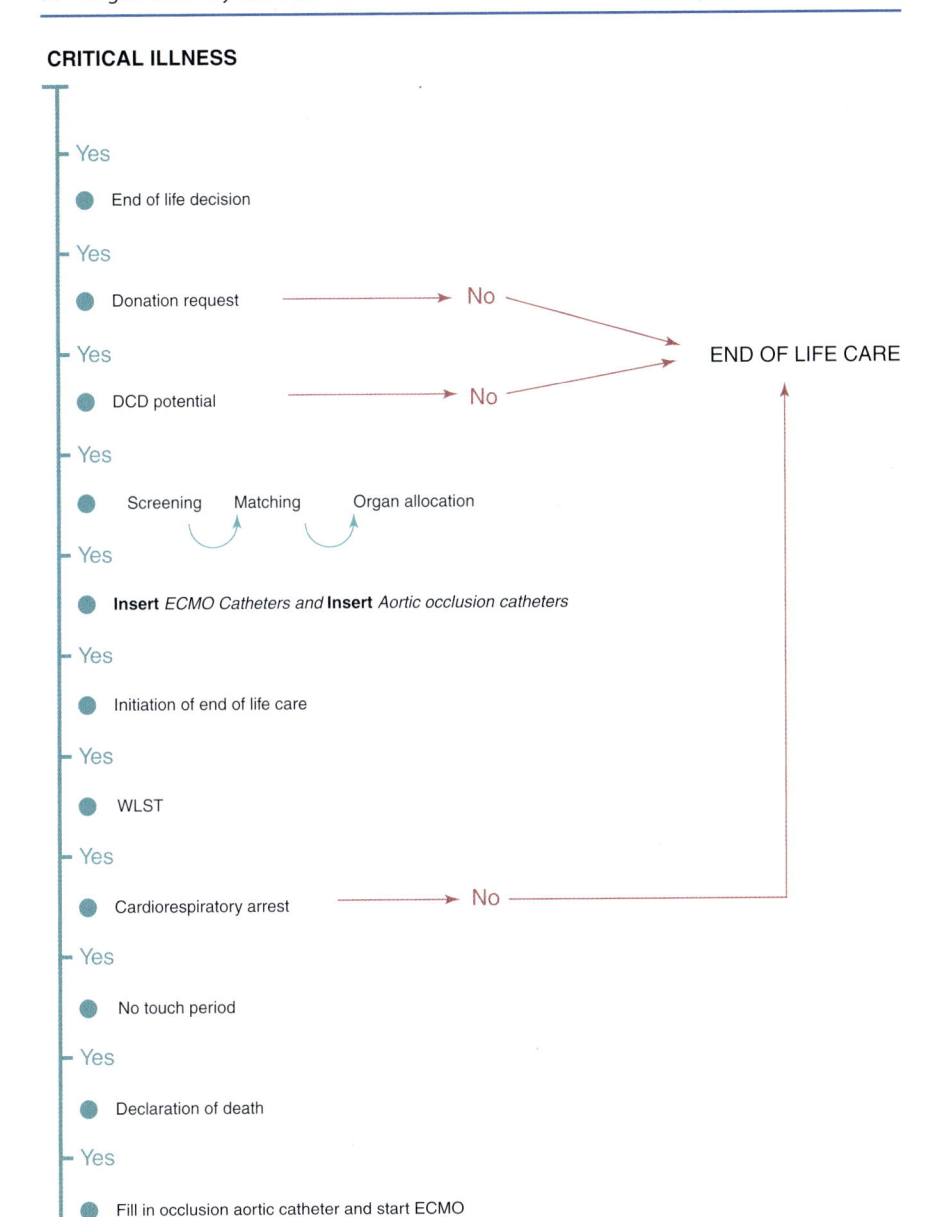

Fig. 38.3 Controlled donation after circulatory death (DCD) pathway. *ECMO* extracorporeal membrane oxygenation, *WLST* withdrawal of life-sustaining therapies

regional perfusion, the arterial pressure from the left radial artery should disappear with adequate blocking of the thoracic aorta while the pressure from the femoral arterial cannula is maintained as a continuous, non-pulsatile pressure. If arterial pressure is detected from the left radial artery during normothermic regional perfusion, this should be immediately stopped. The correct position or filling of the catheter must then be checked and normothermic regional perfusion reinitiated after another period of no-touch.

If antemortem cannulation of femoral vessels is not performed, once death has been confirmed, postmortem cannulation can be undertaken and normothermic regional perfusion initiated. A midline incision (from xiphoid process to pubic symphysis) is undertaken. The distal infrarenal aorta is identified and slung using a vascular snugger. The distal aorta is cross-clamped or ligated. The aortic cannula is inserted, checking the proximal position of the tip. The cannula is secured in place with the vascular snugger and connected to the arterial limb of the circuit. The infrarenal inferior vena cava is then dissected and encircled using a vascular snugger. The distal end is clamped or ligated. The venous cannula is inserted into the inferior vena cava. The tip should sit just below the diaphragm to allow clamping of the suprahepatic inferior vena cava without compromising the venous return in the circuit. The venous limb of the circuit is then connected to the cannula. A rapid sternotomy is carried out using either a power saw or a Gigli saw. The thoracic aorta is clamped below the level of the left subclavian artery. At this point, the normothermic regional perfusion circuit can be started. An alternative approach would be to insert an aortic endo-clamp in the descending thoracic aorta and commence normothermic regional perfusion before undertaking the sternotomy. This approach would enable the cardiothoracic team to undertake the sternotomy, mobilize the lung, and clamp the descending aorta (if simultaneous lung recovery). Once normothermic regional perfusion is established, meticulous hemostasis must be ensured from the abdominal wound edges, sternotomy, and retroperitoneal tissues disrupted during aortic and inferior vena cava cannulation.

The pump parameters are yet to be fully established but Spanish and UK experience suggests a pump flow of 2–3 l/min, temperature of 35.5–37.5 °C, O_2 of 2–4 l/min (or air/O_2 mix as required to maintain PaO_2), a pH of 7.35–7.45 (administer bicarbonate as required), a PaO_2 >90 mmHg, and a hematocrit >20% [25, 27]. Venous oxygen saturation is a good guide of oxygen delivery and mixed venous oxygen saturation (SvO_2) should be around 60–80%.

During this period, serial blood samples are taken to assess the function of the liver and kidneys. Organ mobilization and preparation for the cold phase can be undertaken, following the same steps as a donation after brain death recovery. Once normothermic regional perfusion is completed, cold *in situ* perfusion is instituted and organ recovery continues (Fig. 38.3). Although experience of using normothermic regional perfusion in donation after controlled circulatory death is still limited, published data support these theoretical benefits and report promising results in terms of numbers of organs recovered and transplantation outcomes [25, 26, 29] (Fig. 38.4).

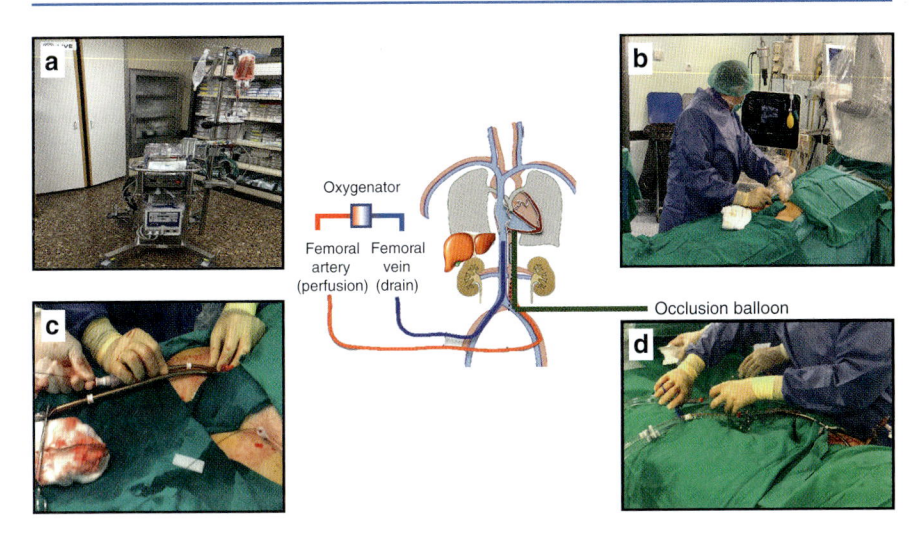

Fig. 38.4 Scheme for extracorporeal membrane oxygenation (ECMO) for donation after circulatory death. In the different pictures, different key elements of the procedure are displayed: (**a**) priming the ECMO; (**b**) using ultrasound for vessel detection; (**c**) inserting arterial and venous cannulas; and (**d**) inflation of occlusion balloon and de-clamping cannulas to start extracorporeal abdominal perfusion

38.3 Liver Transplantation

Two large multicenter studies have described the benefits that may be achieved with postmortem normothermic regional perfusion in liver transplantation from donation after controlled circulatory death [30, 31]. First, a Spanish national study compared the results of 95 donations after controlled circulatory death liver transplants performed with postmortem normothermic regional perfusion with those of 117 liver transplants performed with super rapid recovery. Median donor age in the study was relatively high (57 years [25–75% interquartile range, IQR, 45–65] in the normothermic regional perfusion group, 56 years [25–75% IQR 47–64] in the super rapid recovery group). With a median follow-up of 20 months, the use of postmortem normothermic regional perfusion appeared to significantly reduce rates of postoperative biliary complications (overall 8% normothermic regional perfusion vs. 31% super rapid recovery, $p < 0.001$; ischemic type biliary lesions 2% normothermic regional perfusion vs. 13% super rapid recovery, $p = 0.008$) and graft loss (12% normothermic regional perfusion vs. 24% super rapid recovery, $p = 0.008$) [30]. Similarly, a combined experience from centers in Cambridge and Edinburgh in the United Kingdom compared the results of 43 liver transplants from donation after controlled circulatory death performed with postmortem normothermic regional perfusion with those of a contemporary cohort of 187 liver transplants from donation after controlled circulatory death performed with super rapid recovery. Median donor age was less for normothermic regional perfusion compared to super rapid recovery livers: 41 years (25–75% IQR 33–57) vs. 54 years (25–75% IQR 38–63), respectively. Reported rates of anastomotic biliary strictures were 7% vs. 27% ($p = 0.004$), ischemic type biliary lesions 0 vs. 27% ($p < 0.001$), and 90-day graft loss 2% vs. 10% ($p = 0.102$) [31].

Considered together, the results of these two studies are remarkably consistent and provide a rather clear indication that the use of postmortem normothermic regional perfusion in liver transplantation from donation after controlled circulatory death can help reduce rates of biliary complications, ischemic type biliary lesions, and graft loss, and allow for the successful transplantation of livers from donors after controlled circulatory death even from donors of advanced age.

38.4 Lung Transplantation

Early and intermediate survival rates after lung transplantation from donation after circulatory death were comparable to donation after brain death in two updated meta-analyses [32, 33]. Donation after circulatory death appears to be a safe and effective method to expand the donor pool. Overall, 17 studies with 995 donations after circulatory death recipients and 38,579 donations after brain death recipients were included. The pooled analysis showed comparable 1-year overall survival between the cohorts (RR 0.89, 95% CI [0.74, 1.07], $p = 0.536$, $I^2 = 0\%$). The airway anastomotic complication rate in the donation after circulatory death cohort was higher than that in donation after brain death cohort (RR 2.00, 95% CI [1.29, 3.11], $p = 0.002$, $I^2 = 0\%$). There was no significant difference between donation after circulatory death and donation after brain death in terms of occurrence of primary graft dysfunction grade 2/3, bronchiolitis obliterans syndrome, acute transplantation rejection, or length of stay. The stability of the included studies was strong. These studies add to the body of evidence and support the use of lungs from donation after circulatory death for transplantation.

However, the utilization of lungs from donation after controlled circulatory death remains poor for several reasons, including less experience with the process procurement and inadequate lung management in the ICU [34]. The lungs are recovered in donation after controlled circulatory death donors using the super rapid recovery technique, decreasing the lung temperature with topical cooling as quickly as possible, whereas normothermic regional perfusion seems to be the ideal method for liver grafts. This combined method was first described as a single case report by two UK groups [35, 36].

A variant of the technique, using premortem interventions, in which the risk of potential transdiaphragmatic cooling of the liver is minimized, has been proposed [37]. Once death has been determined and normothermic regional perfusion initiated, the thoracic surgeon performs a quick sternotomy. At the same time, the donor is reintubated and ventilated for 5 min after normothermic regional perfusion with 100% oxygen and positive end-expiratory pressure (PEEP) of 5 cmH$_2$O. The pulmonary artery is cannulated for cold flush perfusion with Perfadex® (50 ml/kg). Only 1 liter of 4 °C saline is delivered in both hemithoraxes for topical cooling. Finally, the superior vena cava is ligated to separate the thoracic and abdominal compartments once the lungs have been preserved with Perfadex® solution, and pulmonary extraction is initiated using the same technique as in donation after brain death donors. This combined method offers an outstanding recovery rate and liver and lung recipient survival comparable with those transplanted with organs harvested after brain death [37].

38.5 Kidney Transplantation

Marked reductions in delayed graft function have been seen in normothermic regional perfusion donation after circulatory death cohorts, suggesting that this is one of the main advantages of this approach to kidney transplantation [38]. Reducing delayed graft function remains an important goal because of the greater risk of graft failure and rejection and the associated costs of additional hemodialysis and hospital stays.

The use of kidneys from donation after controlled circulatory death is increasing for older patients and patients with comorbidity. Short-term graft outcomes are similar for donors meeting expanded and standard criteria for donation after controlled circulatory death, so these donors constitute an acceptable source of kidneys to improve the options of kidney transplantation wait-listed patients [39].

38.6 Pancreas Transplantation

In recent years, normothermic regional perfusion in the donation after controlled circulatory death donor has attracted increasing interest in pancreas transplantation [40]. This process aims to restore cellular energetics and substrates, reducing the damaging ischemic effect on the pancreas. There is very little reported experience in the pancreas: this has now been reported by three centers and has resulted in just four pancreas–kidney transplants, all with good outcomes [25–27]. Clearly, further work is needed to assess the potential benefits of normothermic regional perfusion in pancreas transplantation.

38.7 Heart Transplantation

Due to the difficulties in the heart pool for heart donation, current data suggest that donor hearts from donation after circulatory death that meet the selection criteria and are successfully transplanted lead to outcomes equal to those performed with traditional donation after brain death organs. Donation after circulatory death heart transplantation is being performed only in a few established centers worldwide, not only in adults [41] but also in the pediatric population [42].

In the world of adult heart transplantation, successful donation after circulatory death transplantation with the direct procurement and *ex vivo* perfusion technique was first reported in three patients in 2015 from Sydney, Australia [43]. All three patients had normal cardiac function within 7 days of transplantation. Donor criteria in this study were strict with donor age limited up to 40 years of age and cold ischemic time of less than 30 min. Since publishing, there have been a total of 12 transplants from donations after circulatory death performed at this center with favorable outcomes of 0% mortality as of April 2017 [44]. By utilizing appropriately vetted donation after circulatory death donor hearts, transplant rates were increased by 45% [45].

Ninety-day and one-year survival in 28 donations after circulatory death transplants were found to be equivalent with no significant differences in rejection, graft function, or hospital stay when compared to matched donation after brain death transplants—this included hearts donated after circulatory death both using direct procurement and perfusion and using normothermic regional perfusion [46]. This program at the Royal Papworth Hospital NHS Foundation Trust has now performed 39 donations after circulatory death heart transplants with 91% survival to discharge with only 13% of patients requiring postoperative ECMO [44].

Recently, normothermic regional perfusion has been implemented with successful results [45]. The inability to evaluate donor cardiac function prior to procurement represents an unnecessary risk to the patient. Furthermore, should procurement and resuscitation be begun with *ex vivo* perfusion and the organ then be deemed functionally ineligible for transplant this presents a large preventable financial loss. The assessment of cardiac function during procurement with normothermic regional perfusion enables the age range of donors to be extended (less than 50 years vs. less than 40 years) and has resulted in a greater conversion to actual transplantation than hearts procured with alternative methods [46].

After declaration of death, a sternotomy is rapidly performed and the pericardium opened. The three aortic arch vessels are then clamped to exclude the cerebral circulation before full-flow normothermic regional perfusion is established and the patient is reventilated. A goal of flow index >2.5 l/min/m^2, a MAP of at least 50 mmHg, a core temperature of >35 °C, and a hematocrit of 30% are needed. If necessary, the MAP is supported by infusion of norepinephrine up to a maximum of 0.5 mg/kg/min. Infusions of dobutamine at 5 mg/kg/min, and of isoproterenol at 12–20 mg/kg/min, are also started to support heart automaticity and contractility. After 30 min of normothermic regional perfusion, ECMO is weaned and heart function assessed using both transesophageal echocardiography (TEE) ultrasound and Swan–Ganz catheter. The criteria for performing organ retrieval are as follows: left ventricular ejection fraction >50%; normal size and function of the right ventricle; cardiac index >2.5 l/min/m^2; pulmonary artery occlusion pressure <12 mmHg; and MAP >60 mmHg, with no arrhythmia. These parameters have to remain stable for at least 30 min after ECMO weaning before the decision to transplant is finalized. Cardiectomy is then carried out in a similar fashion to donation after brain death heart procurement. The kidneys and liver are also retrieved [47].

38.8 Conclusion

Donation after circulatory death is a much-needed addition to donation after brain death when we consider the persisting worldwide shortage of donor organs and the need for countries to progress towards self-sufficiency in transplantation.

The field of donation after controlled circulatory death is rapidly evolving, with an increasing number of countries participating in this type of deceased donation that poses particular challenges. Criteria for donor selection are expanding as the results of transplants from donation after controlled circulatory death are becoming more favorable. Current developments in normothermic regional perfusion are contributing to a greater use of organs per donor, better quality of organs, and improved posttransplant outcomes. Kidney, liver, pancreas, lung, and, recently, heart donations are eligible for transplant after controlled circulatory death.

References

1. Global observatory on donation and transplantation. http://www.transplant-observatory.org/. Accessed 2 Sept 2019.
2. Documents produced by the Council of Europe European Committee (partial agreement) on organ transplantation (CD-P-TO). https://www.edqm.eu/en/reports-and-publications. Accessed 2 Sept 2019.
3. Smith M, Citerio G. Death determined by neurological criteria: the next steps. Intensive Care Med. 2017;43:1383–5.
4. Kootstra G, Daemen JH, Oomen AP. Categories of non-heart-beating donors. Transplant Proc. 1995;27:2893–4.
5. Thuong M, Ruiz A, Evrard P, et al. New classification of donation after circulatory death donors definitions and terminology. Transpl Int. 2016;29:749–59.
6. Manyalich M, Nelson H, Delmonico FL. The need and opportunity for donation after circulatory death worldwide. Curr Opin Organ Transplant. 2018;23:136–41.
7. General Medical Council. Treatment and care towards the end of life: good practice in decision making, 2010. Available as 'End of life care guidance' at https://www.gmc-uk.org/ethical-guidance/ethical-guidance-for-doctors/treatment-and-care-towards-the-end-of-life. Accessed 01 Sept 2019.
8. Hulme W, Allen J, Manara AR, Murphy PG, Gardiner D, Poppitt E. Factors influencing the family consent rate for organ donation in the UK. Anaesthesia. 2016;71:1053–63.
9. Mitro G, Warnock R, Wiederhold P, Jiles K, Ortiz J. Consistency of DCD procurement procedures across organ procurement organizations—preliminary findings [abstract]. American Transplant Congress Archives—ATC Abstracts 2018. https://atcmeetingabstracts.com/abstract/consistency-of-dcd-procurement-procedures-across-organ-procurement-organizations-preliminary-findings/. Accessed 27 Aug 2019.
10. Siminoff LA, Gordon N, Hewlett J, Arnold RM. Factors influencing families' consent for donation of solid organs for transplantation. JAMA. 2001;286:71–7.
11. Cao Y, Shahrestani S, Chew HC, et al. Donation after circulatory death for liver transplantation: a meta-analysis on the location of life support withdrawal affecting outcomes. Transplantation. 2016;100:1513–24.
12. Citerio G, Cypel M, Dobb GJ, et al. Organ donation in adults: a critical care perspective. Intensive Care Med. 2016;42:305–15.
13. Pérez-Villares JM, Rubio JJ, Del Río F, Miñambres E. Validation of a new proposal to avoid donor resuscitation in controlled donation after circulatory death with normothermic regional perfusion. Resuscitation. 2017;117:46–9.

14. Reich DJ, Mulligan DC, Abt PL, et al. ASTS recommended practice guidelines for controlled donation after cardiac death organ procurement and transplantation. Am J Transplant. 2009;9:2004–11.
15. Dhanani S, Hornby L, Ward R, Shemie S. Variability in the determination of death after cardiac arrest: a review of guidelines and statements. J Intensive Care Med. 2012;27:238–52.
16. Neyrinck A, Van RD, Monbaliu D. Donation after circulatory death: current status. Curr Opin Anaesthesiol. 2013;26:382–90.
17. Bernat JL, Capron AM, Bleck TP, et al. The circulatory-respiratory determination of death in organ donation. Crit Care Med. 2010;38:963–70.
18. Andrews PA, Burnapp L, Manas D. British Transplantation Society. Summary of the British Transplantation Society guidelines for transplantation from donors after deceased circulatory death. Transplantation. 2014;97:265–70.
19. Kotsopoulos AMM, Boing-Messing F, Jansen NE, Vos P, Abdo WF. External validation of prediction models for time to death in potential donors after circulatory death. Am J Transplant. 2018;18:890–6.
20. Summers DM, Watson CJ, Pettigrew GJ, et al. Kidney donation after circulatory death (DCD): state of the art. Kidney Int. 2015;88:241–9.
21. Smith M, Dominguez-Gil B, Greer DM, Manara AR, Souter MJ. Organ donation after circulatory death: current status and future potential. Intensive Care Med. 2019;45:310–21.
22. Fondevila C, Hessheimer AJ, Flores E, et al. Applicability and results of Maastricht type 2 donation after cardiac death liver transplantation. Am J Transplant. 2012;12:162–70.
23. Ausania F, White SA, Pocock P, Manas DM. Kidney damage during organ recovery in donation after circulatory death donors: data from UK National Transplant Database. Am J Transplant. 2012;12:932–6.
24. Summers DM, Johnson RJ, Hudson A, Collett D, Watson CJ, Bradley JA. Effect of donor age and cold storage time on outcome in recipients of kidneys donated after circulatory death in the UK: a cohort study. Lancet. 2013;381:727–34.
25. Miñambres E, Suberviola B, Domínguez-Gil B, et al. Improving the outcomes of organs obtained from controlled donation after circulatory death donors using abdominal normothermic regional perfusion. Am J Transplant. 2017;17:2165–72.
26. Rojas-Peña A, Sall LE, Gravel MT, et al. Donation after circulatory determination of death: The University of Michigan experience with extra-corporeal support. Transplantation. 2014;98:328–34.
27. Oniscu GC, Randle LV, Muiesan P, et al. In situ normothermic regional perfusion for controlled donation after circulatory death: the United Kingdom experience. Am J Transplant. 2014;14:2846–54.
28. Miñambres E, Rubio JJ, Coll E, Domínguez-Gil B. Donation after circulatory death and its expansion in Spain. Curr Opin Organ Transplant. 2018;23:120–9.
29. Ruiz P, Gastaca M, Bustamante FJ, et al. Favorable outcomes after liver transplantation with normothermic regional perfusion from donors after circulatory death: a single-center experience. Transplantation. 2019;103:938–43.
30. Hessheimer AJ, Coll E, Torres F, et al. Normothermic regional perfusion vs. super-rapid recovery in controlled donation after circulatory death liver transplantation. J Hepatol. 2019;70:658–65.
31. Watson C, Hunt F, Messer S, et al. In situ normothermic perfusion of livers in controlled circulatory death donation may prevent ischemic cholangiopathy and improve graft survival. Am J Transplant. 2019;19:1745–58.
32. Krutsinger D, Reed RM, Blevins A, et al. Lung transplantation from donation after cardiocirculatory death: a systematic review and meta-analysis. J Heart Lung Transplant. 2015;34:675–84.
33. Zhou J, Chen B, Liao H, et al. The comparable efficacy of lung donation after circulatory death and brain death: a systematic review and meta-analysis. Transplantation. 2019;103:2624–33.
34. Mooney JJ, Hedlin H, Mohabir PK, et al. Lung quality and utilization in controlled donation after circulatory determination of death within the United States. Am J Transplant. 2016;16:1207–15.

35. Oniscu GC, Siddique A, Dark J, et al. Dual temperature multi-organ recovery from a Maastricht category III donor after circulatory death. Am J Transplant. 2014;14:2181–6.
36. Perera MT, Clutton-Brock T, Muiesan P. One donor, two types of preservation: first description of a donation after circulatory death donor with normothermic abdominal perfusion and simultaneous cold perfusion of lungs. Liver Transpl. 2014;20:1012–5.
37. Miñambres E, Ruiz P, Ballesteros MA, et al. Combined lung and liver procurement in controlled donation after circulatory death using normothermic abdominal perfusion. Initial experience in two Spanish centers. Am J Transplant. 2020;20:231–40.
38. Farney AC, Singh RP, Hines MH, et al. Experience in renal and extrarenal transplantation with donation after cardiac death donors with selective use of extracorporeal support. J Am Coll Surg. 2008;206:1028–37.
39. Pérez-Sáez MJ, Lafuente Covarrubias O, Hernández D, et al. GEODAS Group. Early outcomes of kidney transplantation from elderly donors after circulatory death (GEODAS study). BMC Nephrol. 2019;20:233.
40. Kopp WH, Lam HD, Schaapherder AFM, et al. Pancreas transplantation with grafts from donors deceased after circulatory death: 5 years single-center experience. Transplantation. 2018;102:333–9.
41. Beaupré RA, Morgan JA. Donation after cardiac death: a necessary expansion for heart transplantation. Semin Thorac Cardiovasc Surg. 2019;31:721–5.
42. Khushnood A, Butt TA, Jungschleger J, et al. Paediatric donation after circulatory determined death heart transplantation using donor normothermic regional perfusion and ex situ heart perfusion: a case report. Pediatr Transplant. 2019;23:e13536.
43. Dhital KK, Iyer A, Connellan M, et al. Adult heart transplantation with distant procurement and ex-vivo preservation of donor hearts after circulatory death: a case series. Lancet. 2015;385:2585–91.
44. Page A, Messer S, Large SR. Heart transplantation from donation after circulatory determined death. Ann Cardiothorac Surg. 2018;7:75–81.
45. Messer SJ, Axell RG, Colah S, et al. Functional assessment and transplantation of the donor heart after circulatory death. J Heart Lung Transplant. 2016;35:1443–52.
46. Messer S, Page A, Axell R, et al. Outcome after heart transplantation from donation after circulatory-determined death donors. J Heart Lung Transplant. 2017;36:1311–8.
47. Tchana-Sato V, Ledoux D, Detry O, et al. Successful clinical transplantation of hearts donated after circulatory death using normothermic regional perfusion. J Heart Lung Transplant. 2019;38:593–8.

Part XIII

Oncology

Admitting Adult Critically Ill Patients with Hematological Malignancies to the ICU: A Sisyphean Task or Work in Progress?

E. N. van der Zee, E. J. O. Kompanje, and J. Bakker

39.1 Introduction

Approximately 40% of the world's population will be diagnosed with a malignancy at some point during their life [1]. In 2012, one-quarter of the global burden of cancer was observed in Europe whereas the total population of Europe represented only 9% of the world's population [2]. In 2015, malignancies were still a major cause of death across the European Union with an average of 261 deaths per 100,000 inhabitants [3]. However, due to progress in early detection and treatment, long-term survival from malignancy has increased over the past decades [4]. Between 2011 and 2016 cancer mortality decreased in both men (8%) and women (3%) [5]. In 2018, there were an estimated 3.91 million new cases of malignancy and 1.93 million deaths from cancer in Europe [2]. The most common malignancies were female breast cancer and colorectal cancer [2]. Over the last decades, the incidence of hematological malignancies has increased as well [6–8]. Approximately 2.2% of the population will be diagnosed with a non-Hodgkin's lymphoma and 1.6% with leukemia [1]. The incidence of hematological malignancies is expected to grow in the future as a result of the aging population and the inability to prevent most cases [6]. As the mortality rate has been decreasing during the past decades [5, 9, 10] and the probability of infiltrative, infectious, or toxic life-threatening events related to therapy has been increasing [11], the burden of these malignancies to healthcare systems is likely to increase. This is especially the case when considering the role of the intensive care unit (ICU) in both the initial treatment and the treatment of these complications. A historical reluctance to admit patients with malignancies to the ICU, especially hematological malignancies, exists [12–15]. However, given the new therapies available, the encouraging survival data, and the possible benefits of an ICU admission, ICU admission should be considered.

The aim of this clinical review is to describe the development of the prognosis of adult patients with a hematological malignancy and the role of the ICU over the past years and in the future.

39.2 Survival and Prognosis of Patients with Hematological Malignancies

As is currently the case, the survival of patients with hematological malignancies varied in the past, depending on the type of hematological malignancy. The literature showed a dramatically low 5-year survival for most leukemias in 1974–1976, especially for acute myeloid leukemia (only 6%) [16]. In contrast, 71% of patients with Hodgkin's lymphoma survived 5 years in this period. Between 1974 and 1996, the 5-year survival for leukemias, myelomas, and lymphomas increased [6, 16]. In the subsequent years (1996–2012), the 5-year survival for these hematological malignancies also improved, varying from a still relatively poor prognosis for acute myeloid leukemia (15–21%) to a very acceptable outcome for Hodgkin's lymphoma (86–92.8%) [1, 10, 16–20]. All of the hematological malignancies described above have shown stabilized or improved 5-year survival rates for the period 2008–2012. Therefore, the outcome of patients with a hematological type of cancer may further improve in the future.

There are several reasons for this increasing survival rate of patients with hematological malignancies [6, 10, 11, 16, 17, 20]: improvements in diagnostic methods, diagnosis being made earlier than before, and more effective treatments. Moreover, advances in molecular biology make it possible to recognize low-grade malignancies with good prognosis. In addition, effective high-dose treatment regimens and targeted treatments have been introduced. Lastly, the complications observed after therapy are better understood and consequently there has been an increase in adequate treatment of these complications. However, despite this encouraging change, improvements in survival for hematological malignancies have not been uniform across Europe [10, 17]. Substantial regional differences in survival rates are seen for different types of hematological cancer. Data show variation across countries and between northern, southern, western, and eastern Europe. On average, survival in eastern European countries is lower compared to the rest of Europe. This difference could be explained by inequalities in provision of care concerning diagnostics and therapy or heterogeneity in case definition. Unsurprisingly, age at diagnosis is a strong prognostic factor [5, 10, 17, 20]. Elderly patients experience limitations of (aggressive and curative) treatment due to the prevalence of comorbidities and frailty. Furthermore, after adjustment for age and country, the data show a significant difference in survival between men and women [5, 10, 20]. Possible explanations are a lesser impact of comorbidities, as well as behavioral and biological factors [10].

39.3 ICU Admission Practices for Patients with Hematological Malignancies: Historical Perspective

Historically, the mortality of patients with a hematological malignancy requiring ICU admission was high. In 1983, Schuster et al. [15] reported an 80% hospital mortality in 77 critically ill patients with a hematological malignancy admitted to the ICU; survival was particularly low when patients required mechanical ventilation. In 1988, Lloyd-Thomas et al. [13] reported a mortality rate of 78% in 60 patients with a hematological type of cancer admitted to the ICU. The mortality rate was consistently higher than predicted from a large validation study of the APACHE II score in a mixed population of critically ill patients. In 1990, Brunet et al. [12] published an ICU mortality rate of 43% and a 1-year survival rate of 19% in 260 patients with a hematological malignancy. Patients who required mechanical ventilation or renal replacement therapy (RRT) showed an increased ICU mortality rate. They concluded that life support should be initiated, but that the combination of RRT and mechanical ventilation was associated with a poor prognosis. With an ICU mortality of 80–90% between 1984 and 1993, Ewig et al. [21] expressed their concerns about the low survival rates of patients with pulmonary complications admitted to the ICU. In the same time period (1980–1992), Rubenfeld et al. noted a mortality rate of 94% in 865 mechanically ventilated patients after bone marrow transplantation [14]. Of the patients with lung injury requiring mechanical ventilation combined with hemodynamic instability, hepatic failure, or renal failure, no one survived. However, the survival rate of critically ill bone marrow transplant patients increased over time, from 5% in 1980 to 16% in 1992. In summary, mortality rates of patients with a hematological type of cancer who required admission to the ICU were high in all five studies [12–15, 21].

In subsequent years, between 1990 and 2005, the hospital mortality rate ranges from 41% to 85% [22–26]. A high risk of refusal of ICU admission for critically ill cancer patients in this period is still seen [27]. This could be explained due to the discouraging mortality rates of previous studies and due to the recommendations of the North American and European Societies of Critical Care Medicine for ICU admission, discharge, and triage [28, 29] in which it is stated that oncologists and intensivists should reserve ICU admission for select cancer patients with a "reasonable prospect of substantial recovery."

39.4 ICU Admission Practices for Patients with Hematological Malignancies: The Modern Area

Large numbers of patients with a malignancy are nowadays admitted to the ICU (15–20% of all patients) [30–32]. Despite a substantial improvement in the survival of critically ill patients with cancer [8, 33, 34], the recent literature concerning critically ill patients with a hematological malignancy is heterogeneous and survival rates differ considerably [8]. ICU and hospital survival vary from 0% to 88% [35–40] and from 0% to 72% [35, 38, 39, 41], respectively. The literature shows that short-term mortality is related to the severity of illness (and organ dysfunction) rather than the underlying malignant diagnosis [8]. Although 1-year mortality may be good (almost 50%) [40], long-term mortality is still limited with a reported 8-year survival rate of only 9% [36]. Data show a decrease in long-term survival of patients admitted to the ICU, in comparison to patients who did not require admission to the ICU [36, 42]. Nonetheless, the ICU mortality rate has decreased impressively compared to the past [41, 43], with an annual decrease of 4–7% between 2003 and 2015 [43]. Based on this improvement in survival and the possible benefits of intensive care treatment, ICU admission should be considered in every patient. Thiéry et al. [27] conducted a study of cancer patients for whom ICU admission was requested. They found that 20% of patients who were not admitted because they were considered "too well" died before hospital discharge, and 25% of the patients who were not admitted because they were considered "too sick" survived. Thus, the clinical evaluation was neither sensitive nor specific for selecting patients for ICU admission. Denial of ICU admission solely on a patient having cancer is not supported by recent outcome data.

The striking difference in survival of critically ill patients with a hematological malignancy across studies and hospitals may be explained by several factors. First, studies reporting high survival rates usually originate from high-volume centers and so the external validity of these data may be limited [11]. Second, the performance status of the patient is a strong predictor of mortality and may differ between studies [8]. Third, timing of admission of patients to the ICU may differ across hospitals. Up to 50% of patients referred to the ICU are not admitted immediately [27]. Early admission is recommended, because improved outcomes associated with early admission have been found in several studies [8, 11, 33]. Bed availability may be an issue in some hospitals, thereby negatively influencing the outcome [8].

Azoulay et al. generated several hypotheses regarding the causes of delayed ICU admission and its relationship to mortality [11] (Box 39.1):

1. Patient related: Patients may interpret acute symptoms as inevitable manifestations of their malignancy or may lack the social support or financial resources needed to obtain medical advice. As a consequence, hospitalization may be delayed and, in case of critical illness, ICU admission may be delayed as well.
2. Disease related: Acute illnesses could develop in a fulminant way in patients with severe immunodeficiency. Subsequently, fast deterioration may occur, with severe (multiple) organ dysfunction. As a result, ICU treatment might be too late to prevent death.

Box 39.1 Causes of delayed ICU admission in patients with hematological malignancy and recommendations for change

Factor	Causes of delayed ICU admission	Recommendations
Patient related	Misinterpretation of acute symptoms Lack of social support or financial resources (delayed hospitalization)	Education regarding alarm symptoms Explanation of relevance of social support Health insurance
Disease related Ward related	Fast deterioration of immunocompromised patients Suboptimal patient evaluation Unclear (poor) prognosis	Use of the modified early warning score and rapid response system Use of the modified early warning score and rapid response system Close collaboration between hematology department and intensive care
ICU related	Unclear (poor) prognosis Ill-equipped ICU with inexperienced healthcare providers Bed availability in ICU	Close collaboration between hematology department and intensive care Close collaboration between experienced hospitals and less experienced hospitals Early aggressive treatment outside the ICU Time-limited or intensity-limited ICU trials

3. Ward related: First, suboptimal patient evaluation on the wards may result in an underestimation of disease severity followed by an unexpected clinical deterioration. Second, when the prognosis is unclear and possibly poor, ICU referral may be difficult and subsequently delayed.
4. ICU related: Likewise, ICU admission decisions could be difficult and delayed in case of an unclear (poor) prognosis. In addition, a delay in optimal care may arise from the initial admission to an ICU ill equipped to manage patients with hematological malignancies with healthcare providers inexperienced in caring for hematological patients. Finally, bed availability may be an issue in some hospitals, resulting in delayed admission.

Some of the causes described above are amendable (Box 39.1). First, to reduce patient-related factors, education concerning alarm signals may improve patient knowledge [11]. The relevance of social support should be explained as well. Although individual financial problems are difficult to solve, national healthcare policies could play an important role in this.

Second, to improve ICU-related factors, good communication and close collaboration between different specialties and different hospitals are recommended [8, 11, 33]. For example, daily formal meetings between the attending hematologists and intensivists [8], advice from intensivists at centers managing large numbers of hematological patients to less experienced intensivists [11], and help from nurse consultants of the hematology department concerning hematological care [8] can be beneficial. In hospitals where ICU bed availability is limited, early aggressive treatment can be initiated outside the ICU [8, 11]. Furthermore, an ICU bed could be used for time-limited or intensity-limited trials, thus improving the chance of survival [8, 11]. Admittance to the ICU for end-of-life care is not recommended, because avoidance of ICU admissions within 30 days of death and death occurring outside the hospital were associated with perceptions of better end-of-life care [44].

Third, concerning the suboptimal evaluation of critically ill patients on the hematological ward, early detection of patient deterioration using the modified early warning score (MEWS) and a rapid response system has proven to be effective in enhancing ICU admission [8].

In summary, although ICU survival rates have been a major reason to deny admission in the past, steadily improving ICU survival rates have been observed in recent years. Denial of ICU admission solely based on the presence of a hematological malignancy is no longer supported by recent outcome data.

39.5 Quality of Life of Patients with a Hematological Malignancy Following ICU Admission

With the improvement in (long-term) survival of patients with a hematological malignancy, questions concerning the quality of life of these patients arise. Literature shows impairment of quality of life, measured by validated questionnaires, compared to their previous state or to the general population [45, 46]. Studies report either physical symptoms, such as fatigue, pain and reduction of vitality, or psychosocial symptoms, including increased levels of anxiety and depression. Mostly, data show a combination of both. A subset of patients with hematological malignancy treated with chemotherapy experience cognitive impairment [47].

Recent literature concerning the quality of life of patients with a malignancy after admission to an ICU is scarce. Oeyen et al. [48] conducted a study to assess long-term outcomes and quality of life in critically ill patients with hematological or solid malignancies, which included quality of life at 3 months and 1 year after discharge, compared to the quality of life before ICU admission. Initially, quality of life declined at 3 months. At 1 year after ICU discharge, quality of life did improve; however it remained under the baseline quality of life. Ehooman et al. showed a strongly impaired quality of life in patients with a hematological malignancy compared to general ICU patients with septic shock at 3 months and 1 year after ICU discharge [39].

By contrast, van Vliet et al. [49] compared patients with hematological malignancies admitted to the ICU with matched patients not admitted to the ICU. Eighteen months after admission, no significant difference in quality of life was found between those groups, other than a lower physical functioning score. Similarly, Azoulay et al. [50] conducted a prospective, multicenter cohort study including 1011 critically ill patients with a hematological malignancy. On day 90, 80% of survivors had no quality-of-life alterations (physical and mental health similar to that of the overall cancer population). After 6 months, 80% of survivors had no change in treatment intensity compared with similar patients not admitted to the ICU.

Patients with a hematological malignancy may experience a decline in quality of life after ICU admission. However, some studies showed no difference in quality of life of patients admitted to the ICU compared to that of patients without ICU admission. Therefore, the benefits of ICU admission for a patient with a hematological malignancy should be considered individually. Denial of ICU admission solely based on a prejudice about quality of life is no longer justified.

39.6 Conclusion

The incidence of hematological malignancies has increased over the past decades with an increasing (long-term) survival rate. Subsequently, the burden to the healthcare system and also referrals to the ICU will probably increase. Where meager ICU survival rates in the past have been a major reason to deny admission, current survival rates no longer justify this general approach. On the contrary, ICU admission of critically ill patients with a hematological malignancy should be considered and tailored to patient-specific characteristics. Thus, where the admission of patients with a hematological malignancy may have been a Sisyphean task in the past, recent outcome data of these patients suggest a work in progress.

Acknowledgment We would like to express our gratitude to Dr. Jelle L. Epker for his valuable and constructive suggestions while writing this clinical review. His help is very much appreciated.

References

1. National Cancer Institute 2016 (Updated 13 September 2018). https://seer.cancer.gov/statfacts/html/all.html. Accessed 9 Nov 2019.
2. Ferlay J, Colombet M, Soerjomataram I, et al. Cancer incidence and mortality patterns in Europe: Estimates for 40 countries and 25 major cancers in 2018. Eur J Cancer. 2018;103:356–87.
3. Eurostat Statistics 2015 (Updated 7 September 2018). http://ec.europa.eu/eurostat/statistics-explained/index.php/Causes_of_death_statistics. Accessed 9 Nov 2019
4. Allemani C, Matsuda T, Di Carlo V, et al. Global surveillance of trends in cancer survival 2000-14 (CONCORD-3): analysis of individual records for 37 513 025 patients diagnosed with one of 18 cancers from 322 population-based registries in 71 countries. Lancet. 2018;391:1023–75.
5. Malvezzi M, Carioli G, Bertuccio P, et al. European cancer mortality predictions for the year 2016 with focus on leukaemias. Ann Oncol. 2016;27:725–31.
6. Lichtman MA. Battling the hematological malignancies: the 200 years' war. Oncologist. 2008;13:126–38.
7. Cancer Research UK 2014 (Updated 3 July 2017). http://www.cancerresearchuk.org/health-professional/cancer-statistics/statistics-by-cancer-type/leukaemia/incidence#ref-2. Accessed 9 Nov 2019.
8. Azoulay E, Schellongowski P, Darmon M, et al. The Intensive Care Medicine research agenda on critically ill oncology and hematology patients. Intensive Care Med. 2017;43:1366–82.

9. Bosetti C, Bertuccio P, Malvezzi M, et al. Cancer mortality in Europe, 2005–2009, and an overview of trends since 1980. Ann Oncol. 2013;24:2657–71.
10. De Angelis R, Minicozzi P, Sant M, et al. Survival variations by country and age for lymphoid and myeloid malignancies in Europe 2000–2007: results of EUROCARE-5 population-based study. Eur J Cancer. 2015;51:2254–68.
11. Azoulay E, Pene F, Darmon M, et al. Managing critically ill hematology patients: Time to think differently. Blood Rev. 2015;29:359–67.
12. Brunet F, Lanore JJ, Dhainaut JF, et al. Is intensive care justified for patients with haematological malignancies? Intensive Care Med. 1990;16:291–7.
13. Lloyd-Thomas AR, Wright I, Lister TA, Hinds CJ. Prognosis of patients receiving intensive care for lifethreatening medical complications of haematological malignancy. Br Med J. 1988;296:1025–9.
14. Rubenfeld GD, Crawford SW. Withdrawing life support from mechanically ventilated recipients of bone marrow transplants: a case for evidence-based guidelines. Ann Intern Med. 1996;125:625–33.
15. Schuster DP, Marion JM. Precedents for meaningful recovery during treatment in a medical intensive care unit. Outcome in patients with hematologic malignancy. Am J Med. 1983;75:402–8.
16. Wigmore TJ, Farquhar-Smith P, Lawson A. Intensive care for the cancer patient—unique clinical and ethical challenges and outcome prediction in the critically ill cancer patient. Best Pract Res Clin Anaesthesiol. 2013;27:527–43.
17. Sant M, Minicozzi P, Mounier M, et al. Survival for haematological malignancies in Europe between 1997 and 2008 by region and age: results of EUROCARE-5, a population-based study. Lancet Oncol. 2014;15:931–42.
18. Integraal Kankercentrum Nederland Survival 2017. http://www.cijfersoverkanker.nl/selecties/Dataset_2/img59b682b776106. Accessed 9 Nov 2019.
19. Gatta G, Capocaccia R, Botta L, et al. Burden and centralised treatment in Europe of rare tumours: results of RARECAREnet—a population-based study. Lancet Oncol. 2017;18:1022–39.
20. Visser O, Trama A, Maynadie M, et al. Incidence, survival and prevalence of myeloid malignancies in Europe. Eur J Cancer. 2012;48:3257–66.
21. Ewig S, Torres A, Riquelme R, et al. Pulmonary complications in patients with haematological malignancies treated at a respiratory ICU. Eur Respir J. 1998;12:116–22.
22. Azoulay E, Pochard F, Chevret S, et al. Compliance with triage to intensive care recommendations. Crit Care Med. 2001;29:2132–6.
23. Benoit DD, Hoste EA, Depuydt PO, et al. Outcome in critically ill medical patients treated with renal replacement therapy for acute renal failure: comparison between patients with and those without haematological malignancies. Nephrol Dial Transplant. 2005;20:552–8.
24. Cherif H, Martling CR, Hansen J, Kalin M, Bjorkholm M. Predictors of short and long-term outcome in patients with hematological disorders admitted to the intensive care unit for a lifethreatening complication. Support Care Cancer. 2007;15:1393–8.
25. Pene F, Aubron C, Azoulay E, et al. Outcome of critically ill allogeneic hematopoietic stem-cell transplantation recipients: a reappraisal of indications for organ failure supports. J Clin Oncol. 2006;24:643–9.
26. Rabbat A, Chaoui D, Lefebvre A, Ret a. Is BAL useful in patients with acute myeloid leukemia admitted in ICU for severe respiratory complications? Leukemia. 2008;22:1361–7.
27. Thiery G, Azoulay E, Darmon M, et al. Outcome of cancer patients considered for intensive care unit admission: a hospital-wide prospective study. J Clin Oncol. 2005;23:4406–13.
28. Guidelines for intensive care unit admission, discharge, and triage. Task Force of the American College of Critical Care Medicine, Society of Critical Care Medicine. Crit Care Med. 1999;27:633–8.
29. Consensus statement on the triage of critically ill patients. Society of Critical Care Medicine Ethics Committee. JAMA. 1994;271:1200–3.
30. Soares M, Caruso P, Silva E, et al. Characteristics and outcomes of patients with cancer requiring admission to intensive care units: a prospective multicenter study. Crit Care Med. 2010;38:9–15.

31. Taccone FS, Artigas AA, Sprung CL, Moreno R, Sakr Y, Vincent JL. Characteristics and outcomes of cancer patients in European ICUs. Crit Care. 2009;13:R15.
32. Bos MM, de Keizer NF, Meynaar IA, Bakhshi-Raiez F, de Jonge E. Outcomes of cancer patients after unplanned admission to general intensive care units. Acta Oncol. 2012;51:897–905.
33. Kostakou E, Rovina N, Kyriakopoulou M, Koulouris NG, Koutsoukou A. Critically ill cancer patient in intensive care unit: issues that arise. J Crit Care. 2014;29:817–22.
34. Darmon M, Bourmaud A, Georges Q, et al. Changes in critically ill cancer patients' short-term outcome over the last decades: results of systematic review with meta-analysis on individual data. Intensive Care Med. 2019;45:977–87.
35. Corcia Palomo Y, Knight Asorey T, Espigado I, Martin Villen L, Garnacho Montero J. Mortality of oncohematological patients undergoing hematopoietic stem cell transplantation admitted to the intensive care unit. Transplant Proc. 2015;47:2665–6.
36. Schellongowski P, Staudinger T, Kundi M, et al. Prognostic factors for intensive care unit admission, intensive care outcome, and post-intensive care survival in patients with de novo acute myeloid leukemia: a single center experience. Haematologica. 2011;96:231–7.
37. Ahmed T, Koch AL, Isom S, et al. Outcomes and changes in code status of patients with acute myeloid leukemia undergoing induction chemotherapy who were transferred to the intensive care unit. Leuk Res. 2017;62:51–5.
38. Belenguer-Muncharaz A, Albert-Rodrigo L, Ferrandiz-Selles A, Cebrian-Graullera G. Ten-year evolution of mechanical ventilation in acute respiratory failure in the hematological patient admitted to the intensive care unit. Med Int. 2013;37:452–60.
39. Ehooman F, Biard L, Lemiale V, et al. Long-term health-related quality of life of critically ill patients with haematological malignancies: a prospective observational multicenter study. Ann Intensive Care. 2019;9:2.
40. Saillard C, Elkaim E, Rey J, et al. Early preemptive ICU admission for newly diagnosed high-risk acute myeloid leukemia patients. Leuk Res. 2018;68:29–31.
41. Algrin C, Faguer S, Lemiale V, et al. Outcomes after intensive care unit admission of patients with newly diagnosed lymphoma. Leuk Lymphoma. 2015;56:1240–5.
42. Mokart D, Granata A, Crocchiolo R, et al. Allogeneic hematopoietic stem cell transplantation after reduced intensity conditioning regimen: Outcomes of patients admitted to intensive care unit. J Crit Care. 2015;30:1107–13.
43. de Vries VA, Muller MCA, Sesmu Arbous M, et al. Time trend analysis of long term outcome of patients with haematological malignancies admitted at Dutch intensive care units. Br J Haematol. 2018;181:68–76.
44. Wright AA, Keating NL, Ayanian JZ, et al. Family perspectives on aggressive cancer care near the end of life. JAMA. 2016;315:284–92.
45. Allart-Vorelli P, Porro B, Baguet F, Michel A, Cousson-Gelie F. Haematological cancer and quality of life: a systematic literature review. Blood Cancer J. 2015;5:e305.
46. Braamse AM, Gerrits MM, van Meijel B, et al. Predictors of health-related quality of life in patients treated with auto- and allo-SCT for hematological malignancies. Bone Marrow Transplant. 2012;47:757–69.
47. Williams AM, Zent CS, Janelsins MC. What is known and unknown about chemotherapy-related cognitive impairment in patients with haematological malignancies and areas of needed research. Br J Haematol. 2016;174:835–46.
48. Oeyen SG, Benoit DD, Annemans L, et al. Long-term outcomes and quality of life in critically ill patients with hematological or solid malignancies: a single center study. Intensive Care Med. 2013;39:889–98.
49. van Vliet M, van den Boogaard M, Donnelly JP, Evers AW, Blijlevens NM, Pickkers P. Long-term health related quality of life following intensive care during treatment for haematological malignancies. PLoS One. 2014;9:e87779.
50. Azoulay E, Mokart D, Pene F, et al. Outcomes of critically ill patients with hematologic malignancies: prospective multicenter data from France and Belgium—a groupe de recherche respiratoire en reanimation onco-hematologique study. J Clin Oncol. 2013;31:2810–8.

Onco-Nephrology: Acute Kidney Injury in Critically Ill Cancer Patients

N. Seylanova, J. Zhang, and M. Ostermann

40.1 Introduction

Acute kidney injury (AKI) is a frequent and serious complication in patients with cancer. The epidemiology varies, depending on the type and stage of cancer, anti-cancer therapy, and patient-related factors [1]. As the number of patients with cancer has increased worldwide and the chances of survival have improved due to advances in therapeutic options and general supportive care, the prevalence of AKI has increased. As a result, onco-nephrology has emerged as a new sub-specialty, focusing particularly on the recognition and management of renal complications in cancer patients.

N. Seylanova
Department of Critical Care, King's College London, Guy's & St Thomas' Hospital NHS Foundation Trust, London, UK

Sechenov Biomedical Science and Technology Park, Sechenov First Moscow State Medical University, Moscow, Russian Federation

J. Zhang
Department of Critical Care, King's College London, Guy's & St Thomas' Hospital NHS Foundation Trust, London, UK

Department of Critical Care Medicine, Zhongnan Hospital of Wuhan University, Wuhan, China

M. Ostermann (✉)
Department of Critical Care, King's College London, Guy's & St Thomas' Hospital NHS Foundation Trust, London, UK
e-mail: Marlies.Ostermann@gstt.nhs.uk

40.2 Epidemiology

The incidence of AKI in cancer patients varies depending on the setting, type and severity of malignancy, type of anticancer therapy, patient demographics, acute and chronic comorbid conditions, and criteria used to define AKI [2–5] (Table 40.1). In a 7-year study from Denmark including 37,267 patients with cancer, the 1-year risk of AKI as defined by the Risk, Injury, Failure, Loss of kidney function, and End-stage kidney disease (RIFLE) classification was 17.5% [6]. AKI was most common among patients with kidney cancer (44%), liver cancer (33%), and myeloma (32%). Furthermore, 5.1% of patients with AKI required long-term dialysis within 1 year. A study from Canada including 163,071 patients undergoing systemic cancer therapy between 2007 and 2014 showed an overall AKI incidence of 9.3% at 1 year [7]. The risk was highest in those with myeloma (26%), bladder cancer (19%), and leukemia (15.4%). A study from China surveyed over seven million patients from 44 academic and local hospitals and demonstrated an incidence of cancer-related AKI (defined as at least a 50% increase in baseline serum creatinine) of 14–20% depending upon the hospital type (community versus academic,

Table 40.1 Definitions of AKI

Classification	Stage	Creatinine or GFR criteria	Urine output criteria
RIFLE [29]	RIFLE Risk	Increase in serum creatinine to ≥1.5-fold to 2-fold from baseline, or GFR decrease by >25%	<0.5 ml/kg/h for >6 h
	RIFLE Injury	Increase in creatinine to >2-fold to 3-fold from baseline, or GFR decrease by >50%	<0.5 ml/kg/h for >12 h
	RIFLE Failure	Increase in creatinine to >3-fold from baseline, or to ≥354 µmol/l (4 mg/dl) with an acute rise of at least 44 µmol/l (0.5 mg/dl), or GFR decrease by >75%	<0.3 ml/kg/h for 24 h or more, or anuria for 12 h
AKIN [30]	Stage I	Increase in serum creatinine by ≥26 µmol/l (0.3 mg/dl) or increase to ≥1.5-fold to 2-fold from baseline	<0.5 ml/kg/h for >6 h
	Stage II	Increase in serum creatinine to >2-fold to 3-fold from baseline	<0.5 ml/kg/h for >12 h
	Stage III	Increase in serum creatinine to >3-fold from baseline, or to ≥354 µmol/l (4 mg/dl) with an acute rise of at least 44 µmol/l (0.5 mg/dl), or treatment with RRT	<0.3 ml/kg/h for 24 h or more, or anuria for 12 h
KDIGO [31]	Stage I	Increase in serum creatinine by ≥26.4 µmol/l (0.3 mg/dl) in 48 h or less or increase to 1.5–1.9 times from baseline	<0.5 ml/kg/h for >6 h
	Stage II	Increase in serum creatinine 2.0–2.9 times from baseline	<0.5 ml/kg/h for >12 h
	Stage III	Increase in serum creatinine three times from baseline, or increase to ≥354 µmol/l (4 mg/dl) with an acute rise of at least 44 µmol/l (0.5 mg/dl), or treatment with RRT	<0.3 ml/kg/h for 24 h or more, or anuria for 12 h

AKIN Acute Kidney Injury Network, *KDIGO* Kidney Disease: Improving Global Outcomes, *RIFLE* Risk, Injury, Failure, Loss of kidney function, and End-stage kidney disease, *RRT* renal replacement therapy, *GFR* glomerular filtration rate respectively) [4]. The incidence was higher in affluent regions, elderly patients, and groups with higher per capita gross domestic product.

In cancer patients requiring admission to the intensive care unit (ICU), the risk of AKI is up to 70% [8–14]. Prognosis is significantly worse in patients with more severe AKI, especially if renal replacement therapy (RRT) is required [11].

40.3 Risk Factors

Risk factors associated with the development of AKI in cancer patients are both cancer specific and patient specific. Advanced cancer stage, chronic kidney disease, and diabetes are associated with an increased risk of AKI in general cancer patients [7]. The risk is particularly increased in the 90-day period following systemic therapy. In patients with hematological malignancies admitted to the ICU, older age, high Sequential Organ Failure Assessment (SOFA) score, hypertension, tumor lysis syndrome, exposure to nephrotoxic agents, and myeloma are independently associated with the development of AKI [8]. Risk factors for AKI in patients with solid tumors include severity of illness, abdominal or pelvic cancer, nephrotoxic chemotherapy within the previous 3 months, and sepsis [12].

40.4 Causes of AKI

AKI in critically ill cancer patients is often multifactorial, similar to AKI seen in non-cancer patients, but there are cancer-specific factors that may contribute (Fig. 40.1). In solid tumors, the main causes of AKI are drug nephrotoxicity, metabolic disturbances, sepsis, tumor infiltration, vascular compression, and obstruction, whereas sepsis, volume depletion, nephrotoxins, and tumor lysis syndrome are the most common causes of AKI in patients with hematological malignancies [15].

40.4.1 AKI Directly Related to Underlying Malignancy

The kidneys are the most common extrareticular site of leukemic and lymphomatous infiltration [16]. Although AKI is common in patients with lymphoma and leukemia, the incidence of AKI caused by tumor cell infiltration is not greater than 1% [17]. The pathogenesis of AKI in this setting includes interstitial expansion and compression of renal tubules and microvasculature, resulting in intrarenal obstruction and ischemia [16]. Kidney function usually rapidly improves after appropriate chemotherapy [1].

Patients with multiple myeloma represent another important cohort of cancer patients who are very susceptible to develop AKI (20–50%). The most common cause is cast nephropathy [18]. This condition develops when free light chains, which are freely filtered by the glomerulus, bind to Tamm-Horsfall protein (uromodulin) in the thick ascending limb of the loop of Henle and form insoluble casts

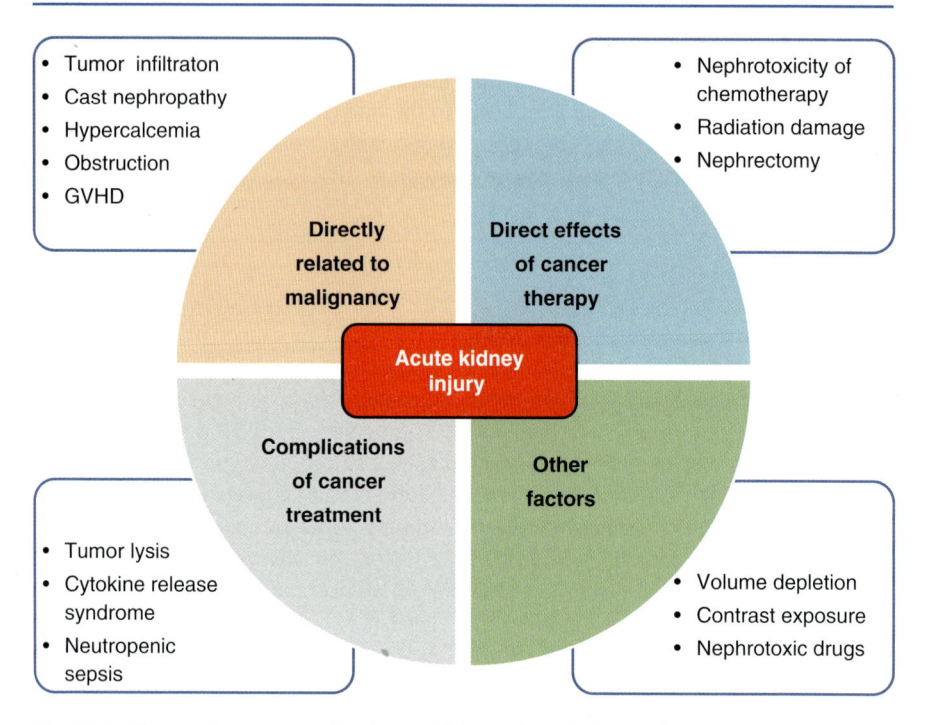

Fig. 40.1 Causes of cancer-associated acute kidney injury. *GVHD* graft-versus-host disease

that obstruct the tubular lumen. This leads to the activation of pro-inflammatory pathways, and intrarenal inflammation. Urinary tract obstruction due to intrinsic or extrinsic causes is another cause of AKI in cancer patients and may be seen in patients with solid tumors and hematological malignancies.

Hypercalcemia accompanies various types of malignancies, most commonly in patients with multiple myeloma and squamous cell carcinomas. It may cause AKI by blocking arginine vasopressin activity in the collecting duct, resulting in hypovolemia due to increased loss of sodium and water [15]. In severe cases of hypercalcemia, AKI can also occur due to nephrocalcinosis (i.e., calcium-phosphate deposition in renal tubules) with potential risk of chronic kidney disease if the duration is prolonged [19].

40.4.2 AKI Due to Direct Effects of Cancer Treatment

Nephrotoxicity from cancer therapies is common and can be a serious limitation for continuation of effective chemotherapy. The main mechanisms of injury include direct toxicity on renal microvasculature, glomeruli, and segments of the tubules (Table 40.2, Fig. 40.2). Entering the tubular cells, these agents can also induce mitochondrial damage and oxidative stress, and initiate apoptosis [20]. Cisplatin, a common drug in the treatment of various solid tumors, is well recognized for its nephrotoxicity [21]. Other forms of AKI that can be caused by chemotherapy are thrombotic microangiopathy (TMA), crystalline nephropathy, and interstitial

Table 40.2 Mechanisms involved in immunosuppressive-induced nephrotoxicity

Site of injury	Mechanism of nephrotoxicity	Examples
Intrarenal blood vessels	Thrombotic microangiopathy	Gemcitabine Mitomycin C Bleomycin Cisplatin 5-Fluorouracil Calcineurin inhibitor
	Vasculitis of renal vessels	Penicillamine
Glomeruli	Minimal change disease	Gold
	Focal segmental glomerulosclerosis	Interferon VEGF inhibitors Sirolimus
	Membranous nephropathy	Gold Penicillamine
Tubules	Acute tubular injury	Cisplatin Methotrexate Trabectedin Pemetrexed Calcineurin inhibitors Ifosfamide
Interstitium	Interstitial nephritis	Ifosfamide Carboplatin Doxorubicin Immune checkpoint inhibitors
Tubular lumen	Formation of intratubular crystals	Methotrexate

VEGF vascular endothelial growth factor

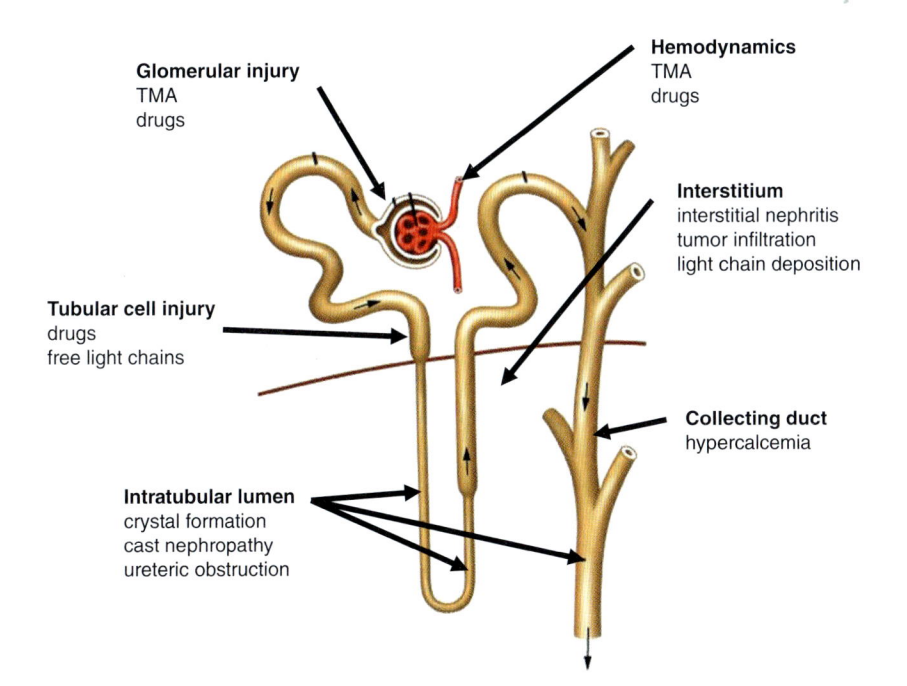

Fig. 40.2 Sites of renal injury in cancer-associated acute kidney injury. *TMA* thrombotic microangiopathy

nephritis [20]. TMA is a dangerous complication, characterized by formation of fibrin microthrombi in glomerular capillaries, arterioles, and arteries.

Over the past decade, cancer therapies have advanced with a more targeted approach specifically against tumor cells. Targeted therapies include agents which target specific gene mutations in cancer cells and inhibit oncogenic signaling pathways that are essential for tumor growth [22, 23]. This class consists of various drugs, such as agents directed at vascular endothelial growth factor (VEGF) or VEGF receptor(s) (VEGFR), epidermal growth factor receptor (EGFR), human epidermal growth factor receptor 2 (HER2), anaplastic lymphoma kinase (ALK), receptor activator of nuclear factor kappa-B ligand (RANKL), and mammalian target of rapamycin (mTOR). Although they are effective therapies, the actions of targeted agents may involve pathways that are also essential for the growth of normal tissue. Injury from targeted agents can occur in all nephron segments and involve different mechanisms.

Immune checkpoint inhibitors are monoclonal antibodies that enhance tumor killing by preventing dendritic cells and tumor antigen ligand binding to cytotoxic T-lymphocyte-associated protein and programmed death receptors, respectively. Chimeric antigen receptor (CAR)-T-cell therapy involves the genetic modification of a patient's autologous T cells to express a CAR specific for a tumor antigen, followed by *ex vivo* cell expansion and reinfusion back into the patient. Both therapies are promising, offering tumor-specific individualized treatment. However, both result in a robust immune response characterized by the release of inflammatory cytokines and the potential risk of severe cytokine release syndrome. A meta-analysis including 48 trials on 11,482 patients treated with immune checkpoint inhibitors reported a pooled relative risk of AKI of 4.19 and a pooled incidence of AKI of 2.1% [24]. The risk of AKI was increased in patients receiving a combination of different checkpoint inhibitors [25]. Others reported that the incidence of nephrotoxicity related to immune checkpoint inhibitors may be up to 29% [26]. After CAR-T-cell therapy, AKI from tumor lysis syndrome and cytokine release syndrome are common complications. Acute cardiomyopathy from cytokine release syndrome may promote hypotension and further exacerbate kidney injury.

40.4.3 AKI Due to Complications of Cancer Treatment

Neutropenic sepsis and tumor lysis syndrome are common causes of cancer-induced AKI. Tumor lysis syndrome is characterized by the release of cellular contents from tumor cells that either have died spontaneously or were damaged by chemotherapy. These cellular contents can lead to hyperuricemia, hyperkalemia, hyperphosphatemia, and hypocalcaemia. AKI may occur due to a combination of acute uric acid/xanthine nephropathy, acute nephrocalcinosis due to an elevated calcium-phosphate product, and cytokine release with inflammatory tubular injury leading to tubulointerstitial inflammation.

Risk factors for the development of tumor lysis syndrome include highly chemosensitive malignancies, large tumor burden, effective cytolytic chemotherapeutic agents, and underlying chronic kidney disease. The most common malignancies associated with tumor lysis syndrome include non-Hodgkin's lymphoma, acute leukemia, and various solid tumors.

40.5 Management

The management of AKI in cancer patients is symptomatic and consists of management of the underlying cause, in addition to hemodynamic resuscitation, correction of intravascular hypovolemia, and discontinuation of potentially nephrotoxic drugs if possible. In the setting of AKI due to severe cytokine release syndrome, treatment with an interleukin (IL)-6 receptor blocker and/or steroids may reduce adverse effects but will also impact the effectiveness of the anticancer therapy. In case of hyperuricemia and tumor lysis syndrome, recombinant urate oxidase (rasburicase) may be employed.

40.6 Outcomes

AKI in cancer patients has numerous deleterious consequences, including increased mortality, a longer stay in hospital, high healthcare costs, and a lower rate of cancer remission [8, 13]. Mortality is particularly high in patients with more severe AKI or those requiring RRT [11]. Salahudeen et al. demonstrated a decrease in survival in cancer patients with AKI [3]. Using modified RIFLE criteria, 12% of patients admitted to the hospital had AKI, with rates in the risk, injury, and failure categories of 68%, 21%, and 11%, respectively. Dialysis was required in 4% of patients. In patients with AKI, length of stay (100%), cost (106%), and odds for mortality (4.7-fold) were significantly greater. In addition, AKI in patients with newly diagnosed hematological malignancies was associated with a lower 6-month complete remission rate (39.4% in patients with AKI vs. 68.3% in patients without AKI), and 14.6% of patients with AKI received suboptimal chemotherapy [9]. Interestingly, a recent meta-analysis concluded that hospital mortality of critically ill cancer patients had steadily decreased over time after adjustment for patients' characteristics and severity of illness except for allogeneic stem cell transplant recipients and patients requiring RRT [27].

The development of AKI negatively impacts the decision about current or future chemotherapeutic regimens. Furthermore, it often excludes patients from potentially beneficial clinical trials. The long-term consequences of AKI in the patient with cancer are highly variable and confounded by the overall severity of illness, age, and functional status of these patients. The impact of AKI on long-term kidney function has been rarely reported in this subset of patients but appears to be variable. Some studies demonstrated that chronic RRT was required in only 6% of patients whilst other studies reported long-term dialysis dependence in 12.9–23% of patients with hematological malignancies and dialysis-requiring AKI [8, 10, 28].

40.7 Conclusion

Advances in cancer therapy have led to better survival in cancer patients. However, AKI remains a serious complication and may adversely affect prognosis, including the chances for complete remission. Anticancer therapies play an important role in the development of AKI, including recent novel treatment strategies involving immune checkpoint inhibitors and CAR-T-cell therapy. Due to scarcity of possible measures to manage AKI, maximal attention should be paid to prevention and early recognition. A multidisciplinary approach from nephrologists, oncologists, intensivists, pharmacists, and allied specialties is required to achieve this goal and optimize the chances of success.

References

1. Rosner MH, Perazella MA. Acute kidney injury in patients with cancer. N Engl J Med. 2017;376:1770–81.
2. Uchida M, Kondo Y, Suzuki S, Hosohata K. Evaluation of acute kidney injury associated with anticancer drugs used in gastric cancer in the Japanese Adverse Drug Event Report Database. Ann Pharmacother. 2019;53:1200–6.
3. Salahudeen AK, Doshi SM, Pawar T, Nowshad G, Lahoti A, Shah P. Incidence rate, clinical correlates, and outcomes of AKI in patients admitted to a comprehensive cancer center. Clin J Am Soc Nephrol. 2013;8:347–54.
4. Jin J, Wang Y, Shen Q, Gong J, Zhao L, He Q. Acute kidney injury in cancer patients: a nationwide survey in China. Sci Rep. 2019;9:3540.
5. Lahoti A, Kantarjian H, Salahudeen AK, et al. Predictors and outcome of acute kidney injury in patients with acute myelogenous leukemia or high-risk myelodysplastic syndrome. Cancer. 2010;116:4063–8.
6. Christiansen CF, Johansen MB, Langeberg WJ, Fryzek JP, Sørensen HT. Incidence of acute kidney injury in cancer patients: a Danish population-based cohort study. Eur J Intern Med. 2011;22:399–406.
7. Kitchlu A, McArthur E, Amir E, et al. Acute kidney injury in patients receiving systemic treatment for cancer: a population-based cohort study. J Natl Cancer Inst. 2019;111:727–36.
8. Darmon M, Vincent F, Canet E, et al. Acute kidney injury in critically ill patients with haematological malignancies: results of a multicentre cohort study from the Groupe de Recherche en Réanimation Respiratoire en Onco-Hématologie. Nephrol Dial Transplant. 2015;30:2006–13.
9. Canet E, Zafrani L, Lambert J, et al. Acute kidney injury in patients with newly diagnosed high-grade hematological malignancies: impact on remission and survival. PLoS One. 2013;8:e55870.
10. Soares M, Salluh JIF, Carvalho MS, Darmon M, Rocco JR, Spector N. Prognosis of critically ill patients with cancer and acute renal dysfunction. J Clin Oncol. 2006;24:4003–10.
11. Libório AB, Abreu KLS, Silva GB Jr, et al. Predicting hospital mortality in critically ill cancer patients according to acute kidney injury severity. Oncology. 2011;80:160–6.
12. Kemlin D, Biard L, Kerhuel L, et al. Acute kidney injury in critically ill patients with solid tumours. Nephrol Dial Transplant. 2018;33:1997–2005.
13. Córdova-Sánchez BM, Herrera-Gómez Á, Ñamendys-Silva SA. Acute kidney injury classified by serum creatinine and urine output in critically ill cancer patients. Biomed Res Int. 2016;2016:1–7.
14. Azoulay E, Mokart D, Pène F, et al. Outcomes of critically ill patients with hematologic malignancies: prospective multicenter data from France and Belgium—A Groupe de Recherche Respiratoire en Réanimation Onco-Hématologique Study. J Clin Oncol. 2013;31:2810–8.

15. Rosner MH, Perazella MA. Acute kidney injury in the patient with cancer. Kidney Res Clin Pract. 2019;38:295–308.
16. Lommatzsch SE, Bellizzi AM, Cathro HP, Rosner MH. Acute renal failure caused by renal infiltration by hematolymphoid malignancy. Ann Diagn Pathol. 2006;10:230–4.
17. Luciano RL, Brewster UC. Kidney involvement in leukemia and lymphoma. Adv Chronic Kidney Dis. 2014;21:27–35.
18. Nasr SH, Valeri AM, Sethi S, et al. Clinicopathologic correlations in multiple myeloma: a case series of 190 patients with kidney biopsies. Am J Kidney Dis. 2012;59:786–94.
19. Rosner MH, Dalkin AC. Onco-nephrology: the pathophysiology and treatment of malignancy-associated hypercalcemia. Clin J Am Soc Nephrol. 2012;7:1722–9.
20. Perazella MA. Onco-nephrology: renal toxicities of chemotherapeutic agents. Clin J Am Soc Nephrol. 2012;7:1713–21.
21. Ozkok A, Edelstein CL. Pathophysiology of cisplatin-induced acute kidney injury. Biomed Res Int. 2014;2014:967826.
22. Porta C, Cosmai L, Gallieni M, Pedrazzoli P, Malberti F. Renal effects of targeted anticancer therapies. Nat Rev Nephrol. 2015;11:354–70.
23. Launay-Vacher V, Aapro M, De Castro G, et al. Renal effects of molecular targeted therapies in oncology: a review by the Cancer and the Kidney International Network (C-KIN). Ann Oncol. 2015;26:1677–84.
24. Manohar S, Kompotiatis P, Thongprayoon C, Cheungpasitporn W, Herrmann J, Herrmann SM. Programmed cell death protein 1 inhibitor treatment is associated with acute kidney injury and hypocalcemia: meta-analysis. Nephrol Dial Transplant. 2019;34:108–17.
25. Cortazar FB, Marrone KA, Troxell ML, et al. Clinicopathological features of acute kidney injury associated with immune checkpoint inhibitors. Kidney Int. 2016;90:638–47.
26. Wanchoo R, Karam S, Uppal NN, et al. Adverse renal effects of immune checkpoint inhibitors: a narrative review. Am J Nephrol. 2017;45:160–9.
27. Darmon M, Bourmaud A, Georges Q, et al. Changes in critically ill cancer patients' short-term outcome over the last decades: results of systematic review with meta-analysis on individual data. Intensive Care Med. 2019;45:977–87.
28. Park MR, Jeon K, Song JU, et al. Outcomes in critically ill patients with hematologic malignancies who received renal replacement therapy for acute kidney injury in an intensive care unit. J Crit Care. 2011;26:107.e1–6.
29. Bellomo R, Ronco C, Kellum JA, Mehta RL, Palevsky P. Acute Dialysis Quality Initiative workgroup. Acute renal failure - definition, outcome measures, animal models, fluid therapy and information technology needs: the Second International Consensus Conference of the Acute Dialysis Quality Initiative (ADQI) Group. Crit Care. 2004;8:R204–12.
30. Mehta RL, Kellum JA, Shah SV, et al. Acute Kidney Injury Network: report of an initiative to improve outcomes in acute kidney injury. Crit Care. 2007;11:R31.
31. Kidney Disease. Improving Global Outcomes (KDIGO) Acute Kidney Injury Work Group KDIGO Clinical Practice Guideline for Acute Kidney Injury. Kidney Int Suppl. 2012;2:1–138.

Part XIV

Severe Complications

41
A Clinician's Guide to Management of Intra-abdominal Hypertension and Abdominal Compartment Syndrome in Critically Ill Patients

I. E. De laet, M. L. N. G. Malbrain, and J. J. De Waele

41.1 Introduction

Intra-abdominal hypertension (IAH) and abdominal compartment syndrome (ACS) are established causes of morbidity and mortality in critically ill patients [1]. When interest in postoperative IAH after major vascular, trauma, and general surgery arose in the 1980s, overt ACS was the only clinical syndrome recognized and decompressive laparotomy the only definitive treatment [2]. Since then, less extreme elevations in intra-abdominal pressure (IAP), defined as IAH, have been recognized to be highly prevalent among all types of patients admitted to the intensive care unit (ICU) [3].

Significant advances in the understanding of the pathophysiology, diagnosis, and management of IAH and ACS have occurred over the last few decades. The importance of IAH has been studied specifically in critically ill patients, leading to a better understanding of the mechanisms of organ dysfunction due to increased IAP and earlier opportunities for therapeutic intervention. Further, medical and minimally invasive techniques have been developed and reported to be potentially effective in small studies [4].

The World Society for the Abdominal Compartment Syndrome (WSACS, recently renamed as WSACS—the Abdominal Compartment Society [5]) was

---

I. E. De laet
Intensive Care Unit and High Care Burn Unit, Ziekenhuis Netwerk Antwerpen, ZNA Stuivenberg, Antwerp, Belgium

M. L. N. G. Malbrain
Department of Intensive Care Medicine, University Hospital Brussels (UZB), Jette, Belgium

Faculty of Medicine and Pharmacy, Vrije Universiteit Brussel (VUB), Campus Jette, Jette, Belgium

J. J. De Waele (✉)
Department of Critical Care Medicine, Ghent University Hospital, Ghent, Belgium
e-mail: Jan.DeWaele@UGent.be

founded in 2004 to "promote research, foster education and improve the survival of patients with IAH/ACS." Consensus papers on IAP measurement and diagnosis and management of IAH/ACS were first published in 2006 and 2007 [1, 6] and a medical management algorithm in 2009 [7]. Subsequently, in 2013, the WSACS published an updated evidence-based version of the definitions, guidelines, and medical management algorithm using GRADE methodology (Box 41.1) [8]. In this last manuscript, the definitions relating to IAP were updated.

Box 41.1 Definitions Related to Intra-abdominal Pressure (IAP) According to the World Society for the Abdominal Compartment Syndrome (WSACS) 2013 Guidelines (Adapted from [8] Under the Terms of the Creative Commons Attribution Noncommercial License)

No.	Definition
1.	IAP is the steady-state pressure concealed within the abdominal cavity
2.	The reference standard for intermittent IAP measurements is via the bladder with a maximal instillation volume of 25 ml of sterile saline
3.	IAP should be expressed in mmHg and measured at end expiration in the supine position after ensuring that abdominal muscle contractions are absent and with the transducer zeroed at the level of the midaxillary line
4.	IAP is approximately 5–7 mmHg in critically ill adults
5.	IAH is defined by a sustained or repeated pathological elevation in IAP ≥ 12 mmHg
6.	ACS is defined as a sustained IAP >20 mmHg (with or without an APP <60 mmHg) that is associated with new organ dysfunction/failure
7.	IAH is graded as follows: Grade I, IAP 12–15 mmHg Grade II, IAP 16–20 mmHg Grade III, IAP 21–25 mmHg Grade IV, IAP >25 mmHg
8.	Primary IAH or ACS is a condition associated with injury or disease in the abdominal pelvic region that frequently requires early surgical or interventional radiological intervention
9.	Secondary IAH or ACS refers to conditions that do not originate in the abdominopelvic region
10.	Recurrent IAH or ACS refers to the condition in which IAH or ACS redevelops following previous surgical or medical treatment of primary or secondary IAH or ACS
11.	APP = MAP – IAP
12.	A polycompartment syndrome is a condition where two or more anatomical compartments have elevated compartmental pressures
13.	Abdominal compliance is a measure of the ease of abdominal expansion, which is determined by the elasticity of the abdominal wall and diaphragm. It should be expressed as the change in intra-abdominal volume per change in IAP
14.	The open abdomen is one that requires a temporary abdominal closure due to the skin and fascia not being closed after laparotomy
15.	Lateralization of the abdominal wall is the phenomenon where the musculature and fascia of the abdominal wall, most exemplified by the rectus abdominis muscles and their enveloping fascia, move laterally away from the midline with time

ACS abdominal compartment syndrome, *MAP* mean arterial pressure, *IAH* intra-abdominal hypertension, *APP* abdominal perfusion pressure

IAH / ACS MEDICAL MANAGEMENT ALGORITHM

- The choice (and success) of the medical management strategies listed below is strongly related to both the etiology of the patient's IAH / ACS and the patient's clinical situation. The appropriateness of each intervention should always be considered prior to implementing these interventions in any individual patient.
- The interventions should be applied in a stepwise fashion until the patient's intra-abdominal pressure (IAP) decreases.
- If there is no response to a particular intervention, therapy should be escalated to the next step in the algorithm.

Patient has IAP ≥12 mmHg
Begin medical management to reduce IAP
(GRADE 1C)

Measure IAP at least every 4-6 hours or continuously.
Titrate therapy to maintain IAP ≤ 15 mmHg (GRADE 1C)

	Evacuate intraluminal contents	Evacuate intra-abdominal space occupying lesions	Improve abdominal wall compliance	Optimize fluid administration	Optimize systemic / regional perfusion
Step 1	Insert nasogastric and/or rectal tube	Abdominal ultrasound to identify lesions	Ensure adequate sedation & analgesia (GRADE 1D)	Avoid excessive fluid resuscitation (GRADE 2C)	Goal-directed fluid resuscitation
	Initiate gastro-/colo-prokinetic agents (GRADE 2D)		Remove constrictive dressings, abdominal eschars	Aim for zero to negative fluid balance by day 3 (GRADE 2C)	
Step 2	Minimize enteral nutrition	Abdominal computed tomography to identify lesions	Consider reverse Trendelenborg position	Resuscitate using hypertonic fluids, colloids	Hemodynamic monitoring to guide resuscitation
	Administer enemas (GRADE 1D)	Percutaneous catheter drainage (GRADE 2C)		Fluid removal through judicious diuresis once stable	
Step 3	Consider colonoscopic decompression (GRADE 1D)	Consider surgical evacuation of lesions (GRADE 1D)	Consider neuro-muscular blockade (GRADE 1D)	Consider hemodialysis/ ultrafiltration	
	Discontinue enteral nutrition				

Step 4: If IAP > 20 mmHg and new organ dysfunction/ failure is present, patient's IAH/ACS is refractory to medical management. Strongly consider surgical abdominal decompression (GRADE ID).

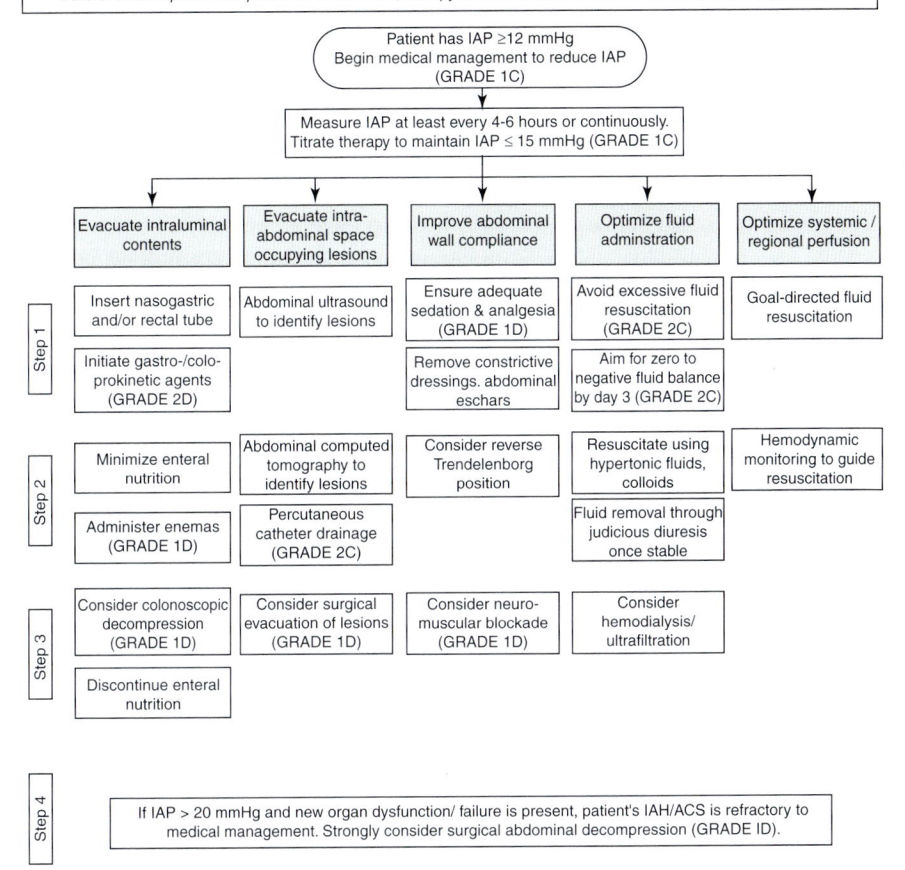

Fig. 41.1 WSACS medical management algorithm as presented in the 2013 guidelines. *IAH* intra-abdominal hypertension, *ACS* abdominal compartment syndrome, *IAP* intra-abdominal pressure. Adapted from [8] under the terms of the Creative Commons Attribution Noncommercial License

The current medical management algorithm for IAH/ACS still has some limitations (Fig. 41.1). First, there is not enough evidence to support some of the interventions described in the algorithm. Second, the use of the algorithm at the bedside also requires an experienced clinician to select the treatment best suited to an individual patient as it does not provide clear, easy, patient-specific recommendations. Finally, management recommendations are chiefly based on a measured IAP value only, an approach likely to underestimate the importance of the dynamic evolution in the patient's situation. Depending on the course of disease and concomitant organ dysfunction, some cases of ACS can be managed conservatively whereas some cases of IAH may require immediate aggressive treatment including fast decision to proceed to decompressive laparotomy before reaching the value of 20 mmHg of IAP. This is important because use of decompressive laparotomy is associated with a number of potential complications (e.g., massive ventral hernia, enteric fistulae, and intra-abdominal sepsis), increased morbidity, and decreased quality of life, especially in younger patients [9–12].

The philosophy of the WSACS Guidelines has been to publish the best available evidence at the time of writing, with the hope that future research would necessitate ongoing revisions and updating of the Guidelines. The aim of this chapter is to provide the reader with a conceptual framework of how to translate the principles of the formal Consensus Guidelines into a practical approach at the bedside to manage a specific patient with IAH and ACS, taking into account patient physiology, current scientific evidence, and clinical experience.

41.2 Managing IAH and ACS: The Triangle Paradigm

It is important to understand that IAH, in contrast to ACS, is a continuum from (often) asymptomatic elevation of IAP to an immediately life-threatening situation (fulminant ACS), where dynamic evolution in both directions is possible. Therefore, it is difficult to identify triggers for interventions that may lead to complications (e.g., percutaneous drainage) or have adverse effects (e.g., sedation, muscle relaxation). Despite this, the optimal treatment choice for a specific patient with IAH/ACS should take into account three critical elements: (1) the measured IAP value (or the degree/magnitude of IAP increase); (2) organ dysfunction characteristics (or the impact of increased IAP); and (3) nature and course of the underlying disease (Fig. 41.2). Using this triangular treatment paradigm enables us to fully acknowledge the importance of the two other factors in addition to the measured IAP value.

41.2.1 Intra-abdominal Pressure (Culprit)

Although the IAP value has always been considered the most important factor in managing IAH/ACS, it should always be viewed within its context. Factors that need to be considered in an individual patient include the IAP measurement strategy and the context in which IAP is measured, the expected baseline value of IAP, the evolution of IAP over time, and the duration of time that the patient has already been exposed to IAH.

41.2.1.1 IAP Measurement and Interpretation
The reference standard for intermittent IAP measurement is via the bladder with a maximal instillation volume of 25 ml of sterile saline. IAP should be measured at end-expiration in the supine position after ensuring that abdominal muscle contractions are absent and with the transducer zeroed at the level where the midaxillary line

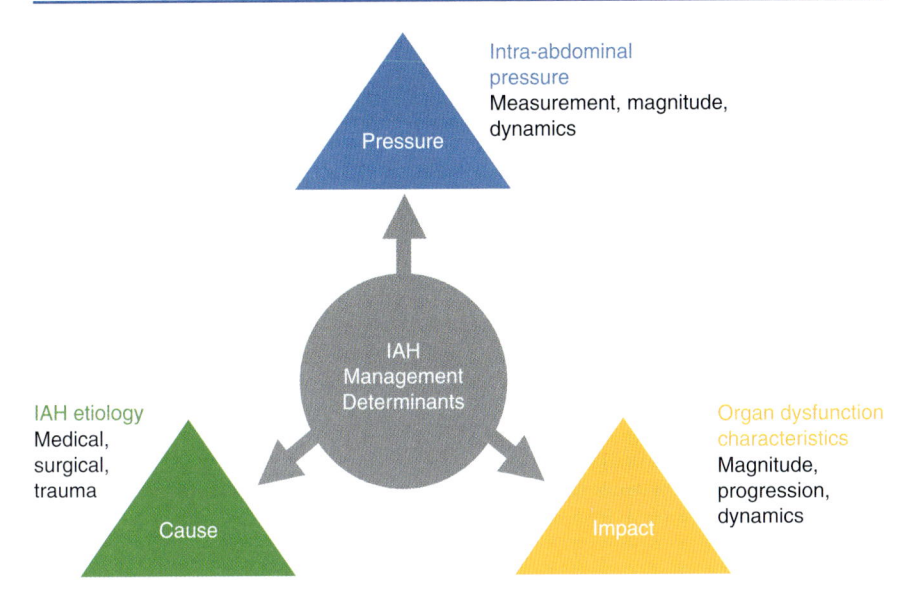

Fig. 41.2 The triangle perspective on the management of intra-abdominal hypertension/abdominal compartment syndrome (IAH/ACS) in the individual patient

crosses the iliac crest [8]. This generally means that IAP measurement is most reliable in completely sedated, mechanically ventilated patients. However, many mechanically ventilated patients in the ICU are at some stage of a weaning process, exhibiting spontaneous breathing movements and possible patient-ventilator asynchrony and pain or distress. Similarly, critically ill patients who are not mechanically ventilated may be managed with noninvasive ventilation or exhibit respiratory failure, forced expiration, and pain or stress. All of the above processes may lead to abdominal wall contraction and increased IAP that may not be reflected by an increase in intra-abdominal volume [13, 14]. Although there are no data as to whether increased IAP due to abdominal muscle activity in these groups of patients has the potential to cause organ dysfunction, it has been reported that in awake, non-critically ill patients without suspicion of IAH, IAP can be as high as 20 mmHg without causing discernible organ dysfunction [15]. The impact of high positive end-expiratory pressure (PEEP; >12 cmH$_2$O) on IAP is considered to be mild and adds 1–2 mmHg at most [16]. As deepening of sedation or using neuromuscular blocking agents may help to decrease IAP and control IAH for a limited period of time, it needs to be considered that deepening of sedation may have deleterious effects on hemodynamics. Switching from assisted to controlled mechanical ventilation may sometimes result in a significant increase in intrathoracic pressure even with muscle relaxation and the expected positive effect on IAP will be negligible compared to its negative effects.

41.2.1.2 Baseline IAP Value and Dynamics

The baseline IAP may vary in individual patients. Obese patients in particular have higher baseline IAP values [17], which in some cases may be higher than the threshold for IAH. One review found that IAP in individuals with a normal weight was around 5–6 mmHg, whereas it was much higher in obese patients with values above 12 mmHg and even above 14 mmHg in morbid obesity [16]. Other conditions associated with "physiologically" increased IAP include pregnancy [18] and liver cirrhosis with ascites [19]. Although this chronic IAP elevation may contribute to chronic forms of organ failure, including chronic kidney failure in patients with congestive heart disease and obesity [20] or pseudotumor cerebri in patients with obesity [21], slight increases from a higher starting value may have limited implications in critically ill patients. As such, an IAP of 16 mmHg may be insignificant if the baseline value was 13 mmHg, where it may cause organ injury if the baseline value was 6 mmHg. Unfortunately, the baseline IAP value is usually unknown and this effect is difficult to quantify.

41.2.1.3 Duration of IAH

In situations where exposure to IAH has already been prolonged (e.g., several days, in cases of delayed IAH diagnosis), organ dysfunction may not be reversible as quickly or fully as in more acute situations. We hypothesize that interventions aimed at lowering IAP are unlikely to have an immediate beneficial effect on organ function in this context, especially when IAH has caused or contributed to cellular organ injury (e.g., acute tubular necrosis). This highlights the importance of IAP monitoring in at-risk patients to avoid delayed diagnosis [22]. On the other hand, one measurement of elevated IAP does not constitute a definite diagnosis of IAH/ACS (as highlighted by the definitions in Box 41.1). Repetitive measurements are more likely to ascertain true IAP values and unmask potential measurement errors. Mild elevation of IAP, measured at one time point, is unlikely to cause organ dysfunction and seldom warrant immediate intervention, but should lead to repeated IAP measurement.

41.2.2 Organ (Dys)Function (Impact)

The second element of the triangle to consider is the resultant degree of organ dysfunction thought to be secondary to IAH and the rapidity with which it occurred. Many experimental studies have shown that subclinical organ injury develops at levels of IAP previously deemed to be safe (IAP between 12 and 15 mmHg), but as IAP increases, organ dysfunction will become more pronounced and a dose-dependent relationship between IAP and organ dysfunction has been demonstrated in many studies [23].

41.2.2.1 Severity of Organ Dysfunction

One of the key features of ACS is organ dysfunction and the absence of organ dysfunction should raise doubts about the reliability of the measurement or the interpretation of the IAP value. The most extreme and urgent form of organ dysfunction in patients with ACS is the inability to ventilate, which requires urgent action. Another very frequent form of IAH-induced organ dysfunction is IAH-induced acute kidney injury (AKI) [24]. There is extensive experimental evidence that AKI occurs at IAP levels as low as 12 mmHg [25]. In patients with ACS, AKI is usually firmly established with anuria and need for renal replacement therapy (RRT) unless early intervention is used to prevent this [25]. Organ dysfunction is not limited to the respiratory or renal system and may include hemodynamic instability, metabolic failure, gastrointestinal failure, and even intracranial hypertension [26]. Often multiple organ systems will fail, and the clinical picture can mimic many conditions (e.g., septic shock, hypovolemia) associated with multiple organ dysfunction syndrome (MODS). Compartment pressures can also be increased in more than one compartment and this has been referred to as the polycompartment syndrome [27].

41.2.2.2 Organ Dysfunction Duration and Dynamics

The speed at which organ function deteriorates and the time-dependent relationship with the increase in IAP are important elements to consider. A sudden increase in intra-abdominal volume, causing a sudden increase in IAP with subsequent organ dysfunction, warrants more aggressive treatment than a situation where a condition frequently associated with MODS is diagnosed concurrently with IAH and organ dysfunction. Indeed, in many conditions that are associated with IAH, the pathophysiology of the underlying disease (e.g., severe trauma, severe acute pancreatitis, or burns) may cause severe organ dysfunction and the exact role of increased IAP superimposed on this "primary" organ injury may be difficult to estimate. Baseline organ dysfunction (i.e., before IAH was present) as well as dynamics between concurrent increase in IAP and deterioration of organ function may offer a clue.

41.2.3 Etiology of IAH/ACS (Cause)

The third element to consider in IAH management is the etiology of the elevated IAP, which allows selection of the best possible treatment option. The course of disease also needs to be considered. An initial increase in IAP up to 18 mmHg after elective abdominal hernia repair may be well tolerated [28] and could be just observed, whereas the same value of IAP in a patient with severe acute pancreatitis and shock still needing massive fluid resuscitation to preserve organ perfusion presents a high risk for developing ACS and needs immediate attention and measures (e.g., sedation, muscle relaxation) to control the IAP.

All reasonable attempts should be made to ascertain the underlying disease leading to elevated IAP before starting treatment. Knowledge of the patient's medical history and present condition and a full general and abdominal clinical examination usually offer the first clues. Directed imaging, such as ultrasound or computed tomography (CT), may also be necessary. A plethora of risk factors for IAH/ACS has been described, but they can be largely divided into three categories: increased intra-abdominal volume, decreased abdominal compliance, and a combination of both [13].

41.2.3.1 Increased Intra-abdominal Volume

This can be caused by increased intraluminal or extraluminal volume within the abdominal cavity. The presence of increased intraluminal volume can be suspected based on the clinical circumstances and diagnosed with medical imaging techniques if indicated (e.g., gastric distention after gastroscopy due to gas insufflation, added colonic volume in *Clostridium difficile* colitis [29], or severe constipation). Increased extraluminal volume may accumulate freely in the abdominal cavity or localized in abdominal collections. Free abdominal air, fluid, or blood can be diagnosed easily by bedside ultrasound and can be evacuated by percutaneous catheter drainage. Extraluminal abdominal collections are mostly associated with underlying abdominal diseases (e.g., pancreatitis, abdominal sepsis, or abdominal hematoma) and usually require abdominal ultrasound or CT imaging for accurate diagnosis and treatment. Tissue edema—often in a context of resuscitation or fluid overload—may be another cause of increased extraluminal volume, without any discernible collections. In rare cases, IAH/ACS may be caused by increased native solid organ volume (e.g., splenomegaly or in solid organ transplants [30], e.g., in children receiving adult organs [31]).

41.2.3.2 Decreased Abdominal Wall Compliance

Abdominal wall compliance is a measure of the ease of abdominal expansion, which is determined by the elasticity of the abdominal wall and diaphragm [32]. When abdominal wall compliance is decreased, any increase in intra-abdominal volume is much more likely to produce a significant increase in IAP. Risk factors for decreased abdominal wall compliance can be divided into three categories, including those related to (1) body anthropomorphism and habitus (e.g., age, morbid obesity); (2) abdominal wall (e.g., burn eschars, rectus sheath hematoma, tight sutures or bandages, ventral hernia repair, prone positioning); and (3) comorbidities (e.g., capillary leak due to sepsis, burns, trauma, or pancreatitis) [33]. Large-volume fluid resuscitation, usually related to systemic inflammatory syndrome and biomediator activation, is one of the most important risk factors for the development of IAH/ACS, due to its combined effects of increased intra-abdominal volume (both intra- and extraluminal due to ascites formation, gut edema, and ileus) and decreased abdominal wall compliance due to tissue edema of the abdominal wall. Respiratory cycle-related variations in IAP have been found to linearly increase with end-expiratory IAP and reflect abdominal wall compliance [34].

41.3 A Practical Approach Based on the IAH Triangle

The first two elements of the triangle (pressure and impact) will determine whether or not active attempts to decrease IAP should be considered, in what timeframe these attempts should produce a clinically relevant result, and what level or invasiveness (and possibility of complications) is required. The third element (cause) will determine which treatment option will most likely produce the desired result. At the bedside, three critical questions should be asked once IAH/ACS has been diagnosed (Fig. 41.3).

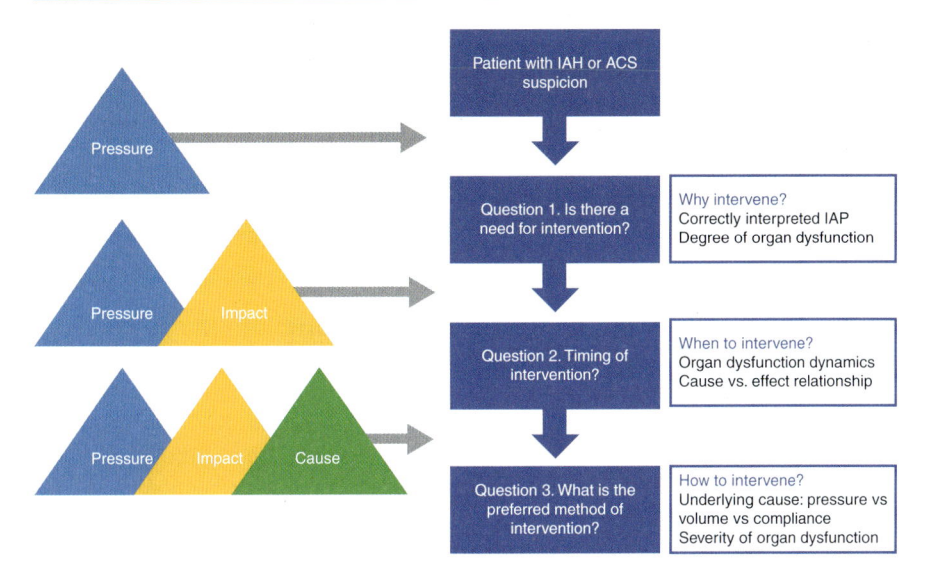

Fig. 41.3 Elements to be considered in decision-making for management of intra-abdominal hypertension (IAH). *ACS* abdominal compartment syndrome, *IAP* intra-abdominal pressure

41.3.1 Is an Intervention Required?

Why intervene: The decision to intervene will be guided by the presence of organ dysfunction caused by a relevant increase in IAP in a patient who has been diagnosed with a condition that may be associated with IAH and in which an intervention is expected to have a beneficial impact on IAP as well as on organ function. The IAP value, the evolution of IAP over time, and the degree of organ dysfunction are the most important considerations. However, the measured IAP value should be interpreted carefully. If IAP is elevated in semiconscious or fully awake patients and organ function is normal or improving, techniques to reduce IAP are probably less warranted and may cause unnecessary complications. If IAP is normal after analgesia/sedation, IAH is unlikely to be a contributing factor to organ dysfunction. If IAP remains increased, an underlying cause of IAH is likely and additional diagnostic and/or therapeutic interventions are warranted.

41.3.2 How Urgent Is the Effect of the Intervention Required?

When to intervene: The urgency of an intervention in the setting of IAH/ACS depends on the measured IAP value, the rate of IAP increase, and the degree of organ dysfunction. In most situations, starting stepwise management should not be delayed and some situations require immediate invasive intervention. In general, in patients with primary ACS, intervention is more urgent than in patients with secondary ACS where the clinician has more time to intervene. If adequate oxygenation and/or ventilation cannot be maintained despite optimal ventilator settings, or circulation is severely compromised despite adequate fluid resuscitation and vasopressor support, immediate decompression may be required—irrespective of the other interventions. If organ function is slowly deteriorating along with a gradually increasing IAP, using a technique expected to have a slower effect on IAP may be considered, if the potential for serious complications can be avoided by this strategy.

41.3.3 What Is the Best Method of Intervention?

How to intervene: The method of choice for treating IAH will be guided by both the cause that led to the IAH and the degree of organ dysfunction. Knowing the cause of IAH can help predict the effect of a specific intervention on IAP, both in magnitude and time to effect. The degree and dynamics of organ dysfunction should be considered to determine the desired decrease in IAP and the time allowed to achieve it. Many techniques to decrease IAP have been described and interventions may be aimed at lowering intra-abdominal volume (intra- or extraluminal volume), improving abdominal compliance, or both.

41.3.3.1 Reducing Intraluminal Volume

Evacuation of excess volume from the gastrointestinal tract can be accomplished by prokinetics and/or enemas. Decompression of the gastrointestinal tract by nasogastric and/or rectal tubes or endoscopic decompression can be performed quickly and safely, but only the most proximal and distal parts of the gastrointestinal tract are accessible for easy intervention [8], thereby limiting their expected effectiveness in some patients. IAH/ACS due to small bowel dilatation may be difficult to treat noninvasively. Even if surgery is not required for treatment of the underlying condition, decompressive laparotomy may be necessary, especially as the combination of abdominal visceral edema and increased IAP poses a significant risk for bacterial translocation or even bowel ischemia [35].

41.3.3.2 Reducing Extraluminal Volume

Percutaneous catheter drainage can be used as a definitive treatment in some cases (e.g., ascites in liver cirrhosis [36], burn patients with ACS [37]), but can also be used as a temporary measure in cases where investigation of the underlying disease is ongoing but organ dysfunction requires urgent decompression (e.g., decompression of pneumoperitoneum before evaluation for gastrointestinal tract perforation [38]) or after definitive treatment of the underlying condition to treat any residual IAH/ACS (e.g., evacuation of free abdominal blood after endovascular aortic reconstruction for ruptured aortic aneurysm). This is a direct challenge to the classical adage that a diagnosis of overt ACS equals the need for decompressive laparotomy while, even in extreme circumstances, the etiology of ACS should be considered. As an example, several cases of ACS due to acute massive pneumoperitoneum, successfully treated with needle decompression, have been published [38].

41.3.3.3 Improving Abdominal Wall Compliance

Some conditions associated with impaired abdominal wall compliance can be easily corrected and enable fast and significant decrease in IAP. Burn eschars can be treated with escharotomy [39], tight bandages can be released, and body position can be changed [13]. For other causes of decreased abdominal wall compliance, fast release is not possible or not desirable (e.g., release of a tight hernia repair). In these cases, other techniques to improve abdominal wall compliance can be attempted (such as analgesia and/or sedation [40], neuromuscular blockers [41], and changing body position [42]) when indicated. Since small changes in intra-abdominal volumes can lead to significant changes in IAP in patients with decreased abdominal wall compliance, bedside ultrasound and removal of moderate amounts of ascites may offer relief of IAH/ACS, even if the main etiology of IAH is decreased abdominal wall compliance not amenable to nonsurgical treatment.

41.3.3.4 Decompressive Laparotomy

Decompressive laparotomy will decrease intra-abdominal volume in relation to the abdominal cavity and abdominal wall compliance and is as such the ultimate treatment for ACS. However, the consequences are considerable and even with improved open abdomen management techniques this should—based on current knowledge—only be reserved for treatment failures [10–12]. However, treatment failures should be identified swiftly when they occur and both the decision to proceed to decompressive laparotomy and the execution of that decision should not be delayed if the patient's condition warrants urgent intervention. The anesthesiologist and/or intensivist should be aware that decompressive laparotomy can be a severe ischemia-reperfusion event, especially when IAP has been elevated for some time, and patients may require supportive measures to tolerate the intervention. After decompressive laparotomy, patients should still be treated according to the medical management principles, especially in terms of controlling fluid balance and improving abdominal compliance, in order to facilitate primary fascial closure. The success of this approach has been demonstrated by Cheatham et al. [43]. IAP should be monitored closely after decompressive laparotomy in order to prevent recurrent ACS [44].

41.4 Supportive Management of the Patient with IAH/ACS

This chapter focuses on the treatment of IAH/ACS in terms of treatment aimed at reducing IAP. It is important to realize that the presence of IAH/ACS may lead to changes in general ICU management [45]. Respiratory management is affected since studies have shown that higher ventilation pressures (both PEEP and plateau pressures) can be used safely in patients with increased IAP and may be warranted in order to maintain alveolar recruitment [46]. Elevated IAP has profound effects on the cardiovascular system and the microcirculation; it changes normal values for hemodynamic monitoring and can mimic a state of fluid responsiveness [47]. Administration of a fluid bolus may temporarily improve tissue perfusion although fluid resuscitation is a major risk factor for (progression of) IAH/ACS [48]. Since IAH/ACS can have an impact on practically all organ systems, it should be a consideration in all aspects of supportive ICU management [49], although a complete discussion on this topic is beyond the scope of this manuscript. Secondary IAH/ACS is mainly an iatrogenic disease related to fluid overload after resuscitation; therefore, a more restrictive fluid management approach with limitation of fluid intake or fluid removal with diuretics or RRT with net ultrafiltration may have a beneficial effect on outcomes [50].

41.5 Conclusion

In 2013, the WSACS published evidence-based guidelines on the definitions, diagnosis, and treatment of IAH and ACS. Even with the implementation of these guidelines, making bedside decisions regarding the management of individual patients with IAH/ACS remains difficult, because of the wide variety of conditions associated with IAH/ACS, the broad spectrum of associated organ dysfunction, and the large number of treatment options available to decrease IAP. In this chapter, we provide a clinical framework that provides insight into how to use the guidelines when managing a specific patient in daily practice. The key message is that treatment should not be based solely on the degree of IAH, but also on the severity and dynamics of organ dysfunction as well as the etiology of IAH/ACS.

In general, the higher the IAP, the faster and more pronounced the rise in IAP and the more severe or deteriorating the organ dysfunction, the prompter and more aggressive treatment of IAH that is warranted. Therefore, frequent re-evaluation, taking into account the progression of IAH and course of disease and organ dysfunction, is necessary. If the underlying cause is well controlled and general condition is improving, the further course of IAH can usually be observed before initiating aggressive treatment. If there is underlying ongoing inflammation and fluid resuscitation continues, it is unlikely that IAH will decrease and more aggressive measures should be considered early.

Acknowledgment The authors would like to thank Drs. Bart De Keulenaer, Chialka Ejike, Adrian Regli, Annika Reintam, Andrew Kirkpatrick, and Derek Roberts for their contributions to this manuscript.

References

1. Malbrain ML, Cheatham ML, Kirkpatrick A, et al. Results from the International conference of experts on intra-abdominal hypertension and abdominal compartment syndrome. I. Definitions. Intensive Care Med. 2006;32:1722–32.
2. Kron IL, Harman PK, Nolan SP. The measurement of intra-abdominal pressure as a criterion for abdominal re-exploration. Ann Surg. 1984;199:28–30.
3. Reintam Blaser A, Regli A, De Keulenaer B, et al. Incidence, risk factors, and outcomes of intra-abdominal hypertension in critically ill patients-a prospective multicenter study (IROI Study). Crit Care Med. 2019;47:535–42.

4. De Keulenaer B, Regli A, De Laet I, Roberts D, Malbrain ML. What's new in medical management strategies for raised intra-abdominal pressure: evacuating intra-abdominal contents, improving abdominal wall compliance, pharmacotherapy, and continuous negative extra-abdominal pressure. Anaesthesiol Intensive Ther. 2015;47:54–62.
5. De Waele JJ, Malbrain ML, Kirkpatrick AW. The abdominal compartment syndrome: evolving concepts and future directions. Crit Care. 2015;19:211.
6. Cheatham ML, Malbrain ML, Kirkpatrick A, et al. Results from the International conference of experts on intra-abdominal hypertension and abdominal compartment syndrome. II. Recommendations. Intensive Care Med. 2007;33:951–62.
7. Cheatham ML. Nonoperative management of intra-abdominal hypertension and abdominal compartment syndrome. World J Surg. 2009;33:1116–22.
8. Kirkpatrick AW, Roberts DJ, De Waele J, et al. Intra-abdominal hypertension and the abdominal compartment syndrome: updated consensus definitions and clinical practice guidelines from the World Society of the Abdominal Compartment Syndrome. Intensive Care Med. 2013;39:1190–206.
9. Struck MF, Reske AW, Schmidt T, Hilbert P, Steen M, Wrigge H. Respiratory functions of burn patients undergoing decompressive laparotomy due to secondary abdominal compartment syndrome. Burns. 2014;40:120–6.
10. De Waele JJ, Hoste EA, Malbrain ML. Decompressive laparotomy for abdominal compartment syndrome—a critical analysis. Crit Care. 2006;10:R51.
11. Van Damme L, De Waele JJ. Effect of decompressive laparotomy on organ function in patients with abdominal compartment syndrome: a systematic review and meta-analysis. Crit Care. 2018;22:179.
12. De Waele JJ, Kimball E, Malbrain M, et al. Decompressive laparotomy for abdominal compartment syndrome. Br J Surg. 2016;103:709–15.
13. Malbrain ML, De Laet I, De Waele JJ, et al. The role of abdominal compliance, the neglected parameter in critically ill patients—a consensus review of 16. Part 2: measurement techniques and management recommendations. Anaesthesiol Intensive Ther. 2014;46:406–32.
14. Malbrain ML, Roberts DJ, De Laet I, et al. The role of abdominal compliance, the neglected parameter in critically ill patients—a consensus review of 16. Part 1: definitions and pathophysiology. Anaesthesiol Intensive Ther. 2014;46:392–405.
15. Chionh JJL, Wei BPC, Martin JA, Opdam HI. Determining normal values for intra-abdominal pressure. ANZ J Surg. 2006;76:1106–9.
16. De Keulenaer BL, De Waele JJ, Powell B, Malbrain ML. What is normal intra-abdominal pressure and how is it affected by positioning, body mass and positive end-expiratory pressure. Intensive Care Med. 2009;35:969–76.
17. Frezza EE, Shebani KO, Robertson J, Wachtel MS. Morbid obesity causes chronic increase of intra-abdominal pressure. Dig Dis Sci. 2007;52:1038–41.
18. Lozada MJ, Goyal V, Osmundson SS, Pacheco LD, Malbrain MLNG. It's high time for intra-abdominal hypertension guidelines in pregnancy after more than 100 years of measuring pressures. Acta Obstet Gynecol Scand. 2019;98:1486–8.
19. Umgelter A, Reindl W, Franzen M, Lenhardt C, Huber W, Schmid RM. Renal resistive index and renal function before and after paracentesis in patients with hepatorenal syndrome and tense ascites. Intensive Care Med. 2008;35:152–6.
20. Verbrugge FH, Dupont M, Steels P, et al. Abdominal contributions to cardiorenal dysfunction in congestive heart failure. J Am Coll Cardiol. 2013;62:485–95.
21. Depauw PRAM, Groen RJM, Van Loon J, Peul WC, Malbrain MLNG, De Waele JJ. The significance of intra-abdominal pressure in neurosurgery and neurological diseases: a narrative review and a conceptual proposal. Acta Neurochir. 2019;161:855–64.
22. Kyoung KH, Hong SK. The duration of intra-abdominal hypertension strongly predicts outcomes for the critically ill surgical patients: a prospective observational study. World J Emerg Surg. 2015;10:22.
23. De Waele JJ, De Laet I, Kirkpatrick AW, Hoste E. Intra-abdominal hypertension and abdominal compartment syndrome. Am J Kidney Dis. 2011;57:159–69.

24. Dalfino L, Tullo L, Donadio I, Malcangi V, Brienza N. Intra-abdominal hypertension and acute renal failure in critically ill patients. Intensive Care Med. 2008;34:707–13.
25. De laet I, Malbrain ML, Jadoul JL, Rogiers P, Sugrue M. Renal implications of increased intra-abdominal pressure: are the kidneys the canary for abdominal hypertension? Acta Clin Belg Suppl. 2007;62(Suppl 1):119–30.
26. De Laet IE, Malbrain M. Current insights in intra-abdominal hypertension and abdominal compartment syndrome. Med Int. 2007;31:88–99.
27. Malbrain ML, Roberts DJ, Sugrue M, et al. The polycompartment syndrome: a concise state-of-the-art review. Anaesthesiol Intensive Ther. 2014;46:433–50.
28. Petro CC, Raigani S, Fayezizadeh M, et al. Permissible intra-abdominal hypertension following complex abdominal wall reconstruction. Plast Reconstr Surg. 2015;136:868–81.
29. Thai H, Guerron AD, Bencsath KP, Liu X, Loor M. Fulminant Clostridium difficile enteritis causing abdominal compartment syndrome. Surg Infect. 2014;15:821–5.
30. Ball CG, Kirkpatrick AW, Yilmaz S, Monroy M, Nicolaou S, Salazar A. Renal allograft compartment syndrome: an underappreciated postoperative complication. Am J Surg. 2006;191:619–24.
31. Gupte GL, Haghighi KS, Sharif K, et al. Surgical complications after intestinal transplantation in infants and children-UK experience. J Pediatr Surg. 2010;45:1473–8.
32. Malbrain ML, Peeters Y, Wise R. The neglected role of abdominal compliance in organ-organ interactions. Crit Care. 2016;20:67.
33. Blaser AR, Björck M, De Keulenaer B, Regli A. Abdominal compliance: a bench-to-bedside review. J Trauma Acute Care Surg. 2015;78:1044–53.
34. Ahmadi-Noorbakhsh S, Malbrain ML. Integration of inspiratory and expiratory intra-abdominal pressure: a novel concept looking at mean intra-abdominal pressure. Ann Intensive Care. 2012;2(Suppl 1):S18.
35. Al-Bahrani AZ, Darwish A, Hamza N, et al. Gut barrier dysfunction in critically ill surgical patients with abdominal compartment syndrome. Pancreas. 2010;39:1064–9.
36. Umgelter A, Reindl W, Wagner KS, et al. Effects of plasma expansion with albumin and paracentesis on haemodynamics and kidney function in critically ill cirrhotic patients with tense ascites and hepatorenal syndrome: a prospective uncontrolled trial. Crit Care. 2008;12:R4.
37. Latenser BA, Kowal-Vern A, Kimball D, Chakrin A, Dujovny N. A pilot study comparing percutaneous decompression with decompressive laparotomy for acute abdominal compartment syndrome in thermal injury. J Burn Care Rehabil. 2002;23:190–5.
38. Bunni J, Bryson PJ, Higgs SM. Abdominal compartment syndrome caused by tension pneumoperitoneum in a scuba diver. Ann R Coll Surg Engl. 2012;94:237–9.
39. Oda J, Ueyama M, Yamashita K, et al. Effects of escharotomy as abdominal decompression on cardiopulmonary function and visceral perfusion in abdominal compartment syndrome with burn patients. J Trauma. 2005;59:369–74.
40. Tasdogan M, Memis D, Sut N, Yuksel M. Results of a pilot study on the effects of propofol and dexmedetomidine on inflammatory responses and intra-abdominal pressure in severe sepsis. J Clin Anesth. 2009;21:394–400.
41. De Laet I, Hoste E, Verholen E, De Waele JJ. The effect of neuromuscular blockers in patients with intra-abdominal hypertension. Intensive Care Med. 2007;33:1811–4.
42. Cheatham ML, De Waele JJ, De Laet I, et al. The impact of body position on intra-abdominal pressure measurement: a multicenter analysis. Crit Care Med. 2009;37:2187–90.
43. Cheatham ML, Safcsak K. Is the evolving management of intra-abdominal hypertension and abdominal compartment syndrome improving survival. Crit Care Med. 2010;38:402–7.
44. Duchesne JC, Baucom CC, Rennie KV, Simmons J, McSwain NE Jr. Recurrent abdominal compartment syndrome: an inciting factor of the second hit phenomenon. Am Surg. 2009;75:1193–8.
45. Regli A, De Keulenaer B, De Laet I, Roberts D, Dabrowski W, Malbrain ML. Fluid therapy and perfusional considerations during resuscitation in critically ill patients with intra-abdominal hypertension. Anaesthesiol Intensive Ther. 2015;47:45–53.

46. Regli A, Pelosi P, Malbrain MLNG. Ventilation in patients with intra-abdominal hypertension: what every critical care physician needs to know. Ann Intensive Care. 2019;9:52.
47. Beurton A, Teboul JL, Girotto V, et al. Intra-abdominal hypertension is responsible for false negatives to the passive leg raising test. Crit Care Med. 2019;47:e639–47.
48. Malbrain MLNG, Van Regenmortel N, Saugel B, et al. Principles of fluid management and stewardship in septic shock: it is time to consider the four D's and the four phases of fluid therapy. Ann Intensive Care. 2018;8:66.
49. De Laet I, Malbrain ML. ICU management of the patient with intra-abdominal hypertension: what to do, when and to whom? Acta Clin Belg Suppl. 2007;62(Suppl 1):190–9.
50. Malbrain ML, Marik PE, Witters I, et al. Fluid overload, de-resuscitation, and outcomes in critically ill or injured patients: a systematic review with suggestions for clinical practice. Anaesthesiol Intensive Ther. 2014;46:361–80.

Update on the Management of Iatrogenic Gas Embolism

N. Heming, M.-A. Melone, and D. Annane

42.1 Introduction

Gas embolism remains a poorly known medical problem albeit it is often of iatrogenic origin and is associated with an unacceptably high rate of morbidity and mortality. In this chapter, we will summarize the physiopathology, diagnosis, and management of iatrogenic gas embolism.

42.2 Definition and Epidemiology

Gas embolism results from a vascular breach leading to the entry of gas into the circulation. Gas embolism is defined by the onset of clinical manifestations resulting from circulating gas. Gas embolism occurs in three main circumstances: pregnancy, trauma, and following medical or surgical procedures, i.e., iatrogenic gas embolism. In this chapter, we will focus on iatrogenic gas embolism. According to where gas enters into the circulation, the terms venous or arterial gas embolism are used. Gas embolism is a potentially catastrophic complication of numerous medical or surgical procedures [1]. The prevalence of iatrogenic gas embolism is estimated to be at least 2.6/100,000 hospitalizations [2]. Gas embolism is likely underdiagnosed, undertreated, and thus underreported. Its mortality rate in the short-term is approximately

---

N. Heming · D. Annane (✉)
General Intensive Care Unit, Raymond Poincaré Hospital, AP-HP Paris Saclay, Garches, France

INSERM U1173 Lab Inflammation & Infection, School of Medicine Simone Veil, Université Paris Saclay—Université de Versailles SQY, Montigny-le-Bretonneux, France
e-mail: djillali.annane@aphp.fr

M.-A. Melone
General Intensive Care Unit, Raymond Poincaré Hospital, AP-HP Paris Saclay, Garches, France

Table 42.1 Mortality and neurological sequelae of gas embolism

First author [ref]	Number of patients	Hyperbaric oxygen therapy	Death (%)	Neurological sequelae (%)
Murphy [3]	16	One session at 6 ATA (US Navy 6A)	12.5	37.5
Bitterman [31]	5	One session at 6 ATA (US Navy 6A)	20	20
Massey [32]	14	One session at 6 ATA (US Navy 6A)	21.4	71.4
Kol [33]	6	One session at 6 ATA (modified US Navy 6A) One patient was treated for 90 min at 2.8 ATA	33	17
Muskat [34]	4	One session at 6 ATA (US Navy 6A)	25	0
Ziser [4]	17	One session at 6 ATA (US Navy 6A) One patient was treated for 90 min at 2.8 ATA	18	35
Blanc [5]	86	One session at 6 ATA (US Navy 6A)	8	33
Bessereau [2]	125	One session at 4 ATA for 15 min with a decompression plateau pressure at 2.8 ATA for 90 min	21	33
Beevor [35]	36	One session at 6 ATA (US Navy 6A)	9	36

ATA atmospheres absolute

8–12% [2–5]. Severe sequelae affect 9–35% of survivors (Table 42.1) [2–5]. The diagnosis is challenging in particular during general anesthesia. Indeed, visualization of gas in the circulation on its own may not mean that there will be clinical consequences and is not sufficient to confirm the diagnosis of gas embolism.

42.3 Physiopathology

There are two main mechanisms by which gas embolism may cause organ damage: mechanical obstruction and inflammation. First, the gas embolus interrupts flow when reaching a vessel with a smaller diameter causing ischemia in corresponding tissues. A venous gas embolus originates before the pulmonary filter and progresses to the right cardiac cavities. When the volume of the bubble is sufficiently large, acute cardiac obstruction may occur [6]. Moderate size bubbles lodged in the pulmonary arteries increase pulmonary vascular resistance and cause pulmonary hypertension [7], abnormal ventilation/perfusion ratios, and subsequently hypoxemia [8]. Small-sized bubbles may remain *asymptomatic* and clear through the pulmonary alveoli without causing any circulatory disorder. The brisk increase in right ventricular pressure may promote the migration of bubbles originating in the venous system into the arterial system, causing a paradoxical embolism. A paradoxical embolism occurs through the existence of a right-left shunt, including patent foramen ovale, a condition present in 20–30% of the adult population [9]. Mechanical ventilation, particularly with positive end-expiratory pressure (PEEP), promotes bubble progression through right-to-left shunting. Gas entering the systemic circulation may affect multiple organs, sometimes simultaneously. In experimental models of arterial gas embolism, there was evidence of gas in the cerebral, mesenteric, femoral, and coronary arteries [10].

A bubble of gas entering the systemic circulation will travel until the caliber of the vessel is too small, forcing the bubble to slow down and then to stop, leading to end-organ ischemia. During this process, a bubble will break up into smaller entities leading to multiple sites of ischemia. Owing to natural dissolution of gas into blood, the diameter of the intravascular bubbles decreases enabling the bubble to progress downstream to a vessel with a smaller diameter. As a result, ischemia-reperfusion injuries may occur. In addition, bubbles interact with the endothelium, triggering activation of platelets, leukocytes, complement system, coagulation cascade, fibrinolysis, and kinin systems [11–13]. The gas embolus may then become covered with fibrin and inflammatory cells or even lead to the formation of a blood clot. This will prevent the natural dissolution of the gas into the blood and prolong tissue ischemia.

A number of factors contribute to the severity of gas embolism. First, the type of gas will determine the speed of the natural dissolution of the bubbles into the blood with nitrogen being less soluble in the blood than oxygen or carbon dioxide. Intravascular gas volume of >50 ml may cause cardiac arrest, and administration of 90 ml/s of air may be lethal in man. In case of venous air embolism, the gradient of pressure between the vessel breach and the right atrium is a major determinant of the volume and flow of air entering the circulation. Typically, the sitting position during neurosurgery or during manipulation of a central venous line is an important risk factor for serious cerebral air embolism [14]. Thus, maintaining the gradient of pressure at zero (supine position) or even negative (Trendelenburg position) usually prevents eruption of gas into the venous circulation. In addition to patient position, hypovolemia and early phase of inspiration in spontaneously breathing patients may also contribute to a positive gradient of pressure between the vessel's hole and the right atrium.

42.4 Diagnosis

Sometimes entry of gas (usually air) into the vessels is directly seen, particularly following extracorporeal circulation or intravascular radiographic procedures. In this context, the diagnosis is immediate and does not require any further investigations. Likewise, clinical manifestations in circumstances such as a disconnected central venous line are sufficient to confirm the diagnosis of air embolism.

42.4.1 Conditions with Risk of Iatrogenic Gas Embolism

42.4.1.1 Venous Gas Embolism

A number of surgical procedures are particularly at risk of gas embolism. They include procedures requiring gas insufflation in a virtual cavity such as the pleura or the peritoneum [15] or in the gastroduodenal tract [16]. High-frequency jet ventilation during surgery is also a common cause of venous air embolism. Surgical procedures in areas of no collapsible veins (i.e., epiploic and emissary veins and dural venous systems) may also promote gas entry into the circulation. For example, neurosurgery of the posterior fossa in a patient in the sitting position is associated with gas embolism in 39% of cases [17]. Hysteroscopy or self-inflicted abortions, through damage to the veins of the myometrium is often associated with gas embolism.

Placement, manipulation, or removal of central venous lines, Swan-Ganz catheters, and dialysis catheters is the primary cause of iatrogenic air embolism [18] with a prevalence of 1/750 to 1/3000 [2, 19]. Gas embolism may also occur following invasive chest procedures, such as thoracoscopy and transthoracic punctures, and during mechanical ventilation with dynamic hyperinflation-induced alveolar breach.

42.4.1.2 Arterial Gas Embolism
Cardiopulmonary bypass (CPB) exposes to arterial gas embolism, and transcranial Doppler monitoring shows the presence of cerebral microbubbles in almost all patients [20]. Gas embolism-related death or major brain injuries may occur in 1/2500 to 1/8000 cases [21]. There are many other procedures, particularly invasive radiography, that may be complicated by gas embolism [2, 22] (Table 42.2).

42.4.2 Clinical Manifestations

Symptoms of gas embolism are of sudden onset during procedures at risk. Sometimes symptoms may be delayed after the procedure, for example, following mobilization of the patient, or during recovery from general anesthesia. Symptoms are usually nonspecific signs of ischemia and/or inflammation.

A precordial "millwheel murmur" can occasionally be heard at the time of gas embolism, indicating gas in the cardiac chambers. More common are cardiac signs of obstruction of the pulmonary arteries, including pulmonary artery hypertension, reduced right ventricular preload, which may lead to lower left ventricular preload and reduced cardiac output, or signs of myocardial ischemia including chest pain, faintness, hypotension, cardiovascular collapse, bradycardia, tachyarrhythmia, or asystole. Neurological signs are related to cerebral ischemia, cerebral edema, and intracranial hypertension, and include headaches, coma, focal neurological signs (anosognosia, hemiparesis, or hemiplegia, ataxia), pyramidal signs, visual anomalies (cortical blindness, hemianopsia), and seizures.

During general anesthesia for at-risk surgery, gas embolism can be diagnosed by a sudden decrease in end-tidal CO_2 indicating a fall in cardiac output. Delayed awakening following surgery may be related to gas embolism of the pons or both hemispheres.

42.4.3 Laboratory Investigations

The diagnosis of gas embolism is often straightforward in the context of sudden onset of neurological and/or cardiorespiratory symptoms during a medical or

Table 42.2 Procedures at risk for iatrogenic gas embolism

Procedures	Mechanisms
Cardiac and vascular surgery	Arterial air embolism
Valve repair	
Coronary artery bypass grafting	
Inter-cavity communication closure	
Aortic aneurysm repair	
Interventional radiology	Arterial air embolism
Coronary angiogram	
Arteriography	
Transarterial chemo-embolization	Arterial air embolism
Neurosurgery	Venous air embolism
Posterior fossa	
Spinal surgery	
Endovascular intervention (e.g., thrombectomy)	Arterial air embolism
Extracorporeal circulation	Arterial air embolism
Arterio-venous ECMO	
Veno-venous ECMO	Venous air embolism
Hemodialysis	
Central vascular access	Venous air embolism
Placement, manipulation, removal of central line	
Cardiac catheterization	
Pacemaker placement	
Peripheral venous access	Venous air embolism
Thoracic procedures	Venous air embolism
Pleural puncture/drainage	
Transparietal puncture/biopsy	
Bronchoscopy	
Laser treatment of the airways	
Thoracoscopy/pleuroscopy	Venous CO_2 embolism
Mechanical ventilation	Venous air embolism
High positive end-expiratory pressure	
Jet ventilation	
High frequency oscillatory ventilation	
Endoscopic procedures requiring gas insufflation	Venous CO_2 embolism
Laparoscopy	
Coelioscopy	
Endoscopic retrograde cholangio-pancreatography	

ECMO extracorporeal membrane oxygenation

surgical procedure at risk. There is no biomarker of gas embolism and electrophysiological studies, whether cerebral or cardiac, are useless and only provide evidence of nonspecific brain injuries or cardiac ischemia. During surgery, monitoring of end-tidal CO_2, or monitoring by transesophageal echocardiography or transcranial Doppler allows early detection of gas embolism. In cases such as delayed awakening from general anesthesia, brain computed tomography (CT) scan may show gas in cerebral vessels (Fig. 42.1). Likewise, presence of gas in intrathoracic vessels or the cardiac cavity can also be demonstrated on chest X-ray, echocardiography, or CT scan.

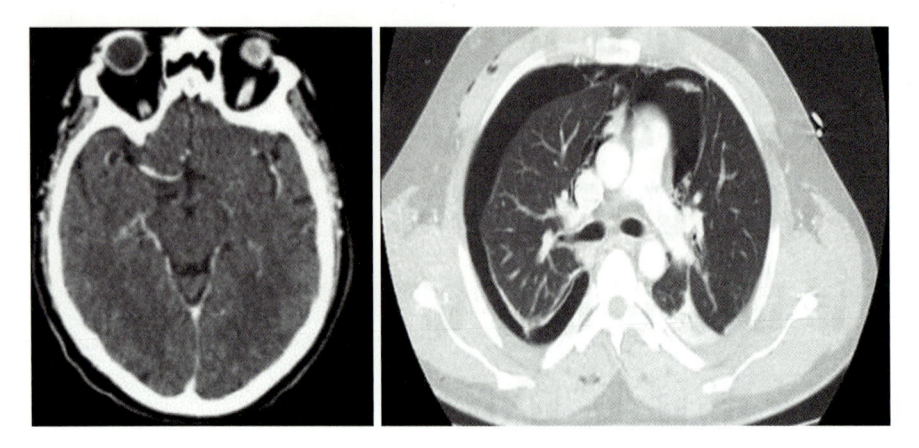

Fig. 42.1 Computed tomography (CT) scan of the brain (left panel) and the thorax (right panel), in a 38-year-old woman who presented suddenly with headaches, bilateral blindness, and chest pain 4 h after coelioscopy for ovarian resection. CT scan showed multiple air-density areas in both cerebral hemispheres (left panel) and a right pneumothorax and air in the intrathoracic vessels (right panel)

42.5 Treatment

42.5.1 Immediate Interventions

Any suspicion of gas embolism should prompt specific management. First, the invasive procedure should be terminated without delay and the patient be placed in the supine or Trendelenburg position. Whenever possible, gas should be removed from the right atrium and or the superior vena cava through the central venous line, and sometimes chest compression may help split a large embolus obstructing the heart [23, 24]. To further reduce the gradient pressure between a vessel's breach and the right atrium, rapid volume expansion or shockproof trousers may be used [1]. Patients should be breathing at a fraction of inspired oxygen of 100%, and mechanical ventilation may help accelerate the clearance of gas from the cerebral circulation [25].

42.5.2 Hyperbaric Oxygen Therapy

Hyperbaric oxygen therapy is the gold standard treatment of gas embolism, and patients should be referred to the hyperbaric center without delay [1, 26, 27]. The administration of hyperbaric oxygen therapy is based on solid rationale. First, according to gas physics, increasing atmospheric pressure will mechanically reduce the volume of bubbles in the body. The Boyle and Marriote law states that for a given mass of confined gas, and as long as the temperature is constant, the product of pressure and volume is constant. As shown in Fig. 42.2, increase of absolute pressure to

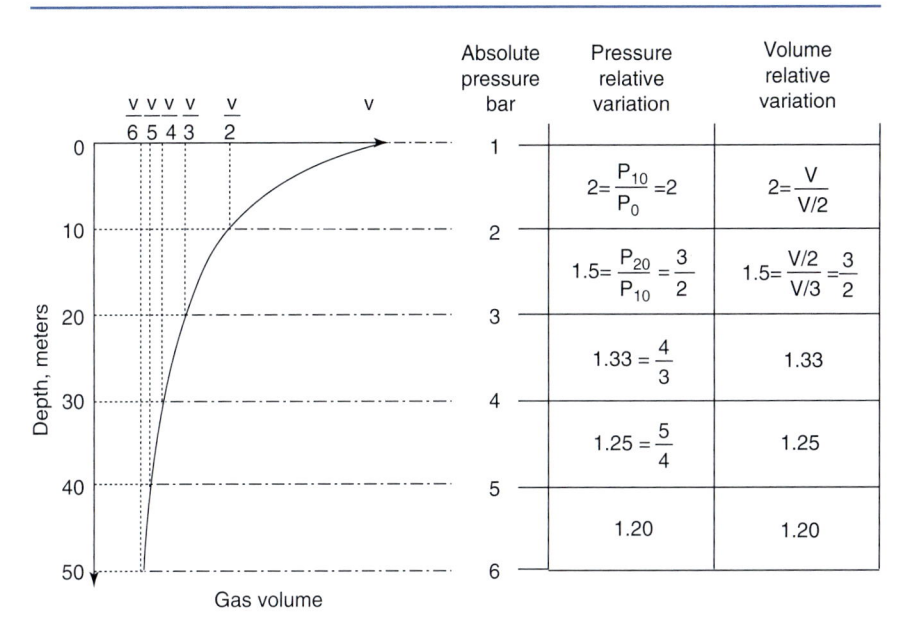

Fig. 42.2 Relationship between atmospheric pressure (P) and volume (V) of gas

Table 42.3 Relationship between atmospheric pressure, alveolar oxygen pressure (P_AO_2), and arterial oxygen content (CaO_2)

Atmospheric pressure ATA	P_AO_2 FiO$_2$: 21% mmHg	P_AO_2 FiO$_2$: 100% mmHg	CaO_2 FiO$_2$: 21% Vol (%)	CaO_2 FiO$_2$: 100% Vol (%)
1	760	102	673	0.32	2.09
2	1520	262	1053	0.81	3.26
3	2280	422	1433	1.31	6.80
4	3040	582	1813	1.80	9.34
6	4560	902	2193	2.80	14.53

FiO_2 inspired fraction of oxygen, *ATA* atmospheres absolute

2 and 3 bars reduced the volume of gas by two- and threefold, respectively. The magnitude of the reduction in the size of bubbles is much less above 3 bar, suggesting that in medical practice there is limited added value of high pressurization (i.e., above 2.8 bar). Second, according to the Dalton law, increase in absolute pressure increases blood oxygen content with denitrogenation accelerating the dissolution of nitrogen into the blood and subsequently diminishing the size of circulating air bubbles [21, 24]. Table 42.3 illustrates the relationship between increase in atmospheric pressure and alveolar oxygen pressure and arterial oxygen content. Finally, hyperbaric oxygen therapy contributes to reducing brain vascular permeability, edema, and intracranial pressure improving the cerebral perfusion pressure [28, 29].

In patients, the evidence supporting hyperbaric oxygen therapy comes from cohort studies (Table 42.1). The most recent and largest cohort study found that 1 year after one session of hyperbaric oxygen therapy, 78/119 patients had survived severe iatrogenic gas embolism free of sequelae [2]. Long-term major neurological sequelae, i.e., a Glasgow outcome scale of three or lower, were seen in only 12/119 patients. Risk factors for mortality at 1 year included an initial cardiac arrest and a Babinski sign. Likewise, a Babinski sign upon ICU admission was a strong and independent predictor of major neurological sequels at 1 year. There is no randomized trial comparing hyperbaric oxygen therapy versus normobaric oxygen therapy. Such a trial would be ethically challenging owing to the iatrogenic nature of gas embolism, the strong rationale and the consistency in the results of cohort studies. One large cohort study found that when hyperbaric oxygen therapy was delivered within 6 h from gas embolism, the recovery rate was dramatically better than if this treatment was delayed (38/56 versus 12/30) [5]. Furthermore, with appropriate preventative measures for oxygen neurotoxicity and barotrauma, hyperbaric oxygen therapy has consistently been reported to be safe with infrequent undesirable effects [30]. Nevertheless, a number of issues have not been addressed so far, including which absolute pressure, which duration, and how many hyperbaric sessions are optimal.

42.6 Conclusion

Gas embolism is an underestimated and potentially cataclysmic complication of invasive procedures. Physicians should suspect gas embolism whenever there is sudden onset of cardiac, neurological, or respiratory symptoms during an at-risk procedure. Whenever suspected, gas embolism should prompt termination of the procedure and rapid management of patients, including positioning and breathing high oxygen concentrations, while being referred to the hyperbaric center. Iatrogenic gas embolism remains associated with an unacceptably high morbidity and mortality.

References

1. Muth CM, Shank ES. Gas embolism. N Engl J Med. 2000;342:476–82.
2. Bessereau J, Genotelle N, Chabbaut C, et al. Long-term outcome of iatrogenic gas embolism. Intensive Care Med. 2010;36:1180–7.
3. Murphy BP, Harford FJ, Cramer FS. Cerebral air embolism resulting from invasive medical procedures. Treatment with hyperbaric oxygen. Ann Surg. 1985;201:242–5.
4. Ziser A, Adir Y, Lavon H, Shupak A. Hyperbaric oxygen therapy for massive arterial air embolism during cardiac operations. J Thorac Cardiovasc Surg. 1999;117:818–21.
5. Blanc P, Boussuges A, Henriette K, Sainty JM, Deleflie M. Iatrogenic cerebral air embolism: importance of an early hyperbaric oxygenation. Intensive Care Med. 2002;28:559–63.
6. Adornato DC, Gildenberg PL, Ferrario CM, Smart J, Frost EA. Pathophysiology of intravenous air embolism in dogs. Anesthesiology. 1978;49:120–7.
7. Gottdiener JS, Papademetriou V, Notargiacomo A, Park WY, Cutler DJ. Incidence and cardiac effects of systemic venous air embolism. Echocardiographic evidence of arterial embolization via noncardiac shunt. Arch Intern Med. 1988;148:795–800.

8. Hlastala MP, Robertson HT, Ross BK. Gas exchange abnormalities produced by venous gas emboli. Respir Physiol. 1979;36:1–17.
9. Thackray NM, Murphy PM, McLean RF, deLacy JL. Venous air embolism accompanied by echocardiographic evidence of transpulmonary air passage. Crit Care Med. 1996;24:359–61.
10. Kunlin J, Benitte AC, Richard S. Study of experimental air embolism and its treatment. Rev Pathol Gen Physiol Clin. 1959;59:891–6.
11. Perkett EA, Brigham KL, Meyrick B. Granulocyte depletion attenuates sustained pulmonary hypertension and increased pulmonary vasoreactivity caused by continuous air embolization in sheep. Am Rev Respir Dis. 1990;141:456–65.
12. Ritz-Timme S, Eckelt N, Schmidtke E, Thomsen H. Genesis and diagnostic value of leukocyte and platelet accumulations around "air bubbles" in blood after venous air embolism. Int J Legal Med. 1998;111:22–6.
13. Warren BA, Philp RB, Inwood MJ. The ultrastructural morphology of air embolism: platelet adhesion to the interface and endothelial damage. Br J Exp Pathol. 1973;54:163–72.
14. Durant TM, Long J, Oppenheimer MJ. Pulmonary (venous) air embolism. Am Heart J. 1947;33:269–81.
15. Yacoub OF, Cardona I, Coveler LA, Dodson MG. Carbon dioxide embolism during laparoscopy. Anesthesiology. 1982;57:533–5.
16. Lanke G, Adler DG. Gas embolism during endoscopic retrograde cholangiopancreatography: diagnosis and management. Ann Gastroenterol. 2019;32:156–67.
17. Fathi A-R, Eshtehardi P, Meier B. Patent foramen ovale and neurosurgery in sitting position: a systematic review. Br J Anaesth. 2009;102:588–96.
18. Heckmann JG, Lang CJ, Kindler K, Huk W, Erbguth FJ, Neundörfer B. Neurologic manifestations of cerebral air embolism as a complication of central venous catheterization. Crit Care Med. 2000;28:1621–5.
19. Feliciano DV, Mattox KL, Graham JM, Beall AC, Jordan GL. Major complications of percutaneous subclavian vein catheters. Am J Surg. 1979;138:869–74.
20. Borger MA, Feindel CM. Cerebral emboli during cardiopulmonary bypass: effect of perfusionist interventions and aortic cannulas. J Extra Corpor Technol. 2002;34:29–33.
21. Tovar EA, Del Campo C, Borsari A, Webb RP, Dell JR, Weinstein PB. Postoperative management of cerebral air embolism: gas physiology for surgeons. Ann Thorac Surg. 1995;60:1138–42.
22. McCarthy CJ, Behravesh S, Naidu SG, Oklu R. Air embolism: diagnosis, clinical management and outcomes. Diagn Basel Switz. 2017;7(1):5.
23. De Angelis J. A simple and rapid method for evacuation of embolized air. Anesthesiology. 1975;43:110–1.
24. Moon RE, de Lisle Dear G, Stolp BW. Treatment of decompression illness and iatrogenic gas embolism. Respir Care Clin N Am. 1999;5:93–135.
25. Annane D, Troché G, Delisle F, et al. Effects of mechanical ventilation with normobaric oxygen therapy on the rate of air removal from cerebral arteries. Crit Care Med. 1994;22:851–7.
26. Leach RM, Rees PJ, Wilmshurst P. ABC of oxygen: hyperbaric oxygen therapy. BMJ. 1998;317:1140–3.
27. Mathieu D, Marroni A, Kot J. Tenth European consensus conference on hyperbaric medicine: recommendations for accepted and non-accepted clinical indications and practice of hyperbaric oxygen treatment. Diving Hyperb Med. 2017;47:24–32.
28. Miller JD, Ledingham IM, Jennett WB. Effects of hyperbaric oxygen on intracranial pressure and cerebral blood flow in experimental cerebral oedema. J Neurol Neurosurg Psychiatry. 1970;33:745–55.
29. Mink RB, Dutka AJ. Hyperbaric oxygen after global cerebral ischemia in rabbits reduces brain vascular permeability and blood flow. Stroke. 1995;26:2307–12.
30. Bessereau J, Aboab J, Hullin T, et al. Safety of hyperbaric oxygen therapy in mechanically ventilated patients. Int Marit Health. 2017;68:46–51.
31. Bitterman H, Melamed Y. Delayed hyperbaric treatment of cerebral air embolism. Isr J Med Sci. 1993;29:22–6.

32. Massey E, Moon R, Shelton D, Camporesi E. Hyperbaric oxygen therapy of iatrogenic air embolism. J Hyperb Med. 1990;5:15–21.
33. Kol S, Ammar R, Weisz G, Melamed Y. Hyperbaric oxygenation for arterial air embolism during cardiopulmonary bypass. Ann Thorac Surg. 1993;55:401–3.
34. Mushkat Y, Luxman D, Nachum Z, David MP, Melamed Y. Gas embolism complicating obstetric or gynecologic procedures. Case reports and review of the literature. Eur J Obstet Gynecol Reprod Biol. 1995;63:97–103.
35. Beevor H, Frawley G. Iatrogenic cerebral gas embolism: analysis of the presentation, management and outcomes of patients referred to The Alfred Hospital Hyperbaric Unit. Diving Hyperb Med. 2016;46:15–21.

Alcohol Withdrawal Syndrome in the ICU: Preventing Rather than Treating?

M. Geslain and O. Huet

43.1 Introduction

Alcohol use disorders are a major health issue worldwide as they are a component of many diseases and injuries. The health burden of alcohol consumption has been well reported by the World Health Organization (WHO), and it is now acknowledged that pathologic consumption of alcohol is an independent cause of health frailty [1]. Because of this acquired frailty, patients with alcohol use disorders are more prone to be admitted to hospital general wards and also to intensive care units (ICU) [2, 3]. Chronic alcohol consumption leads to well-known diseases, but the effects of alcohol withdrawal on short- and long-term outcomes are less acknowledged. ICU admission of a patient suffering from an alcohol use disorder may lead to a forced and unplanned withdrawal. Alcohol withdrawal will have a wide range of clinical manifestation with its extreme represented by delirium tremens [4]. Delirium tremens was first described by Dr. Sutton in England in 1813. He reported 16 cases of delirium tremens, which he treated with opium and was the first practitioner to link delirium tremens to alcohol withdrawal.

Alcohol withdrawal is an independent factor for disease severity with an increased morbidity and risk of mortality for ICU patients [5, 6]. Moreover, alcohol withdrawal will worsen the severity of the disease requiring ICU admission. Despite its severity, there are only a few studies that have tested strategies to avoid and treat alcohol withdrawal. Therefore, acute alcohol withdrawal is often poorly diagnosed and treated in hospitalized patients, and this is even more obvious for ICU patients. The lack of evidence leads to non-standardized treatment and follow-up with a significant risk of negative consequences on patient outcome.

M. Geslain · O. Huet (✉)
Département d'Anesthésie Réanimation, Hôpital la Cavale Blanche, CHRU de Brest, France

UFR de Médecine, Université de Bretagne Occidentale, Brest, France
e-mail: olivier.huet@chu-brest.fr

In this chapter, we will address definition and epidemiology of alcohol use disorders, and the diagnosis and treatment of acute alcohol withdrawal with a special focus on ICU patients.

43.2 Alcohol Use Disorders: Definition and Epidemiology

Alcohol use disorders are defined in the Statistical Manual of Mental Disorders (DSM-5) [7]. Initially, the DSM-4 definition included 11 criteria to define alcohol abuse and alcohol dependence. In DSM-5, these are now grouped under the name of alcohol use disorders as soon as a patient meets 2 of the 11 criteria. This definition is based on the relationship between the patient and the substance he/she is addicted to. Alcohol addiction is diagnosed by the presence of cognitive, behavioral, and psychological symptoms linked to the consumption of alcohol independent of the amount of alcohol consumed daily. Three stages of disorders are described, from mild to severe. Although this definition is suitable for long-term assessment of patients, it is hard to use in daily clinical practice to detect patients at risk of alcohol use disorders and alcohol withdrawal syndrome, especially in the ICU.

Another approach to evaluate the impact of alcohol consumption on public health has been suggested by the WHO [1]. This definition is based on a continuum between recreational alcohol consumption and addiction (Fig. 43.1). It is correlated to the amount of alcohol consumption by the individual. Therefore, the definition of alcohol use disorders by the WHO includes harmful alcohol use and alcohol dependence. Harmful alcohol use occurs when the daily alcohol consumption may or will lead to negative consequences for the patient or his/her environment. For example, the French society of alcoholology defines harmful alcohol use as occurring as soon as the daily alcohol consumption is greater than two glasses of wine for females and three glasses for men (with a glass containing 10 g of alcohol) every day. Although this threshold may vary among patients depending on medical history, it draws a line between normal and pathologic behavior. This definition may be helpful for clinicians and researchers.

Fig. 43.1 Continuum between recreational alcohol consumption and alcohol use disorders

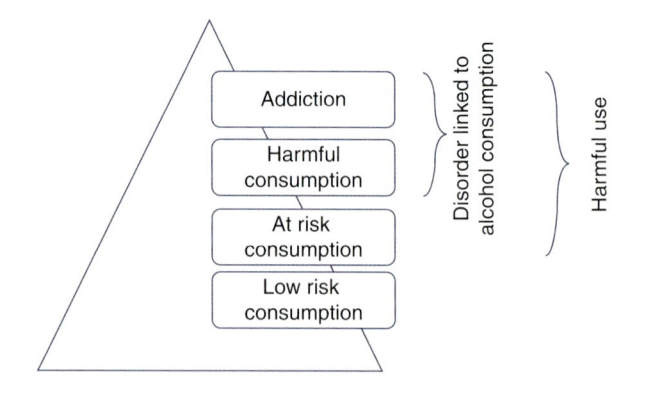

43 Alcohol Withdrawal Syndrome in the ICU: Preventing Rather than Treating? 571

The epidemiological study from the WHO shows that 4.1% of the world population has an alcohol use disorder [1]. There is a major geographic disparity as Europe is the region where the incidence of alcohol use disorders is the highest. Currently, 7.5% of the adult population suffers from alcohol use disorders in Europe, and the average consumption is the highest in the world with 12.5 liters of pure alcohol per year per person older than 15 years of age.

Mortality caused by alcohol use disorders is considerable as, in 2012, 3.3 million deaths were estimated to be caused by alcohol consumption. This represents 1 in every 20 deaths in the world. The highest numbers of deaths are due to cardiovascular disease, followed by injuries, gastrointestinal disease, and cancers. The health burden is also critical as in 2012, 5.1% of the global burden of health and injury was attributable to alcohol.

The severity of disease related to alcohol use disorders is likely to lead patients to require ICU admission at some point. Up to 20% of patients currently admitted to ICUs have an alcohol use disorder, making this one of the most common medical history conditions in ICU patients [2, 8]. Despite this fact, alcohol use disorders are often underestimated or ignored by clinicians compared to other chronic diseases such as cardiovascular diseases.

43.3 Alcohol Withdrawal Syndrome: Pathophysiology and Definition

Although it is acknowledged that a wide range of chronic diseases can be attributed to alcohol use disorders, the impact of alcohol withdrawal syndrome on short- and long-term outcome is less known [9, 10]. Any emergency hospital admission of a patient suffering from an alcohol use disorder involves an unplanned interruption of alcohol consumption exposing the patient to the risk of an acute withdrawal. The effect of alcohol on the central nervous system (CNS) is mainly mediated by gamma aminobutyric acid (GABA) receptors and N-methyl-D-aspartate (NMDA) receptors. During chronic alcohol consumption, GABA receptors are activated and NMDA receptors inhibited. Alcohol's GABA-like effect explains the clinical signs observed during alcohol intake (drunkenness, drowsiness). On the other hand, chronic alcohol consumption leads to a decrease in GABA-related activity and a compensatory increase in NMDA activity. When an equilibrium is reached, a patient's tolerance to the effects of alcohol increases. This acquired tolerance to alcohol's effects leads the patient to increase his/her consumption. The combination of chronic alcohol/acute withdrawal-induced increases in NMDA receptor function and acute alcohol-induced NMDA receptor inhibition during the early stages of withdrawal is likely to generate a hyperexcitable state. This can increase brain activity and lead to withdrawal symptoms [11]. Generally, this excitotoxicity during alcohol withdrawal contributes to alcohol-related neuronal loss in the brain.

The symptoms of alcohol withdrawal syndrome develop within a few hours to a few days after an individual stops drinking [12, 13]. These can include the following: insomnia (trouble sleeping); autonomic symptoms (including sweating or racing heart); increased hand tremors (known as "the shakes"); nausea and/or vomiting; psychomotor agitation (feeling physically restless, inability to stop moving); anxiety; seizures (typically the generalized tonic-clonic type, which is characterized by rhythmic, yet jerking movement, especially of the limbs); and hallucinations, or perceptual disturbances of the auditory, tactile, or visual type (the rarest of alcohol withdrawal symptoms).

The diagnosis of acute alcohol withdrawal can be made if there is evidence of the interruption of alcohol consumption and if at least two of the clinical signs are observed. Clinical manifestations of alcohol withdrawal can be more or less severe, and up to 50% of patients with alcohol use disorders will suffer from withdrawal. The most severe and spectacular clinical manifestation of alcohol withdrawal is delirium tremens. Delirium tremens is defined by the following symptoms: impaired consciousness, severe cognitive disorders, acute withdrawal symptoms fluctuating over time and no other cause of delirium.

Up to 20% of patients suffering from acute withdrawal syndrome will have delirium tremens with major acute and long-term consequences. The acute consequences of delirium tremens can easily be recognized (seizure, aggressiveness, exposure to sedative medication and physical restraints, increased hospital length of stay), but long-term consequences are poorly known. Chronic alcohol exposure progressively damages the CNS leading to dementia, but the occurrence of alcohol withdrawal syndrome also induces neuron damage, increasing and accelerating the risk of long-term CNS damage. It also has a cumulative effect.

Therefore, alcohol withdrawal syndrome is a severe and acute disease that often occurs in the ICU and needs to be carefully assessed and not underestimated. Better knowledge of this disease is critical and considering a prophylactic approach seems relevant.

43.4 Current Guidelines for Alcohol Withdrawal Syndrome

There are several recent guidelines regarding alcohol withdrawal syndrome [13–15]. These guidelines draw almost the same conclusions regarding the treatment for alcohol withdrawal: benzodiazepines [16] are the first line of treatment as they decrease the severity of the withdrawal symptoms and reduce the onset of seizures and delirium tremens. The following environmental measures should also be combined with prescription of a benzodiazepine: inform the patient about the symptoms he/she may experience; reassure the patient and provide comfort care; provide a safe and quiet environment; restore diurnal rhythm; early mobilization; provide patients with their glasses, dental prostheses, earing devices; provide free access to water. Measures should also be taken to correct fluid and electrolyte disturbances and provide B1 vitamin supplementation to prevent Gayet-Wernicke encephalopathy.

However, all these guidelines stress the weakness of the available evidence. The studies referred to in these guidelines are old and have a low level of proof, small sample sizes, and a wide range of studied treatments and endpoints, which make them difficult to compare. This finding made Dr Clark, president of the American Society of Addiction Medicine, state, "There is a current lack of guidance around alcohol withdrawal management that has led to inadequate clinical practices, particularly in inpatient medical and surgical units, and patients are suffering as a result" [14].

43.5 Alcohol Withdrawal in the ICU

In the ICU, up to 20% of patients have an alcohol use disorders, and up to 50% of these patients are at risk of severe alcohol withdrawal syndrome depending on the study [3, 17]. Thus, alcohol use disorders represent an independent frailty even in the absence of symptoms of withdrawal. In fact, alcohol use disorder is independently associated with an increased ICU length of stay, ICU mortality, and incidence of sepsis compared to the overall ICU population. The occurrence of alcohol withdrawal syndrome during the ICU stay is also an independent factor for severity as it increases ICU length of stay, complication rates, and increases costs of care [18, 19]. Although the data come from early studies, it is striking to note that the mortality of untreated alcohol withdrawal syndrome can reach 15–20%, but only 2% when appropriately treated.

Only a few studies have tested medical interventions to prevent alcohol withdrawal in the ICU. The treatments tested were alcohol prescription, benzodiazepines, alpha-2 agonists, and neuroleptics. Alcohol prescription has been compared to benzodiazepines to prevent acute withdrawal syndrome [20]. The primary outcome was a difference in the sedation agitation scale; there was no difference between the groups. Therefore, alcohol prescription is not recommended to prevent alcohol withdrawal as it seems inefficient and may expose patients to adverse effects.

Benzodiazepines are considered to be the first line of treatment for alcohol withdrawal [21]. A large range of medications is available with various delays of onset of action and half-life. No superiority has been found between the different available molecules regarding efficacy. Second-line treatments such as neuroleptics, alpha-2 agonists, propofol, and barbituric have also been tested [22, 23]. Unfortunately, most of the studies have a low level of evidence.

Clonidine has been tested in association with other treatments and was not associated with any advantage. Mueller et al. tested the addition of dexmedetomidine to lorazepam in the treatment of alcohol withdrawal [24]. In this randomized, double-blind, placebo-controlled trail enrolling 24 patients with severe alcohol withdrawal symptoms (Clinical Institute Withdrawal Assessment [CIWA] > 15), the adjunction of dexmedetomidine reduced short-term (day 1) lorazepam exposure but not long term (up to day 7). Bielka et al. reported comparable results [25]. Therefore, more studies are needed to confirm these results. Evidence for the use of neuroleptics is scarce as they have not been tested against benzodiazepines.

On the other hand, it has been demonstrated that the titration of treatment to the symptoms is better than systematic administration, regardless of the intensity of the symptoms. This approach seems to be beneficial. DeCarolis et al. reported that a symptom-driven protocol for the treatment of severe alcohol withdrawal in ICU patients significantly decreased the amount of medication required to control withdrawal symptoms [26]. The study also demonstrated that a symptom-driven protocol decreased the duration of withdrawal symptoms, ICU and hospital length of stay. Other studies have since confirmed the positive results of this approach.

Thus, it seems critical to be able to quantify the intensity of withdrawal symptoms. For non-intubated patients, the revised CIWA for alcohol (CIWA-ar) is available (Table 43.1) [27]. The CIWA-ar score is a specific score allowing the severity of withdrawal to be staged from mild (CIWA-ar <8) to moderate (9< CIWA-ar <15) to severe (CIWA-ar >15). It can easily be performed by any care team member. For intubated patients, the usual scores for agitation, such as the Riker Sedation-Agitation scale or the Richmond Agitation-Sedation Scale (RASS), can be used [28, 29].

Some patients may suffer from acute withdrawal syndrome resistant to benzodiazepines. This severe form of withdrawal is only encountered in the ICU, as the amount of benzodiazepine reached to control the symptoms requires continuous medical supervision. The amount of benzodiazepine requiring this supervision has arbitrarily been defined as >40 mg of diazepam given in 1 h, and salvage treatment is then required [30]. The management of severe resistant alcohol withdrawal has been reported by Wong et al. in a multicenter observational study [30]. In this study, propofol was the most used adjunct sedative treatment (57%), followed by anti-psychotics (27.5%) and dexmedetomidine (14%) [30]. The study also pointed out a great heterogeneity in the prescriptions and combination of drugs. The use of midazolam in continuous infusion seems of interest because of its pharmacodynamics as midazolam is a fast acting molecule with a short half-life. Another interesting result of this study was the lower rate of complications in the benzodiazepine-alone patients compared to patients receiving a combination of drugs.

Severe resistant withdrawal syndrome may lead to delirium tremens. Complications of delirium tremens in the ICU are poorly described; however, patients are at high risk of uncontrollable agitation requiring deep sedation and mechanical ventilation. The need for mechanical ventilation during severe alcohol withdrawal syndrome varies from 10% to 50% of patients depending on the study, but it seems that it occurs more frequently in benzodiazepine-resistant withdrawal with up to 73% of the patients requiring mechanical ventilation [23]. Other complications are mainly traumatic with falls, pulling out central lines and tubes, etc. The prevalence of these self-inflicted traumas reported in one study was 50%.

The difficulty of alcohol withdrawal syndrome management in the ICU lies in the fact that not all patients with a medical history of alcohol use disorders will present with clinically significant alcohol withdrawal syndrome. Therefore, it is not ethically possible to administer a prophylactic treatment to all patients with a

Table 43.1 The revised Clinical Institute Withdrawal Assessment for alcohol [28]

Clinical Institute Withdrawal Assessment of Alcohol Scale, Revised (CIWA-Ar)	
Patient: .... Date: .... Time: .... (24 h clock, midnight = 00:00)	
Pulse or heart rate, taken for 1 min: .... Blood pressure:	
NAUSEA AND VOMITING—Ask "Do you feel sick to your stomach? Have you vomited?" Observation. 0- no nausea and no vomiting 1- mild nausea with no vomiting 2- 3- 4- intermittent nausea with dry heaves 5- 6- 7- constant nausea, frequent dry heaves, and vomiting	**TACTILE DISTURBANCES**—Ask "Have you any itching, pins and needles sensations, any burning, any numbness, or do you feel bugs crawling on or under your skin?" Observation. 0- none 1- very mild itching, pins and needles, burning or numbness 2- mild itching, pins and needles, burning or numbness 3- moderate itching, pins and needles, burning or numbness 4- moderately severe hallucinations 5- severe hallucinations 6- extremely severe hallucinations 7- continuous hallucinations
TREMOR—Arms extended and fingers spread apart. Observation. 0- no tremor 1- not visible, but can be felt fingertip to fingertip 2- 3- 4- moderate, with patient's arms extended 5- 6- 7- severe, even with arms not extended	**AUDITORY DISTURBANCES**—Ask "Are you more aware of sounds around you? Are they harsh? Do they frighten you? Are you hearing anything that is disturbing to you? Are you things you know are not there?" Observation. 0- not present 1- very mild harshness or ability to frighten 2- mild harshness or ability to frighten 3- moderate harshness or ability frighten 4- moderately severe hallucinations 5- severe hallucinations 6- extremely severe hallucinations 7- continuous hallucinations
PAROXYSMAL SWEATS—Observation. 0- no sweat visible 1- barely perceptible sweating, palms moist 2- 3- 4- beads of sweat obvious on forehead 5- 6- 7- drenching sweats	**VISUAL DISTURBANCES**—Ask "Does the light appear to be too bright? Is its color different? Does it hurt your eyes? Are you seeing anything that is disturbing to you? Are you seeing things you know are not there?" Observation. 0- not present 1- very mild sensitivity 2- mild sensitivity 3- moderate sensitivity 4- moderately severe hallucinations 5- severe hallucinations 6- extremely severe hallucinations 7- continuous hallucinations

(continued)

Table 43.1 (continued)

ANXIETY—Ask "Do you feel nervous?" Observation. 0- no anxiety, at ease 1- mild anxious 2- 3- 4- moderately anxious, or guarded, so anxiety is inferred 5- 6- 7- equivalent to acute panic states as seen in severe delirium or acute schizophrenic reactions	**HEADACHE, FULLNESS IN HEAD**—Ask "Does your head feel different? Does it feel like there is a band around your head? Do not rate for dizziness or lightheadedness. Otherwise, rate severity." Observation. 0- not present 1- very mild 2- mild 3- moderate 4- moderately severe 5- severe 6- very severe 7- extremely severe
AGITATION—Observation. 0- normal activity 1- somewhat more than normal activity 2- 3- 4- moderately fidgety and restless 5- 6- 7- paces back and forth during most of the interview, or constantly thrashes about	**ORIENTATION AND CLOUDING OF SENSORIUM**—Ask "What day is this? Where are you? Who am I?" 0- oriented and can do serial additions 1- cannot do serial additions or is uncertain about date 2- disoriented for date by no more than 2 calendar days 3- disoriented for date by more than 2 calendar days 4- disoriented for place/or person Total CIWA-Ar Score: .... Rater's Initials: .... Maximum Possible Score 67

history of an alcohol use disorder. This would expose a large number of patients to unnecessary prophylaxis, which could lead to several adverse effects, including delirium, falls, sedation, or respiratory depression. Therefore, a key to improving standard of care is to be able to detect patients at risk of severe alcohol withdrawal before clinical signs occur. Once this screening has been performed, a standardized protocol to prevent alcohol withdrawal syndrome should improve patient outcome.

Wood et al. performed a systematic review of rational clinical examinations to assess whether some clinical signs had good likelihood ratios, sensitivity, and specificity to detect patients at risk of severe alcohol withdrawal syndrome [31]. A history of delirium tremens and a systolic blood pressure >140 mmHg on admission were associated with an increased likelihood of severe alcohol withdrawal syndrome, but the authors reported that no single symptom or sign could exclude severe alcohol withdrawal syndrome.

However, they isolated six high-quality studies evaluating combinations of clinical findings that were useful for identifying patients at risk of alcohol severe

Table 43.2 The Prediction of Alcohol Withdrawal Severity Scale (PAWSS)

Part A: Threshold Criteria:	("+" or "−," no point)
Have you consumed any amount of alcohol (i.e., been drinking) <u>within the last 30 d</u>? Or did the patient have a "+" BAL upon admission?	…………
If the answer to either is YES, proceed with test:	(1 point each)
PART B: Based on patient interview:	(1 point each)
1. Have you been recently intoxicated/drunk <u>within the last 30 d</u>?	…………
2. Have you <u>ever</u> undergone alcohol use disorder rehabilitation treatment or treatment for alcoholism? (i.e., inpatient or outpatient treatment programs or AA attendance)	…………
3. Have you <u>ever</u> experienced any previous episodes of alcohol withdrawal, regardless of severity?	…………
4. Have you <u>ever</u> experienced blackouts?	…………
5. Have you <u>ever</u> experienced alcohol withdrawal seizures?	…………
6. Have you <u>ever</u> experienced delirium tremens or DTs?	…………
7. Have you combined alcohol with other "downers" like benzodiazepines or barbiturates <u>during the last 90 d</u>?	…………
8. Have you combined alcohol with any other substance of abuse <u>during the last 90 d</u>?	…………
PART C: Based on clinical evidence:	(1 point each)
Was the patient's blood alcohol level (BAL) <u>on presentation</u> ≥200?	…………
Is there evidence of increased autonomic activity? (e.g., HR > 120 bpm, tremor, sweating, agitation, nausea)	…………
	Total Score: …………

From [32] with permission
Notes: maximum score = 10. This instrument is intended as a SCREENING TOOL. The greater the number of positive findings, the higher the risk for the development of alcohol withdrawal syndromes. A score of ≥4 suggests HIGH RISK for moderate to severe alcohol withdrawal syndrome; prophylaxis and/or treatment may be indicated

withdrawal syndrome. Among them the Prediction of Alcohol Withdrawal Severity Scale (PAWSS) seemed to be the most useful.

The PAWSS (Table 43.2) was prospectively developed by Maldonado et al. in patients from general medicine and surgery units [32]. They separated patients into two groups: patients with a PAWSS <4 and patients with a PAWSS ≥4. This cutoff enabled identification of patients at risk of severe alcohol withdrawal syndrome with a specificity of 99.5% and a sensitivity of 93.1%. Despite the fact that the score was only tested on a relatively small sample size (403 patients), the results seem encouraging.

By using a score, it therefore seems possible to detect patients at risk of alcohol withdrawal syndrome. This early detection should enable us to change our current approach. Instead of starting to treat patients when they show the first signs of withdrawal, it is possible to have a prophylactic approach. Knowing the impact of alcohol withdrawal syndrome on short- and long-term prognosis of patients with alcohol use disorders, a prophylactic approach, when possible, seems more clinically and ethically relevant. Prophylaxis of alcohol withdrawal syndrome would include a bundle of environmental measures and a prophylactic treatment.

The molecule used for prophylaxis should meet the following criteria: effective on symptoms of alcohol withdrawal syndrome, fast acting, and easily reversible. Therefore, a benzodiazepine should be the medication to use, and among them midazolam seems to meet all the criteria. Once initiated, treatment efficacy could be assessed using the CIWA-ar and treatment tolerance by assessing the RASS or the Riker Sedation-Agitation scale. An example of a prophylactic approach to prevent alcohol withdrawal syndrome in ICU patients is shown in Fig. 43.2.

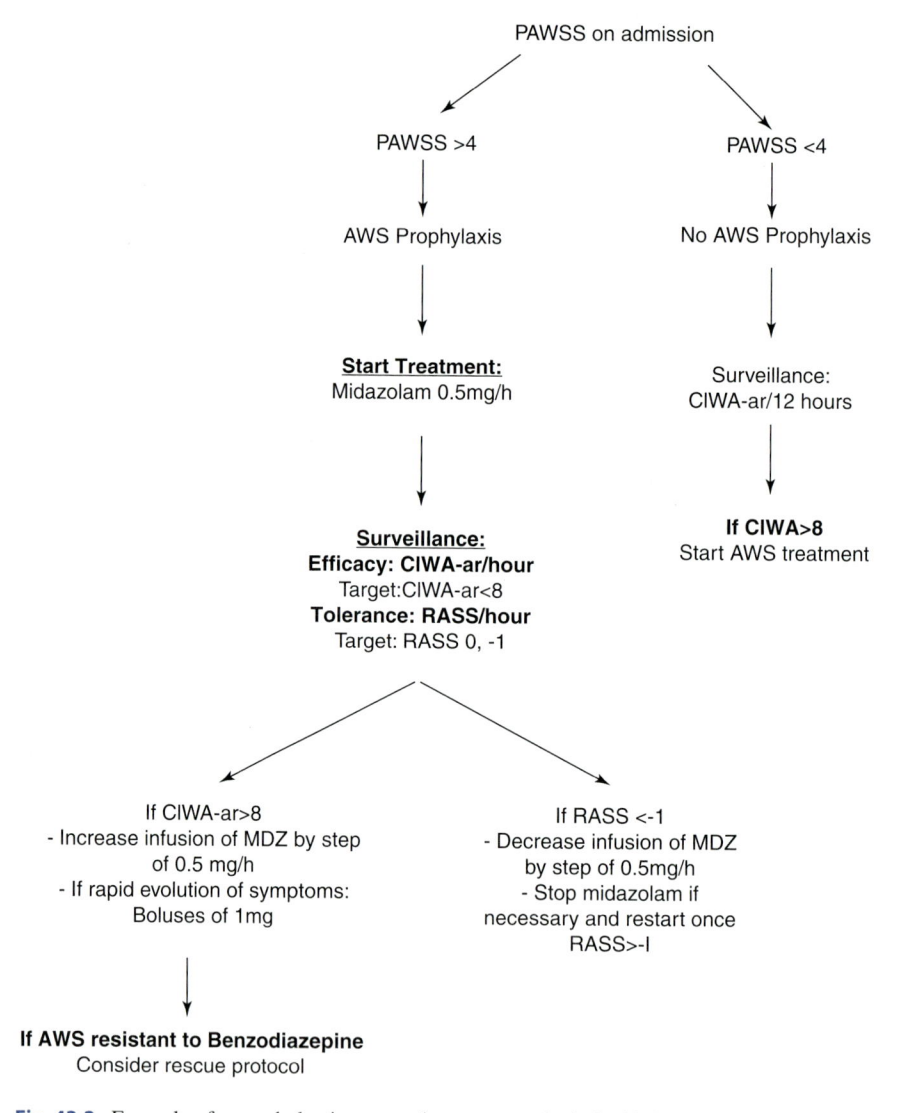

```
                        PAWSS on admission
                       ↙              ↘
              PAWSS >4                  PAWSS <4
                 ↓                         ↓
          AWS Prophylaxis            No AWS Prophylaxis
                 ↓                         ↓
          Start Treatment:             Surveillance:
          Midazolam 0.5mg/h           CIWA-ar/12 hours
                 ↓                         ↓
            Surveillance:              If CIWA>8
       Efficacy: CIWA-ar/hour       Start AWS treatment
          Target:CIWA-ar<8
         Tolerance: RASS/hour
          Target: RASS 0, -1
              ↙         ↘
    If CIWA-ar>8              If RASS <-1
- Increase infusion of MDZ     - Decrease infusion of MDZ
   by step of 0.5 mg/h           by step of 0.5mg/h
- If rapid evolution of         - Stop midazolam if
   symptoms:                    necessary and restart once
   Boluses of 1mg                     RASS>-I
         ↓
If AWS resistant to Benzodiazepine
   Consider rescue protocol
```

Fig. 43.2 Example of a prophylactic approach to prevent alcohol withdrawal syndrome (AWS). *CIWA* Clinical Institute Withdrawal Assessment, *MDZ* midazolam, *PAWSS* Prediction of Alcohol Withdrawal Severity Scale, *RASS* Richmond agitation and sedation scale Agitation-Sedation Scale

43.6 Conclusion

It is well acknowledged that alcohol use disorders represent a worldwide health burden. Therefore, alcohol use disorder is common in the medical history of hospitalized patients. On admission, patients are exposed to an acute and unplanned withdrawal which may lead to an alcohol withdrawal syndrome.

Although alcohol withdrawal syndrome is known to be an independent factor for worse short- and long-term outcomes, very little evidence is available in the literature to help the clinician.

Although treating alcohol withdrawal syndrome when clinical signs appear tends to be the current clinical practice, a prophylactic approach seems more relevant as it should decrease the impact of alcohol withdrawal syndrome on outcome and decrease hospital and ICU length of stay. Albeit this approach seems reasonable, more evidence is needed to confirm its efficacy and its safety.

References

1. World Health Organization. Management of substance abuse unit. Global status report on alcohol and health, 2014. Geneva: World Health Organization; 2014.
2. Uusaro A, Parviainen I, Tenhunen J, et al. The proportion of intensive care unit admissions related to alcohol use: a prospective cohort study. Acta Anaesthesiol Scand. 2005;49:1236–40.
3. McKenny M, O'Beirne S, Fagan C, et al. Alcohol-related admissions to an intensive care unit in Dublin. Ir J Med Sci. 2010;179:405–8.
4. Schuckit MA. Recognition and management of withdrawal delirium (delirium tremens). N Engl J Med. 2014;371:2109–13.
5. Guérin S, Laplanche A, Dunant A, et al. Alcohol-attributable mortality in France. Eur J Pub Health. 2013;23:588–93.
6. Salottolo K, McGuire E, Mains CW, et al. Occurrence, predictors, and prognosis of alcohol withdrawal syndrome and delirium tremens following traumatic injury. Crit Care Med. 2017;45:867–74.
7. American Psychiatric Association, American Psychiatric Association. Diagnostic and statistical manual of mental disorders: DSM-5. 5th ed. Washington: American Psychiatric Association; 2013.
8. Awissi DK, Lebrun G, Coursin DB, et al. Alcohol withdrawal and delirium tremens in the critically ill: a systematic review and commentary. Intensive Care Med. 2013;39:16–30.
9. Bard MR, Goettler CE, Toschlog EA, et al. Alcohol withdrawal syndrome: Turning minor injuries into a major problem. J Trauma. 2006;61:1441–5.
10. Broyles LM, Colbert AM, Tate JA, et al. Clinicians' evaluation and management of mental health, substance abuse, and chronic pain conditions in the intensive care unit. Crit Care Med. 2008;36:87–93.
11. Roberto M, Varodayan FP. Synaptic targets: Chronic alcohol actions. Neuropharmacology. 2017;122:85–99.
12. Behnke RH. Recognition and management of alcohol withdrawal syndrome. Hosp Pract. 1976;11:79–84.
13. Alcohol-use disorders: diagnosis and management of physical complications. https://www.nice.org.uk/guidance/cg100. Accessed 9 Nov 2019.
14. ASAM Commences Clinical Practice Guideline on Alcohol Withdrawal Management. https://www.asam.org/resources/publications/magazine/read/article/2017/11/01/asam-commences-clinical-practice-guideline-on-alcohol-withdrawal-management. Accessed 9 Nov 2019.

15. Société Française d'Alcoologie. Alcohol misuse: screening, diagnosis and treatment; 2015. http://www.sfalcoologie.asso.fr/. Accessed 9 Nov 2019.
16. Amato L, Minozzi S, Vecchi S, et al. Benzodiazepines for alcohol withdrawal. Cochrane Database Syst Rev. 2010;2010:CD005063.
17. de Wit M, Jones DG, Sessler CN, et al. Alcohol-use disorders in the critically ill patient. Chest. 2010;138:994–1003.
18. de Wit M, Best AM, Gennings C, et al. Alcohol use disorders increase the risk for mechanical ventilation in medical patients. Alcohol Clin Exp Res. 2007;31:1224–30.
19. O'Brien JM, Lu B. Ali NA at al. Alcohol dependence is independently associated with sepsis, septic shock, and hospital mortality among adult intensive care unit patients. Crit Care Med. 2007;35:345–50.
20. Weinberg JA, Magnotti LJ, Fischer PE, et al. Comparison of intravenous ethanol versus diazepam for alcohol withdrawal prophylaxis in the trauma ICU: results of a randomized trial. J Trauma. 2008;64:99–104.
21. Mayo-Smith MF. Pharmacological management of alcohol withdrawal. A meta-analysis and evidence-based practice guideline. American Society of Addiction Medicine Working Group on Pharmacological Management of Alcohol Withdrawal. JAMA. 1997;278:144–51.
22. Adinoff B. Double-blind study of alprazolam, diazepam, clonidine, and placebo in the alcohol withdrawal syndrome: preliminary findings. Alcohol Clin Exp Res. 1994;18:873–8.
23. Brotherton AL, Hamilton EP, Kloss HG, et al. Propofol for treatment of refractory alcohol withdrawal syndrome: a review of the literature. Pharmacotherapy. 2016;36:433–42.
24. Mueller SW, Preslaski CR, Kiser TH, et al. A randomized, double-blind, placebo-controlled dose range study of dexmedetomidine as adjunctive therapy for alcohol withdrawal. Crit Care Med. 2014;42:1131–9.
25. Bielka K, Kuchyn I, Glumcher F. Addition of dexmedetomidine to benzodiazepines for patients with alcohol withdrawal syndrome in the intensive care unit: a randomized controlled study. Ann Intensive Care. 2015;5:33.
26. DeCarolis DD, Rice KL, Ho L, et al. Symptom-driven lorazepam protocol for treatment of severe alcohol withdrawal delirium in the intensive care unit. Pharmacotherapy. 2007;27:510–8.
27. Sullivan JT, Sykora K, Schneiderman J, et al. Assessment of alcohol withdrawal: the revised clinical institute withdrawal assessment for alcohol scale (CIWA-Ar). Br J Addict. 1989;84:1353–7.
28. Sessler CN, Gosnell MS, Grap MJ, et al. The Richmond agitation-sedation scale: validity and reliability in adult intensive care unit patients. Am J Respir Crit Care Med. 2002;166:1338–44.
29. Riker RR, Picard JT, Fraser GL. Prospective evaluation of the Sedation-Agitation Scale for adult critically ill patients. Crit Care Med. 1999;27:1325–9.
30. Wong A, Benedict NJ, Kane-Gill SL. Multicenter evaluation of pharmacologic management and outcomes associated with severe resistant alcohol withdrawal. J Crit Care. 2015;30:405–9.
31. Wood E, Albarqouni L, Tkachuk S, et al. Will this hospitalized patient develop severe alcohol withdrawal syndrome? The Rational Clinical Examination Systematic Review. JAMA. 2018;320:825–33.
32. Maldonado JR, Sher Y, Das S, et al. Prospective validation study of the Prediction of Alcohol Withdrawal Severity Scale (PAWSS) in medically ill inpatients: a new scale for the prediction of complicated alcohol withdrawal syndrome. Alcohol Alcohol. 2015;50:509–18.

Part XV

Prolonged Critical Illness

Muscle Dysfunction in Critically Ill Children

44

T. Schepens and H. Mtaweh

44.1 Introduction

Increasing numbers of children require admission to a pediatric intensive care unit (PICU) annually, including more admissions for children with complex health conditions [1]. With the decline in mortality, ICU morbidities have increased; among them two entities that involve muscle weakness: ICU-acquired weakness and critical illness-associated diaphragm weakness [2, 3]. Evidence on the incidence of muscle weakness in children admitted to the PICU is limited, and the effect of muscle weakness on mortality and long-term functional outcome is not well defined. A total of 10–36% of children can experience functional impairment after an episode of critical illness, persisting in 10–13% of survivors 2 years after discharge [4, 5]. Children often exit the ICU with functional impairment, occurring in 47% of those with normal baseline [6].

Recent studies have started to focus on the precise elements that define these entities, and the association between muscle weakness and worse ICU outcome has started to emerge. Diaphragm weakness strongly impacts the potential to liberate adults from mechanical ventilation [7], and recent evidence shows that this entity exists in mechanically ventilated children as well [8, 9].

In this chapter, we will discuss the various types of muscle dysfunction in critically ill children, with a specific focus on recent evidence of diaphragm dysfunction.

T. Schepens (✉)
Department of Critical Care Medicine, Antwerp University Hospital, Edegem, Belgium
e-mail: tom.schepens@uza.be

H. Mtaweh
Department of Critical Care Medicine, Hospital for Sick Children, Toronto, ON, Canada

44.2 Incidence and Risk Factors

ICU-acquired weakness is caused by different pathologies, including critical illness polyneuromyopathy [10]. Compared to the available evidence in adult patients with critical illness, the data regarding muscle weakness in children is limited. One of the first prospective trials that reported an incidence of pediatric ICU-acquired weakness was by Banwell and colleagues, documenting confirmed pediatric ICU-acquired weakness in 1.7% (2–30) of all admitted patients [11]. A recent study by Choong and colleagues showed an incidence of 6.7% with confirmed diagnoses but reports that the incidence was closer to 30% when accounting for "suspected" cases as well, stating the challenges of confirming this diagnosis by electrophysiologic testing and muscle biopsies in children [12]. Still, both these incidences are much lower than what is usually reported in the adult ICU [13].

Multiple factors could explain this difference. First, the detection of muscle weakness in critically ill children is more difficult. The Medical Research Council (MRC) scale grades muscle strength and is the gold standard in adults but has proven to be difficult to use in a pediatric setting [14]. Second, the lack of awareness of this entity results in poor screening strategies. A recent retrospective study of a PICU database crossing 107 institutions found that critical illness neuropathy and myopathy were reported only in 55 patients for a total of over 200,000 PICU admissions, resulting in an incidence of 0.02% [15]. This level of under-reporting reflects the low level of suspicion and poor recognition of pediatric ICU-acquired weakness. It is reasonable to think that pediatric ICU-acquired weakness is an underestimated problem with highly underreported incidences.

Children admitted to an ICU often encounter very similar disease processes and ICU-related elements that are known to result in muscle wasting and weakness in adults. These risk factors include sepsis, shock and multiple organ dysfunction, acute lung injury and mechanical ventilation, and endocrine disruption [16]. The limited data that are currently available about pediatric ICU-acquired weakness suggests that the risk factors are similar for children and adults: in a small cohort of patients where critical illness myopathy was diagnosed, the risk factors that were defined included lower age, a primary diagnosis of respiratory and infectious pathology, mechanical ventilation, renal replacement therapy (RRT), and extracorporeal life support [15].

Reported incidences of muscle atrophy in a PICU are much higher than those of ICU-acquired weakness; a recent ultrasound study by Valla and colleagues showed a median decrease in quadriceps thickness of 13% during the stay in a PICU, with interquartile ranges of 9–25% [17]. More importantly, the authors demonstrated atrophy (defined as >10% decrease in thickness) in 59% of all studied patients within 5 days of mechanical ventilation.

44.3 Impact of Muscle Dysfunction on Outcome

Increasing numbers of children are admitted to PICUs with underlying chronic health conditions. Even though no good data exist about muscle weakness on ICU admission, a large number of patients have an abnormal baseline physical status [1], including generalized muscle weakness.

As mentioned, muscle atrophy is much more frequently reported than pediatric ICU-acquired weakness. This is an important observation, as decreased (baseline) muscle thickness is associated with worse outcome in a PICU population [18], and some evidence shows that muscle atrophy during ICU stay is associated with worse outcome in children as well [15].

The effect of muscle atrophy on long-term functional outcome is not well studied in the pediatric population. In adults, ICU-acquired weakness is directly associated with worse functional capacity and quality of life [19]. Some case series have described persistent electromyographic (EMG) findings indicative of chronic partial denervation in children 1 year after ICU discharge [20].

Transient physical impairment is of no major concern if children recover from it after the ICU stay, whereas prolonged impairment impacts both the patient and the family. The scarce evidence that exists in children shows that, when compared to age-matched controls, children with congenital heart disease who reach adulthood have impaired skeletal and respiratory muscle strength, potentially implying long-lasting ICU-related effects [21]. In a large post-ICU follow-up study, 38% of ICU survivors had symptoms of fatigue 5 months after ICU discharge [22]. After traumatic brain injury (TBI), this number is even higher, with incidences reported up to 47% [23]. Although this is obviously multifactorial, muscle weakness presumably is involved as well.

44.4 Diagnostic Techniques

The MRC score is the gold standard in awake and cooperative patients. It includes formal testing of three muscle groups in each limb on a scale of 1–5, thus with a maximal score of 60. Critical illness polyneuropathy/critical illness myopathy is diagnosed if the score is less than 48, or an average score of less than four across all muscles [24].

In a study evaluating its feasibility as a screening tool, Siu and coworkers were able to successfully conduct the MRC in 43% of attempts [14]. Uncooperative patients (usually as a result of sedation), lack of cognitive ability, or baseline neurological deficits were among the most frequent reasons for MRC exam failure. This limits the MRC score to be used in a select group of alert and cooperative children where maximal volatile contractions can be elicited, excluding the patients at highest risk for pediatric ICU-acquired weakness.

Electrophysiological studies (EMG or nerve conduction studies) are suggested as an alternative bedside method to diagnose critical illness polyneuromyopathy, but are rarely used in a pediatric setting because of the time-consuming factor or its invasiveness. Furthermore, it is unclear whether formal diagnosis of critical illness polyneuromyopathy by electrophysiological tests has an impact on outcome [24]. Of interest, when muscle weakness is only related to deconditioning, i.e., when no electrophysiologic abnormalities are seen, prognosis is generally better [25].

As the MRC scores and clinical tests frequently underestimate muscle weakness [26], and as electrophysiological studies are not frequently used, alternatives have been tested and proposed. Muscle biopsies are excellent in diagnosing myopathy and neuropathy, but their practical use outside of a research setting is limited. Bedside limb ultrasound measurements in a PICU have been shown to be reliable [27].

44.4.1 Ultrasound

Muscle ultrasound has been evaluated to diagnose critical illness polyneuromyopathy, and the change in thickness over time can be used to diagnose ICU-acquired atrophy. As muscle thinning is a marker of ICU-acquired weakness, muscle atrophy predicts muscle weakness and thus ICU-acquired weakness.

44.4.2 Echogenicity

In a recent trial in adult patients, muscle ultrasound echogenicity had a sensitivity of 82% and specificity of 57% to detect critical illness polyneuromyopathy [28]. This was a similar result to that achieved with single nerve conduction studies, and it was associated with increased ICU mortality. Abnormal echogenicity was associated with a reduced likelihood of discharge to home (9% vs. 50%), fewer ICU-free days (median 3 days vs. 16 days), and increased ICU mortality (42% vs. 12%).

44.4.3 Limb Muscle Thickness

The recommended technique to measure limb muscle thickness is with extended extremities, supinated arms, with relaxed muscles. Measuring locations are those that correspond with maximal muscle diameter. For the quadriceps femoris, which is the most commonly used muscle in this setting, this is halfway along the line from the anterior superior iliac spine to the superior aspect of the patella. When repeated measures are taken, the position of the ultrasound probe needs to be marked so that the exact same spot can be used each time. Usually, transverse images are obtained, although it has also been suggested to combine longitudinal and transverse images. The transducer must be placed perpendicularly while applying minimal pressure. The quadriceps femoris thickness is defined as the sum of the anterior thickness of the rectus femoris and vastus intermedius muscle heads.

44.5 Limb and Respiratory Muscle Weakness

Patients who are diagnosed with ICU-acquired weakness frequently have difficulty being liberated from the ventilator [24], and it has recently been shown that one of the muscles that is frequently affected during critical illness is the diaphragm. Many elements that result in limb muscle weakness also affect the diaphragm, and limb and diaphragm muscle weakness are often simultaneously present. Dres and colleagues demonstrated that (in an adult ICU), at the moment when patients were assessed for extubation readiness, 63% had diaphragm dysfunction, 34% had limb muscle weakness, and 21% had a combination of both [2]. Furthermore, diaphragm dysfunction at the moment of extubation impacts survival [7].

There are multiple intertwined factors related to critical illness, including ICU stay, pharmacological therapies, and mechanical ventilation, which are causing this weakness. The combination of all these mechanisms that result in diaphragm weakness in the ICU is now called critical illness-associated diaphragm weakness. These elements that affect diaphragm strength in the ICU have been summarized in a recent review [3]. Even though there is some overlap between critical illness-associated diaphragm weakness and critical illness polyneuromyopathy/ICU-acquired weakness, multiple differences exist, and several observations suggest that critical illness polyneuromyopathy is not the main cause of diaphragm weakness in ventilated patients. Some histological features that are typically seen in critical illness polyneuromyopathy, like the selective loss of thick filaments and patchy necrosis and regeneration, are not present in the diaphragm of ventilated patients. Moreover, whereas the effect of critical illness polyneuromyopathy on inactive limb muscles usually takes days or weeks to develop, the observed injury and weakness of diaphragm muscle occurs very early (hours to days) after initiating mechanical ventilation [29, 30]. Recently, the presence of diaphragm atrophy has been demonstrated in mechanically ventilated children as well. In a study by Glau et al. [31], the decrease in diaphragm thickness was about 14%, lower than the 20% which is usually seen in adults [8, 29].

44.6 Diaphragm Dysfunction

The diaphragm is the most important (inspiratory) respiratory muscle, accounting for about 70% of respiratory activity in adults. In young children, the diaphragm is even more important, as their accessory respiratory muscle strength is limited. Shortening of diaphragm muscle fibers results in a piston-like action, drawing the lungs downwards. The diaphragm has a great level of adaptation to physiologic needs, with increasing caudal displacement during exercise. Expiration is normally a passive motion, but active expiration is possible by the contraction of abdominal muscles, frequently seen in children when the load on the respiratory system is increased, and when expiratory airflow is limited (e.g., during asthma exacerbations).

44.6.1 Dysfunction Pre-ICU

Even before the effect of ICU stay has become apparent, patients who are admitted to an adult ICU frequently exhibit diaphragm dysfunction [32]. Many factors that are present before ICU admission and the start of mechanical ventilation (e.g., sepsis) impact muscle function, including the diaphragm. Little is known about diaphragm dysfunction before ICU admission in children, although the time from onset of illness to admission is usually shorter compared to adults, so diaphragm dysfunction on PICU admission may be less present.

44.6.2 Mechanical Ventilation and the Diaphragm

It is now well established that mechanical ventilation itself results in structural injury, atrophy, and weakness of the diaphragm of critically ill adult and pediatric patients [33]. In fact, the first report of diaphragm atrophy after long-term ventilatory support in humans was in infants and neonates [34]. Mechanical ventilation results in diaphragm injury through a variety of mechanisms referred to as myotrauma [33]. Recent evidence suggests that four separate forms of myotrauma may occur. These include ventilator over-assistance, ventilator under-assistance, eccentric (pliometric) diaphragm contractions, and excessive end-expiratory shortening.

The mechanism that is arguably best documented is that the lack of muscle activity results in diaphragm atrophy, called over-assist myotrauma. Around 50% of mechanically ventilated children experience diaphragm atrophy [31], similar to what is seen in adults. Furthermore, this hypothesis is supported by the fact that both in adults and in children a certain degree of diaphragm activity during mechanical ventilation has the potential to attenuate atrophy and dysfunction [31].

Second, under-assistance myotrauma develops when insufficient unloading results in excessive respiratory effort. Experimental and clinical studies have demonstrated sarcomere disruption, tissue inflammation, and muscle fatigue during resistive loading [35]. Sepsis renders the diaphragm muscle tissue particularly susceptible to this form of injury. This injury could reflect itself in the observed increase in thickness of the diaphragm of some ventilated patients who have increased inspiratory effort [7]. The precise effect of increased work of breathing before or after the start of mechanical ventilation in the pediatric population needs further attention.

Recent evidence suggests that appropriate (neither excessive nor absence of) diaphragm activity during mechanical ventilation has the potential to prevent diaphragmatic injury [7]. Currently, a trial aiming to prevent diaphragm injury in ventilated children by incorporating parameters of respiratory effort is being conducted (ClinicalTrials.gov Identifier: NCT03266016).

Eccentric diaphragm contractions, during the ventilator's expiratory phase and thus during muscle fiber lengthening, may also cause injury. This is called eccentric myotrauma, and in adults it is demonstrated that this can result from increased post-inspiratory diaphragm activity in the expiratory phase (expiratory braking), patient-ventilator dyssynchrony, or even excessive accessory respiratory muscle activity moving the diaphragm cranially during inspiration [36]. This mechanism of injury is of particular interest in children, as asynchrony is much more common in the PICU than in the adult ICU [37]. Interestingly, in a recent study by Johnson and colleagues, the authors discovered both atrophy and increases in thickness in a cohort of mechanically ventilated critically ill children [9], suggesting that similar mechanisms and risks for diaphragm injury are at play in PICU patients.

As a final mechanism of diaphragm injury, some evidence suggests that elevated positive end-expiratory pressure (PEEP) may cause muscle fiber "dropout," resulting in longitudinal atrophy [38]. Its existence in a pediatric setting and its clinical relevance is uncertain to date.

44.6.3 Monitoring Diaphragm Activity and Function

Several techniques are available to monitor the diaphragm, although some of them are more difficult to use in the pediatric population. Depending on the conditions under which they are measured, these techniques can quantify both function (strength) and contractile activity. The European Respiratory Society (ERS) has recently updated their guidelines on respiratory muscle testing [39]. We will briefly focus on some details specific to the pediatric population.

Esophageal (P_{es}) and transdiaphragmatic pressures (P_{di}) can be monitored in children, and low values are seen in children with myopathies.

Maximal inspiratory pressure measurements are usually possible only in cooperative children, and reference values are summarized in Table 44.1. Alternatives have been trialed in younger children, with airway pressure during crying as a potential surrogate for maximal voluntary inspiratory peak pressure of the respiratory system. In intubated children, maximal efforts can likely be elicited during an airway occlusion maneuver with a one-way valve, allowing for expiration (the Marini maneuver).

Sniff nasal inspiratory pressures (SNIP) have proven to be reliable in children of >2 years old [40], but their use in the ICU is limited, albeit technically possible. To measure maximal expiratory force, mouth whistle and cough pressures or gastric cough pressures ($P_{ga,cough}$) can be recorded [41]. Visualization of the P_{ga} on a screen is a playful way to motivate a child to generate maximal pressures.

The gold standard in monitoring diaphragm strength, P_{di} monitoring after bilateral magnetic phrenic nerve stimulation ($P_{di,tw}$), is not often used in children but can be done in a similar way. Reference values are available for neonates [42] and children [43] and are summarized in Table 44.1. As maximal pressures vary with age, we refer to the manuscript by Rafferty and colleagues for age-specific reference values [43]. Low $P_{di,tw}$ values are seen in neonates with diaphragmatic paralysis and in children with neuromuscular disorders.

The one method that has recently become increasingly popular is diaphragm ultrasound. As a noninvasive technique with excellent reproducibility, it is the technique of choice in the PICU to measure diaphragm activity by assessing thickening or downward movement during inspiration. In infants, the unilateral subcostal approach to measure downward movement can be replaced by a subxiphoid transverse view, bringing both sides simultaneously into view.

Finally, measurement of the EMG activity of the diaphragm through a neurally adjusted ventilatory assist (NAVA) catheter is straightforward in infants and children.

Table 44.1 Pressure-based monitoring tools, electrophysiological and ultrasound parameters to evaluate diaphragm and respiratory system function (strength)

	Test	Cutoff defining weakness	Refs.
Clinical parameters	MRC	Sum score <48 (cooperative children)	[24]
Pressure-derived parameters			
Respiratory system	MIP	<68 cmH$_2$O in men, <58 cmH$_2$O in women (children)	[48]
	SNIP	<80 cmH$_2$O in men, <70 cmH$_2$O in women (children)	[40]
Diaphragm	$P_{di,max}$	<80 cmH$_2$O in men, <70 cmH$_2$O in women (adults)	
	$P_{di,tw}$	<5 cmH$_2$O (infant)	[42]
	$P_{aw,tw}$	<11.5 cmH$_2$O (children)	[43]
Electrophysiology	NCS	No consensus	[24]
	EMG	No consensus	[24]
Ultrasound	TFdi,max	<20% (adults)	
	EXdi	<1 cm (adults)	
	EXdi,max	<3.6 (female)/<4.7 (male) (adults)	
	Sniff EXdi	<1.6 (female)/<1.8 (male) (adults)	

MRC Medical Research Council, *MIP* maximal inspiratory pressure, *SNIP* sniff nasal inspiratory pressure, $P_{di,max}$ maximal transdiaphragmatic pressure, $P_{di,tw}$ twitch transdiaphragmatic pressure, $P_{aw,tw}$ twitch airway pressure, *NCS* nerve conduction studies, *EMG* electromyography, *TFdi* thickening fraction of the diaphragm, *Exdi* caudal excursion of the diaphragm

44.7 Prevention of Weakness: Therapeutic Strategies

As muscle weakness in the PICU has only recently gained more attention, the number of specific preventive strategies in children are limited, and some of them based on what is known from the adult literature. Only a single study has thus far evaluated the factors that have an impact on recovery after functional impairment acquired in a PICU, demonstrating that persistent functional impairment 24 months after PICU admission was higher in children with chronic diseases.

44.7.1 Early Mobilization

Several studies have demonstrated the feasibility and effectiveness of early mobilization in critically ill adults to decrease muscle weakness, most of them through a multimodal, interdisciplinary approach. The evidence in children is much less clear, although several studies have shown that early mobilization in a PICU is feasible. Choong and colleagues were able to implement an early mobilization protocol in the first 48 h of PICU admission in 10–15% of admitted patients. In the patients that were able to receive early mobilization, ICU length of stay, delirium scores, duration of mechanical ventilation, and vasoactive drug infusions were lower [44]. Increasing activity levels within 72 h after admission, Wieczorek and colleagues did not see a change in clinical outcome parameters [45]. Two practice recommendations have been published to date, but the efficacy of early mobilization in the pediatric cohort is thus far not determined.

44.7.2 Nutritional Support

Critically ill children have an increased protein turnover with increased breakdown and synthesis. As a result, many believe that in order to have a neutral or positive protein balance, dietary protein requirements are high in the PICU [46]. However, the negative effects of higher protein loads, including uremia and acidosis, should be taken into account. A *post hoc* analysis of data from the PEPaNIC trial (early versus late parenteral nutrition in the PICU) showed that a high protein intake, but not glucose or lipids, during the acute phase (before day 4) of critical illness resulted in poorer outcome [47]. This suggests that the negative effects of a high nitrogen intake surpassed the potential benefit of protein synthesis, although this hypothesis was not confirmed by measuring nitrogen excretion in this cohort.

Nutritional demands vary during the course of critical illness, and nutritional demands can surpass double the resting energy expenditure during the recovery phase. Further evidence will need to demonstrate what amount of protein supplementation is required to optimally preserve muscle mass and function, and delineate the precise timing in an episode of critical illness when protein supplementation is beneficial or disadvantageous regarding muscle mass and function.

44.7.3 Prevention of Diaphragm Dysfunction

The mechanisms that link mechanical ventilation to diaphragm injury have been detailed previously (see earlier). Of particular interest for the clinician is that these mechanisms have the potential to be targeted by specific ventilation strategies, potentially mitigating the occurrence or severity of diaphragm myotrauma. Patients who were successfully weaned from ventilation had an amount of effort that is similar to what would correlate with diaphragm activity during normal tidal breathing during their weaning trial. Furthermore, in a recent study, respiratory morbidity (prolonged ventilation and reintubation), and also mortality, was lowest in patients whose inspiratory effort during the first 3 days of ventilation was similar to that of healthy subjects breathing at rest [7]. Even though the exact effects of increased diaphragm activity during mechanical ventilation in children need further attention, avoiding diaphragm inactivity or excessive inspiratory effort during mechanical ventilation seems a prudent lung- and diaphragm-protective approach.

44.7.4 Transcutaneous Electrical Muscle Stimulation

Transcutaneous electrical muscle stimulation (TEMS) has been tested in the adult ICU to reduce muscle atrophy in critically ill adults and in children with neuromuscular disease outside of the ICU. Although potentially promising, no trials have tested its potential to mitigate muscle dysfunction in the PICU.

44.8 Conclusion

Evidence of the impact of critical illness and ICU therapies on muscle strength in children is starting to emerge. Limb muscles and respiratory muscles are at risk of dysfunction, and muscle weakness has an impact on outcome. Novel diagnostic tools, including ultrasound, have improved and attracted more attention and can easily be used at the bedside. Several strategies have been proposed to mitigate weakness, including preserving muscle activity and nutrition optimization. Monitoring muscle function and individualization of therapies to address muscle weakness have the potential to further improve long-term outcomes for the increasing number of PICU survivors.

References

1. Cremer R, Leclerc F, Lacroix J, Ploin D. GFRUP/RMEF chronic diseases in PICU Study Group. Children with chronic conditions in pediatric intensive care units located in predominantly French-speaking regions: Prevalence and implications on rehabilitation care need and utilization. Crit Care Med. 2009;37:1456–62.
2. Dres M, Dubé BP, Mayaux J, et al. Coexistence and impact of limb muscle and diaphragm weakness at time of liberation from mechanical ventilation in medical intensive care unit patients. Am J Respir Crit Care Med. 2017;195:57–66.
3. Dres M, Goligher EC, Heunks LMA, Brochard LJ. Critical illness-associated diaphragm weakness. Intensive Care Med. 2017;43:1441–52.
4. Butt W, Shann F, Tibballs J, et al. Long-term outcome of children after intensive care. Crit Care Med. 1990;18:961–5.
5. Taylor A, Butt W, Ciardulli M. The functional outcome and quality of life of children after admission to an intensive care unit. Intensive Care Med. 2003;29:795–800.
6. Bone MF, Feinglass JM, Goodman DM. Risk factors for acquiring functional and cognitive disabilities during admission to a PICU. Pediatr Crit Care Med. 2014;15:640–8.
7. Goligher EC, Dres M, Fan E, et al. Mechanical ventilation-induced diaphragm atrophy strongly impacts clinical outcomes. Am J Respir Crit Care Med. 2018;197:204–13.
8. Lee EP, Hsia SH, Hsiao HF, et al. Evaluation of diaphragmatic function in mechanically ventilated children: an ultrasound study. PLoS One. 2017;12:e0183560.
9. Johnson RW, Ng KWP, Dietz AR, et al. Muscle atrophy in mechanically-ventilated critically ill children. PLoS One. 2018;13:e0207720.
10. Stevens RD, Marshall SA, Cornblath DR, et al. A framework for diagnosing and classifying intensive care unit-acquired weakness. Crit Care Med. 2009;37:S299–308.
11. Banwell BL, Mildner RJ, Hassall AC, Becker LE, Vajsar J, Shemie SD. Muscle weakness in critically ill children. Neurology. 2003;61:1779–82.

12. Choong K, Al-Harbi S, Siu K, et al. Functional recovery following critical illness in children: the "wee-cover" pilot study. Pediatr Crit Care Med. 2015;16:310–8.
13. De Jonghe B, Sharshar T, Lefaucheur J-P, et al. Paresis acquired in the intensive care unit: a prospective multicenter study. JAMA. 2002;288:2859–67.
14. Siu K, Al-Harbi S, Clark H, et al. Feasibility and reliability of muscle strength testing in critically ill children. J Pediatr Intensive Care. 2015;4:218–24.
15. Field-Ridley A, Dharmar M, Steinhorn D, McDonald C, Marcin JP. ICU-acquired weakness is associated with differences in clinical outcomes in critically ill children. Pediatr Crit Care Med. 2016;17:53–7.
16. Hermans G, Van den Berghe G. Clinical review: intensive care unit acquired weakness. Crit Care. 2015;19:274.
17. Valla FV, Young DK, Rabilloud M, et al. Thigh ultrasound monitoring identifies decreases in quadriceps femoris thickness as a frequent observation in critically ill children. Pediatr Crit Care Med. 2017;18:e339–47.
18. Weijs PJM, Looijaard WGPM, Dekker IM, et al. Low skeletal muscle area is a risk factor for mortality in mechanically ventilated critically ill patients. Crit Care. 2014;18:R12–7.
19. Batt J, Santos dos CC, Cameron JI, Herridge MS. Intensive care unit-acquired weakness: clinical phenotypes and molecular mechanisms. Am J Respir Crit Care Med. 2013;187:238–46.
20. Vondracek P, Bednarik J. Clinical and electrophysiological findings and long-term outcomes in paediatric patients with critical illness polyneuromyopathy. Eur J Paediatr Neurol. 2006;10:176–81.
21. Greutmann M, Le TL, Tobler D, et al. Generalised muscle weakness in young adults with congenital heart disease. Heart. 2011;97:1164–8.
22. Als LC, Picouto MD, Hau S-M, et al. Mental and physical well-being following admission to pediatric intensive care. Pediatr Crit Care Med. 2015;16:e141–9.
23. Gagner C, Landry-Roy C, Lainé F, Beauchamp MH. Sleep-wake disturbances and fatigue after pediatric traumatic brain injury: a systematic review of the literature. J Neurotrauma. 2015;32:1539–52.
24. Fan E, Cheek F, Chlan L, et al. An Official American Thoracic Society clinical practice guideline: the diagnosis of intensive care unit–acquired weakness in adults. Am J Respir Crit Care Med. 2014;190:1437–46.
25. Hermans G, Van Mechelen H, Bruyninckx F, et al. Predictive value for weakness and 1-year mortality of screening electrophysiology tests in the ICU. Intensive Care Med. 2015;41:2138–48.
26. Berek K, Margreiter J, Willeit J, Berek A, Schmutzhard E, Mutz NJ. Polyneuropathies in critically ill patients: a prospective evaluation. Intensive Care Med. 1996;22:849–55.
27. Ng KWP, Dietz AR, Johnson R, Shoykhet M, Zaidman CM. Reliability of bedside ultrasound of limb and diaphragm muscle thickness in critically ill children. Muscle Nerve. 2019;59:88–94.
28. Kelmenson DA, Quan D, Moss M. What is the diagnostic accuracy of single nerve conduction studies and muscle ultrasound to identify critical illness polyneuromyopathy: a prospective cohort study. Crit Care. 2018;22:342–9.
29. Schepens T, Verbrugghe W, Dams K, Corthouts B, Parizel PM, Jorens PG. The course of diaphragm atrophy in ventilated patients assessed with ultrasound: a longitudinal cohort study. Crit Care. 2015;19:422.
30. Puthucheary ZA, Rawal J, McPhail M, et al. Acute skeletal muscle wasting in critical illness. JAMA. 2013;310:1591–600.
31. Glau CL, Conlon TW, Himebauch AS, et al. Progressive diaphragm atrophy in pediatric acute respiratory failure. Pediatr Crit Care Med. 2018;19:406–11.
32. Demoule A, Jung B, Prodanovic H, et al. Diaphragm dysfunction on admission to icu: prevalence, risk factors and prognostic impact—a prospective study. Am J Respir Crit Care Med. 2013;188:213–9.
33. Goligher EC, Brochard LJ, Reid WD, et al. Diaphragmatic myotrauma: a mediator of prolonged ventilation and poor patient outcomes in acute respiratory failure. Lancet Respir Med. 2019;7:90–8.

34. Knisely AS, Leal SM, Singer DB. Abnormalities of diaphragmatic muscle in neonates with ventilated lungs. J Pediatr. 1988;113:1074–7.
35. Reid WD, Huang J, Bryson S, Walker DC, Belcastro AN. Diaphragm injury and myofibrillar structure induced by resistive loading. J Appl Physiol. 1994;76:176–84.
36. Tobin MJ, Perez W, Guenther SM, Lodato RF, Dantzker DR. Does rib cage-abdominal paradox signify respiratory muscle fatigue? J Appl Physiol. 1987;63:851–60.
37. Mortamet G, Larouche A, Ducharme-Crevier L, et al. Patient-ventilator asynchrony during conventional mechanical ventilation in children. Ann Intensive Care. 2017;7:122.
38. Lindqvist J, van den Berg M, van der Pijl R, et al. Positive end-expiratory pressure ventilation induces longitudinal atrophy in diaphragm fibers. Am J Respir Crit Care Med. 2018;198:472–85.
39. Laveneziana P, Albuquerque A, Aliverti A, et al. ERS statement on respiratory muscle testing at rest and during exercise. Eur Respir J. 2019;53:1801214.
40. Stefanutti D, Fitting JW. Sniff nasal inspiratory pressure. Reference values in Caucasian children. Am J Respir Crit Care Med. 1999;159:107–11.
41. Aloui S, Khirani S, Ramirez A, et al. Whistle and cough pressures in children with neuromuscular disorders. Respir Med. 2016;113:28–36.
42. Rafferty GF, Greenough A, Dimitriou G, et al. Assessment of neonatal diaphragm function using magnetic stimulation of the phrenic nerves. Am J Respir Crit Care Med. 2000;162:2337–40.
43. Rafferty GF, Greenough A, Manczur T, et al. Magnetic phrenic nerve stimulation to assess diaphragm function in children following liver transplantation. Pediatr Crit Care Med. 2001;2:122–6.
44. Choong K, Foster G, Fraser DD, et al. Acute rehabilitation practices in critically ill children: a multicenter study. Pediatr Crit Care Med. 2014;15:e270–9.
45. Wieczorek B, Ascenzi J, Kim Y, et al. PICU Up!: Impact of a quality improvement intervention to promote early mobilization in critically ill children. Pediatr Crit Care Med. 2016;17:e559–66.
46. Coss-Bu JA, Hamilton-Reeves J, Patel JJ, Morris CR, Hurt RT. Protein requirements of the critically ill pediatric patient. Nutr Clin Pract. 2017;32:128S–41S.
47. Vanhorebeek I, Verbruggen S, Casaer MP, et al. Effect of early supplemental parenteral nutrition in the paediatric ICU: a preplanned observational study of post-randomisation treatments in the PEPaNIC trial. Lancet Respir Med. 2017;5:475–83.
48. Heinzmann-Filho JP, Vasconcellos Vidal PC, Jones MH, Donadio MVF. Normal values for respiratory muscle strength in healthy preschoolers and school children. Respir Med. 2012;106:1639–46.

Respiratory Muscle Rehabilitation in Patients with Prolonged Mechanical Ventilation: A Targeted Approach

B. Bissett, R. Gosselink, and F. M. P. van Haren

45.1 Introduction

Early and proactive rehabilitation of intensive care unit (ICU) patients is essential to reverse or minimize the impact of ICU-acquired weakness [1]. While ICU clinicians have largely focused on whole-body exercise to address limb muscle weakness (e.g., early mobilization), we now know that respiratory muscle weakness is twice as prevalent as limb muscle weakness in ICU patients [2]. Moreover, respiratory muscle weakness is associated with a higher risk of extubation failure [3], a longer duration of ventilator-dependence [4] and worse outcomes in terms of hospital mortality [2] and mortality within 1 year [3]. While ventilator-weaning failure is complex, and respiratory muscle weakness is only one contributing factor [5], this weakness is modifiable and can respond to targeted training. In this context, it is surprising that respiratory muscle rehabilitation is not yet standard practice in many ICUs around the world.

Drawing on recent and emerging evidence, we will give an overview of the impact of respiratory muscle weakness in ICU patients (both at the physiological and patient level), and summarize the current evidence regarding the effects of respiratory muscle training. We will also outline strategies for identifying respiratory muscle weakness in ICU patients, as well as an evidence-based and pragmatic approach to providing targeted and individualized respiratory muscle rehabilitation in the ICU. Finally, we will describe the newest technological

---

B. Bissett
Discipline of Physiotherapy, University of Canberra, Bruce, ACT, Australia

R. Gosselink
Department of Rehabilitation Sciences, KU Leuven, Health Science Campus Gasthuisberg O&N IV, Leuven, Belgium

F. M. P. van Haren (✉)
Intensive Care Unit, Canberra Hospital, Garran, ACT, Australia

Australian National University Medical School, Canberra, Australia
e-mail: Frank.Vanharen@act.gov.au

developments that have radically changed the scope of respiratory muscle rehabilitation for even our most profoundly weak ICU patients.

45.2 Respiratory Muscle Weakness in ICU Patients: A Call to Action

There is now compelling evidence that respiratory muscle weakness is a highly likely consequence of prolonged mechanical ventilation. Diaphragm proteolysis is detectable within 18–69 h of controlled mechanical ventilation [6], and rapid atrophy affects respiratory muscles more frequently than limb muscles. Following at least 24 h of mechanical ventilation, respiratory muscle weakness is almost twice as prevalent as limb muscle weakness (63% vs. 34%) [2]. Even patients ventilated primarily with pressure support modes are not immune to these atrophic changes, but they are likely to have respiratory muscle weakness at the point of weaning from mechanical ventilation (e.g., 38% of predicted maximal inspiratory pressure) [7]. While "under-assistance" has been identified as a potential contributor to myotrauma [8], respiratory muscle weakness could be potentially attributable to "over-assistance" from the ventilator in pressure support mode: a recent prospective study of 231 patients in Australian ICUs identified excessive support provided in 41% of patients in pressure support mode [9]. Therefore, inspiratory muscle weakness appears to be a likely consequence of mechanical ventilation, regardless of the mode of ventilation provided.

Far from being merely an inconvenient side effect of mechanical ventilation, respiratory muscle weakness can directly affect a patient's ventilation and ICU outcomes. Recent ultrasound studies of diaphragm thickness (a surrogate measure of inspiratory muscle strength) revealed that by day 4 of mechanical ventilation, reduced diaphragm thickness could be detected in 41% of patients [4, 10]. Reduced diaphragm thickness is associated with reduced likelihood of weaning from mechanical ventilation, higher likelihood of complications, and prolonged ICU admission [4]. Furthermore, low inspiratory muscle strength (maximal inspiratory pressure ≤ 30 cmH$_2$O) at the point of extubation is associated with extubation failure, and is independently associated with 1-year mortality (hazard ratio 4.41, 95% CI 1.5–12.9) [3]. Inspiratory muscle weakness is also associated with higher ICU and hospital mortality [2]. Thus, from an ICU clinician's perspective, inspiratory muscle weakness must be considered as a potentially treatable and reversible component in the matter of life and death.

From a patient perspective, respiratory muscle weakness typically renders patients breathless at rest, let alone during exercise [7]. Yet while ICU physiotherapists now invest considerable energy in providing early mobilization therapy to offset the impact of ICU-acquired weakness [11, 12], the respiratory muscles are frequently neglected in the rehabilitation approach [13]. Clearly respiratory muscle atrophy is an important aspect of ICU-acquired weakness, and we can no longer afford to ignore respiratory muscle rehabilitation as part of holistic recovery for ICU survivors. Identification of respiratory muscle weakness, and early commencement of targeted training, requires effective collaboration of the whole ICU multidisciplinary team, but in particular a cohesive approach between medical, nursing, and physiotherapy staff [14].

45.3 Identifying Respiratory Muscle Weakness in ICU Patients

While researchers have used sophisticated and sometimes invasive methods to study respiratory muscle weakness in ICU patients (e.g., muscle biopsies and nerve stimulation), simple bedside measures of respiratory muscle strength do not have to be complex or invasive. For ventilator-dependent patients, features within the ventilator software can be used to obtain an approximation of maximal inspiratory pressure (e.g., "negative inspiratory force"). In this procedure, the ICU clinician coaches the patient to inhale forcefully against a "closed gate" within the system, with the resultant pressure an indication of inspiratory muscle strength. In our experience it is essential that the patient is warned that they will experience no flow of air during the attempt. While this is not a true measure of maximal inspiratory pressure, as it is not performed from residual volume (due to the presence of positive end-expiratory pressure [PEEP]), a low "negative inspiratory force" score can flag a patient for whom inspiratory muscle weakness should be suspected. Based on both our clinical experience and the data available [3], scores <30 cmH_2O should be cause for concern.

An alternative method of inspiratory muscle strength assessment in ICU patients is the Marini method [15] where the patient exhales for 25 s through a one-way valve to reach true residual volume before maximal inhalation. This approach has been described as a strategy to obtain maximal inspiratory pressure values in ICU patients who are not responsive or cooperative [16]. However, this method has questionable inter-rater reliability in ICU patients [17], and in our clinical practice this procedure can be prohibitively stressful for patients who are conscious.

Instead, we use either the method described above (i.e., ventilator-based assessment) or a handheld manometer (Fig. 45.1). In this latter approach, the patient is briefly disconnected from the ventilator, instructed to "empty their lungs", and the manometer is attached to the endotracheal or tracheostomy tube via a connector. The patient then inhales maximally and the best of three attempts are recorded [18]. While maximal inspiratory pressure scores have not been found to reliably predict weaning failure [18], our experience has been that scores <30 cmH_2O may indicate a degree of inspiratory muscle weakness which could impact on weaning and

Fig. 45.1 Handheld respiratory pressure manometer connected to endotracheal tube for measurement of maximal inspiratory pressure (Reproduced from [14] with permission)

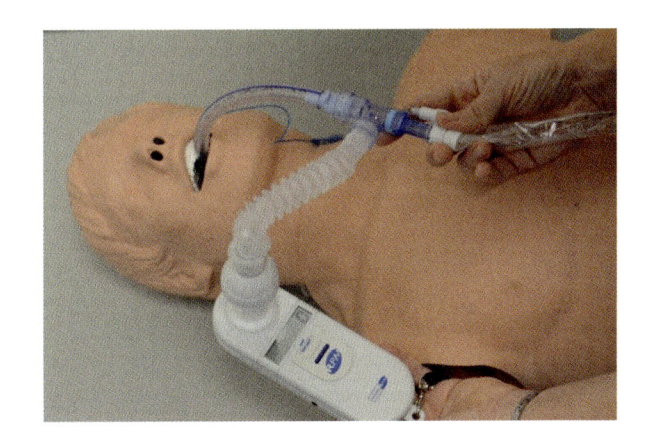

> **Box 45.1: Calculating Normal Values of Respiratory Muscle Strength** [19]
>
> Male MIP = 120 − (0.41 × age), and male MIP LLN = 62 − (0.15 × age)
> Male MEP = 174 − (0.83 × age), male MEP LLN = 117 − (0.83 × age)
> Female MIP = 108 − (0.61 × age), and female MIP LLN = 62 − (0.50 × age)
> Female MEP = 131 − (0.86 × age), and female MEP LLN = 95 − (0.57 × age)
>
> MIP = maximal inspiratory pressure; MEP = maximal expiratory pressure; age in years; LLN = lower limit of normal

recovery. To obtain an estimate of the patient's inspiratory muscle strength as a percentage of predicted values (that accommodate variance due to age and sex), we recommend the normalization equations provided by Evans et al. [19] (Box 45.1).

For cooperative patients recently weaned from mechanical ventilation, measurement of maximal inspiratory pressure can be feasibly done through either the mouth or a tracheostomy using a handheld manometer [14]. However, even if ICU clinicians do not have access to this device, lack of measurement does not preclude appropriate therapy. Any patient who has recently weaned from invasive mechanical ventilation of more than 7 days duration should be regarded as at high-risk of inspiratory muscle weakness [7], and proactive targeted therapy should commence as soon as possible. This therapy is specific respiratory muscle training.

45.4 Specific Respiratory Muscle Training: Can It Make a Difference to ICU Patients?

The availability and quality of evidence regarding inspiratory and expiratory muscle training in ICU patients differs, and we will address each in turn.

There is now convincing evidence that specific inspiratory muscle training can increase inspiratory muscle strength in ventilator-dependent ICU patients, measured as changes in maximal inspiratory pressure. Three systematic reviews and meta-analyses [20–22] have revealed that inspiratory muscle training results in higher maximal inspiratory pressure scores compared to usual care (e.g., 15 studies; pooled mean difference, 6 cmH_2O; 95% CI, 5–8 cm [22]). A study of inspiratory muscle training in ICU patients recently weaned from mechanical ventilation [23] similarly showed significant improvements in maximal inspiratory pressure in the training group compared to the control (mean difference 11% of predicted values). Clearly, we can strengthen inspiratory muscles in ICU patients at various points in their recovery journey.

However, improvements in strength measures alone are unlikely to drive practice change. Far more relevant are the changes in patient-centered outcomes that have accompanied strength improvements in numerous studies. These include reduced duration of weaning from ventilation (five trials; pooled mean difference, 3.2 days; 95% CI 0.6–5.8 days [22]); increased likelihood of liberation from the ventilator within 28 days (71% vs. 47%) [24]; and improved quality of life [23]. While most studies have not been powered for these important outcomes, or have not measured patient-centered outcomes such as quality of life or dyspnea, these promising results indicate that the benefits of inspiratory muscle training extend beyond strength alone.

The evidence regarding the impact of expiratory muscle training in ICU patients is currently more limited. Indeed, the expiratory muscles have been described as the "neglected component" of the respiratory system in a recent comprehensive review that describes expiratory muscle physiology in ICU patients [25]. In the most recent systematic review of respiratory muscle training in ICU patients [22], four studies of expiratory muscle training (comprising 153 participants) were meta-analyzed, revealing a mean difference of 9 cmH_2O (95% CI 5–14) in favor of the training group relative to control. However, the effect of expiratory muscle training on patient outcomes requires further exploration in an ICU context. In this light, the remainder of this chapter will focus on the implementation of inspiratory muscle training in ICU patients.

45.5 Current Practice: Inspiratory Muscle Training in the ICU—Not All Approaches Are Equal

While we have been using inspiratory muscle training in our ICU for the past 15 years [14], we are aware that such training is a relatively new approach for many ICU clinicians. Moreover, where inspiratory muscle training is being used around the world, a wide variety of approaches is being employed, and not all of these are evidence-based. For example, a survey of French physiotherapists revealed that 83% considered controlled diaphragmatic breathing (without resistance) to be a form of inspiratory muscle training, and only 16% measured inspiratory muscle strength [26]. More recently, a meta-analysis of 28 studies of inspiratory muscle training in ICU patients described a broad range of training strategies, including strength-based and endurance-based loading (through a removable threshold device or through manipulating ventilator settings), and also more general strategies such as upper limb exercises, mobility training, and biofeedback [22]. However, to understand the strengths and limitations of the different approaches, it is essential to appreciate the importance of titratable loading with regard to muscle training.

In respiratory muscle training, "resistive loading" usually refers to patients breathing through a small aperture connector to provide a training load. A limitation of this resistive loading is that the amount of resistance (and therefore load) depends on the flow rate generated by the patient. If the patient breathes slowly enough, the load can be very low or negligible. In contrast, "threshold loading," typically using a removable device, requires patients to generate a specific resistance as they initiate a breath to open the valve and generate flow. An important advantage of this threshold loading is that a specific, reliable, and reproducible load can be titrated and applied to the respiratory muscles [27], which can be increased over time to generate a training effect. As with all strength training, gradual increases over time are the key to muscle fiber proliferation and hypertrophy. If the load is unreliable or variable, then our ability to deliver an efficient and effective training regime is hampered, and our patients may waste valuable effort with suboptimal training. Thus, inspiratory muscle training strategies that use a titratable load are more likely to result in effective training.

Threshold loading in ICU patients is usually achieved in one of two ways: manipulating the ventilator settings (i.e., reducing the pressure trigger sensitivity, such that the patient has to increase their effort to trigger an augmented breath); or through a removable threshold device which is intermittently applied to the endotracheal tube or tracheostomy. While theoretically both approaches should result in reliable training, the outcomes are contrasting. Studies of ventilator manipulations have failed to show significant benefits in terms of either breathing muscle strength or weaning duration, despite applying training loads for up to 30 min at loads up to 40% of maximal inspiratory pressure [28]. In contrast, as outlined earlier, several studies of threshold loading (using removable devices) have demonstrated significant gains in inspiratory muscle strength and ventilator-weaning success rates [24, 29–31]. While these contrasting results may be challenging, there is a key feature differentiating the approaches: in the training with removable devices, patients must actively participate in their therapy and, if only for a short time, consciously tolerate breathing without the ventilator support. In addition to physiological adaptations, there may be a psychological dimension to this training (i.e., development of tolerance to the sensations of unsupported breathing) that would be absent in the ventilator-based approach. Future studies are needed to better elucidate the potential psychological dimensions of respiratory muscle training, but psychological factors may be key to the success of the therapy.

There is no evidence that coached deep breathing exercises (without resistance) make any difference to respiratory muscle strength or weaning outcomes in ICU patients. In fact, there is scarce evidence that deep breathing exercises (without resistance) confer any benefit in acutely unwell patients, for example, in the postoperative phase [32, 33]. Upper limb exercises and mobilization are important aspects of whole-body strengthening and rehabilitation and will also induce, via increased ventilation, an endurance type of training to the respiratory muscles. However, it is our view that ICU clinicians should be wary of classifying these as respiratory muscle strength training *per se*. Instead, focused and targeted respiratory muscle strengthening should be achieved using titratable resistance, individualized to the patient's current level of weakness, and followed by sufficient rest periods to allow recovery as in athletic training [34]. Based on the available evidence, an international shift toward titratable loading for respiratory muscle training in ICU patients is now overdue.

45.6 Practicalities of Inspiratory Muscle Training in ICU Patients

The most common device used to apply intermittent threshold loading in ICU patients is a simple mechanical spring-loaded one-way valve [22], where resistance can be titrated (e.g., between 9 and 41 cmH_2O). In this approach, the patient is briefly removed from the ventilator, and the inspiratory muscle trainer is connected to the endotracheal tube or tracheostomy for training (i.e., breathing through the valve). The intensity is increased over time simply by winding the spring more tightly [14]. This device has been shown to be safe for inspiratory muscle training in selected ventilator-dependent ICU patients, with a negligible rate of adverse events [35].

Typically, this training is prescribed and supervised by the ICU physiotherapist or respiratory therapist. Whether the therapist should use a "strength" (high intensity, low repetition) or "endurance" (low intensity, longer duration) approach to prescribing training parameters is still somewhat open to debate. In the recent systematic review of inspiratory muscle training in ICU patients [22], where "strength" and "endurance" regimes were analyzed separately, both favored inspiratory muscle training relative to control groups. It could be argued that as the inspiratory muscles are primarily muscles of endurance, an endurance-based approach would be sensible [36]. However, in our experience, the highly limited window of patient effort (frequently compromised by fatigue, inattention, or delirium), coupled with the relative disadvantage of potential lung decruitment during sustained training (e.g., secondary to prolonged loss of PEEP), makes strength training a more realistic option for the ICU patient. A patient may be willing to attempt six high-resistance breaths, whereas the prospect of breathing against a low resistance for several minutes can appear prohibitively daunting. From this perspective, the best respiratory muscle training approach may be the one that the ventilator-dependent patient can successfully achieve.

Indeed, there may be psychological benefits to successfully completing short bursts of achievable work. Anecdotally, our patients often report pride and excitement when they observe, for example, that last week they could only train at 17 cmH_2O, but this week they can train at 29 cmH_2O. At a time in recovery when progress of any kind can feel extraordinarily slow, recovery of inspiratory muscle strength may be tangible and therapeutic at many levels. Again, this deserves more in-depth exploration from a psychological perspective.

If we are to use a strength-focused approach to training ICU patients, we should draw on the wealth of research in inspiratory muscle training in other populations (e.g., chronic obstructive pulmonary disease [COPD] [37, 38], heart failure [39], athletes [40–43]) where intensity is crucial. Early studies in COPD patients often failed to detect benefits of inspiratory muscle training where intensity was less than 30% of maximal inspiratory pressure [44, 45]. In contrast, later systematic reviews and meta-analyses which included studies with intensities great then 30% of maximal inspiratory pressure were more favorable not just for inspiratory muscle strength but also for exercise tolerance and quality of life [37, 46]. In athletes, inspiratory muscle training intensity is typically prescribed between 50% and 80% of maximal inspiratory pressure, across endurance sports such as swimming [42], cycling [41], rowing [40], and running [43]. With high-intensity training, athletes improve not just inspiratory muscle strength but frequently exercise performance as well (e.g., 2.6% increase in 25 km cycling time trial performance [41]; 3.5% increase in 6-min rowing time trial performance [40]). In studies of inspiratory muscle training in ICU patients, high-intensity training (6 repetitions per set, >50% of maximum, 30 breaths per day) has resulted in improvements in inspiratory muscle strength [24, 30], and in the postweaning period has improved quality of life [23]. Therefore, wherever possible, a high-intensity approach to strength training should be used to optimize inspiratory muscle training in ICU patients.

Acknowledging the relative advantages of the simple mechanical threshold device (including its low cost and accessibility), we have experienced some limitations of this device in an ICU context. First, the floor effect of this spring-loaded device can be problematic for a patient who is profoundly weak (e.g., maximal inspiratory pressure <18 cmH$_2$O). If the lowest setting of the device is only 9 cmH$_2$O, patients may struggle to open the valve at its lowest setting. Second, we have also noted a ceiling effect. Toward the end of training, several of our patients have comfortably exceeded the 41 cmH$_2$O upper limit of the device and would be capable of training at much higher intensities. While for most patients this might not be necessary, for those returning to a more active lifestyle, continuing to improve their inspiratory muscle strength may be a vehicle to better tolerance of endurance exercise. To better suit the needs of our ICU patients, we require devices with a broader training spectrum.

45.7 Emerging Strategies for Inspiratory Muscle Training in ICU Patients

In the past few years there have been crucial developments in the sophistication of inspiratory muscle training devices. Electronic devices provide a much wider training spectrum (e.g., from 1 to 200 cmH$_2$O), and although they are more expensive than the disposable spring-loaded device, they have other advantages, including the capacity to measure performance within the device (e.g., maximal inspiratory pressure, tidal volume, work and energy of breathing during the training session). As a handheld, chargeable device, they are ideally suited for bedside treatment in the ICU and can be adapted to interface with either a tracheostomy or an endotracheal tube via a simple connector (Fig. 45.2).

The most important difference in the design of these devices is the incorporation of a tapered flow resistance load. The advantages of a tapered flow resistance load have been well-described in patients with COPD [47] but may also be advantageous for ICU patients. Briefly, whereas a traditional threshold load requires the patient to generate a preset pressure, beyond which they can "coast" through the rest of the breath, the tapered flow resistance load provides a tapered load beyond the threshold

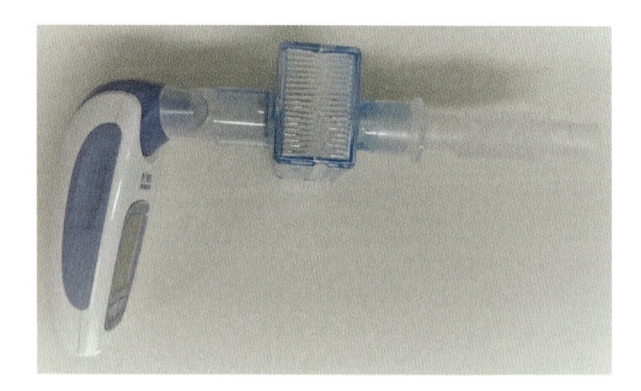

Fig. 45.2 Attachment of electronic inspiratory muscle training device to filter and connector

point, meaning that patients continue to work throughout the duration of the breath, rather than "coasting." The result is that for each breath at the specified intensity, the patient generates more work (at a guaranteed achievable resistance). Thus, the total workload (and therefore potential training effect achievable) is considerably higher with tapered flow resistance load compared to traditional threshold loading. The following graph from a study of tapered flow resistance load in a ventilator-dependent ICU patient captures this difference (Fig. 45.3).

So far, there has been one randomized trial of tapered flow resistance load inspiratory muscle training in ICU patients, where it was compared with a sham treatment of intermittent nebulization [29]. Although this was a small study, capturing 21 patients, the results were encouraging: while the sham intervention group had a

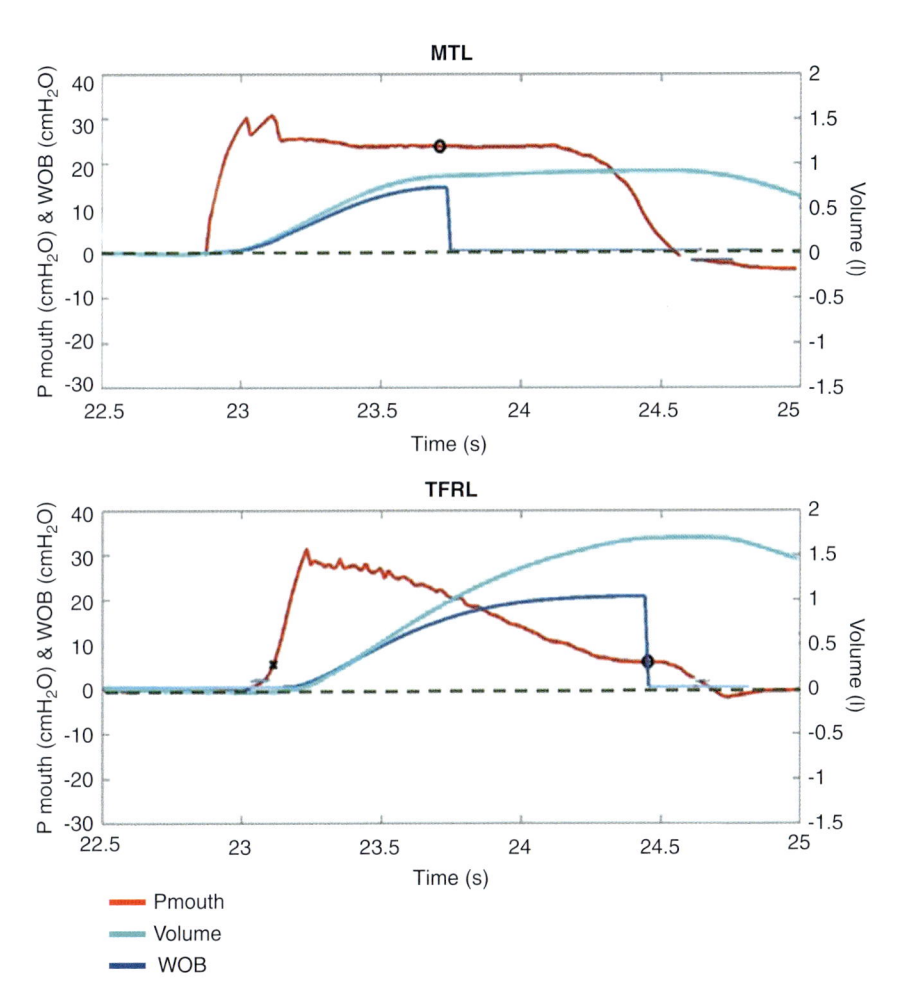

Fig. 45.3 A single respiratory cycle, comparing mechanical threshold loading (MTL) with tapered flow resistive loading (TFRL) in a ventilator-dependent patient. *Pmouth* pressure at the mouth, *WOB* work of breathing

mean ventilatory weaning time of 9.4 days, the tapered flow resistance load training group's mean weaning time was 3.5 days, and this difference was statistically significant ($p = 0.0192$) [29]. Clearly, we need more studies in different patient cohorts to confirm these findings and elucidate the optimal training approach. Another major randomized trial is underway, using tapered flow resistance load and comparing both strength and endurance approaches [48]. We await the results of this study with keen interest. Meanwhile our clinical experience of tapered flow resistance load training (Fig. 45.4) is that it is well-tolerated by ICU patients and

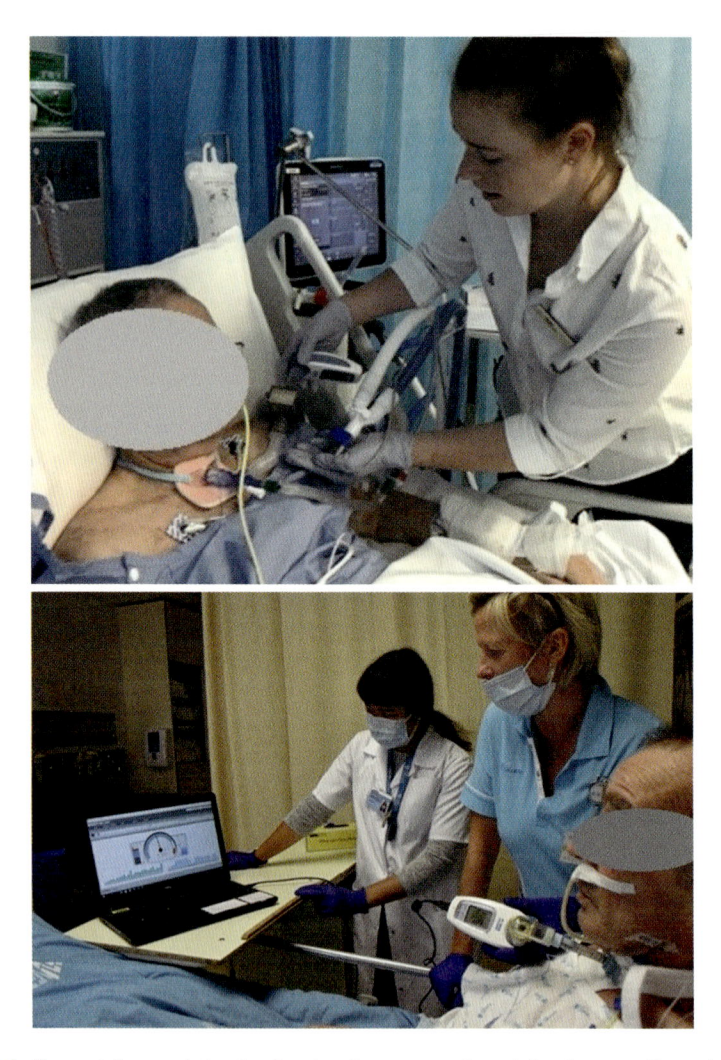

Fig. 45.4 Tapered flow resistive loading inspiratory muscle training in a ventilator-dependent patient (upper panel). Visual feedback provided during tapered flow resistive loading in a ventilator-dependent patient (lower panel)

readily captures considerably more data for analysis by the treating clinicians (including maximal inspiratory pressure, work of breathing, tidal volume).

Furthermore, this new technology can provide visual feedback of the training on a computer screen (Fig. 45.4 lower panel). This information allows better guidance of the training by the physiotherapist, while the visual feedback on the screen stimulates the patient to achieve large tidal volumes to ensure loading of the inspiratory muscles over full range of motion.

45.8 Barriers to Respiratory Muscle Rehabilitation in ICU Patients

Potential contraindications to inspiratory muscle training in ICU patients have been identified and include pre-existing neuromuscular disease, hemodynamic instability (arrhythmia, decompensated heart failure, coronary insufficiency), hemoptysis, use of any type of home mechanical ventilatory support prior to hospitalization, any skeletal pathology that impairs chest wall movements such as severe kyphoscoliosis, congenital deformities or contractures, poor general prognosis, or anticipated fatal outcome [48].

One major barrier to effective inspiratory muscle training in ICU patients is that this approach requires the patient to be awake and actively participating in their training. Patients need to be capable of understanding and tolerating an increased resistance for short periods, without being overly distressed by it. If patients are too sedated, they cannot benefit. In the landscape of reducing sedation to facilitate early rehabilitation in the ICU [1], this provides yet another imperative to minimize (or eliminate) sedation as early as possible.

In our recent practice guideline for inspiratory muscle training in ICU patients [14], we outlined criteria for suitability (Fig. 45.5) and identified patients for whom inspiratory muscle training is not appropriate, including those who require high levels of PEEP (e.g., >15 cmH$_2$O), those with high respiratory rates (e.g., >25 breaths per minute) or deteriorating respiratory or cardiovascular stability. From a purely practical perspective, inspiratory muscle training is also not feasible in patients experiencing extreme pain or dyspnea, and these will need to be addressed to facilitate effective treatment.

It is likely that some ICU patients will not be able to participate in inspiratory muscle training while ventilator-dependent, due to a combination of factors that may include sedation, delirium, or physiologic instability. Given the very high likelihood that these patients will have significant respiratory muscle weakness when they are eventually weaned from the ventilator, is there any advantage to commencing respiratory muscle training after liberation from the ventilator? The good news is that these patients can still benefit from training in the postweaning period. In a study of inspiratory muscle training in recently weaned ICU patients (invasively ventilated for 7 days or more), 70 patients were randomized to either usual care or additional daily threshold-based inspiratory muscle training [23]. Two weeks of

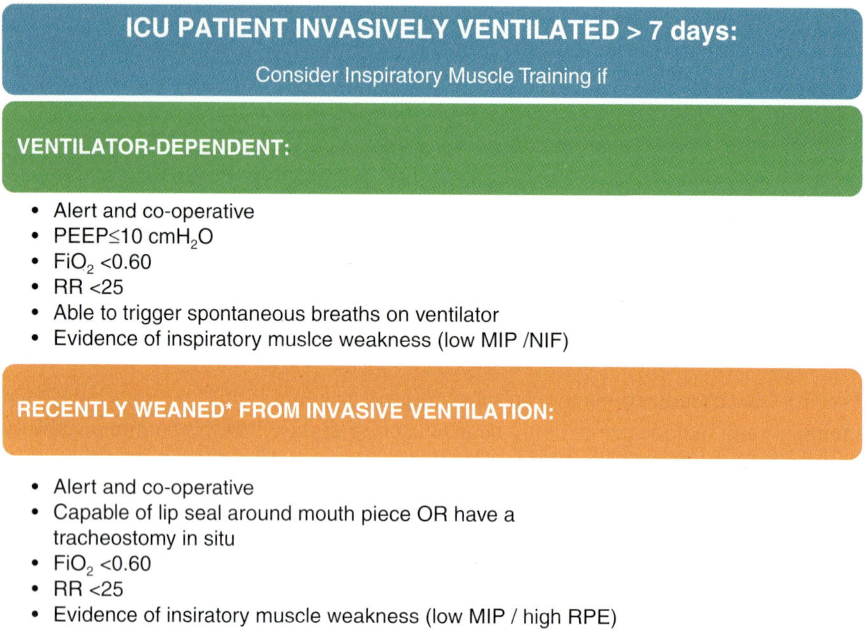

ICU PATIENT INVASIVELY VENTILATED > 7 days:
Consider Inspiratory Muscle Training if

VENTILATOR-DEPENDENT:

- Alert and co-operative
- PEEP≤10 cmH$_2$O
- FiO$_2$ <0.60
- RR <25
- Able to trigger spontaneous breaths on ventilator
- Evidence of inspiratory muslce weakness (low MIP /NIF)

RECENTLY WEANED* FROM INVASIVE VENTILATION:

- Alert and co-operative
- Capable of lip seal around mouth piece OR have a tracheostomy in situ
- FiO$_2$ <0.60
- RR <25
- Evidence of insiratory muscle weakness (low MIP / high RPE)

Fig. 45.5 Criteria for suitability for inspiratory muscle training for ICU patients. *PEEP* positive end-expiratory pressure, *FiO$_2$* fraction of inspired oxygen, *RR* respiratory rate, *MIP* maximum inspiratory pressure, *NIF* negative inspiratory force (measured on the ventilator). *Recently weaned means independently breathing 24 hours per day without any invasive ventilatory support. (Reproduced from [14] with permission)

daily training improved inspiratory muscle strength (maximal inspiratory pressure) as well as quality of life. Patients were most likely to benefit if they had at least moderate inspiratory muscle strength (28 cmH$_2$O or more) [49]. Therefore, a targeted approach to inspiratory muscle training in recently weaned ICU patients appears to be a worthwhile investment.

45.9 Future Directions for Respiratory Muscle Rehabilitation in ICU Patients

While inspiratory muscle training is effective in strengthening inspiratory muscles and accelerating ventilator weaning in ICU patients, we are yet to elucidate the optimal training parameters. Current and future studies will guide clinicians regarding the relative value of strength or endurance approaches to training, but in the short term it appears that strength training (high-intensity low repetition loading) is feasible and effective, both for ventilator-dependent patients and in the postweaning phase of recovery. While mechanical threshold loading can be effective in patients with moderate inspiratory muscle weakness, electronic inspiratory training may be better suited to profoundly weak ICU patients.

Although this chapter has focused on the physical and physiological aspects of respiratory muscle rehabilitation, future research needs to also consider the contribution of psychological factors to ventilatory weaning and rehabilitation. As has been described most eloquently with respect to patients with COPD, dyspnea is best understood as a complex and individual phenomenon, highly modified by emotional, cognitive, and contextual factors [50]. In an ICU environment, these factors could include fear and anxiety, as well as cognitive challenges around attention, catastrophizing, and perceived lack of control. A better understanding of the psychological dimension of dyspnea in ICU patients could further inform our approach to optimized ventilatory weaning and respiratory muscle rehabilitation. We hope that future studies of ICU patients will incorporate these patient-centered perspectives and shape our understanding of how best to facilitate holistic recovery.

45.10 Conclusion

Early and proactive rehabilitation of the respiratory muscles is feasible and effective in ICU patients. As respiratory muscle weakness clearly affects outcomes within and beyond the ICU, the multidisciplinary team should implement targeted and individualized training of respiratory muscles to optimize patient recovery. Inspiratory muscle training can facilitate ventilator liberation, while potentially improving patients' quality of life. Given the return on investment of this relatively low-cost therapy, respiratory muscle rehabilitation should be considered a priority in the modern approach to the management of ICU-acquired weakness.

References

1. Hodgson CL, Capell E, Tipping CJ. Early mobilization of patients in intensive care: organization, communication and safety factors that influence translation into clinical practice. Crit Care. 2018;22:77.
2. Dres M, Dube BP, Mayaux J, Delemazure J, Reuter D, Brochard L, et al. Coexistence and impact of limb muscle and diaphragm weakness at time of liberation from mechanical ventilation in medical intensive care unit patients. Am J Respir Crit Care Med. 2017;195:57–66.
3. Medrinal C, Prieur G, Frenoy E, et al. Respiratory weakness after mechanical ventilation is associated with one-year mortality - a prospective study. Crit Care. 2016;20:231.
4. Goligher EC, Dres M, Fan E, et al. Mechanical ventilation-induced diaphragm atrophy strongly impacts clinical outcomes. Am J Respir Crit Care Med. 2018;197:204–13.
5. Doorduin J, van der Hoeven JG, Heunks LM. The differential diagnosis for failure to wean from mechanical ventilation. Curr Opin Anaesthesiol. 2016;29:150–7.
6. Levine S, Nguyen T, Taylor N, et al. Rapid disuse atrophy of diaphragm fibers in mechanically ventilated humans. N Engl J Med. 2008;358:1327–35.
7. Bissett B, Leditschke IA, Neeman T, Boots R, Paratz J. Weaned but weary: one third of adult intensive care patients mechanically ventilated for 7 days or more have impaired inspiratory muscle endurance after successful weaning. Heart Lung. 2015;44:15–20.
8. Goligher EC, Brochard LJ, Reid WD, et al. Diaphragmatic myotrauma: a mediator of prolonged ventilation and poor patient outcomes in acute respiratory failure. Lancet Respir Med. 2019;7:90–8.

9. Al-Bassam W, Dade F, Bailey M, et al. "Likely overassistance" during invasive pressure support ventilation in patients in the intensive care unit: a multicentre prospective observational study. Crit Care Resusc. 2019;21:18–24.
10. Dres M, Goligher EC, Dube BP, et al. Diaphragm function and weaning from mechanical ventilation: an ultrasound and phrenic nerve stimulation clinical study. Ann Intensive Care. 2018;8:53.
11. Green M, Marzano V, Leditschke I, Mitchell I, Bissett B. Mobilization of intensive care patients: a multidisciplinary practical guide for clinicians. J Multidiscip Healthc. 2016;9:247–56.
12. Hodgson CL, Bailey M, Bellomo R, et al. A binational multicenter pilot feasibility randomized controlled trial of early goal-directed mobilization in the ICU. Crit Care Med. 2016;44:1145–52.
13. Gosselink R, Langer D. Recovery from ICU-acquired weakness; do not forget the respiratory muscles! Thorax. 2016;71:779–80.
14. Bissett B, Leditschke IA, Green M, Marzano V, Collins S, Van Haren F. Inspiratory muscle training for intensive care patients: A multidisciplinary practical guide for clinicians. Aust Crit Care. 2018;32:249–55.
15. Marini JJ, Rodriguez RM, Lamb V. Bedside estimation of the inspiratory work of breathing during mechanical ventilation. Chest. 1986;89:56–63.
16. Tzanis G, Vasileiadis I, Zervakis D, Karatzanos E, Dimopoulos S, Pitsolis T, et al. Maximum inspiratory pressure, a surrogate parameter for the assessment of ICU-acquired weakness. BMC Anesthesiol. 2011;11:14.
17. Multz AS, Aldrich TK, Prezant DJ, Karpel JP, Hendler JM. Maximal inspiratory pressure is not a reliable test of inspiratory muscle strength in mechanically ventilated patients. Am Rev Respir Dis. 1990;142:529–32.
18. Laveneziana P, Albuquerque A, Aliverti A, et al. ERS statement on respiratory muscle testing at rest and during exercise. Eur Respir J. 2019;53:1801214.
19. Evans JA, Whitelaw WA. The assessment of maximal respiratory mouth pressures in adults. Respir Care. 2009;54:1348–59.
20. Moodie L, Reeve J, Elkins M. Inspiratory muscle training increases inspiratory muscle strength in patients weaning from mechanical ventilation: a systematic review. J Physiother. 2011;57:213–21.
21. Elkins M, Dentice R. Inspiratory muscle training facilitates weaning from mechanical ventilation among patients in the intensive care unit: a systematic review. J Physiother. 2015;61:125–34.
22. Vorona S, Sabatini U, Al-Maqbali S, Bertoni M, Dres M, Bissett B, et al. Inspiratory muscle rehabilitation in critically ill adults: a systematic review and meta-analysis. Ann Am Thorac Soc. 2018;15:735–44.
23. Bissett BM, Leditschke IA, Neeman T, Boots R, Paratz J. Inspiratory muscle training to enhance recovery from mechanical ventilation: a randomised trial. Thorax. 2016;71:812–9.
24. Martin AD, Smith BK, Davenport PD, et al. Inspiratory muscle strength training improves weaning outcome in failure to wean patients: a randomized trial. Crit Care. 2011;15:R84.
25. Shi ZH, Jonkman A, de Vries H, et al. Expiratory muscle dysfunction in critically ill patients: towards improved understanding. Intensive Care Med. 2019;45:1061–71.
26. Bonnevie T, Villiot-Dangerd J, Graviera F, Dupuisf J, Prieurc G, Médrinalc C. Inspiratory muscle training is used in some intensive care units, but many training methods have uncertain efficacy: a survey of French physiotherapists. J Physiother. 2015;61:204–9.
27. Gosselink R, Wagenaar RC, Decramer M. Reliability of a commercially available threshold loading device in healthy subjects and in patients with chronic obstructive pulmonary disease. Thorax. 1996;51:601–5.
28. Caruso P, Denari SD, Ruiz SA, et al. Inspiratory muscle training is ineffective in mechanically ventilated critically ill patients. Clinics (Sao Paulo). 2005;60:479–84.
29. Tonella RM, Ratti L, Delazari LEB, et al. Inspiratory muscle training in the intensive care unit: a new perspective. J Clin Med Res. 2017;9:929–34.

30. Cader SA, Vale RG, Castro JC, et al. Inspiratory muscle training improves maximal inspiratory pressure and may assist weaning in older intubated patients: a randomised trial. J Physiother. 2010;56:171–7.
31. Condessa RL, Brauner JS, Saul AL, Baptista M, Silva AC, Vieira SR. Inspiratory muscle training did not accelerate weaning from mechanical ventilation but did improve tidal volume and maximal respiratory pressures: a randomised trial. J Physiother. 2013;59:101–7.
32. Mackay MR, Ellis E, Johnston C. Randomised clinical trial of physiotherapy after open abdominal surgery in high risk patients. Aust J Physiother. 2005;51:151–9.
33. Brasher PA, McClelland KH, Denehy L, Story I. Does removal of deep breathing exercises from a physiotherapy program including pre-operative education and early mobilisation after cardiac surgery alter patient outcomes? Aust J Physiother. 2003;49:165–73.
34. American College of Sports Medicine. American College of Sports Medicine position stand. Progression models in resistance training for healthy adults. Med Sci Sports Exerc. 2009;41:687–708.
35. Bissett B, Leditschke IA, Green M. Specific inspiratory muscle training is safe in selected patients who are ventilator-dependent: a case series. Intensive Crit Care Nurs. 2012;28:98–104.
36. Schellekens WJ, van Hees HW, Doorduin J, et al. Strategies to optimize respiratory muscle function in ICU patients. Crit Care. 2016;20:103.
37. Shoemaker MJ, Donker S, Lapoe A. Inspiratory muscle training in patients with chronic obstructive pulmonary disease: the state of the evidence. Cardiopulm Phys Ther J. 2009;20:5–15.
38. Gosselink R, De Vos J, van den Heuvel SP, Segers J, Decramer M, Kwakkel G. Impact of inspiratory muscle training in patients with COPD: what is the evidence? Eur Respir J. 2011;37:416–25.
39. Dall'Ago P, Chiappa GR, Guths H, Stein R, Ribeiro JP. Inspiratory muscle training in patients with heart failure and inspiratory muscle weakness: a randomized trial. J Am Coll Cardiol. 2006;47:757–63.
40. Volianitis S, McConnell AK, Koutedakis Y, McNaughton L, Backx K, Jones DA. Inspiratory muscle training improves rowing performance. Med Sci Sports Exerc. 2001;33:803–9.
41. Johnson MA, Sharpe GR, Brown PI. Inspiratory muscle training improves cycling time-trial performance and anaerobic work capacity but not critical power. Eur J Appl Physiol. 2007;101:761–70.
42. Kilding AE, Brown S, McConnell AK. Inspiratory muscle training improves 100 and 200 m swimming performance. Eur J Appl Physiol. 2010;108:505–11.
43. Edwards AM, Wells C, Butterly R. Concurrent inspiratory muscle and cardiovascular training differentially improves both perceptions of effort and 5000 m running performance compared with cardiovascular training alone. Br J Sports Med. 2008;42:823–7.
44. Lisboa C, Munoz V, Beroiza T, Leiva A, Cruz E. Inspiratory muscle training in chronic airflow limitation: comparison of two different training loads with a threshold device. Eur Respir J. 1994;7:1266–74.
45. Smith K, Cook D, Guyatt GH, Madhavan J, Oxman AD. Respiratory muscle training in chronic airflow limitation: a meta-analysis. Am Rev Respir Dis. 1992;145:533–9.
46. Lotters F, van Tol B, Kwakkel G, Gosselink R. Effects of controlled inspiratory muscle training in patients with COPD: a meta-analysis. Eur Respir J. 2002;20:570–6.
47. Langer D, Charususin N, Jacome C, et al. Efficacy of a novel method for inspiratory muscle training in people with chronic obstructive pulmonary disease. Phys Ther. 2015;95:1264–73.
48. Hoffman M, Van Hollebeke M, Clerckx B, et al. Can inspiratory muscle training improve weaning outcomes in difficult to wean patients? A protocol for a randomised controlled trial (IMweanT study). BMJ Open. 2018;8:e021091.
49. Bissett B, Wang J, Neeman T, Leditschke I, Boots R, Paratz J. Which ICU patients benefit most from inspiratory muscle training? Retrospective analysis of a randomized trial. Physiother Theory Pract. 2019;9:1–6.
50. Hayen A, Herigstad M, Pattinson KT. Understanding dyspnea as a complex individual experience. Maturitas. 2013;76:45–50.

Post-Intensive Care Syndrome and Chronic Critical Illness: A Tale of Two Syndromes

46

H. Bailey and L. J. Kaplan

46.1 Introduction

Approximately 15% of the 5.7 million US patients receiving critical care require mechanical ventilation [1]. While the United States Agency for Healthcare Reporting and Quality has noted that hospital-acquired conditions have decreased over the past 4 years, there are two conditions that are not surveilled, but occur with greatest frequency in patients supported with mechanical ventilation [2]. One condition occurs only in survivors of critical illness and is termed the post-intensive care syndrome (PICS). The other condition is chronic critical illness, and it occurs in both survivors and decedents. There is overlap in that those with chronic critical illness are at high risk for PICS but not *vice versa*. It is relevant to understand the defining features of each syndrome in order to identify the at-risk patient populations, establish epidemiologic baselines, and articulate a platform from which to launch intervention.

46.2 Post-intensive Care Syndrome Features

PICS is characterized by new cognitive dysfunction, persistent muscle weakness, and disorder of psychosocial interactions [3] (Fig. 46.1). When the effects of the syndrome also impact family members, it is denoted as PICS family (PICS-F).

H. Bailey (✉)
Department of Emergency Medicine, Durham VAMC, Durham, NC, USA
e-mail: President@SCCM.org

L. J. Kaplan
Perelman School of Medicine, University of Pennsylvania, Philadelphia, PA, USA

Department of Surgery, Division of Trauma, Surgical Critical Care and Emergency Surgery, University of Pennsylvania Hospital Systems, Philadelphia, PA, USA

© Springer Nature Switzerland AG 2020
J.-L. Vincent (ed.), *Annual Update in Intensive Care and Emergency Medicine 2020*, Annual Update in Intensive Care and Emergency Medicine, https://doi.org/10.1007/978-3-030-37323-8_46

Triggers

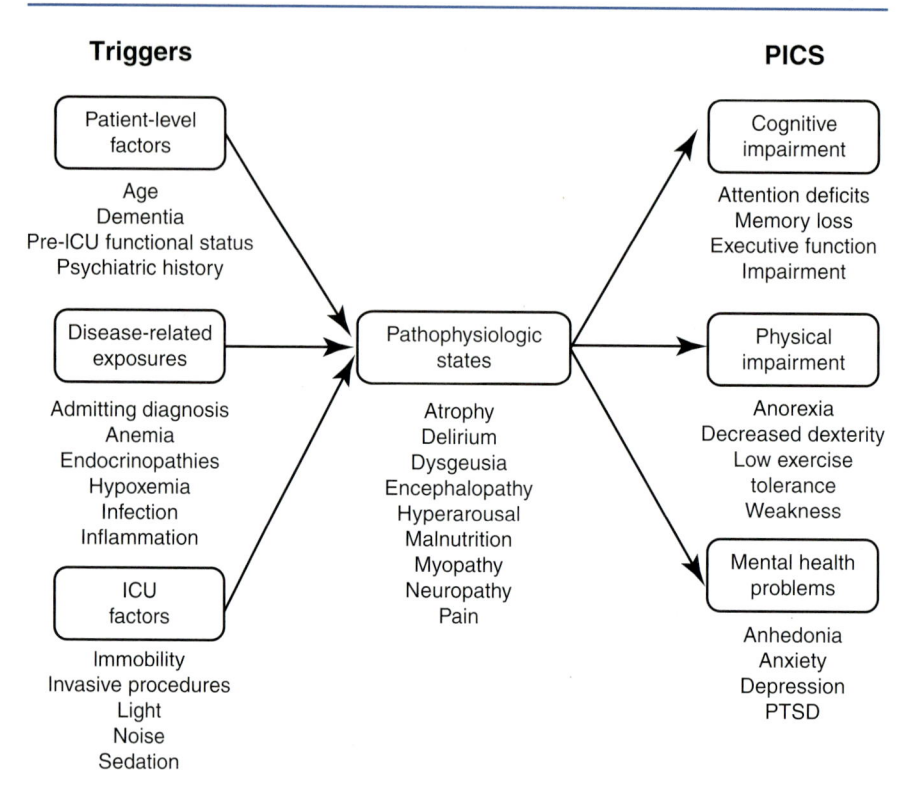

PICS

```
Patient-level factors
```
Age
Dementia
Pre-ICU functional status
Psychiatric history

```
Disease-related exposures
```
Admitting diagnosis
Anemia
Endocrinopathies
Hypoxemia
Infection
Inflammation

```
ICU factors
```
Immobility
Invasive procedures
Light
Noise
Sedation

```
Pathophysiologic states
```
Atrophy
Delirium
Dysgeusia
Encephalopathy
Hyperarousal
Malnutrition
Myopathy
Neuropathy
Pain

```
Cognitive impairment
```
Attention deficits
Memory loss
Executive function
Impairment

```
Physical impairment
```
Anorexia
Decreased dexterity
Low exercise tolerance
Weakness

```
Mental health problems
```
Anhedonia
Anxiety
Depression
PTSD

Fig. 46.1 Potential triggers and outcome features of the post-intensive care syndrome (PICS). *PTSD* post-traumatic stress disorder (Reproduced from [4] with permission)

Affected family members are less likely to return to work and are transformed into *de facto* care givers, generally without specific training, and may not receive appropriate financial or material support [5]. Additionally, family members are apt to experience anxiety, post-traumatic stress disorder (PTSD), and for those whose loved one has died, complicated grief [6].

Critical illness survivors afflicted with PICS demonstrate impaired memory and executive function to a greater extent than with attention, visuospatial competency, or processing speed [7]. Persistent skeletal muscle weakness is a prominent feature that reinforces dependence, especially when it is not addressed with dedicated physical therapy coupled with nutritional support. The perception of being "shut-in" amplifies disordered psychosocial interactions. The expectation that once out of the acute care or rehabilitation facility normal life will resume is often not realizable. Loss of pride, confidence, and joy often stem from altered body habitus and body image, all of which are reinforced by being unable to engage in typical interpersonal dynamics. Overall, each of these elements degrades quality of life for critical illness survivors [4, 8]. While many risk factors have been identified, we are unable to pinpoint a specifically high-risk group other than those receiving ICU care who require mechanical ventilation, develop delirium, and have been treated for sepsis or septic shock [9].

46.3 PICS In-Hospital Interventions

Having identified a broad target group, interventions designed to reduce ICU length of stay, mechanical ventilation duration, avoid delirium, and rapidly diagnose and treat sepsis or septic shock could be anticipated to reduce PICS incidence. Two such interventions are the ICU Liberation bundle and the Surviving Sepsis Campaign. The latter is well covered elsewhere and will not be further discussed [10]. The ICU Liberation bundle, on the other hand, merits specific exploration. This particular bundle uses an A through F metric to help guide care (Fig. 46.2) [6]. Importantly, this bundle deliberately incorporates the family into the bundle elements providing an integrated approach to patient- and family-centered care.

Bundle deployment as an aid in managing the critically ill accrues specific benefits. In one study assessing bundle compliance, hospital survival clearly correlated

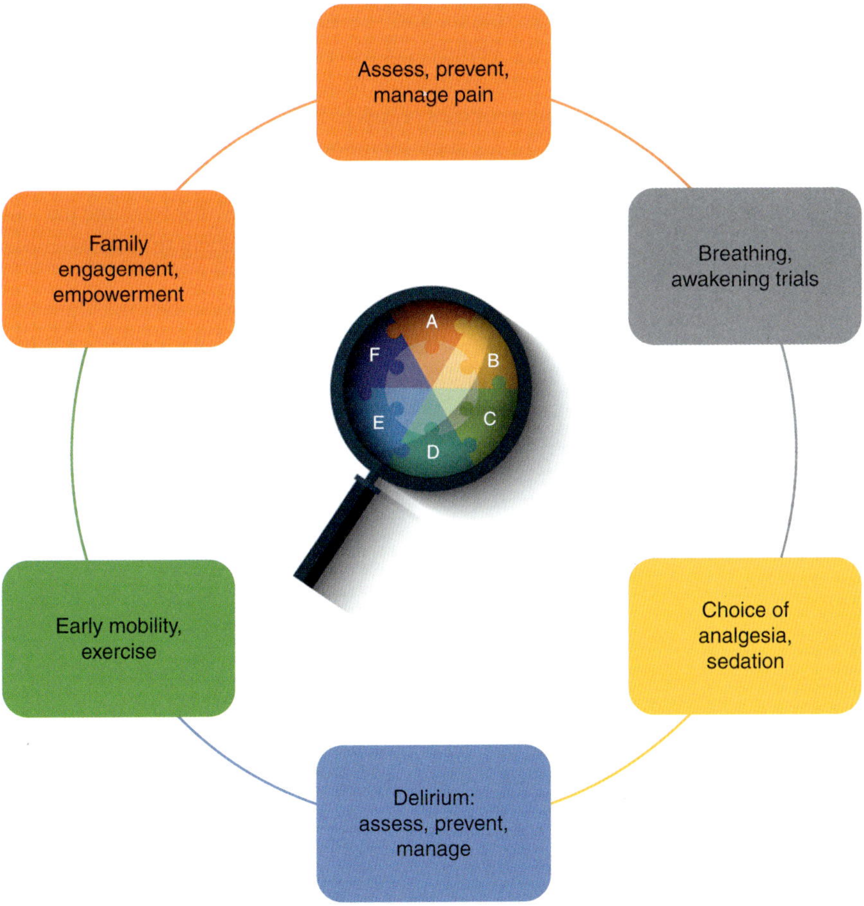

Fig. 46.2 The A-B-C-D-E-F elements of the ICU Liberation Bundle

with progressive application of bundle elements; the greatest survival was noted for those in whom all elements were applied [11]. Similar benefits were noted when assessing delirium-free and coma-free days as well. A larger follow-up study also documented improved survival, as well as decrease ICU and hospital LOS with progressive application of bundle elements [12]. Detailed analysis noted decreases in delirium, coma, restraint use, and mechanical ventilation. These benefits were accompanied by a surprising but anticipatable outcome—increased pain reporting. Patients who are more awake and interactive are able to specify their pain scores while those deeply sedated are not. It is likely that a multimodal approach to analgesia will also support bundle deployment by avoiding opioid or sedative-induced respiratory depression [13].

Regardless of care efficacy, PTSD is a prominent feature of family members whose loved one has survived critical illness, especially if the patient was previously healthy [14]. Incorporating family members into the daily rounding process improves their knowledge of the care plan, improves nursing satisfaction, embraces goals of therapy discussions on rounds and substantially decreases the need for after-rounds family meetings [15]. Family members—when accompanied by a staff member—also appear to derive benefit from being present during resuscitation events [16]. Chronicling the course of care seems to help patients "recover" the time lost in the ICU and recreate a linear representation of their life; staff and family entries both demonstrate value during patient recovery [17]. Guidelines for diary entries have been established to help shape how data is entered and to frame the lost time in a fashion that supports recovery when the patient is ready to read what has been recorded.

Patients transferred from outlying and perhaps critical access facilities into tertiary or quaternary facilities may be particularly vulnerable as the plethora of support services that encircle major hospitals are notoriously absent in more remote regions. Home repatriation is a critical event for survivors of critical illness as well as for their family members [18]. This is in part because the development of PICS occurs in the hospital, but screening for it and its untoward sequelae occur after discharge. In this way, there is high reliance on primary care physicians and advanced practice providers to identify those with PICS. Such activities will benefit from focused communication from ICU clinicians to those who will continue care after discharge—a feature that may leverage the interconnectedness of the electronic health record. Once PICS is identified, three overlapping approaches may help enhance recovery.

46.4 PICS Out-of-Hospital Interventions

Recovery efforts focus on three main interventions: physical rehabilitation, peer support groups, and post-ICU clinics. It is clear that rehabilitation addresses persistent weakness. Recent data suggest that a guided course of rehabilitation leads to more sustained gains, especially with regard to independence (and quality of life) than when rehabilitation activities are self-directed [19]. While rehabilitation addresses the physical impairments associated with PICS, peer support groups appear effective at addressing the psychosocial elements. Peer support groups, such as those developed and deployed by the SCCM Thrive collaborative, engage survivors as part of a new team [20]. A variety of models exist, including those run by ICU staff, a psychologist, or a survivor as well as those existing solely online. Of course, a cross-over model that links survivors with patients actively receiving care in the ICU has been articulated, and may ideally provide family support when patients are unable to participate in dialog.

Post-ICU clinics are well established in the United Kingdom and have been since 1985 [21]. Key features of these clinics include an endurance assessment with a 6-minute walk test, symptom query, medication assessment and reconciliation, discussion of impediments to recovery, and modification or elaboration of plans for rehabilitation. Such clinics are relatively new in the USA but are steadily gaining momentum. Barriers to establishing a post-ICU clinic include finding space, clinician time, and a mechanism for remuneration for care. Unexpectedly, the post-ICU clinic and peer support space also help drive improvements in the ICU [22]. Notable benefits include identifying new targets for quality improvement, creating new roles for survivors, improved understanding of the patient experience, improving ICU staff morale and inviting colleagues to participate in post-ICU activities.

46.5 Chronic Critical Illness Features

Chronic critical illness was also previously termed the persistent inflammation, immunosuppression, catabolism syndrome [23]. Now that grouping of findings is identified as the pathophysiology that underpins chronic critical illness. Those with chronic critical illness share common features including care in an ICU, ICU length of stay (LOS) more than 14 days, and ongoing organ dysfunction. This is often manifested as prolonged mechanical ventilation, ongoing renal replacement techniques, as well as recurrent or recrudescent infection. Indeed, chronic critical illness—compared to rapid recovery—strongly impacts survival and functional outcome in survivors of sepsis in the surgical ICU population [24, 25]. The impact of this pathophysiology on outcome is presented in Fig. 46.3. Relatedly, a scheme of immune mediator cells that drive the proliferation of myeloid-derived suppressor cells with subsequently induced T-cell dysfunction has been advanced [27]. This pathway incudes a host of feature that result in immune paralysis, in large part explaining defective host defense and susceptibility to infection as a driver of organ failure (Fig. 46.4). There are increasing data that the elderly may be more susceptible on the basis of accumulated oxidative stress and damage, autophagy failure, and preadmission malnutrition [28]. In this way, the foundations of chronic critical illness are better understood from a mechanistic perspective than are those for PICS.

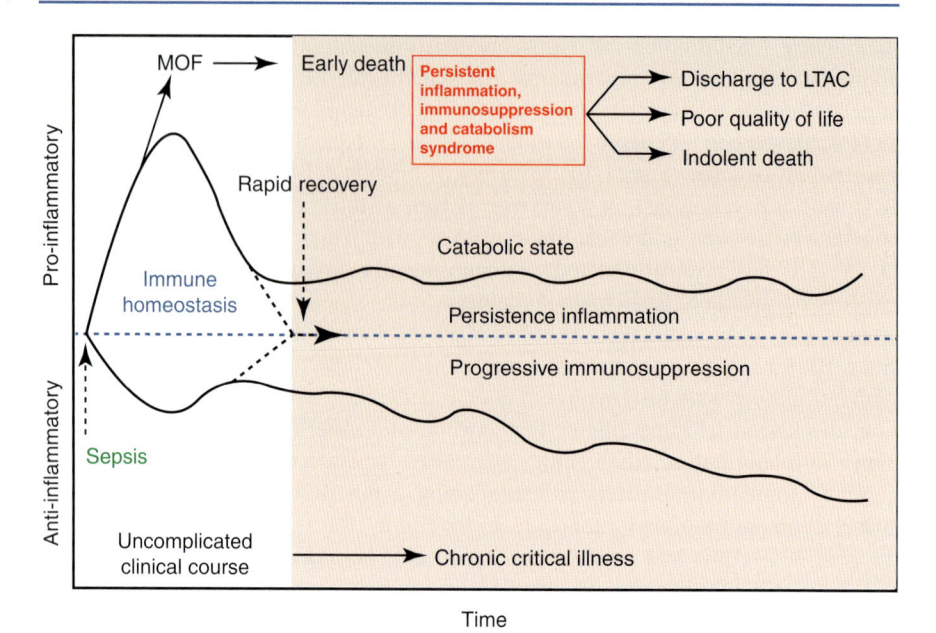

Fig. 46.3 Graphic demonstrating time frames and trajectories of patients with the persistent inflammation, immunosuppression, catabolism syndrome, which is the pathophysiology underlying chronic critical illness. *LTAC* long-term acute care facility (Reproduced from [26] under the terms of the Creative Commons license)

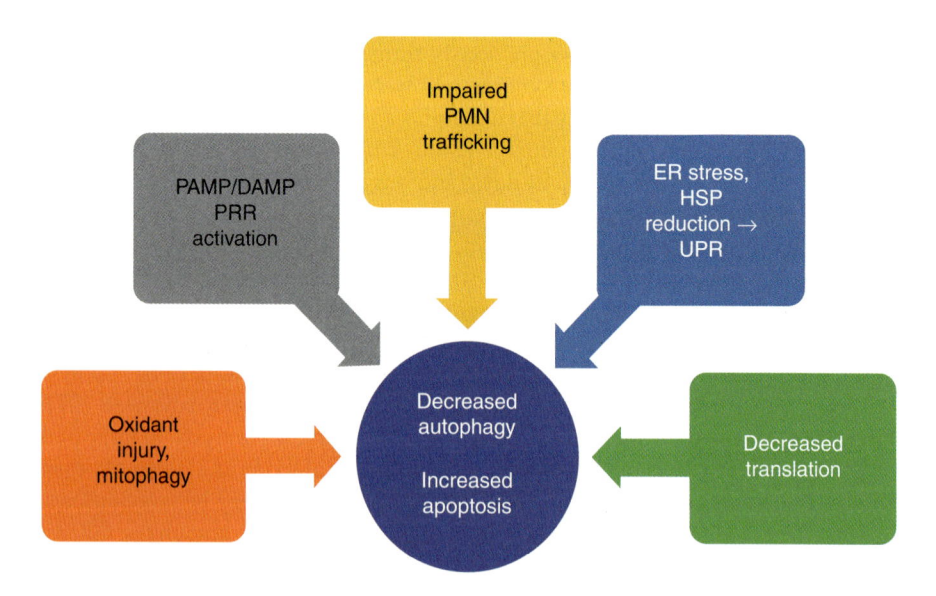

Fig. 46.4 This graphic illustrates the key features of innate immune paralysis. *PAMP* pathogen-associated molecular pattern, *DAMP* damage-associated molecular pattern, *PRR* pattern-recognition receptor, *HSP* heat shock protein, *UPR* unfolded protein response, *ER* endoplasmic reticulum

46.6 Unanticipated Survivor Sequelae

New chronic health conditions appear more common in critical illness survivors [29]. It is likely that those with chronic critical illness are overrepresented in this observation. Unsurprisingly, men appear to be more greatly afflicted than are women—at least in this particular study. As a result, the financial burden addressing chronic health expenditure is also increased in ICU survivors, never returning to the pre-illness baseline healthcare cost [30]. Relatedly, care recidivism after surviving chronic critical illness exceeds that of ICU survivors who did not develop chronic critical illness. Sepsis and septic shock as index diagnoses appear to be the main drivers of this observation [31, 32]. Indeed, physical performance, independence, and quality of life are all degraded by developing chronic critical illness, perhaps reflecting persistence of abnormal physiology past the time when recovery has been assumed to have occurred [24].

46.7 Syndromic Overlap

While not specifically examined, it is highly likely that there is syndromic overlap between those afflicted with PICS and those with chronic critical illness. The duration of critical care, organ dysfunction, and observations with regard to physical performance and quality of life make those with chronic critical illness at particularly high risk for PICS. Indeed, those with chronic critical illness should be deliberately queried for PICS symptomatology. Syndromic overlap may prove to be a fertile domain for future investigation in order to target interventions in an especially high-risk group of patients with accelerated healthcare financial burdens.

46.8 Conclusion

Both PICS and chronic critical illness demonstrate distinct clinical criteria. However, the two syndromes also share important elements demonstrating syndromic overlap. While the prevalence of PICS seems to exceed that of chronic critical illness, our understanding of the genesis and pathophysiology of chronic critical illness outstrips that for PICS. In-hospital as well as out-of-hospital interventions have been identified for PICS mitigation, many of which may also serve to favorably impact the occurrence and impact of chronic critical illness. Both syndromes merit focused inquiry, as well as dedicated surveillance following acute care discharge and after home repatriation.

References

1. Mikkelson ME, Jackson JC, Hopkins RO, et al. Peer support as a novel strategy to mitigate post-intensive care syndrome. AACN Adv Crit Care. 2016;27:221–9.
2. Agency for Healthcare Research and Quality. AHRQ National Scorecard on Hospital-Acquired Conditions. https://www.ahrq.gov/sites/default/files/wysiwyg/professionals/quality-patient-safety/pfp/hac-cost-report2017.pdf. Accessed 29 Aug 2019.

3. Desai S, Lawa T, Needham DM. Long-term complications of critical care. Crit Care Med. 2011;39:371–9.
4. Lane-Fall MB, Kuza CM, Fakhry S, Kaplan LJ. The lifetime effects of injury: post-intensive care syndrome (PICS) and post-traumatic stress disorder (PTSD). Anesthesiol Clin. 2019;37:135–50.
5. Haines KJ, Quasim T, McPeake J. Family and support networks following critical illness. Crit Care Clin. 2018;34:609–23.
6. Harvey MA, Davidson JE. Post-intensive care syndrome: right care right now … and later. Crit Care Med. 2016;44:381–5.
7. Ramona O, Girard TD. Medical and economic implications of cognitive and psychiatric disability of survivorship. Semin Respir Crit Care Med. 2012;33:348–56.
8. Bein T, Weber-Carstens S, Apfelbacher C. Long-term outcome after the acute respiratory distress syndrome: different from general critical illness? Curr Opin Crit Care. 2018;24:35–40.
9. Davidson JE, Harvey MA, Bemis-Dougherty A, et al. Implementation of the pain, agitation, and delirium clinical practice guidelines and promoting patient mobility to prevent post-intensive care syndrome. Crit Care Med. 2013;41(9 Suppl):S136–45.
10. Levy MM, Evans LE, Rhodes A. The surviving sepsis campaign bundle: 2018 update. Intensive Care Med. 2018;44:925–8.
11. Barnes-Daly MA, Phillips G, Ely EW. Improving hospital survival and reducing brain dysfunction at seven California community hospitals: implementing PAD Guidelines via the ABCDEF bundle in 6,064 patients. Crit Care Med. 2017;45:171–8.
12. Pun BT, Balas MC, Barnes-Daly MA, et al. Caring for critically ill patients with the ABCDEF bundle: results of the ICU Liberation Collaborative in over 15,000 adults. Crit Care Med. 2019;47:3–14.
13. Ayad S, Khanna AK, Iqbal SU, Singla N. Characterisation and monitoring of postoperative respiratory depression: current approaches and future considerations. Br J Anesth. 2019;123:378–91.
14. Lee RY, Engelberg RA, Curtis JR, Hough CL, Kross EK. Novel risk factors for posttraumatic stress disorder symptoms in family members of acute respiratory distress syndrome survivors. Crit Care Med. 2019;47:934–41.
15. Allen SR, Pascual JL, Martin N, et al. A novel method of optimizing patient and family centered care in the ICU. J Trauma Acute Care Surg. 2017;82:582–6.
16. Davidson JE, Aslakson RA, Long AC, et al. Guidelines for family-centered care in the neonatal, pediatric and adult ICU. Crit Care Med. 2017;45:103–28.
17. Levine SA, Reilly KM, Nedder MM, Avery KR. The patient's perspective of the intensive care unit diary in the cardiac intensive care unit. Crit Care Nurse. 2018;38:28–37.
18. Cameron JL, Chu LM, Matte A, et al. One-year outcomes in caregivers of critically ill patients. N Engl J Med. 2016;374:1831–41.
19. Walker W, Wright J, Danjoux G, Howell SJ, Martin D, Bonner S. Project post intensive care eXercise (PIX): a qualitative exploration of intensive care unit survivors' perceptions of quality of life post-discharge and experience of exercise rehabilitation. J Int Care Soc. 2015;16:37–44.
20. McPeake J, Hirshberg EL, Christie LM, et al. Models of peer support to remediate post-intensive care syndrome: a report developed by the society of critical care medicine thrive international peer support collaborative. Crit Care Med. 2019;47:e21–7.
21. Colbenson GA, Johnson A, Wilson ME. Post-intensive care syndrome: impact, prevention and management. Breathe. 2019;15:98–101.
22. Haines KJ, Sevin CM, Hibbert E, et al. Key mechanisms by which post-ICU activities can improve in-ICU care: results of the international THRIVE collaboratives. Intensive Care Med. 2019;45:939–47.
23. Stortz JA, Mira JC, Raymond SL, et al. Benchmarking clinical outcomes and the immunocatabolic phenotype of chronic critical illness after sepsis in surgical intensive care unit patients. J Trauma Acute Care Surg. 2018;84:342–9.

24. Gardner AK, Ghita GL, Wang Z, et al. The development of chronic critical illness determines physical function, quality of life, and long-term survival among early survivors of sepsis in surgical ICUs. Crit Care Med. 2019;47:566–73.
25. Martin ND, Ramaswamy T, Moin E, et al. The critical illness inflection point during prolonged surgical ICU length of stay. Pulm Crit Care Med. 2018;3:2–7.
26. Loftus TJ, Mira JC, Ozrazgat-Baslanti T, et al. Sepsis and critical illness research center investigators: protocols and standard operating procedures for a prospective cohort study of sepsis in critically ill surgical patients. BMJ Open. 2007;7:e015136.
27. Stortz JA, Murphy TJ, Raymond SL, et al. Evidence for persistent immune suppression in patients who develop chronic critical illness after sepsis. Shock. 2018;49:249–58.
28. Nomellini V, Kaplan LJ, Sims C, Caldwell CC. Chronic critical illness and persistent inflammation: what can we learn from the elderly, injured, septic, and malnourished? Shock. 2018;49:4–14.
29. van Beusekom I, Bakhshi-Raiez F, van der Shaaf, Busschers WB, de Keizer NF, Dongelmans DA. ICU survivors have a substantial higher risk of developing new chronic conditions compared to a population-based control group. Crit Care Med. 2019;47:324–30.
30. Koster-Brouwer ME, van de Groep K, Pasma W, et al. Chronic healthcare expenditure in survivors of sepsis in the intensive care unit. Intensive Care Med. 2016;42:1641.
31. Giurgis FW, Brakenridge SC, Sutchu S, et al. The long-term burden of severe sepsis and septic shock: Sepsis recidivism and organ dysfunction. J Trauma Acute Care Surg. 2016;81:525–32.
32. Brakenridge SC, Efron PA, Cox MC, et al. Current epidemiology of surgical sepsis: discordance between inpatient mortality and 1-year outcomes. Ann Surg. 2019;270:502–10.

Part XVI

Organizational and Ethical Aspects

Sepsis as Organ and Health System Failure

P. Dickmann and M. Bauer

47.1 Introduction: Introducing Sepsis—Reframing Risks and Relevance

47.1.1 The Biomedical Lens: The Dogma

From a biomedical lens, broad awareness, early diagnosis and fast treatment are the key narratives that drive debate and progress in biomedical sciences. Leading within the traditional biomedical focus have been three interconnected key narratives and their respective rationales:

1. Inflammation—and the respective administration of antibiotic treatment following a "bug-focused" approach
2. *Early* administration of antibiotics—which suggests early broad-spectrum antibiotics vs. empirical use of antibiotics after blood cultures and antibiograms.
3. "Golden hour"—adopting a classic health economics performance parameter for quality control measurement (time) and a set of decisions and actions (bundles) to be undertaken within the first hour of entering the health system.

P. Dickmann (✉)
Department of Anesthesiology and Intensive Care Medicine, Jena University Hospital, Jena, Germany

Center for Sepsis Control and Care (CSCC), Jena University Hospital, Jena, Germany

Dickmann Risk Communication drc, London, UK
e-mail: petra.dickmann@med.uni-jena.de

M. Bauer
Department of Anesthesiology and Intensive Care Medicine, Jena University Hospital, Jena, Germany

Center for Sepsis Control and Care (CSCC), Jena University Hospital, Jena, Germany

These three aspects have formed key pillars of public awareness campaigns, such as "Think Sepsis" and "Ask: Could It Be Sepsis" [1, 2].

The landmark paper by Kumar et al. in 2006, albeit monocenter and retrospective, set the orthodoxy in the care for critically ill patients with infection [3]. According to their analyses, a delay of 1 h to initiate appropriate antibiotics was allegedly associated with an increase of approximately 7% in attributable mortality. Quality initiatives almost immediately adopted the intuitive concept of a need to act immediately within the "golden hour" of sepsis. Terms such as "early," "aggressive," and "pre-emptive" strategies were coined in particular in the context of antimicrobial therapy and cardiovascular support to seemingly compensate for the lack of rapid diagnostics and lack of understanding of the molecular mechanisms of a host response that went out of control.

In addition, these concepts were well suited to be applied in simple "bundles" that could be enforced through regulatory actions requiring hospitals to follow protocols for the early identification and treatment of sepsis. Hospitals can actually be fined if they do not meet the sepsis targets [4]. Consequently, a "1-h bundle" formed the core of the Surviving Sepsis Campaign's quality improvement efforts. According to the campaign, applying the sepsis bundle "simplifies the complex processes of the care of patients with sepsis." The bundle is based on the 2016 guideline recommendations integrating identified decision points and largely relying on early administration of broad-spectrum antibiotics and a standardized fluid bolus if lactate levels suggest impaired tissue perfusion.

Increased awareness of sepsis along with standardized treatment procedures ("bundles") has to some extent improved care for patients with life-threatening infections and organ dysfunction by advocating a high level of attention from patients, health professionals, and health policy makers. The contribution of the single components of the bundle to this effect, however, remains at best controversial [5].

47.1.2 Controversy

The controversy touches upon almost every aspect of these three interconnected narratives leading to inconclusive implications for health policy decision making and treatment guidelines. Data sets evaluating timing of antibiotics in sepsis have shown mixed results and very ambitious timing thresholds of less than 1 h for antibiotic administration in sepsis have led to overuse of broad-spectrum antibiotics and increased resistance pressure. Thus, a potential benefit for the patient being treated must be weighed against health system concerns about increasing antimicrobial resistance. In the light of a better understanding of off-target effects of broad-spectrum antibiotics on the microbiome or on mitochondrial function, the liberal administration of antibiotic has come under scrutiny [6].

A recent study analyzing approximately 35,000 patients treated within a contemporary multicenter quality improvement program for sepsis documented that increased time to antibiotics after emergency department presentation was associated with mortality in all sepsis severity groups [7], but this effect was substantially below the 7% per hour originally described by Kumar and colleagues [3]. A prospective study by Bloos et al. studied the impact of a continuous medical education program on 28-day mortality in a cluster-randomized protocol with special emphasis on time to antibiotics and source control [8]. Median time to antimicrobial therapy was approximately 1.5 h in the intervention group and 2.0 h in controls. The risk of death increased by 2% per hour delay of antimicrobial therapy and 1% per hour delay of source control, independent of group assignment, suggesting a significant but moderate effect of antibiotics on the course of the disease [8]. In particular, the need to combine multiple anti-infective compounds in the light of diagnostic uncertainty might outweigh the benefit of early source control through off-target effects of combined and broad-spectrum antibiotics. In addition to the intuitively negative effects on the (gut) microbiome, adverse effects on mitochondria as "endosymbionts" have been suggested to potentially negatively affect organ integrity and function [9]. As a consequence, controversial data have been reported as to whether or not to postpone antibiotics until diagnostic hints are available and despite strong recommendations to initiate antibiotics early; the database for such guidelines is rather weak. Most importantly, in a before-and-after study by Hranjec et al. the subgroup with least benefit from "calculated" broad-spectrum antibiotics was the group of sickest patients presenting with septic shock, i.e., those in whom the current paradigm would predict the greatest need to initiate early anti-infective therapy [10].

A more restrictive anti-infective approach is requested from a health policy perspective; this restrictive policy could also benefit the individual patient. But more and conclusive prospective data are needed. Moreover, there is broad consensus that culture-independent molecular tests to shorten time to identify the suspected pathogen and its resistance pattern carry potential to improve the outcome of critically ill patients with infection, in particular if embedded in an antibiotic stewardship program [11].

Evidence to support fluid bolus or to standardize resuscitation according to the "early goal-directed therapy" algorithm is even less conclusive [5]. Three large, randomized control trials—ARISE, ProMISe, and ProCESS—all demonstrated no significant difference in patient mortality when comparing usual care versus the protocol [12–14].

Lack of definitive data to support the concept that bundle compliance improves mortality in septic patients and the enforcement of these protocols within regulatory activities leading to consequences regarding reimbursement has led to significant controversy at policy level. Ironically, the 1-h bundle has never been prospectively tested, yet it was recommended globally. In a joint statement, the Society of Critical Care Medicine (SCCM) and the American College of Emergency Physicians (ACEP) advocated for a moratorium of this practice in the United States pending further review. The recommendation to set the bundle on hold was specifically given for a high-end healthcare system rather than for the world-wide campaign. Thus, concerns were raised based on specific issues regarding the bundle elements in the context of a one world policy. Many physicians still believe that the SSC 1-h bundle is efficient in a resource-limited context albeit evidence being correlational, at best.

This prompts the question whether or not such recommendations should be given generally for all strata of healthcare from the emergency department to the ICU across low- and high-income settings. A consensus process that will lead to such a broad recommendation can only reflect a minimum standard and contradicts an individualized precision medicine approach.

47.1.3 The Impact of the Dogma on Research Horizons

The biomedical focus on the three narratives has led to anomalies and substantial controversy over guidelines and policies. It has also narrowed the research horizon, slowing the development of innovative treatment alternatives that are based on new and better understanding of the pathophysiology.

The intuitive concept in acute and critical care of a need to be "fast" and "early" following the motto "time is tissue" has improved outcome in many areas of medicine, such as myocardial infarction or stroke, in which timing of an intervention, typically re-establishing oxygen availability, is of the essence. As discussed above, this concept has been rolled out to other areas in critical care, most notably sepsis. The evidence base, however, to justify this generalization is shaky. Extrapolation of the data from other forms of shock, e.g., hypovolemic shock, to septic shock is not as solid as it may seem at first glance. While this approach will improve oxygen delivery when an inappropriately low preload contributes to anaerobic metabolism, the pathogenesis of hyperlactatemia in sepsis is multifactorial and includes several causes unrelated to an impaired preload, such as mitochondrial uncoupling and Warburg metabolism [15]. Moreover, mandatory fulfillment of a predefined volume load even in those patients that are not volume responsive is wrong. As such, the lack of documented benefit of the volume challenge in healthcare systems in high-income countries does not come as a surprise and is reflected in data that a positive fluid balance is associated with worsening outcome [16].

Similar to the discussed limitations of early and broad-spectrum antibiotics, another dilemma unfolds when looking at the fluid bolus to improve oxygen utilization. In order to establish a "one world" campaign that meets the needs of settings as diverse as low- to high-income healthcare systems or even within the strata, settings as diverse as general wards, emergency rooms, and ICUs, a minimum consensus of 30 ml of crystalloid across the strata was chosen that is difficult to justify [17].

47.1.4 Modifications Within the Paradigm

As more anomalies and substantial controversy arose, modifications within the paradigm led the discussion to a reflection on treatment rationales (e.g., kill bugs) and paved the way for a more modern understanding of sepsis that allows alternative treatment options, such as modulating the immune system. It also led the way to re-defining sepsis (Sepsis-3 definition) [18–20].

Thus, the discussed limitations of the bundle approach determined that the pathophysiological framework of sepsis as derived from clinical studies was oversimplified to the extent of erroneous recommendations. From a philosophy of science perspective, the even broader gap of the currently unfolding basic scientific understanding of pathogen-driven organ dysfunction and clinical care limits the required paradigm shift regarding care for the critically ill. In fact, the recent Sepsis-3 definition advocates for the initiation of the process to close this gap by acknowledging failure of the systemic inflammatory response syndrome (SIRS) concept and by revising the understanding of cellular mechanisms of septic shock.

The most promising current development, however, relies on the discovery of resilience or disease tolerance as a strategy of the host to deal with infection. The characteristic hallmark of this host response pattern is an increased ability to cope with pathogens in otherwise sterile tissues without impairment of host fitness. Thus, while resistance mechanisms rely on reducing the pathogen load, resilience can be achieved even despite a persistently high pathogen load. This would suggest that beyond interventions to reduce the pathogen load, i.e., antibiotics, treatment options can be designed which increase the ability of the host to withstand pathogens, including those that are resistant to antibiotics. Several options that are promising have been reported which include therapeutic use of cholesterol in pneumococcal or apoferritin in polymicrobial sepsis [21, 22]. Interestingly, the therapeutic use of cholesterol was patented as early as 1910 by the Bayer Company, i.e., in the pre-antibiotic era and might become interesting for the post-antibiotic era again.

47.2 Political Science Intermezzo

Sepsis has become a more prominent topic on the global policy agenda, and health decision makers are rightly attentive to further advance the progress in science, policy, and practices. However, there seems to be a tendency to break down big global challenges into smaller manageable chunks that can be achieved by individuals: combatting climate change by flying less, controlling pandemics by washing hands and reducing antimicrobial resistance by taking and prescribing antibiotics more consciously.

This is a double-edged sword: while it is, obviously, a reasonable and sensible policy approach to encourage a responsible lifestyle, modern risk management is not an individual lifestyle choice. By referring policy decisions to individual choices, these smaller manageable parts (e.g., hand washing) become disconnected from the bigger picture, leaving individuals depoliticized with lifestyle choices rather than policy decisions. This individualization mimics economic history: washing hands is, literally, a tiny piece in the conveyor belt process where individuals lose contact and context with the real world and just contribute tiny, mechanic, repetitive moves to running a well-oiled machinery. Individualization (e.g., hand washing), in this regard, is a political driver to refer and defer responsibility.

This individualization mirrors the industrialization process and contributes to the "silo-ing" of problems—a tendency the global community often complains about.

From this political science perspective, medical specialization echoes the distribution of labor, risking the loss of access and ability to understanding the broader picture. Overspecialization could mean not looking at the contexts any longer which have important roles in determining the conditions in which diseases, patients, and health professionals interact. Global challenges, such as climate change, pandemics, and antimicrobial resistance, are about governance and health policy. Antimicrobial resistance, for example, is not just about hand washing. It is also driven by how hospitals are designed, built, operated, staffed, and governed; antimicrobial resistance is about how animals are fed; antimicrobial resistance is about the role of healthcare within society [23].

47.3 Modern Understanding of Risks: Looking at the Contexts

Having re-narrated the progress of sepsis research, policy, and practices, including the paradigm shift that is reflected in the new sepsis definition, we highlight the importance of understanding the various drivers and perspectives that run the discourse of sepsis and other big challenges.

In order to modulate the discourse to include a health system perspective, we review the fundamental re-thinking of sepsis as deterioration at the patient level within a complex system. Our starting point is the concept of risks—and the traditional risk assessment, in particular. In a traditional approach, risks are calculated as a product of probability by impact, resulting in a number ("risks"). Conventional approaches understand the communication of these "risks" as risk communication. We advocate for a more modern understanding of risks that is aligned with the ISO 9001 understanding of risks in modern risk management (ISO 9001: 2015 Risk Management): risk is anything that has an effect on the uncertainty of objectives, meaning that risks deviate from the objectives of an organization or institution. Translating into the risk management of sepsis, the key question is not how big the risk is, but how one can detect the deviation early. In a visual representation, the development of sepsis (red graph) and the health system response (orange graph) is displayed in Fig. 47.1 [24, 25].

Fig. 47.1 The development of sepsis and the health system response (interventions) over time [24, 25] (Modified from [24] with permission)

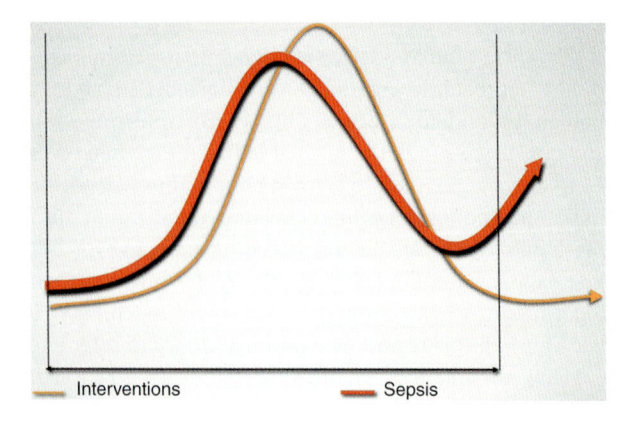

Fig. 47.2 Earlier, faster, smoother, and smarter: risk management in sepsis aims to detect the deviation (escalation of a patient's condition) earlier, respond faster, have smoother coordination, and create a smarter legacy in terms of governance [24, 25] (Modified from [24] with permission)

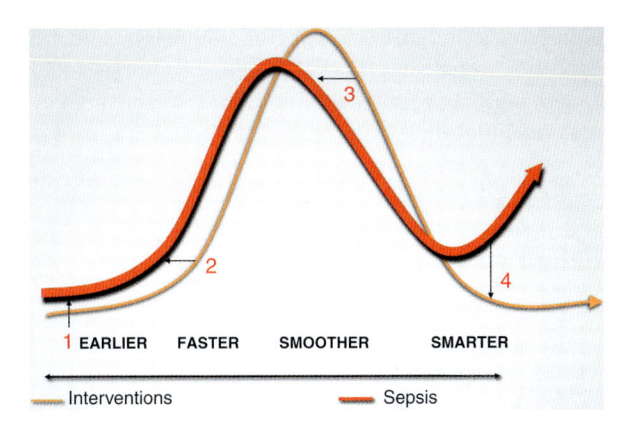

Risk in this new approach is not a number referring to statistics but a deviation that relates to objectives. This reframes risk in a relational approach as a relationship between two dynamics: the dynamic of the deterioration of a patient and the dynamic of the system in which it happens (health system responsiveness). This new approach also modifies the investigation: the key ambition now is to detect the deviation (escalation of a patient's condition) earlier, respond faster, have smoother coordination, and create a smarter legacy in terms of governance (Fig. 47.2).

47.4 Sepsis as Health System Failure

A health system approach looks at sepsis from the context in which it takes place. It reflects the entire process (earlier, faster, smoother, and smarter) and highlights the conditions that enable patients to deteriorate and their influencing factors. Previous research has used this relational risk and the methodology to better understand and speed up the detection time to major public health events [26]. Transferring this approach to sepsis enables application of a radical approach, literally analyzing the root cause by looking at the conditions and their influencing factors.

47.5 Conclusion

We have reviewed two perspectives displaying a similar pattern. Through a biomedical lens, we reviewed the development of powerful policies, general recommendations, and practical guidelines (bundles) that are based on outdated evidence. These strong statements come into conflict with current evidence. Current evidence has been articulated in the new sepsis definition. It is now time to produce strong and stable policies and practices based on a more advanced, better understanding of the pathophysiology.

From a health system perspective, risk management and risk communication are also based on a rather traditional and flawed concept of risk. Innovative thinking points to a better understanding of a more dynamic, relational risk. The conceptual approach investigates the determining conditions and their influencing facts.

Having uncovered a similar pattern of sepsis in organ and health system failure, we advocate for an integrated approach to better care for patients with life-threatening infections.

References

1. Vogel L. Think sepsis to stop deaths, urge advocates. CMAJ. 2017;189:E1219–E20.
2. Voelker R. Act fast and think sepsis. JAMA. 2016;316:1440.
3. Kumar A, Roberts D, Wood KE, et al. Duration of hypotension before initiation of effective antimicrobial therapy is the critical determinant of survival in human septic shock. Crit Care Med. 2006;34:1589–96.
4. Iacobucci G. NHS hospitals could be fined if they miss new sepsis targets. BMJ. 2019;364:l124.
5. Seymour CW, Gesten F, Prescott HC, et al. Time to treatment and mortality during mandated emergency care for sepsis. N Engl J Med. 2017;376:2235–44.
6. Hiensch R, Poeran J, Saunders-Hao P, et al. Impact of an electronic sepsis initiative on antibiotic use and health care facility-onset Clostridium difficile infection rates. Am J Infect Control. 2017;45:1091–100.
7. Liu VX, Fielding-Singh V, Greene JD, et al. The timing of early antibiotics and hospital mortality in sepsis. Am J Respir Crit Care Med. 2017;196:856–63.
8. Bloos F, Ruddel H, Thomas-Ruddel D, et al. Effect of a multifaceted educational intervention for anti-infectious measures on sepsis mortality: a cluster randomized trial. Intensive Care Med. 2017;43:1602–12.
9. Kalghatgi S, Spina CS, Costello JC, et al. Bactericidal antibiotics induce mitochondrial dysfunction and oxidative damage in mammalian cells. Sci Transl Med. 2013;5:192ra85.
10. Hranjec T, Rosenberger LH, Swenson B, et al. Aggressive versus conservative initiation of antimicrobial treatment in critically ill surgical patients with suspected intensive-care-unit-acquired infection: a quasi-experimental, before and after observational cohort study. Lancet Infect Dis. 2012;12:774–80.
11. Banerjee R, Ozenci V, Patel R. Individualized approaches are needed for optimized blood cultures. Clin Infect Dis. 2016;63:1332–9.
12. Peake SL, Delaney A, Bellomo R, et al. Goal-directed resuscitation in septic shock. N Engl J Med. 2015;372:190–1.
13. Mouncey PR, Osborn TM, Power GS, et al. Trial of early, goal-directed resuscitation for septic shock. N Engl J Med. 2015;372:1301–11.
14. Pro CI, Yealy DM, Kellum JA, et al. A randomized trial of protocol-based care for early septic shock. N Engl J Med. 2014;370:1683–93.
15. Cheng SC, Quintin J, Cramer RA, et al. mTOR- and HIF-1alpha-mediated aerobic glycolysis as metabolic basis for trained immunity. Science. 2014;345:1250684.
16. Seymour CW, Kennedy JN, Wang S, et al. Derivation, validation, and potential treatment implications of novel clinical phenotypes for sepsis. JAMA. 2019;321:2003–17.
17. Kress JP, Hall JB. Treating sepsis is complicated: are governmental regulations for sepsis care too simplistic? Ann Intern Med. 2018;168:594–5.
18. Seymour CW, Liu VX, Iwashyna TJ, et al. Assessment of clinical criteria for Sepsis: For the Third International Consensus Definitions for Sepsis and Septic Shock (Sepsis-3). JAMA. 2016;315:762–74.
19. Singer M, Deutschman CS, Seymour CW, et al. The third international consensus definitions for Sepsis and septic shock (Sepsis-3). JAMA. 2016;315:801–10.
20. Dickmann P, Scherag A, Coldewey SM, Sponholz C, Brunkhorst FM, Bauer M. Epistemology in the intensive care unit-what is the purpose of a definition?: paradigm shift in sepsis research. Anaesthesist. 2017;66:622–5.

21. Weis S, Carlos AR, Moita MR, et al. Metabolic adaptation establishes disease tolerance to sepsis. Cell. 2017;169:1263–75.e14.
22. Weber M, Lambeck S, Ding N, et al. Hepatic induction of cholesterol biosynthesis reflects a remote adaptive response to pneumococcal pneumonia. FASEB J. 2012;26:2424–36.
23. Dickmann P, Keeping S, Doring N, et al. Communicating the risk of MRSA: the role of clinical practice, regulation and other policies in five European countries. Front Public Health. 2017;5:44.
24. Dickmann P, McClelland A, Gamhewage GM, Portela de Souza P, Apfel F. Making sense of communication interventions in public health emergencies—an evaluation framework for risk communication. J Commun Healthc. 2015;8:233–40.
25. Dickmann P, Abraham T, Sarkar S, et al. Risk communication as a core public health competence in infectious disease management: development of the ECDC training curriculum and programme. Euro Surveill. 2016;21:30188.
26. Adini B, Singer SR, Ringel R, Dickmann P. Earlier detection of public health risks—health policy lessons for better compliance with the international health regulations (IHR 2005): insights from low-, mid- and high-income countries. Health Policy. 2019;123:941–6.

Burnout and Joy in the Profession of Critical Care Medicine

M. P. Kerlin, J. McPeake, and M. E. Mikkelsen

48.1 Introduction

The intensive care unit (ICU) can be a stressful environment for patients and families, with well-established long-term consequences [1, 2]. The impact that this unique environment can have on healthcare professionals is being increasingly recognized [3–5]. Challenging ethical situations, exposure to high patient mortality and difficult daily workloads can lead to excessive stress for those caring for critically ill patients [3, 6, 7]. A growing body of literature suggests that this excessive stress and resultant moral distress can lead to burnout syndrome.

In this state-of-the-art review, we focus on the epidemiology of burnout syndrome in the ICU and the impact it can have on clinicians, patients, and the health service. Risk factors for burnout syndrome, alongside potential strategies to mitigate burnout and optimize fulfillment, will also be discussed.

48.2 Burnout Syndrome

In 2016, the Critical Care Societies Collaborative, which includes the American Thoracic Society, the American Association of Critical Care Nurses, the American College of Chest Physicians, and the Society of Critical Care Medicine, convened a working group to focus attention on psychological health and well-being for providers of critical care. This official "Call for Action" statement defined burnout syndrome as an "individual response to particular work related events that manifest in people that do not have baseline psychological disorders" [3].

Burnout syndrome, described nearly half a century ago, is defined as a work-related condition characterized by three symptoms: emotional exhaustion, depersonalization, and a reduced sense of personal accomplishment [8, 9]. Burnout syndrome manifests when an individual's perceived self-worth and expectations do not match those of the employers/organization [3, 4]. Although the concept of burnout syndrome, applied to healthcare providers, is still evolving and its causes and manifestations have overlap with other concepts such as compassion fatigue, for the purpose of clarity, this state-of-the-art review will focus on burnout and burnout syndrome.

In general, burnout manifests when one (or more) of six mismatches between individual and job is present: workload, control, reward, community, fairness, and values [9]. The six-mismatch framework has been applied to design interventions at the individual and organization level and, as described below, was simplified and applied to the profession of critical care medicine by the Critical Care Societies Collaborative (Fig. 48.1).

48.3 Prevalence of Burnout Syndrome Among Critical Care Professionals

Multidisciplinary, coordinated care, delivered by caring and compassionate clinicians trained in critical care, is an essential component to high-quality critical care delivery [10]. Relative to other professions, burnout is more common among the "caring" professions [11], which partly explains the burnout epidemic present among healthcare professionals and critical care clinicians, in particular [3, 4, 10–18].

In cross-sectional studies, most critical care clinicians manifest one of the three classic features of burnout [3, 4]. For example, in a United States study of university hospital ICU nurses, 81% of critical care nurses experienced one or more symptoms of burnout [12], and severe burnout syndrome was found in 33% of critical care nurses and nursing assistants studied in a large French survey study [14].

Two large national surveys conducted more than a decade apart reveal the magnitude of what appears to be an enduring epidemic among critical care physicians. In a landmark, 1-day national survey conducted in 189 French ICUs in 2004, a high level of burnout was observed in 46.5% of critical care physicians [17]. In a survey of 15,069 United States physicians conducted in 2019, wherein critical care

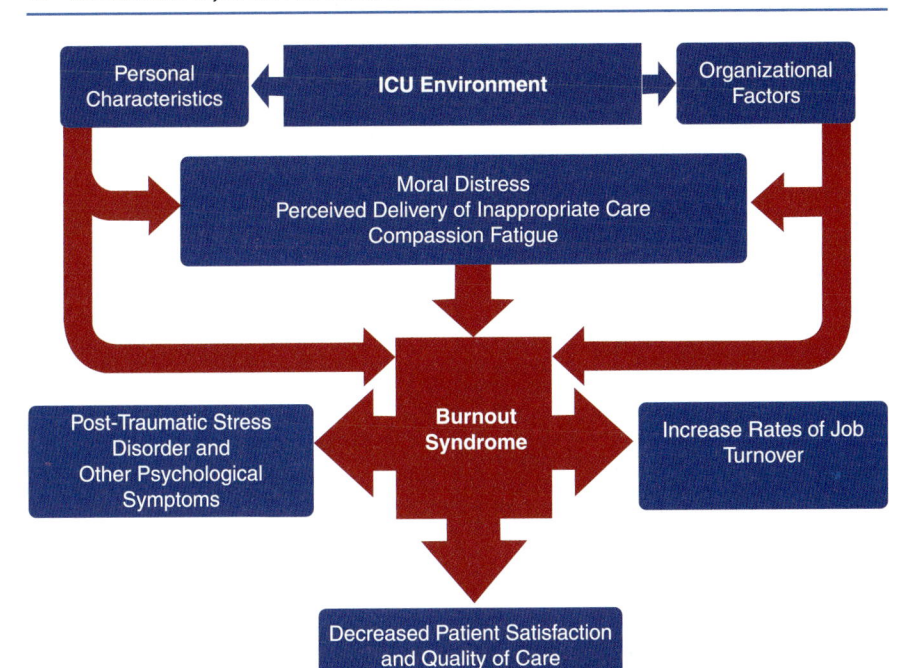

Fig. 48.1 Risk factors associated with burnout syndrome and impact on the provider, care, and the healthcare system (Reprinted from [3] with permission of the American Thoracic Society. Copyright © 2019 American Thoracic Society)

physicians comprised 1% of respondents, 44% of physicians surveyed were burned out, as were 44% of the critical care physicians surveyed [16]. Furthermore, 14% of survey respondents reported that they had thoughts of suicide. Burned out or depressed critical care physicians, who on average reported working longer hours, were less likely to seek professional help [16].

48.4 Burnout and Fulfillment in Critical Care as a Profession

To date, the epidemiology of well-being among critical care professionals has focused on burnout assessed at a single time point. To gain a more complete understanding of critical care professional well-being, in line with the National Academy of Medicine recommendation to improve clinician well-being, which requires a commitment to "measure it, develop and implement interventions, and then re-measure it" [19], one health system implemented an initiative wherein they serially assess critical care provider well-being [18]. At each survey, section critical care physicians complete two, complementary, validated tools to measure burnout and professional fulfillment [18–21]. Notably, the initiative measures well-being when physicians are not on service in the ICU, in addition to measuring well-being when on service. As the investigators hypothesized, an ebb and flow to burnout exists, with burnout peaking at 41% when on service and subsiding to 25% when not attending in the ICU [18]. Burnout varied by rotation, implying role, staffing and ICU culture can impact burnout measures, and, as detailed below, rotation length. Furthermore, in contrast to the ebb and flow of burnout, fulfillment was common whether the physician was off service, at 60%, or during service, at 55% [18]. As context, fulfillment was observed in 34% of physicians in the validation study of the survey instrument [21]. These data suggest that fulfillment, or joy, is common in the profession of critical care medicine. Confirmatory studies engaging the entire multidisciplinary care team are warranted, as are studies designed to elucidate factors associated with professional fulfillment in the field of critical care medicine.

48.5 The Impact of ICU Burnout Syndrome

The effects of clinician burnout syndrome are far reaching. In addition to adversely affecting the well-being of individual clinicians, burnout syndrome can have major adverse consequences for patient-care and the healthcare system [3, 4, 10].

48.5.1 Individual Impact

Burnout syndrome can have a significant impact on the health and well-being of individual clinicians. For example, symptoms of depression and post-traumatic stress disorder (PTSD) are more common in ICU physicians and nurses with burnout syndrome [12, 22, 23]. This can have wide ranging effects on the individual's private life as well as patient safety. In a recent prospective, observational multicenter study of over 1500 staff from 31 ICUs in France, symptoms of depression in healthcare staff were an independent risk factor for medical errors [24]. There is also a negative relationship between individual clinician productivity and burnout. This definition of productivity included an increased number of sick days, intent to continue practicing and intent to change jobs [25]. One study from Europe also demonstrated that physicians with burnout had significantly greater odds of having self-perceived "insufficient" work ability [26]. This lack of confidence in one's ability may have an impact on both the practitioner's mental health and indeed ongoing patient care.

48.5.2 Healthcare System and Patient Safety

International research has demonstrated the relationship between patient-reported experience and staff burnout. For example, in one US-based study of more than 800 nurses and 600 patients from over 20 hospitals, nurse burnout was associated with patient satisfaction. In this particular study, patients who were cared for on units that nurses characterized as having adequate staff, good administrative support for care and good relations between staff groups were more than twice as likely as other patients to report high levels of satisfaction with the care they had received, and the nurses in these units reported significantly lower levels of burnout [27].

Burnout syndrome can have a bi-directional relationship with patient safety. Errors in the clinical setting can cause stress for the individual clinician involved and lead to burnout syndrome. Conversely, burnout syndrome may cause stress, reduce performance, and thus cause more errors [3, 4]. Burnout syndrome can also result in high sickness rates and potential skill drain in organizations if staff members feel they have no option but to leave their jobs prematurely to preserve their own mental and physical health; this may cause problems for the healthcare system, the individual, and also patient safety [28, 29]. Although an easy solution may appear to be to replace staff in these roles, this may not be a straightforward process and may be associated with a reduction in efficiency [29]. A recent estimate suggests that the average costs to replace an ICU nurse in the United States range from $36,657 to $88,000; thus higher turnover can have a significant economic impact for healthcare systems [30]. In more extreme cases, there may be no other suitably qualified candidates to perform the task, which may be a further risk to patient safety [31].

48.6 Risk Factors for Burnout Among ICU Clinicians

Previous surveys of broad populations of physicians and nurses, and of critical care physicians, nurses, nurse assistants, and respiratory therapists specifically, have elucidated several factors associated with stress and burnout, which can be categorized into four broad domains: (1) individual characteristics, (2) workload and organizational issues, (3) quality of working relationships, and (4) clinical care requirements (Fig. 48.1) [3].

The primary individual characteristic associated with increased risk of burnout among physicians is female sex. Women physicians had approximately a 60% increased rate of burnout compared to men in both the Physician Work Life Study, which included almost 6000 physicians across a broad range of medical specialties in the United States [32], and in a survey of almost 1000 French intensivists [17]. Among nurses, female sex has not been consistently associated with the presence of burnout; however, nursing surveys have reported very high percentages of female respondents, perhaps limiting the possibility of testing this association.

Younger age has been associated with burnout among ICU nurses [14, 33]. This may reflect increased perceived stress related to inexperience or self-confidence, or that those nurses who experienced burnout left the specialty or clinical practice altogether at a younger age. Certain personality characteristics may also influence the experience of burnout. For example, among a group of nurses in Spain, neuroticism (as measured by a validated personality inventory) was associated with increased emotional exhaustion, depersonalization, and decreased personal accomplishment. Conversely, extroversion and agreeableness were potentially protective, as they were associated with decreased burnout scores [34].

A number of workload measures and organizational factors have been linked to increased burnout. Notably, the sheer volume of work (as measured by working hours) has not been demonstrated to have a consistent association; however, timing of work has. For example, among ICU nurses, lack of control over one's schedule and rapid patient turnover is associated with increased burnout [14]. On the other hand, having professional activities outside of bedside care, such as involvement in a work group or research team, may be protective against burnout [14, 35, 36]. Among physicians, having more night shifts, more consecutive work days, and less time since the last nonworking week contribute to burnout [17, 18]. Furthermore, ICU physicians who display evidence of psychological distress or depression perceive feeling too much responsibility as a major stressor, suggesting that concurrent and competing clinical demands contribute to burnout [37].

Among physicians and nurses, working relationships have been consistently described as important contributors to job satisfaction. Numerous surveys have demonstrated an association of interpersonal conflicts—between nurses and physicians, with peers and colleagues, with supervisors, and with patients and families—with increased risk of burnout. Interpersonal conflict in the care of critically ill patients can lead to moral distress (that is, the inability of a clinician to act according to his/her values due to internal and external constraints), which has specifically been linked to burnout [38, 39]. Even in the absence of conflicts, higher scores for quality of relationships with nurses as reported by physicians were associated with less burnout [17], suggesting the importance of healthy and positive collaboration as a mechanism to protect clinicians.

Finally, the clinical care that is required of ICU clinicians may contribute to burnout. Taking care of critically ill patients is by nature stressful, fast-paced, and potentially chaotic. Although studies have not shown a consistent independent association between patient severity of illness and risk of burnout, a few studies among ICU nurses have demonstrated higher rates of burnout when caring for dying patients and being involved in decisions about withholding and withdrawing life-sustaining therapies [14, 36].

48.7 Strategies to Mitigate Burnout

The prevalence of burnout among ICU clinicians and its potential consequences warrant immediate action. Given the breadth of risks to clinicians, to quality of care and patient outcomes of today, and to the quality and size of the ICU workforce of tomorrow, we believe that clinicians, hospital administrators, and policy makers must share in the responsibility for taking action.

Unfortunately, there has been limited empirical research thus far to guide us. To our knowledge, there have been no randomized trials of interventions focused on prevention or treatment of burnout in ICU clinicians. We suggest that candidate interventions—focused on recognition of burnout as a common syndrome in ICU clinicians, establishing and maintaining healthy collaborative work environments, and providing flexibility and resources to support clinicians experiencing burnout—should be developed and tested with the same rigor as patient-targeted therapeutic interventions in critical care.

According to the Critical Care Societies Collaborative, in addition to organizational accountability, clinicians should have "individual accountability for maintaining their own emotional and physical health and for building resiliency" [3]. To do so, clinicians must first learn how to identify burnout symptoms in themselves and their colleagues. Then, they must develop healthy strategies to ensure self-care and mitigate fatigue (such as getting adequate sleep, exercise [40], or engaging in mindfulness and meditation practices); for time management; and to optimize integration and balance between personal and professional responsibilities, all of which promote resiliency and may reduce burnout.

Clinicians should also be mindful to avoid unhealthy behaviors that can exacerbate fatigue (e.g., limit alcohol [40]), undermine health and fuel burnout. For example, 41%, 23%, and 19% of physicians in a US survey acknowledged coping with burnout by isolating themselves from others, drinking alcohol, and binge eating, respectively [16]. Rather than distancing oneself from others and disengaging, evidence suggests that engagement and a commitment to deliver compassionate care mitigates burnout, in addition to improving patient outcomes [41].

There are several ways in which organizations can address ICU clinician burnout. In general, these strategies are designed to address one or more of the "individual-to-job mismatches" that contribute to burnout: workload, control, reward, community, fairness, and values [9]. First, to prevent burnout, organizations should prioritize the creation and maintenance of healthy work environments. For example, incorporating team-building and communication training into professional development activities could improve working relationships and conflict management. Use of team debriefings after high-stress team interactions, such as cardiac arrest, can similarly promote increased and improved interpersonal communication and effective collaboration while acknowledging and applauding the team's valuable efforts. Structured communication, such as during interprofessional rounds, can support role clarity and teamwork. Collaborative decision-making and ethical deliberation on critical decisions can also improve the ICU environment and potential mitigate moral distress.

Second, organizations can take steps to address the issues around workload and timing. Providing clinicians with some flexibility and autonomy in scheduling may provide a sense of control that promotes job satisfaction. Furthermore, putting limits on continuous working days may lessen the emotional and physical exhaustion and sleep deprivation that accompanies the high-intensity clinical care. Indeed, studies have demonstrated that changing intensivist rotations from 14 consecutive days to either 7 consecutive days or giving the weekend off in the middle is associated with reduced burnout symptoms [18, 42].

A novel strategy for the prevention of burnout syndrome is the adoption of activities that recognize the long-term recovery trajectory of patients and caregivers following the initial ICU exposure [43]. Recent multicenter work undertaken by the Society of Critical Care Medicine's THRIVE initiative has demonstrated that longitudinal feedback improved staff satisfaction at work, as well as potentially improving patient care in the ICU [44]. This feedback can be obtained through a number of forums including peer support groups, ICU follow-up clinics, and patient and staff celebration events. This novel mechanism is still developing, and more research is required around its relationship with clinician burnout syndrome.

Finally, providing training and resources to build resiliency could improve the ability of ICU clinicians to cope with the stressful ICU environment. For example, in a recent pilot study, ICU nurses participated in a 2-day resilience training workshop on topics such as self-care, mindfulness exercises, and expressive writing therapy. Participants found this workshop acceptable and had decreased PTSD symptom scores afterwards [45]. In another pilot study of physicians, a professional coaching program reduced emotional exhaustion and improved overall quality of life and resiliency [46]. Other resources that organizations could provide include access to cognitive-behavioral therapy, establishment of support groups, and stress-reduction training.

48.8 Conclusion

Burnout is a threat to the profession of critical care medicine, with high prevalence rates across critical care provider disciplines. However, with a robust community response to the call to action, the opportunity exists to mitigate burnout and optimize fulfillment among critical care professionals to ensure that caring, compassionate, high-quality critical care is delivered to all critically ill patients.

Acknowledgement The work was supported in part by the Louis Nayovitz Foundation, in memory of Julian "Jay" Brockway, to honor the delivery of compassionate critical care.

References

1. Herridge MS, Tansey CM, Matte A, et al. Functional disability five years after ARDS. N Engl J Med. 2011;364:1293–304.
2. McPeake JM, Devine H, MacTavish P, et al. Caregiver strain following critical care discharge: an exploratory evaluation. J Crit Care. 2016;35:180–4.
3. Moss M, Good VS, Gozal D, Kleinpell R, Sessler CN. A critical care societies collaborative statement: burnout syndrome in critical care health professional. A call for action. Am J Respir Crit Care Med. 2016;194:106–13.
4. Costa DK, Moss M. The cost of caring: emotion, burnout and psychological distress in critical care clinicians. Ann Am Thoracic Soc. 2018;15:787–90.
5. van Mol MMC, Kompanje EJO, Benoit DD, Bakker J, Nijkamp MD. The prevalence of compassion fatigue and burnout among healthcare professional in intensive care units: a systematic review. PLoS One. 2015;10:e0136955.
6. Dzeng E, Curtis JR. Understanding ethical climate, moral distress and burnout: a novel tool and a conceptual framework. BMJ Qual Saf. 2018;27:766–70.
7. Schwarzkopf D, Ruddel H, Thomas-Ruddel DO, et al. Perceived non-beneficial treatment of patients, burnout and intention to leave the job among ICU nurses and junior and senior physicians. Crit Care Med. 2017;45:e265–73.

8. Maslach C, Leiter MP. The truth about burnout: how organizations cause personal stress and what to do about it. San Francisco: Jossey-Bass; 1997.
9. Maslach C, Leiter MP. Reversing burnout: how to rekindle your passion for your work. Stanf Soc Innov Rev. 2005;2005:43–9.
10. Pastores SM, Kvetan V, Coopersmith CM, et al. Workforce, workload, and burnout among intensivists and advanced practice providers: a narrative review. Crit Care Med. 2019;47:550–7.
11. Brindley PG. Psychological burnout and the intensive care practitioner: a practical and candid review for those who care. J Intensive Care Soc. 2017;18:270–5.
12. Mealer M, Burnham EL, Goode CJ, et al. The prevalence and impact of post traumatic stress disorder and burnout syndrome in nurses. Depress Anxiety. 2009;26:1118–26.
13. Chlan LL. Burnout syndrome among critical care professionals: a cause for alarm. Crit Care Alert. 2013;21:65–8.
14. Poncet MC, Toullic P, Papazian L, et al. Burnout syndrome in critical care nursing staff. Am J Respir Crit Care Med. 2007;175:698–704.
15. Epp K. Burnout in critical care nurses: a literature review. Dynamics. 2012;23:25–31.
16. Kane L. Medscape national physician burnout, depression & suicide report 2019. https://www.medscape.com/slideshow/2019-lifestyle-burnout-depression-6011056. Accessed 5 Sep 2019.
17. Embriaco N, Azoulay E, Barrau K, et al. High level of burnout in intensivists: prevalence and associated factors. Am J Respir Crit Care Med. 2007;175:686–92.
18. Mikkelsen ME, Anderson BJ, Bellini L, et al. Burnout, and fulfillment, in the profession of critical care medicine. Am J Respir Crit Care Med. 2019;200:931–93.
19. National Academy of Medicine Action Collaborative on Clinician Well-Being and Resilience. Validated Instruments to Assess Work-Related Dimensions of Well-Being. https://nam.edu/valid-reliable-survey-instruments-measure-burnout-well-work-related-dimensions/. Accessed 10 Nov 2019.
20. Dyrbye LN, Satele D, Sloan J, Shanafelt TD. Utility of a brief screening tool to identify physicians in distress. J Gen Intern Med. 2013;28:421–7.
21. Trockel M, Bohman B, Lesure E, et al. A brief instrument to assess both burnout and professional fulfillment in physicians: reliability and validity, including correlation with self-reported medical errors, in a sample of resident and practicing physicians. Acad Psychiatry. 2018;42:11–24.
22. Seaman JB, Cohen TR, White DB. Reducing the stress on clinicians working in the ICU. JAMA. 2018;320:1981–2.
23. Mealer M. Burnout syndrome in the intensive care unit. Future directions for research. Ann Am Thorac Soc. 2016;13:997–8.
24. Garrouste-Orgeas M, Perrin M, Soufir L, et al. The latroref study: medical errors are associated with symptoms of depression in ICU staff but not burnout or safety culture. Intensive Care Med. 2015;41:273–84.
25. Dewa CS, Loong D, Bonato S, Thanh NX, Jacobs P. How does burnout affect physician productivity? A systematic literature review. BMC Health Serv Res. 2014;14:325.
26. Ruitenburg MM, Frings-Dresen MHW, Sluiter JK. The prevalence of common mental disorders among hospital physicians and their association with self-reported work ability: a cross-sectional study. BMC Health Serv Res. 2012;12:292.
27. Vahey DC, Aiken LH, Sloane DM, Clarke SP, Vargas D. Nurse burnout and patient satisfaction. Med Care. 2004;42(2 Suppl):II57–ii66.
28. Papazian L, Sylvestre A, Herridge M. Should all ICU clinicians regularly be tested for burnout? Yes. Intensive Care Med. 2018;44:681–3.
29. Hayes LJ, O'Brien-Pallas L, Duffield C, et al. Nurse turnover: a literature review- an update. Int J Nurs Stud. 2012;49:887–905.
30. Kurnat-Thoma E, Ganger M, Peterson K, Channell L. Reducing annual hospital and registered nurse staff turnover—a 10 element onboarding program intervention. SAGE Open Nursing. 2017;3:1–13.

31. Khan N, Jackson D, Stayt L, Walthall H. Factors influencing nurses' intentions to leave adult critical care settings. Nurs Crit Care. 2018;24:24–32.
32. McMurray JE, Linzer M, Konrad TR, Douglas J, Shugerman R, Nelson K. The work lives of women physicians: results from the physician Worklife study. J Gen Intern Med. 2000;15:372–80.
33. Merlani P, Verdon M, Businger A, Domenighetti G, Pargger H, Ricou B. Burnout in ICU caregivers: a multicenter study of factors associated to centers. Am J Respir Crit Care Med. 2011;184:1140–6.
34. Cañadas-De la Fuente GA, Vargas C, San Luis C, García I, Cañadas GR, Emilia I. Risk factors and prevalence of burnout syndrome in the nursing profession. Int J Nurs Stud. 2015;52:240–9.
35. Teixeira C, Ribeiro O, Fonseca AM, Carvalho AS. Burnout in intensive care units-a consideration of the possible prevalence and frequency of new risk factors: a descriptive correlational multicentre study. BMC Anesthesiol. 2013;13:38.
36. Burghi G, Lambert J, Chaize M, et al. Prevalence, risk factors and consequences of severe burnout syndrome in ICU. Intensive Care Med. 2014;40:1785–6.
37. Coomber S, Todd C, Park G, Baxter P, Firth-Cozens J, Shore S. Stress in UK intensive care unit doctors. Br J Anaesth. 2002;89:873–81.
38. Fumis RR, Amarante GA, de Fátima Nascimento A, Junior JM. Moral distress and its contribution to the development of burnout syndrome among critical care providers. Ann Intensive Care. 2017;7:71.
39. Mealer M, Moss M. Moral distress in ICU nurses. Intensive Care Med. 2016;42:1615–7.
40. Henrich N, Ayas NT, Stelfox HT, Peets AD. Cognitive and other strategies to mitigate the effects of fatigue. Lessons from staff physicians working in intensive care units. Ann Am Thorac Soc. 2016;13:1600–6.
41. Trzeciak S, Roberts BW, Mazzarelli AJ. Compassionomics: hypothesis and experimental approach. Med Hypothesis. 2017;107:92–7.
42. Ali NA, Wolf KM, Hammersley J, et al. Continuity of care in intensive care units: a cluster-randomized trial of intensivist staffing. Am J Respir Crit Care Med. 2011;184:803–8.
43. Jarvie L, Robinson C, MacTavish P, et al. Understanding the patient journey: a mechanism to reduce staff burnout? Br J Nurs. 2019;28:396–7.
44. Haines KJ, Sevin C, Hibbert E, et al. Key mechanisms by which post-ICU activities can improve in-ICU care: results of the international THRIVE collaboratives. Intensive Care Med. 2019;45:939–47.
45. Mealer M, Conrad D, Evans J, et al. Feasibility and acceptability of a resilience training program for intensive care unit nurses. Am J Crit Care. 2014;23:e97–105.
46. Dyrbye LN, Shanafelt TD, Gill PR, et al. Effect of a professional coaching intervention on the well-being and distress of physicians: a pilot randomized clinical trial. JAMA Intern Med. 2019;179:1406–14.

Advance Directives in the United Kingdom: Ethical, Legal, and Practical Considerations

V. Metaxa

49.1 Introduction

An advance directive is a statement made by a capacitous person, specifying the treatment they are willing to receive should they become incompetent in the future. In the area of bioethics, advance directives represent the epitome of individual autonomy, as they allow the wishes of the patient to be heard even when decision-making capacity is lost. There are different ways by which a person can form an advance directive: stating (verbal or written) advance decisions (or living wills), granting a lasting power of attorney for health and welfare, completing a do-not-attempt resuscitation form, or enrolling in the organ donor registry are some of the most common ones (Fig. 49.1). Specifically, in critical care, intensivists may come across advance directives in several different situations: first, a patient might have drafted an advance directive for situations where they have temporarily lost consciousness but wish to refuse certain treatments; an example would be an advance directive by a Jehovah's Witness to refuse blood products. Second, a patient might be suffering from a degenerative physical or mental illness that will ultimately render them incompetent and want treatment to be withdrawn when they reach a state that is unacceptable to them (e.g., in motor neuron disease or dementia). Third, patients might have a more general verbal directive discussed with their family, where they express conditions or situations that they would find unacceptable.

However, despite their conceptual advantages, the number of valid advance directives in the UK remains very small, demonstrating an issue with their uptake. In this chapter, the ethical, legal, and practical challenges that surround the use of advance directives are explored, and suggestions for a more effective use are presented.

V. Metaxa (✉)
Critical Care Department, King's College Hospital NHS Foundation Trust, London, UK
e-mail: victoria.metaxa@nhs.net

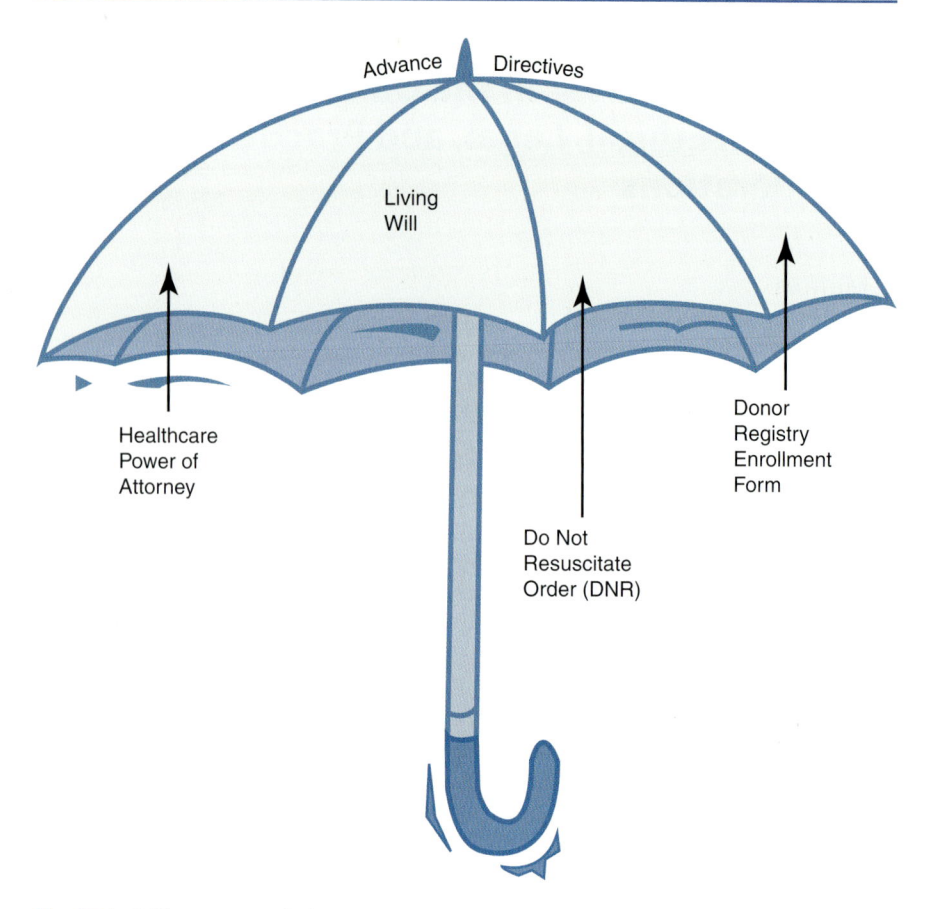

Fig. 49.1 Different types of advance directive

49.2 The Present

Advanced directives are viewed as a celebration of autonomy in UK healthcare and since the Mental Capacity Act they are also legally binding, protecting the anticipatory wishes of the individual [1]. Despite their clear legal status, their number and utilization are limited, with only 8–13% of patients having expressed their wishes in case of future incapacitation and no specific data for intensive care units (ICUs) [2]. The small numbers of advance directives have led authors to write about the "failure of the living will" [3], highlighting that not many people actually know what their wishes are and if they do, they are unable to articulate them clearly. In the SUPPORT trial there was evidence of confusion in the patients' stated wishes, which raised concerns that they either did not know what they really wanted or they could not accurately articulate their wishes [4]. Furthermore, people fear that their advance directives will either be misinterpreted or not be taken into account [3]. Surprisingly, the presence of an advance directive does not ensure its respect by the treating physicians, partly due to doubts regarding its genuineness and partly due to prognostic uncertainties [5]. In one study, only 39% of physicians followed the directions of care stated on a patient's advance directive [6] and only when it was concordant to their own medical plan [7]. Other issues highlighted are the doubt in the ability of individuals to know what they would want in the future, the fear of ignoring a change of mind, and the lack of applicability in urgent scenarios.

49.3 Ethical Issues

The purpose of advance deliberation is to allow a person to maintain control, by encouraging them to determine how they want to be treated in the future, without anyone having to second-guess their wishes. As such, advance directives represent the essence of autonomy, whereby the individual acts freely in accordance with a self-chosen plan, which will be implemented not contemporaneously but in a future scenario when the creator will have lost capacity. As an autonomous action though, it falls under specific moral requirements: it has to be (a) intentional; (b) made with understanding; and (c) made without controlling influences [8]. It is in each of those requirements that moral counterarguments arise, casting doubt on the usefulness of advance directives as a reflection of a person's core values.

One of the most contested points in the area of advanced deliberation is in situations where the person that drafted the advance directive is very different from the person whose fate will be determined by it. Dworkin, in his much-quoted case of Margo, described a patient with an advance directive that stated that if she were to develop Alzheimer's disease, she would not want to receive any life-sustaining treatment [9]. However, when she developed the disease, she appeared perfectly content and requested antibiotics in order to continue to live. The critics of binding decisions in cases of advanced dementia claim that the present and past Margo are two different moral agents, and the connection between them has broken so irrevocably that the applicability of any advance directive no longer exists. In these cases, precommitment with an advance directive is "an impractical and inappropriate strategy for securing humane and dignified death" [10]. Why should the focus on prospective autonomy result in the harm of an individual, who does not even recognize their previous wishes? The indisputable fact is that individuals express different treatment preferences in times of health and illness [11], and hence their advance directives are frequently unclear and should not be followed blindly, especially when they endanger the individual's life [4].

Contrary to the argument above, Dworkin's reasoning for ignoring Margo's request is that if autonomy is to be respected, it is her initial, capacitous wish that should be given priority, as it represents an important core value of her life [9]. By creating an advance directive regarding dementia, the patient has apparently thought about a potential future with the disease and discarded it as unbearable. As dementia is linked with loss of one's personality and not commonly with pain or other form of physical suffering, it would seem plausible that it is this exact situation of de-personalization that the creator of the advance directive wanted to avoid. Being happily or unhappily demented does not alter the fact that one is indeed demented, and this was the situation (and the indignity attached to it) they wanted to avoid all along. The mere existence of an advance directive proves that the individual had thought in advance that a situation might arise, when the preservation of their life would be worse than its termination. Why should someone that felt so strongly about the future treatment they receive not be allowed to set a framework for their medical management? Approaching every end-of-life situation with a preset bias toward the sanctity of life assumes that it is less harmful to erroneously disregard a person's autonomous decision to refuse life-sustaining treatment than it is to conform with such a decision and end a patient's life in error. However, not everyone ascribes such absolute value to preservation of life and it would seem reasonable that the same individuals who made an effort to create a valid and applicable advance directive are those that would also want to be in control of their own death when life is judged to have become unbearable [12].

Further moral issues around self-determination arise from the need for the decisions to be based on firm understanding of the situation in question. No consensus exists about the nature of understanding; however, in the Mental Capacity Act of 2005 the need for the creator to be specific in the treatment and circumstances mentioned points toward (without clearly mentioning) the need for a higher level of understanding of the treatment that is refused [1]. To complicate matters even more, studies on patient preferences have shown that people are quite inaccurate in predicting the intensity and duration of their emotions [13], as well as the stability of their preferences [14]. A poignant question thus arises: how can an individual make a binding decision about a future situation that she/he cannot fully understand in the present? This rationale though would invalidate all prospective decision-making, from blood transfusion to consent for life-saving interventions. Assuming that a patient is incapable of making autonomous decisions relating to healthcare, just because they do not have the breadth and depth of medical knowledge, is a paternalistic stance that disregards the ability of a person to know what is best for themselves. Especially when the patient has had the time to live with a condition or disease, their understanding is deeper, the emotions generated have been reflected upon, and hence the decisions reflect a higher degree of autonomy.

It is essential to highlight that important differences exist between various cultural, religious, social, and geographical populations, and the multicultural character of the UK renders this fact even more obvious. Unlike England and other Western societies, especially North America, in Southern European as well as in Asian countries patient autonomy is not the overriding principle—family ties are still very strong and sometimes take precedent over individual autonomy [15]. Given the very strong family involvement in all important aspects of one's life in these countries, it would be uncommon for an individual to make decisions in isolation about fundamental issues, such as death and dying. It would also be very difficult for physicians to prioritize the written wishes of unconscious patients over those of their family, especially if there was discordance. It follows that the existence of a document that went directly against the values of the patient's relatives would undoubtedly be disbelieved and ultimately ignored. The role of a lasting power of attorney, who would act as a surrogate decision-maker adopting either substituted judgment or a best-interests approach, would be more appropriate in this setting. Even allowing for the criticisms expressed for the proxy role [16], giving legal status to a person chosen by the patient would be more widely accepted than the legal document with pre-stated wishes.

49.4 Legal Issues

The first advance directive was drafted in 1967 in the United States of America by a Chicago attorney, member of a right-to-die organization, who termed it "living will." It was a response to the rapid technological advances in healthcare and patients' concerns that they will "become victims trapped […] after they lose their ability to voice their wishes" [17]. In English common law, the advance directive was first recognized in 1990 by Lord Goff, who stated that "one of the limits on providing treatment without consent in emergency situations, was the existence of some evidence of a pre-existing wish of the patient, expressed at a time when they were competent, which indicated that they may wish to refuse medical treatment for a particular illness or injury" [18]. Since then, the courts' stance toward anticipatory choices has been inconsistent and frequently paternalistic, using uncertainties around the patient's competency at the time of the advance directive, its applicability in specific circumstances, and its validity based on the information provided to justify the decision-making.

The case of *HE v A Hospital Trust* is one of the examples in the common law, before 2005, which demonstrates the difficulty of the courts to rule favorably toward self-determination [19]. The young female, who was born a Muslim, was a Jehovah's Witness in need of a life-saving blood transfusion, with a recent advance directive specifically refusing all such treatment. Her father pertained that she had recently renounced her faith, as she had become engaged to a Muslim man and had not been to church for 2 months. The Judge, J Mundy, decided that there was considerable doubt regarding the validity of the advance directive and granted the father's declaration, noting that the legal burden of proof lay on the person seeking to have an advance directive accepted, and in case of doubt, "convincing" and "inherently reliable" evidence "must be scrutinized with especial care." It is obvious that in the face of uncertainty, a presumption in favor of preserving life was assumed and, instead of demanding equal amounts of scrutiny to evidence provided by each side, the burden of proof was applied only on proving the validity of the advance directive. Mundy J accepted the evidence of HE's father but disregarded the testimony of her mother and brother, as well as the fact that the patient repeated her Jehovah's Witness beliefs only days before in a hospital appointment, opting to protect the sanctity of life.

Along the same lines was the decision in *The NHS Trust v T*, where a patient with borderline personality disorder and history of self-harm created a written advance directive refusing blood transfusion [20]. Her decision was overridden as it was deemed she lacked capacity, presumably because of her mental condition and despite the testimony of three different physicians who pertained she was competent to make that decision. Charles J based the decision on one consultant who disagreed with the rest and created enough uncertainty (like in the case of HE) to overrule the patient's autonomous, written, and supported decision. Once more, it appears that the common law is quick to act paternalistically and with a bias toward life preservation. There was no explanation why evidence disproving the validity and applicability of the advance directive (in both cases) carried more weight than the evidence that upheld it; it would appear that any future decision relating to end-of-life could just be overturned when any individual casts a shadow of doubt.

The essence of the advance directive is evident in *Re AK*, in which a patient who had motor neuron disease and was able to communicate only by blinking his eye, made an advance decision which stated that he wanted artificial nutrition and hydration to be withheld when he lost all powers of communication; the court upheld his request [21]. Apart from the fact that this is a situation where the patient retained capacity until the end and foresaw the exact circumstances of his death, thus negating the grounds for refusals used in the aforementioned cases, it has been suggested that the law will validate advance directives more easily if the decision is considered "objectively rational" or if the patient's welfare is not compromised [22].

The Mental Capacity Act was introduced in 2005, and one of its aims was to simplify the law in respect to advance directives, applying appropriate safeguards that would clarify the situations in which future decisions are binding and, more importantly, where they can be legitimately overridden [1]. It strived to find a balance between the patient's right to self-determination and the need to protect the interests of the future, incompetent person. Although the Act provides freedom from liability to a physician who conforms with the patient's wishes for non-escalating/terminating treatment, it is also very quick to allow decision-makers to override its decisions, if the circumstances are not clearly specified (section 25§4) or if they are not "satisfied that an advance directive […] is valid and applicable to treatment" (section 26§2). There have not been many case laws since the Act was implemented in 2007 and the messages continue to be mixed.

In *A Local Health Authority v E*, the first case after the Act's introduction, a 33-year-old woman with anorexia nervosa created a formal, witnessed advance directive in which she refused tube feeding or life support [23]. Jackson J, against the views of the consulted medical professionals, doubted E's capacity around the time of her drafting the advance directive and ruled in favor of preservation of life, as there was no formal assessment [24]. This decision is problematic but still permissible under the Mental Capacity Act; even though there is no legal obligation to have a formal capacity assessment when creating an advance directive (in an attempt to make them accessible), the safeguard requesting persons to be satisfied of their validity allows them to be easily overridden. The ruling appears to contradict the very essence of the Mental Capacity Act, which is the presumption of capacity, and is very similar to the one in the aforementioned *The NHS Trust v T*, which was decided under the common law. The difficulty of the courts to honor autonomy appears to be persistent, despite the introduction of the new legislation, as is their "tendency to assess the patient's competence on the basis of the outcome of the choice that he or she has made" [22]. Unfortunately, the Code of Practice that accompanies the Mental Capacity Act does not provide any useful guidance regarding assessing capacity; this allows the assessors to vary the requirements depending on the circumstances of the case and their own bias.

A different use of the safeguards can be observed in the case of *X Primary Care Trust v XB and YB*, in which a patient suffering from motor neuron disease created a witnessed advance directive in order to refuse life-sustaining ventilation in the event of further deterioration [25]. Despite the incorrect terms used ("refusal of non-invasive ventilation" when the patient had been receiving invasive ventilation for almost a decade) and an uncertainty around the advance directive's expiry date, Theis J upheld its validity. This appears contradictory not only to the previous ruling by Munby J in *HE v A Hospital Trust* but also his own conclusion remarks that there should be "clarity in relation to what the terms of the advance decision are". Contrary to decisions discussed above where, either by posing the question of capacity or by referring to one of the safeguards, the law appeared quick to contradict an advanced decision, the ruling by Theis J might signify the beginning of an era where patient wishes are not biased in favor of the sanctity of life. The legal implications of the Mental Capacity Act are far from decided, and future cases will determine whether there is change in the direction of the courts.

As a specific form of advance directive, a do-not-attempt cardiopulmonary resuscitation (DNA-CPR) order in case of a cardiac arrest is mentioned in a joint statement by Medical and Nursing Associations, which states, "if the healthcare team is as certain as it can be that a person is dying as an inevitable result of underlying disease or a catastrophic health event, and cardiopulmonary resuscitation (CPR) would not restart the heart and breathing for a sustained period, CPR should not be attempted" [26]. Interestingly, a recent ruling has demanded that patients should be consulted before a DNA-CPR order is put in place, with the only exception being when the doctor thinks that the conversation will result in physical or psychological harm [27]. When the patient lacks capacity, decisions around DNA-CPR should be discussed with the patient's family [28]. It should be noted that the rulings only necessitate that a discussion takes place and not that the patient/family are in agreement with the DNA-CPR decision.

49.5 The Future

When exploring the ethical and legal issues that arise around advance decision-making, the central argument appears to be between the right of the individual for self-determination on one hand and medicolegal paternalism on the other. Even in a society with libertarian tradition, such as the UK, the balance is a very difficult one to strike, as both healthcare professionals and the courts frequently ignore valid advance decisions on treatment refusal, in order to protect the life of the patient. A change of culture is required in both fields, without which the disrespect toward advance deliberation will continue. It may be that the majority of patients do not have strong views regarding their future state of health and are unwilling to think and plan ahead on an individual basis [15]—this should be acknowledged and respected. However, for the individuals who wish to make advanced decisions about situations and interventions they are not prepared to accept, the uncertainty that still surrounds the concept of advance directives sends mixed messages and renders what should be a celebration of free will, an invalidated bureaucratic exercise.

49.6 Conclusion

Advance care planning in the form of advance directives has been proposed as a way to promote self-determination in situations where the individual would have lost decision-making capacity. However, despite the theoretical advantages, there have been important moral reservations regarding their validity and applicability in future scenarios, springing from uncertainties around understanding of the future disability, accuracy in forecasting one's future preferences and potential changes in values and wishes following the occurrence of that disability. These ethical issues are mirrored in contemporary UK case law; there is a far from coherent approach in different legal cases, which depicts the discrepancy between theory and practice. Even though the law gives a patient the absolute right to refuse life-saving treatment, either contemporaneously or in an advance directive, the seemingly unlimited protection of their autonomy only exists as a matter of legal principle; it is frequently overridden especially in order to protect the loss of a life considered worthwhile.

References

1. Department of Health. Mental Capacity Act, 2005. http://www.legislation.gov.uk/ukpga/2005/9/contents. Accessed 10 Nov 2019.
2. Hughes PM, Bath PA, Ahmed N, et al. What progress has been made towards implementing national guidance on end of life care? A national survey of UK general practices. Palliat Med. 2009;24:68–78.
3. Fagerlin A, Schneider CE. Enough: the failure of the living will. Hast Cent Rep. 2004;34:30–42.
4. Teno JM, Licks S, Lynn J, et al. Do advance directives provide instructions that direct care? J Am Geriatr Soc. 1997;45:508–12.
5. Horn R. "I don't need my patients' opinion to withdraw treatment": patient preferences at the end-of-life and physician attitudes towards advance directives in England and France. Med Health Care Philos. 2014;17:425–35.
6. Schiff R, Sacares P, Snook J, et al. Living wills and the mental capacity act: a postal questionnaire survey of UK geriatricians. Age Ageing. 2006;35:116–21.
7. Bond CJ, Lowton K. Geriatricians' views of advance decisions and their use in clinical care in England: qualitative study. Age Ageing. 2011;40:450–6.
8. Beauchamp TL, Childress JF. Principles of biomedical ethics. Oxford: Oxford University Press; 2001.
9. Dworkin R. Life's dominion. New York: Alfred A. Knopf; 1993.
10. Dresser R. Precommitment: a misguided strategy for securing death with dignity. Tex Law Rev. 2003;81:1823–47.

11. Ditto PH, Jacobson JA, Smucker WD, et al. Context changes choices: a prospective study of the effects of hospitalization on life-sustaining treatment preferences. Med Decis Mak. 2006;26:313–22.
12. Michalowski S. Advance refusals of life-sustaining medical treatment: the relativity of an absolute right. Modern Law Rev. 2005;68:958–82.
13. Wilson TDG, Daniel T. Affective forecasting. Adv Exp Soc Psychol. 2003;35:345–411.
14. Ditto PH, Smucker WDD, Joseph H, et al. Stability of older adults' preferences for life-sustaining medical treatment. Health Psychol. 2003;22:605–15.
15. Mallia P. Is there a Mediterranean bioethics? Med Health Care Philos. 2012;15:419–29.
16. Wrigley A. Proxy consent: moral authority misconceived. J Med Ethics. 2007;33:527–31.
17. Capron AM. Advance directives. In: Kuhse H, Singer P, editors. A companion to bioethics. Hoboken: Wiley; 2010. p. 299–311.
18. In Re F (Mental Patient: Sterilisation). 2 AC 1, 1990.
19. HE v A Hospital NHS Trust [2003] EWHC 1017 (Fam) at [46].
20. The NHS v T. [2004] EWHC 1279.
21. Re AK (Adult Patient) (Medical Treatment: Consent) 1 FLR 129, 2001.
22. Maclean AR. Advance directives and the rocky waters of anticipatory decision-making. Med Law Rev. 2008;16:1–22.
23. A Local Health Authority v E. [2004] EWHC 1279.
24. Herring J. Medical law and ethics. 7th ed. Oxford: Oxford University Press; 2018.
25. Voultsos P. The criminal problematic of euthanasia. Komotini: Sakkoulas AN; 2006.
26. British Medical Association. Decisions relating to cardiopulmonary resuscitation. A joint statement from the British Medical Association, the resuscitation council (UK) and the Royal College of nursing. BMA House: Tavistock; 2014.
27. R (Tracey) v Cambridge University Hospitals NHS Foundation Trust and another. EWCA Civ 822, 2014.
28. Winspear v City Hospital Sunderland NHS Foundation Trust. EWHC 3250 (QB), 2015.

Part XVII
Future Aspects

Mobile Devices for Hemodynamic Monitoring

50

L. Briesenick, F. Michard, and B. Saugel

50.1 Introduction

The first iPhone was released in 2007. Since then, mobile technology development has moved at a fast pace, and smartphones have become an integral part of daily life. Smartphones are defined as mobile phones that perform many functions of a computer, typically have a touchscreen interface, internet access, and an operating system capable of running downloadable applications [1]. Smartphones and other mobile devices using wireless internet are now used ubiquitously—to send e-mails, stay updated on the latest news, navigate or use social media applications. Additionally, the "internet of things"—i.e., interconnecting sensors in everyday objects with mobile and other computing devices via the internet, giving access to a multitude of new data sources—now allows data to be transferred within wireless networks. Among the millions of available applications ("apps"), there are numerous digital applications for healthcare and medical use [2]. Most of them have been developed to track physical activity, weight loss, or treatment adherence with a personal mobile device [3]. In this chapter, we discuss how mobile devices may be used for hemodynamic monitoring.

Hemodynamic monitoring is the repeated or continuous observation or measurement of cardiovascular variables to ensure patient safety and guide therapy. Hemodynamic monitoring and management is essential to patient care in perioperative and intensive care medicine. In the operating room and in the intensive care unit (ICU), the monitoring of cardiovascular variables helps to optimize and individualize hemodynamic treatment strategies, thereby promoting patient safety and

---

L. Briesenick · B. Saugel (✉)
Department of Anesthesiology, Center of Anesthesiology and Intensive Care Medicine, University Medical Center Hamburg-Eppendorf, Hamburg, Germany
e-mail: b.saugel@uke.de

F. Michard
MiCo, Switzerland

improving patient-centered outcomes [4–6]. However, hemodynamic monitoring devices and their sensors are often invasive and bulky, not wireless or integrated, expensive and uncomfortable for awake patients. Therefore, continuous hemodynamic monitoring is currently limited to the operating room and the ICU. Monitoring of patients on general medical and surgical wards remains basic and intermittent [7, 8] although physiologic perturbations ultimately leading to life-threatening adverse events on normal wards can often be detected through the deterioration in vital signs in the minutes or hours preceding the critical event [9, 10]. Hence, with current monitoring, abnormalities in vital signs are often missed, leading to "failure to rescue" situations in patients developing life-threatening complications [11]. Outside the hospital, patients are usually not monitored at all [7]. Before and after hospital admission, monitoring is, if at all, only sporadic, and the resulting data are usually not transferred to the hospital patient record.

Mobile technology may have the potential to solve some of these problems of today's hemodynamic monitoring systems. It may create an accessible, integrated, and interconnected platform that has the potential to optimize patient care [12]. With the ubiquitous availability of smartphones and other mobile devices, the possibility to monitor and record physiologic information on mobile devices has led to the development of tools and applications that may capture and authenticate physiologic events to improve patient safety and guide therapy [13].

50.2 Digital Stethoscope

A mobile device can function as a digital stethoscope. The stethoscope membrane can be part of the phone case (e.g., Steth IO, Bothell, WA, USA) or be a handheld, wireless device compatible with a smartphone (e.g., Stethee, M3DICINE, Brisbane, Australia). Digital stethoscope devices are all based on the same method: amplification and digitization of the captured heart sounds allow "visualization" of the heart sounds and a "Shazam-like" identification of potential heart murmurs (Fig. 50.1) [14]. Thus, the assessment and monitoring of heart murmurs could be facilitated with mobile devices that enable recording, replaying, identifying, and sending of heart murmurs to remote experts as well as allowing comparison of the heart murmur over time [15].

50.3 Electrocardiogram

Atrial fibrillation is the most common cardiac arrhythmia and is associated with a significant increase in mortality and cerebrovascular events [16]. At least one-third of patients are asymptomatic, and 25% of patients with a stroke or a transient ischemic attack have an undiagnosed atrial fibrillation [17], stressing the need for primary preventive screening for atrial fibrillation. Smartphones have the potential to function as electrocardiogram (EKG) monitors that allow recording, storing, and transfer of EKGs. One application, Cardiio Rhythm (Cardiio; Cambridge, MA,

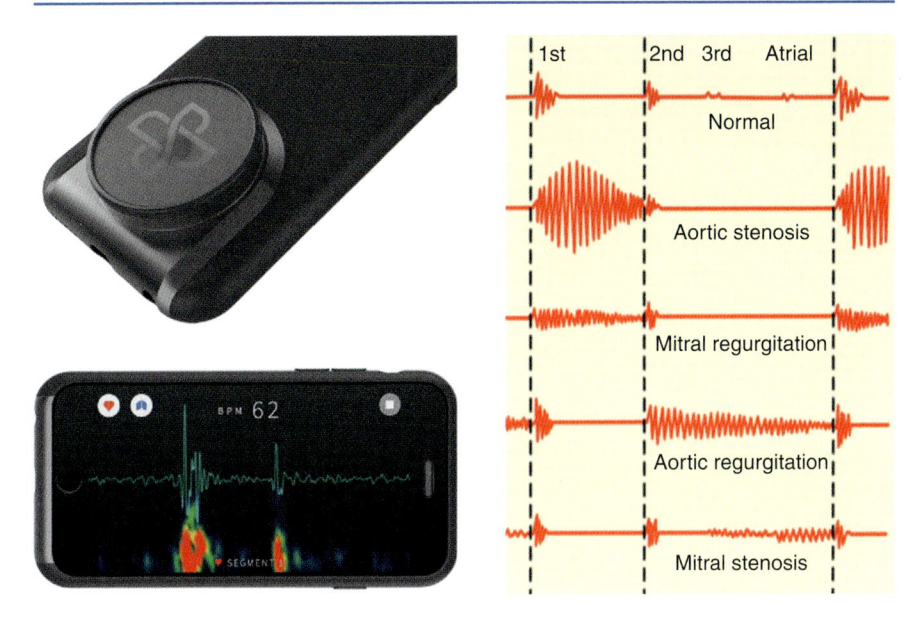

Fig. 50.1 Digital stethoscope. The stethoscope membrane is part of the phone case. The sound is digitized, allowing "visualization" and a "Shazam-like" identification of heart murmurs (From [15] with permission)

USA), uses smartphone camera-based photoplethysmography measurements of the pulse waveform to measure the pulsatile changes in light intensity reflected from a finger placed simultaneously on the LED smartphone flash and on the smartphone camera [18]. In 1013 patients in a primary care outpatient screening setting, it was shown that the Cardiio Rhythm application had a sensitivity of 93% and specificity of 98% for detecting atrial fibrillation [19]. A photoplethysmography measurement only lasted 17 s per patient and was performed under physician supervision to avoid artifacts by improper finger placement or movement resulting in false-positive EKG readings [19]. Future studies need to show the feasibility and reliability for at home self-screening. Integrated into patients' own smartphones without the need for additional hardware, this application could enable population-wide screening for atrial fibrillation [19].

Another randomized controlled trial used the single lead handheld EKG monitor AliveCor Kardia (AliveCor; Mountain View, CA, USA) connected to a WiFi-enabled mobile device with additional sensors embedded into the device's case to screen ambulatory patients ≤65 years of age at an increased risk of stroke for atrial fibrillation [20]. Patients in the control group were followed up as normal by their regular practitioner, whereas the intervention group carried out twice-weekly (and additionally on subjective symptoms) 30-s single lead EKG recordings that were transmitted wirelessly to a secure server for assessment. The primary outcome was the time until diagnosis of atrial fibrillation during a 12-month period. The study showed a significant superiority in the detection probability of atrial fibrillation in patients monitored with the smartphone EKG compared to control group patients. However, smartphone-EKG monitoring resulted in a high rate of false-positive readings. Point-of-care atrial fibrillation screening using the AliveCor Kardia monitor in 772 patients in internal medicine practices was feasible and also showed a high rate of false-positive results [21]. Nevertheless, the authors described a significant educational benefit after the screening, which could help create patient awareness for morbidities associated with atrial fibrillation. Further technological advances and evaluations in larger trials could improve the potential of this monitoring device for screening for atrial fibrillation in patients at risk.

EKG tracking with the AliveCor monitor may even detect myocardial ischemia according to a small pilot study that showed excellent correlation between conventional 12-lead EKG and the smartphone-EKG tracings [22]. Based on these findings, a larger, observational, multicenter trial is currently being conducted [23], comparing the diagnostic accuracy to diagnose ST-elevation myocardial infarction (STEMI) of the single lead smartphone EKG compared to the standard 12-lead EKG. The results will indicate whether smartphone EKG could become a potential point-of-care method to simplify the early detection of STEMI, thereby reducing the time until treatment initiation.

50.4 Blood Pressure

Blood pressure is a key variable of the cardiovascular system. Its serial or continuous measurement is a crucial component of hemodynamic monitoring in many fields of medicine. It is well established that hypotension is associated with organ dysfunction in patients having surgery [4] and critically ill patients [24], stressing the need to prevent even short periods of hypotension [25]. Chronic arterial hypertension, on the other hand, is a modifiable major risk factor for adverse cardiovascular events with a high prevalence in the population [26]. Accurate blood pressure monitoring is essential to diagnose and accurately treat chronic arterial hypertension. Since gold standard measurements using an invasive arterial catheter are restricted to the operating room and ICU, in other settings, blood pressure is usually measured with upper-arm cuff oscillometry, a method with limited accuracy [27]. In addition, ubiquitous periodical blood pressure measurement at home to screen for hypertension is not common practice.

The integration of blood pressure measurements into suitable mobile wireless devices could tackle some of these problems and is currently being promoted, resulting in numerous new applications and tools. The CareTaker (Empirical Technologies Cooperation, Charlottesville, Virginia, USA) is a low-pressure finger cuff connected to a piezoelectric wrist sensor that converts pressure pulsations into a derivative voltage signal and allows wireless recording and display of arterial pressure waveforms on mobile devices [28, 29]. A good correlation was shown between this noninvasive blood pressure measurement method and conventional invasive blood pressure measurement at the radial artery in patients having major abdominal surgery [29]. Future studies need to evaluate how this method can be applied for monitoring blood pressure at home or on general wards, thus potentially improving patient safety by early detection of blood pressure dysregulation.

Another wireless and integrated blood pressure measurement method, the oscillometric finger pressing method [30], is based on photoplethysmography using the preinstalled force sensors in smartphones. The user presses his fingertip against the phone, steadily increasing the external pressure on the underlying artery, thus causing blood volume oscillations and increasing applied pressure to the mobile device, while the mobile device serves as a sensor, calculating blood pressure from the measurement (Fig. 50.2) [30]. The method still needs further improvement to

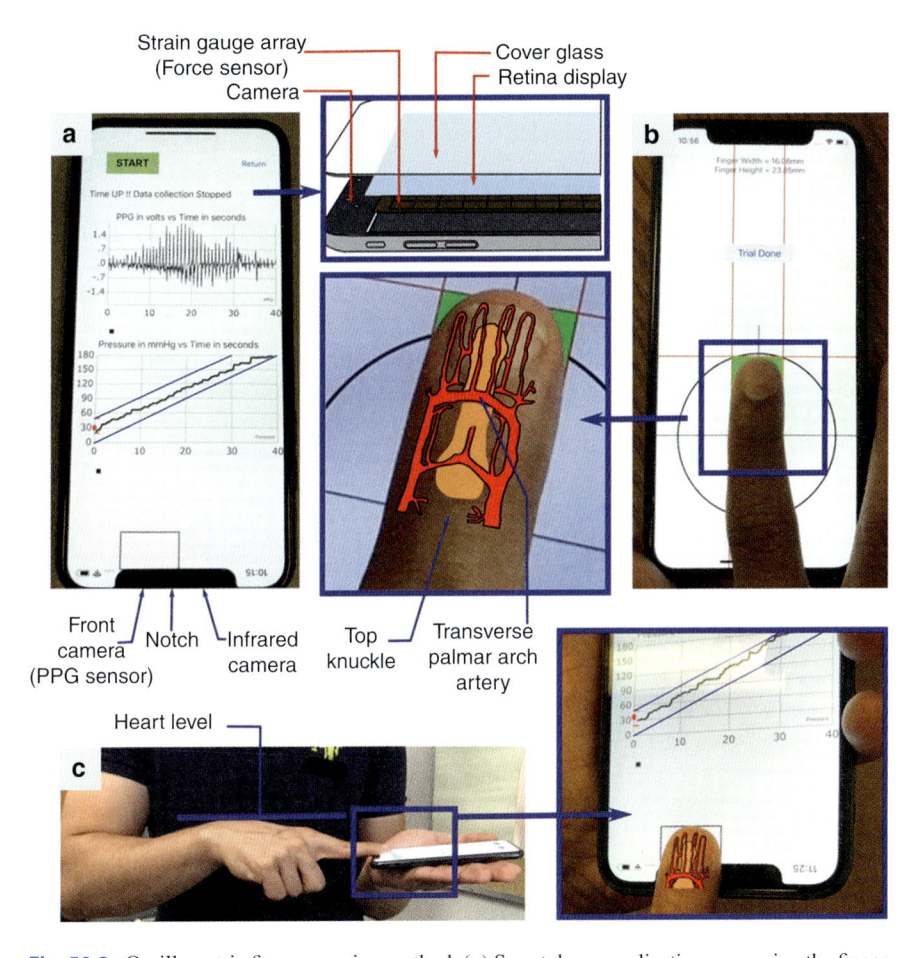

Fig. 50.2 Oscillometric finger pressing method. (**a**) Smartphone application measuring the finger pressure via the force sensor under the smartphone screen and finger blood volume oscillations via the phone front camera. (**b**) Capturing of fingertip width and height during initialization of the measurement. (**c**) Measurement holding the smartphone horizontally at heart level: placing the fingertip within a rectangular box of the previously captured finger width and height, followed by increased pressing to maintain the pressure within the two blue target lines (Modified from [30] under the terms of the Creative Commons license)

generate reliable results as, for example, the position of the mobile device can affect measured blood pressure values significantly [30].

Recently, the transdermal optical imaging method for contactless blood pressure measurements was presented [31]. This method analyzes facial blood flow data from facial videos captured with a smartphone camera using advanced machine learning algorithms. In an observational study including 1328 normotensive adults, the transdermal optical imaging blood pressure measurements showed a clinically acceptable accuracy (defined as a mean of the differences of 5 ± 8 mmHg) compared to the reference method (upper-arm cuff oscillometry) under well-controlled study conditions [31]. Provided that future studies validate the accuracy of transdermal optical imaging in hypo- and hypertensive patients in a self-monitoring setting, this noninvasive, contactless, and integrated tool could improve patient monitoring and treatment adherence.

There is a risk of novelty blindness with many new applications and tools constantly becoming available, making it tempting to integrate them into clinical practice without proper validation of their clinical value [32]. For example more than 140,000 people had already downloaded the blood pressure monitoring application "Instant Blood Pressure," before it was removed from the market 13 months later—likely linked to a publication showing that its measurements were highly inaccurate, and it missed 78% of hypertensive individuals [32].

Nevertheless, ubiquitously available blood pressure monitoring through mobile technology could help create awareness, empower patients to improve their treatment adherence, and potentially reduce the incidence of cardiovascular morbidities.

50.5 Advanced Hemodynamic Monitoring

In surgical and critically ill patients, changes in cardiovascular dynamics need to be recognized instantaneously to identify underlying pathophysiologic causes, optimize hemodynamic status, and eventually improve patient outcome. Assessment of the intravascular fluid status plays a key role in this process, and—besides functional tests—dynamic cardiac preload variables such as pulse pressure variation (PPV) and stroke volume variation (SVV) can be used to assess fluid responsiveness in mechanically ventilated patients in sinus rhythm [33]. The accurate prediction of fluid responsiveness is essential as both complications due to hypervolemia (primarily causing tissue edema) as well as hypovolemia (leading to peripheral hypoperfusion) are detrimental to patient outcome [34]. To assess PPV, advanced hemodynamic monitoring technology is needed because manual PPV calculation is time consuming and visual PPV estimation is not reliable [35]. A new tool, the Capstesia smartphone application (Galenic App, Vitoria-Gasteiz, Spain), was developed to automatically calculate PPV and cardiac output from a digital photograph of any monitor screen displaying invasive arterial pressure waves. In a simulator study, a good correlation between PPV calculated by the Capstesia application and PPV calculated manually was observed [36]. Recent studies showed that PPV calculated by the Capstesia application and PPV obtained from an established pulse contour analysis monitors correlated well in cardiac surgery patients [37] and patients having major oncological surgery (i.e., urogynecological, gastrointestinal, or thoracic) [38]. More studies are needed to investigate the clinical usefulness and the impact of using this application on patient outcome.

The evaluation of global cardiac performance is key in cardiology and perioperative and intensive care medicine. An established variable to assess individual cardiac performance, e.g., cardiac contractility, is to measure the left ventricular ejection fraction (LVEF). Currently this assessment is either done noninvasively with transthoracic echocardiography or (with significantly higher costs) through cardiac magnetic resonance imaging (MRI) or invasively via transesophageal echocardiography or angiography. These procedures take time and are thus not well suited to rapidly assess sudden or unexpected changes in cardiac performance. Hemodynamic variations impeding the LVEF in the intraoperative or ICU setting can be caused by changes in preload and/or afterload [39] and need rapid diagnosis and compensation. A recently developed application for the assessment of the LVEF with a smartphone camera positioned on the carotid artery captures a signal from skin displacement images during the cardiac cycle and analyzes them to extract hidden oscillations (also known as intrinsic frequencies) [40]. An observational comparison study in 72 volunteers, aged 20–92 years, showed a significant correlation ($r = 0.74$) between LVEF computed using the intrinsic frequencies algorithm and cardiac MRI measurement. However, 50% of patients with an LVEF <40% were not detected, and the limits of agreement between the two methods were wide (±19%) [40, 41].

50.6 Blood Transfusion Management

Of further key importance in optimizing cardiovascular dynamics and oxygen delivery are adequate fluid resuscitation and blood transfusion in case of intraoperative blood loss. However, quantifying intraoperative blood loss in an objective and timely manner is challenging, not standardized, and therefore often inaccurate. In the era of patient blood management, it is well established that intraoperative blood transfusions are associated with an increased risk of perioperative morbidity, reinforcing the need to prevent unnecessary intraoperative transfusions [42]. Better objectivity could be achieved with a recently developed application (Triton OR; Gauss Surgical, Palo Alto, CA), quantifying blood loss in surgical sponges and suction canisters. The Triton application analyzes a photograph of the surgical sponges and suction canisters to calculate the hemoglobin mass present and to correspondingly extrapolate an estimated blood loss in real time. In validation studies, the precision to accurately assess blood loss with the Triton application was higher than with established methods like the gravimetric method or visual estimation [43, 44].

50.7 Ultrasound

The use of ultrasound imaging is ubiquitous and indispensable in medical care. Small, handheld, and pocket-sized ultrasound probes offer point-of-care ultrasound at the bedside [45], not only for cardiologists but also in perioperative and intensive care medicine. More widespread implementation of ultrasound may be facilitated by using mobile technology since echo probes can also be directly connected to smartphones or other mobile devices [12] either via cable or via wireless connections. This integration has the potential to minimize costs compared to conventional ultrasound equipment, offers bedside assessment and recording of pathologies, and enables subsequent transfer of images to and evaluation by remote specialists. Access to remote expertise can help guide critical decision-making, e.g., assessing potential organ donors in remote areas at any time [46].

50.8 Sensor Technology

New biosensor materials [47] and other technical developments will—in the near future—enable miniaturized devices to be used for continuous monitoring of hemodynamic and other physiological variables inside and outside the hospital. Innovations in micro- and nanoelectronic mechanical systems may lead to the development of small, adhesive sensors, e.g., able to provide arterial pressure signals [48]. Other sensors, such as noninvasive electromagnetic monitoring systems, may detect changes in lung fluid content to monitor and manage pulmonary congestion in heart failure patients [49].

Technological start-ups and giants like Apple and Google have discovered this potentially interesting market, resulting in competitive efforts to contribute to developing and investigating feasible and smart sensor technology.

50.9 Conclusion

Mobile devices offer noninvasive, small, wireless, and integrated hemodynamic monitoring strategies. Noninvasive mobile devices have the potential to improve patient monitoring, expand the use of real-time hemodynamic monitoring to a broader patient population—and even facilitate ward and home monitoring. Capturing and recording hemodynamic alterations using mobile devices and applications may facilitate objective and timely clinical decisions and improve patient treatment adherence. However, serious validation studies of new applications and tools are a necessity before their clinical adoption. A key challenge is the huge amount of data acquired through continuous monitoring. Data storage and privacy as well as intelligent assessment algorithms to prevent false-alarm fatigue are crucial to reliably implement mobile technology into everyday healthcare.

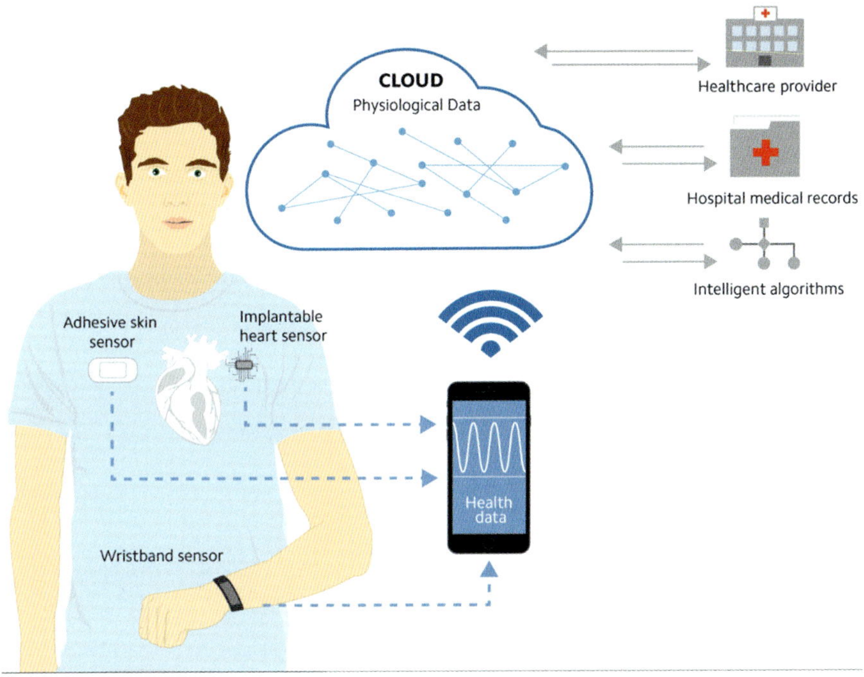

Fig. 50.3 Mobile devices for hemodynamic monitoring. Miniaturized wearable devices and adhesive or implantable sensors can record and transmit physiologic information to a mobile device and applications. Data can be assessed directly on the mobile device or in-app. It can also be sent to the cloud for data storage, where it can be made available to other healthcare providers. In the cloud, the data can be shared with personal health records, hospital information systems, or analyzed by individual physicians or intelligent algorithms

Mobile devices and their ubiquitous availability and connectivity could help to assess, monitor, and record cardiovascular dynamics. By continuously monitoring and identifying patients at risk, mobile devices could become a key element of our patient-centered healthcare (Fig. 50.3).

References

1. Oxford English Dictionary. 3 ed. Internet: Oxford University Press. "smartphone, n."
2. Eapen ZJ, Peterson ED. Can mobile health applications facilitate meaningful behavior change? Time for answers. JAMA. 2015;314:1236–7.
3. Sim I. Mobile devices and health. N Engl J Med. 2019;381:956–68.
4. Sessler DI, Bloomstone JA, Aronson S, et al. Perioperative quality initiative consensus statement on intraoperative blood pressure, risk and outcomes for elective surgery. Br J Anaesth. 2019;122:563–74.
5. Vincent JL, Pelosi P, Pearse R, et al. Perioperative cardiovascular monitoring of high-risk patients: a consensus of 12. Crit Care. 2015;19:224.

6. Vincent JL, Rhodes A, Perel A, et al. Clinical review: update on hemodynamic monitoring—a consensus of 16. Crit Care. 2011;15:229.
7. McGillion MH, Duceppe E, Allan K, et al. Postoperative remote automated monitoring: need for and state of the science. Can J Cardiol. 2018;34:850–62.
8. Vincent JL, Einav S, Pearse R, et al. Improving detection of patient deterioration in the general hospital ward environment. Eur J Anaesthesiol. 2018;35:325–33.
9. Sun Z, Sessler DI, Dalton JE, et al. Postoperative hypoxemia is common and persistent: a prospective blinded observational study. Anesth Analg. 2015;121:709–15.
10. Jones D, Mitchell I, Hillman K, Story D. Defining clinical deterioration. Resuscitation. 2013;84:1029–34.
11. Sessler DI, Saugel B. Beyond 'failure to rescue': the time has come for continuous ward monitoring. Br J Anaesth. 2019;122:304–6.
12. Michard F. Smartphones and e-tablets in perioperative medicine. Korean J Anesthesiol. 2017;70:493–9.
13. Michard F, Barrachina B, Schoettker P. Is your smartphone the future of physiologic monitoring? Intensive Care Med. 2019;45:869–71.
14. Michard F, Badheka A. Toward the 'Shazam-Like' identification of valve diseases with digital auscultation? Am J Med. 2019;132:e595–e6.
15. Michard F. A sneak peek into digital innovations and wearable sensors for cardiac monitoring. J Clin Monit Comput. 2017;31:253–9.
16. Lip GYH, Tse HF, Lane DA. Atrial fibrillation. Lancet. 2012;379:648–61.
17. Sposato LA, Cipriano LE, Saposnik G, Vargas ER, Riccio PM, Hachinski V. Diagnosis of atrial fibrillation after stroke and transient ischaemic attack: a systematic review and meta-analysis. Lancet Neurol. 2015;14:377–87.
18. Scully CG, Lee J, Meyer J, et al. Physiological parameter monitoring from optical recordings with a mobile phone. IEEE Trans Biomed Eng. 2012;59:303–6.
19. Chan PH, Wong CK, Poh YC, et al. Diagnostic performance of a smartphone-based photoplethysmographic application for atrial fibrillation screening in a primary care setting. J Am Heart Assoc. 2016;5:e003428.
20. Halcox JPJ, Wareham K, Cardew A, et al. Assessment of remote heart rhythm sampling using the AliveCor heart monitor to screen for atrial fibrillation: the REHEARSE-AF study. Circulation. 2017;136:1784–94.
21. Rosenfeld LE, Amin AN, Hsu JC, Oxner A, Hills MT, Frankel DS. The Heart Rhythm Society/American College of Physicians Atrial Fibrillation Screening and Education Initiative. Heart Rhythm. 2019;16:e59–65.
22. Muhlestein JB, Le V, Albert D, et al. Smartphone ECG for evaluation of STEMI: results of the ST LEUIS pilot study. J Electrocardiol. 2015;48:249–59.
23. Barbagelata A, Bethea CF, Severance HW, et al. Smartphone ECG for evaluation of ST-segment elevation myocardial infarction (STEMI): design of the ST LEUIS international multicenter study. J Electrocardiol. 2018;51:260–4.
24. Maheshwari K, Nathanson BH, Munson SH, et al. The relationship between ICU hypotension and in-hospital mortality and morbidity in septic patients. Intensive Care Med. 2018;44:857–67.
25. Sudfeld S, Brechnitz S, Wagner JY, et al. Post-induction hypotension and early intraoperative hypotension associated with general anaesthesia. Br J Anaesth. 2017;119:57–64.
26. Lewington S, Clarke R, Qizilbash N, et al. Age-specific relevance of usual blood pressure to vascular mortality: a meta-analysis of individual data for one million adults in 61 prospective studies. Lancet. 2002;360:1903–13.
27. Muntner P, Shimbo D, Carey RM, et al. Measurement of blood pressure in humans: a scientific statement from the American Heart Association. Hypertension. 2019;73:e35–66.
28. Baruch MC, Warburton DE, Bredin SS, Cote A, Gerdt DW, Adkins CM. Pulse decomposition analysis of the digital arterial pulse during hemorrhage simulation. Nonlinear Biomed Phys. 2011;5:1.

29. Gratz I, Deal E, Spitz F, et al. Continuous non-invasive finger cuff CareTaker® comparable to invasive intra-arterial pressure in patients undergoing major intra-abdominal surgery. BMC Anesthesiol. 2017;17:1–11.
30. Chandrasekhar A, Natarajan K, Yavarimanesh M, Mukkamala R. An iPhone application for blood pressure monitoring via the oscillometric finger pressing method. Sci Rep. 2018;8:13136.
31. Luo H, Yang D, Barszczyk A, et al. Smartphone-based blood pressure measurement using transdermal optical imaging technology. Circ Cardiovasc Imaging. 2019;12:e008857.
32. Plante TB, Urrea B, MacFarlane ZT, et al. Validation of the instant blood pressure smartphone app. JAMA Intern Med. 2016;176:700–2.
33. Monnet X, Marik PE, Teboul JL. Prediction of fluid responsiveness: an update. Ann Intensive Care. 2016;6:1–11.
34. Bellamy MC. Wet, dry or something else? Br J Anaesth. 2006;97:755–7.
35. Rinehart J, Islam T, Boud R, et al. Visual estimation of pulse pressure variation is not reliable: a randomized simulation study. J Clin Monit Comput. 2012;26:191–6.
36. Desebbe O, Joosten A, Suehiro K, et al. A novel mobile phone application for pulse pressure variation monitoring based on feature extraction technology: a method comparison study in a simulated environment. Anesth Analg. 2016;123:105–13.
37. Joosten A, Boudart C, Vincent JL, et al. Ability of a new smartphone pulse pressure variation and cardiac output application to predict fluid responsiveness in patients undergoing cardiac surgery. Anesth Analg. 2019;128(6):1145–51.
38. Shah SB, Bhargava AK, Hariharan U, Vishvakarma G, Jain CR, Kansal A. Cardiac output monitoring: a comparative prospective observational study of the conventional cardiac output monitor Vigileo and the new smartphone-based application Capstesia. Indian J Anaesth. 2018;62:584–91.
39. Scolletta S, Bodson L, Donadello K, et al. Assessment of left ventricular function by pulse wave analysis in critically ill patients. Intensive Care Med. 2013;39:1025–33.
40. Pahlevan NM, Rinderknecht DG, Tavallali P, et al. Noninvasive iPhone measurement of left ventricular ejection fraction using intrinsic frequency methodology. Crit Care Med. 2017;45:1115–20.
41. Michard F, Range G, Biais M. Smartphones to assess cardiac function: Novelty blindness or fresh perspectives? Crit Care Med. 2017;45:e1199–e201.
42. Mueller MM, Van Remoortel H, Meybohm P, et al. Patient blood management: recommendations from the 2018 Frankfurt Consensus Conference. JAMA. 2019;321:983–97.
43. Holmes AA, Konig G, Ting V, et al. Clinical evaluation of a novel system for monitoring surgical hemoglobin loss. Anesth Analg. 2014;119:588–94.
44. Saoud F, Stone A, Rahman M, et al. 163: Quantification of blood loss during cesarean delivery using an iPad based application (Triton). Am J Obstet Gynecol. 2019;220:S122–3; (abst)
45. Platz E, Solomon SD. Point-of-care echocardiography in the accountable care organization era. Circ Cardiovasc Imaging. 2012;5:676–82.
46. Scali MC, de Azevedo Bellagamba CC, Ciampi Q, et al. Stress echocardiography with smartphone: real-time remote reading for regional wall motion. Int J Card Imaging. 2017;33:1731–6.
47. Boland CS, Khan U, Ryan G, et al. Sensitive electromechanical sensors using viscoelastic graphene-polymer nanocomposites. Science. 2016;354:1257–60.
48. Michard F. Hemodynamic monitoring in the era of digital health. Ann Intensive Care. 2016;6:15.
49. Amir O, Rappaport D, Zafrir B, Abraham WT. A novel approach to monitoring pulmonary congestion in heart failure: initial animal and clinical experiences using remote dielectric sensing technology. Congest Heart Fail. 2013;19:149–55.

Artificial Intelligence in the Intensive Care Unit

G. Gutierrez

51.1 Introduction

The past century has witnessed a massive increase in our ability to perform complex calculations. The development of the transistor in the 1950s, followed by the silicone integrated circuit, accelerated those capabilities and gave rise to what is commonly known as Moore's Law. According to this principle, the number of transistors packed into a dense integrated circuit doubles every 2 years. The corollary is that computation speed also doubles at 2-year intervals. Figure 51.1 is a graphical interpretation of Moore's Law, showing an exponential increase in computational power, in terms of calculations per second that can be purchased with $1000 (constant US, 2015). According to that graph, computing power has increased by a factor of 10^{18} from the mechanical analytical engine of the early 1900s to today's core I7 Quad chip found in personal laptop computers.

The growth in computing power was made possible by the relentless downsizing of integrated circuits, with some components being produced in the sub-100 nm range. As we approach the physical limits of silicone chip downsizing, other materials are being developed. A likely candidate is the carbon nanotube, composed of a single sheet of carbon atoms arranged in a hexagonal pattern. When rolled into itself, the sheet becomes a tube approximately 2 nm in diameter, capable of forming different circuit elements. This nascent technology, along with the development of quantum computing, assures the durability of Moore's Law well into the future.

As processors grew in power, and personal computers became ubiquitous appliances, the stage was set for the development of the Internet, a digital network that morphed from the ARPANET, a communication structure designed by the U.S. Advanced Research Projects Agency (ARPA) to transfer information among

---

G. Gutierrez (✉)
Pulmonary, Critical Care and Sleep Medicine Division, The George Washington University, Washington, DC, USA
e-mail: ggutierrez@mfa.gwu.edu

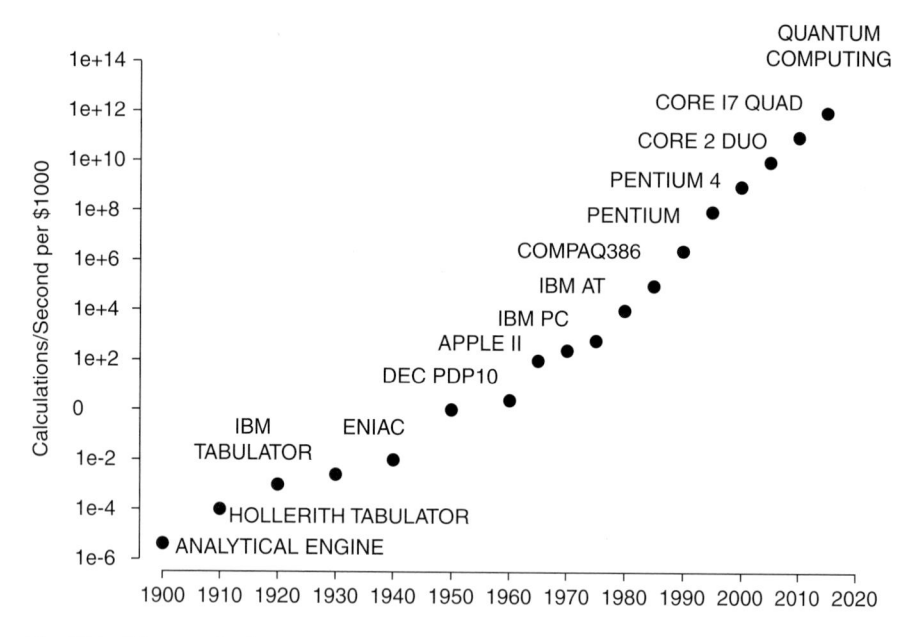

Fig. 51.1 The growth of computer power, based on calculations per second purchased by $1000 USD (constant 2015) during the past century. Also shown are significant developments in technology associated with increases in computer power. Modified from https://www.flickr.com/photos/jurvetson/25046013104 (with license). Original graph in Ray Kurzweil. "The singularity is near: When humans transcend biology," p67, The Viking Press, 2006

computers located at remote distances. The internet promoted the free dissemination of software and provided the impetus for computer scientists to develop powerful algorithms aimed at simulating human intelligence.

According to the Encyclopedia Britannica, artificial intelligence (AI) refers to a system "endowed with the intellectual processes characteristic of humans, such as the ability to reason, discover meaning, generalize, or learn from past experience." AI computer systems are able to perform tasks normally requiring human intelligence and that are considered "smart" by humans. AI systems act on information, such as controlling a self-driving automobile or influencing consumer shopping decisions.

In the area of medicine, AI has been used in drug discovery, personalized diagnostics and therapeutics, molecular biology, bioinformatics, and medical imaging. AI applications are also capable of discerning patterns of disease by scrutinizing and analyzing massive amounts of digital information stored in electronic medical records. In a recent proposal aimed at regulating AI software in medical devices, the U.S. Food and Drug Administration states that "Artificial intelligence-based technologies have the potential to transform healthcare by deriving new and important insights from the vast amount of data generated during the delivery of healthcare every day" [1].

51.2 Machine Learning

Human intelligence is defined by the mental capability to think abstractly, use reason to solve problems, make plans, comprehend complex ideas, and learn from experience [2]. Much of human intelligence involves pattern recognition, a process that matches a visual or other type of stimuli, to similar information stored in our brains. Although endowed with abstract thinking and capable of sublime leaps in imagination, humans have a limited capacity for memory. It is estimated that the brain cannot store more than four "chunks" of short-term memory at any one time [3]. Moreover, humans find it difficult to think in terms of n-dimensional spaces or visualize patterns embedded into large quantities of data. Conversely, computers have vast memory storage, excel at handling multidimensional problems and can discern even small or "fuzzy" associations within massive data collections.

The use of computers to guide the treatment of critically ill patients is not a new concept. With uneven results, computerized systems have been proposed in the past to monitor ICU patients [4], manage patients on mechanical ventilators [5, 6], guide care in patients with acute respiratory distress syndrome (ARDS) [7], and manage arterial oxygenation [8]. These early computer systems were programmed with highly specific and sequential IF/THEN/ELSE logical expressions that assessed the validity of a condition based on accepted physiological principles and/or clinical experience (Fig. 51.2). According to these expressions, IF a given condition was judged to be "true," THEN the program executed instruction 1, ELSE, it executed instruction 2.

AI is based on a fundamentally different approach to traditional computer programming. Instead of instructing the computer to evaluate a given condition, or to perform a specific task according to detailed programmed instructions, AI

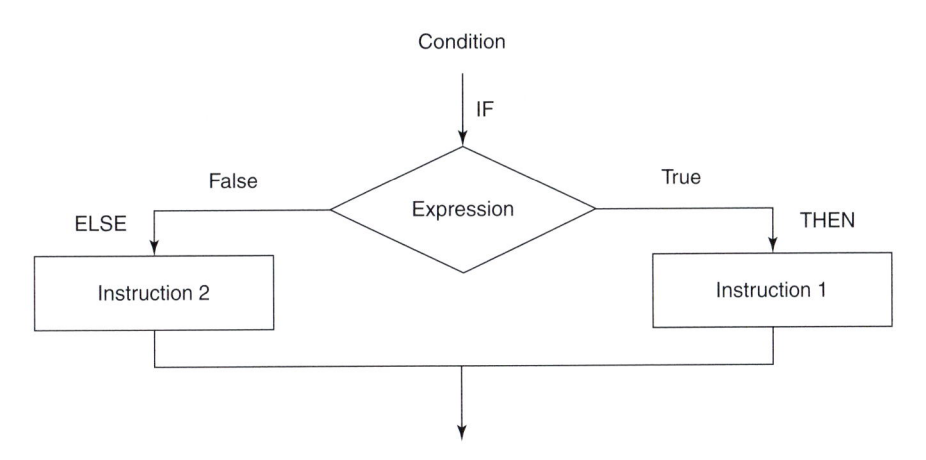

Fig. 51.2 A logical IF expression. The condition is evaluated by the expression, and Instruction 1 is executed if TRUE, otherwise, Instruction 2

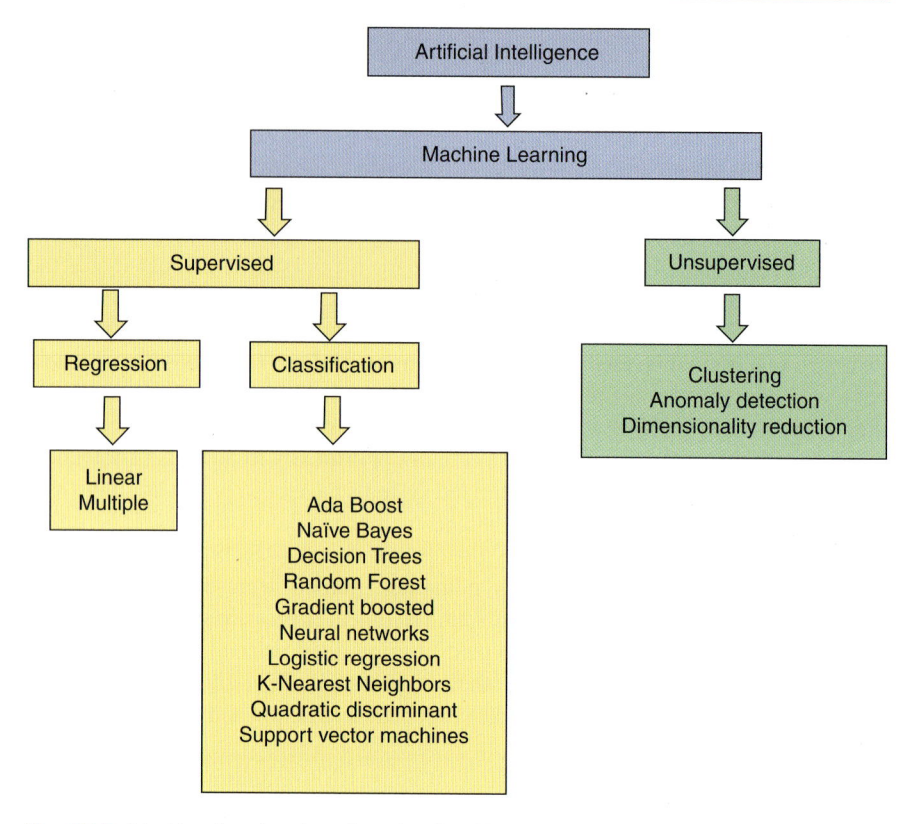

Fig. 51.3 Machine learning is a branch of artificial intelligence encompassing two major approaches: supervised and unsupervised learning. Shown under each branch are algorithm types used in model development

algorithms, in a manner similar to the way children absorb knowledge, learn from exposure to numerous examples. AI algorithms establish their own rules of behavior and can even improve on their "intelligence" by incorporating additional experiences resulting from the application of these rules.

Machine learning is a subset of AI in which machines learn or extract knowledge from the available data, but do not act on the information. Machine learning combines statistical analysis techniques with computer science to produce algorithms capable of "statistical learning." Broadly speaking, there are two types of machine learning structures: supervised and unsupervised (Fig. 51.3).

51.2.1 Supervised Machine Learning

The objective of supervised machine learning is to develop an algorithm capable of predicting a unique output when provided with a specific input. In other words, the machine is shown examples of input (x) and its corresponding output (y), such that

$y = f(x)$. Machine learning is predicated on large sets of data containing myriad examples that relate one or several input variables to a single output. The expectations are that the resulting algorithm will deliver accurate predictions when exposed to new and never before seen data. Supervised learning requires a great deal of human effort when building large datasets to train and test the algorithm. There are two major types of supervised learning: regression and classification.

51.2.1.1 Regression Learning
Most clinicians are familiar with regression analysis, a statistical technique producing a mathematical expression relating one input variable to another (linear regression) or many input variables to one dependent variable (multiple regression). In regression analysis, the output is a continuous function of the input. In other words, the predicted variable will change in concert with the input variables. Regression is used commonly to test hypotheses involving causal relationships, with the choice of model being based on its significance and goodness of fit.

51.2.1.2 Classification Learning
Classification supervised learning is a form of pattern recognition designed to predict a single, nonnumerical output, or "class," from a predefined list of possibilities. Classifier algorithms are trained with many lines of data, with each line having several input variables and one desired output. For example, a model designed to identify a breed of dog may be trained with data listing their traits or characteristics, e.g., height, type of hair, and length of tail. Each line will be associated with a specific breed. Once trained, the model can be asked to predict the dog breed when given new set of input variables. Two important steps are needed to build a classifier model. The first is to establish the number of classes the model will be required to identify. The second is to identify the number of variables required to describe the classes. Fewer variables and classes require less training data and result in simpler and more accurate models. The simplest classification model is the binary kind, in which the model is asked to choose between a "Yes" and a "No" answer.

Classes may consist of physical objects (chair, table, etc.), medical conditions (e.g., sepsis, ARDS, chronic obstructive pulmonary disease [COPD], etc.), clinical or physiological observations (e.g., different types of arrhythmia or ventilator asynchronies). Each class is associated with a number of input variables common to all classes. In machine learning parlance, input variables are known as "features," with each line of data, or "instance," containing several features and a single class.

Let us say we want to develop a classifier algorithm to identify five different kinds of animal (Fig. 51.4). In this example, each line of data has one animal class and several features to describe the animal's characteristic, such as sea or land dwelling, fish or mammal. This is a very simple example having only one instance per class. The model, therefore, would be totally inadequate if its purpose were to differentiate among different dog or cat breeds. In that case, many more instances would be needed to describe different types of dogs and cats. The more specific one wishes to be, the more features are needed to describe the classes. On the other hand, increasing the number of features results in complex models that require

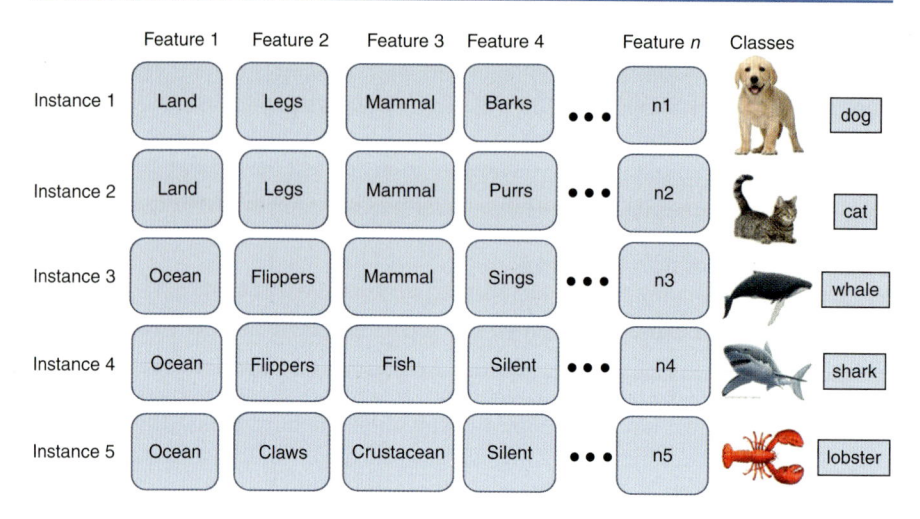

Fig. 51.4 An example of a classification problem showing features describing five classes of animal. Each line represents an instance

greater computing power and longer time to run, a condition termed "the curse of dimensionality." An important guiding principle in machine learning is the truism that "less is best."

In mathematical terms, a feature matrix contains n features and m instances, and it is associated with an m length classification vector:

$$x11 \quad x12... \quad x1n = y1$$
$$x12 \quad x22... \quad x2n = y2$$
$$x1m \quad x2m... \quad xnm = ym.$$

Developing a classifier model: Perhaps the most important step in developing a machine learning model is to have a clear definition of the problem and to determine its suitability for machine learning. The next step is to determine the size of the feature matrix and the classification vector (Fig. 51.5). Whereas humans develop generalized concepts on the basis of just a few examples, training a machine learning algorithm requires large quantities of data. The creation of a large feature matrix with its classification vector is accomplished by gathering as many instances as possible. Once satisfied that we have collected an adequate number of examples to be presented to the computer, we split the feature matrix into a "training" dataset, for model development, and a "test" dataset. The data are split by a random process that assigns instances from the original data to each dataset. A common practice is to use 70% or 80% of the data for training and the remainder for testing.

The purpose of the "test" dataset is to assess the algorithm's accuracy when exposed to never before seen data. Accuracy is defined as the percentage of correct answers made by the algorithm on the unknown "test" dataset. Should accuracy fall below a chosen expected value, we can choose to gather more "training" data or to use another type of machine learning algorithm altogether.

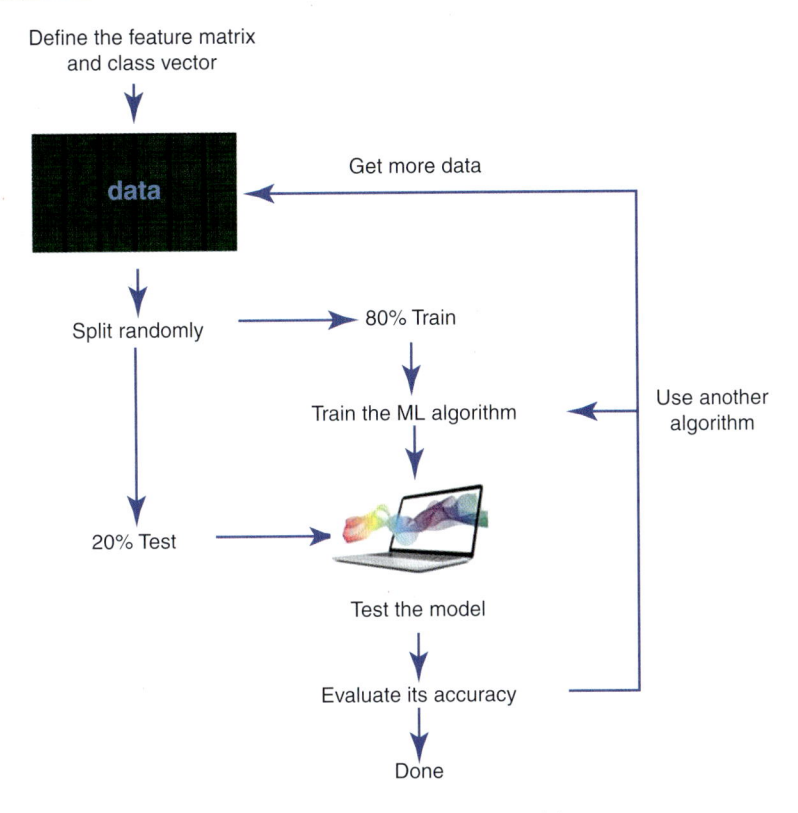

Fig. 51.5 The process of creating a machine learning (ML) model

Several types of classifier algorithms may be used to create the machine learning model. Among them are decision trees, random forests, k-nearest neighbors, and many others (Fig. 51.3). A popular type of classifier algorithm is the neural network, modeled on the way human neurons are thought to process information. The basic element of the neural network, the perceptron, produces a single binary output from several inputs. A neural network results from the interacting of several perceptrons. Advanced machine learning systems encompassing several layers of stacked complex neural networks are called deep learning.

It is beyond the purpose of this chapter to describe the theory and application of these algorithms (listed in Fig. 51.3), but the reader interested in pursuing this line of investigation can access "scikit-learn" (https://scikit-learn.org/stable/), an open source machine learning library written with the Python programming language (https://www.python.org/). This library of programs makes it relatively easy to develop classification supervised machine learning algorithms.

When building a classifier model, it is imperative to generalize its utility to make accurate predictions using both the "training" and the "test" datasets. One should beware of models of high complexity that may conform closely to the "training" set, but have poor accuracy when applied to the "test" dataset, a phenomenon called "overfitting."

51.2.2 Unsupervised Machine Learning

In this type of machine learning, no instructions are given to the algorithm on how to process the data. Instead, the computer is asked to extract knowledge from a large set of unclassified data with no known output or a set of rules. Given the lack of label information, a major challenge for the investigator when evaluating an unsupervised algorithm is how to determine the utility of the results, or whether the right output has been achieved. Unsupervised algorithms, however, can be very useful in exploratory attempts to understand large collections of data. The techniques most commonly used are clustering, anomaly detection, and dimensionality reduction.

In clustering, algorithms are asked to identify or partition large data sets into subsections and patterns sharing similar characteristics. In anomaly detection the algorithm is asked to detect atypical patterns in the dataset, such as searching for outliers. Dimensionality reduction is useful when analyzing data having many features, or dimensions. These algorithms may be able to present the data in a simpler form, summarizing its essential characteristics and making it easier for humans or other machine learning algorithms to understand.

An important point to keep in mind is that no machine learning algorithm, regardless of its accuracy, is the only possible choice for a model. Other algorithms may be capable of providing a good fit and derive additional useful inferences from the data. For those wishing to delve deeper into the development of machine learning models, a good source of information is the book by Müller and Guido [9] and the website (https://www.geeksforgeeks.org/learning-model-building-scikit-learn-python-machine-learning-library/).

51.3 AI Applications in Critical Care

There are numerous opportunities in the hospital setting to apply AI. Unsupervised machine learning techniques have been used to explore massive amounts of data encoded in electronic medical records. Models have been developed to obtain important information in a patient's chart [10] and identify high-cost patients [11]. Supervised machine learning algorithms, given their potential for automated pattern recognition of images, have proven their utility in radiology [12] and histopathology [13]. Machine learning has been used extensively in the fields of surgery, as it pertains to robotics [14], in cardiology [15] for early detection of heart failure [16], and in cancer research to classify tumor types and growth rates [17].

Although the introduction of machine learning to the ICU is in its infancy, several studies have already been published describing the application of this technology in the management of the critically ill patient. Some have used large population datasets to predict length of stay, ICU readmission and mortality rates, and the risks of developing medical complications or conditions such as sepsis and ARDS. Other studies have dealt with smaller datasets of clinical and physiological data to aid in the monitoring of patients undergoing ventilatory support.

51.3.1 Length of Stay

Houthooft et al. [18] trained a support vector machine model to forecast patient survival and length of stay using data from 14,480 patients. The model's area under the curve (AUC) for predicting a prolonged length of stay was 0.82. This is in contrast to a clinical study showing the accuracy of physicians to be only 53% when predicting ICU length of stay [19]. A hidden Markov model framework applied to physiological measurements taken during the first 48 h of ICU admission also predicted ICU length of stay with reasonable accuracy [20]. The problem of ICU readmission was investigated with a neural network algorithm applied to the Medical Information Mart for Intensive Care III (MIMIC-III) database. This is an open source, freely available database collected from patients treated in the critical care units of the Beth Israel Deaconess Medical Center between 2001 and 2012. The algorithm was able to identify patients at risk of ICU readmission with 0.74 sensitivity and AUC of 0.79 [21].

51.3.2 ICU Mortality

Awad et al. [22] applied several machine learning algorithms, including decision trees, random forest, and naïve Bayes to 11,722 first admission MIMIC-II data to predict ICU mortality. Features included demographic, physiological, and laboratory data. These models outperformed standard scoring systems, such as APACHE-II, sequential organ failure assessment (SOFA), and Simplified Acute Physiology Score (SAPS), a finding that was confirmed by the same group in a follow-up study using time-series analysis [23]. A Swedish system using artificial neural networks applied to >200,000 first-time ICU admissions also showed superior performance in predicting the risk of dying when compared to SAPS-3 [24]. Machine learning models have also been proposed to predict mortality in trauma [25] and pediatric ICU patients [26].

The abovementioned ICU survival models, while offering improved performance when compared to standard mortality prediction scoring systems, are somewhat cumbersome to use, require a large number of variables and have yet to be tested prospectively.

51.3.3 Complications and Risk Stratification

Yoon et al. [27] developed a method to predict instability in the ICU based on logistic regression and random forest models of electrocardiogram (EKG) measures of tachycardia, reporting an accuracy of 0.81 and AUC of 0.87. The publication of the study is accompanied by an excellent and highly recommended editorial by Vistisen et al. [28] that thoroughly analyzes the strengths and pitfalls of machine learning methods as predictors of complications in the ICU.

A recent study applied a random forest classifier to over 200,000 electronic health records of hospitalized patients to predict the occurrence of sepsis and septic shock. Although the algorithm was highly specific (98%), it only had a sensitivity of 26%, severely limiting its utility [29]. Other studies have been published describing the use of machine learning models in generating patient-specific risk scores for pulmonary emboli [30], risk stratification of ARDS [31], prediction of acute kidney injury in severely burned patients [32] and in general ICU populations [33], prediction of volume responsiveness after fluid administration [34] and identification of patients likely to develop complicated *Clostridium difficile* infection [35].

51.3.4 Mechanical Ventilation

Whereas present day mechanical ventilators work exceedingly well in delivering air to diseased lungs, they are "feed-forward" or open loop systems where the input signal, or mode of ventilation, is largely unaffected by its output, the adequacy of ventilation. As such, ventilators lack the capacity to assess the patient's response to the delivered breath. A desirable solution is the development of the autonomous ventilator, a device that could monitor the patient's response to ventilation continuously, while adjusting ventilatory parameters to provide the patient with a comfortable, optimally delivered breath. Although we are far from this ideal device, significant strides are being made toward making it into a reality.

Over the past decade, there has been considerable interest in detecting and classifying patient-ventilator asynchrony, a phenomenon indicating the degree of coupling or response of the patient to ventilatory support [36]. Machine learning methods of detecting patient-ventilator asynchrony have been based on morphological changes of the pressure and flow signals. Chen et al. [37] developed an algorithm to identify ineffective efforts from the maximum deflection of the expiratory portion of airway pressure and flow. Ineffective effort was present in 58% of the 24 patients enrolled in their study. Analysis of 5899 breaths yielded sensitivity and specificity for the detection of ineffective efforts >90%. An algorithm developed by Blanch at al [38]. compared a theoretical exponential expiratory flow curve to actual flow tracings. A deviation exceeding 42% was considered indicative of ineffective effort. They compared the predictions of the algorithm in a random selection of 1024 breaths obtained from 16 patients, to those made by five experts and reported 91.5% sensitivity and 91.7% specificity with 80.3% predictive value. As proof-of-concept, this group also reported monitoring airway signals in 51 mechanically ventilated patients and were able to predict the probability of an asynchrony occurring from one breath period to the next using a hidden Markov model [39]. The system used in these trials has been commercialized as Better Care®, and it is capable of acquiring, synchronizing, recording, and analyzing digital signals from bedside monitors and mechanical ventilators [38].

Rhem et al. [40] and Adams et al. [41] developed a set of algorithms to detect two types of asynchrony associated with dynamic hyperinflation, double triggering, and flow asynchrony. Based on a learning database of 5075 breaths from

16 patients, they developed logical operators to recognize double triggering based on bedside clinical rules. Dynamic hyperinflation was identified from the ratio of exhaled to inhaled tidal volume. The algorithms were validated with data drawn from another patient cohort ($n = 17$), resulting in sensitivity and specificity >90%.

Sottile at al. [42] evaluated several types of machine learning algorithms, including random forest, naïve Bayes, and AdaBoost on data recorded from 62 mechanically ventilated patients with or at risk of ARDS. They chose 116 features based on clinical insight and signal description and were able to determine the presence of synchronous breathing, as well as three types of patient-ventilator asynchrony, including double triggering, flow limited and ineffective triggering, with an AUC >0.89. The authors did acknowledge that their algorithm does not identify all types of patient-ventilator asynchrony, in particular premature ventilator terminated breaths, or cycling asynchronies.

Gholami et al. [43] trained a random forest classifier algorithm from a training data set produced by five experts who evaluated 1377 breath cycles from 11 mechanically ventilated patients to evaluate cycling asynchronies. Patients were ventilated with pressure-controlled volume ventilation. The model accurately detected the presence or absence of secondary synchrony with a sensitivity of 89%. Mulqueeny et al. [44] used a naïve Bayes machine learning algorithm with 21 features, including measures of respiratory rate, tidal volume, respiratory mechanics and expiratory flow morphology to a dataset of 5624 breaths manually classified by a single observer, resulting in an accuracy of 84%, but a sensitivity of only 59%. Loo et al. [45] trained a convolutional neural network with 5500 abnormal and 5500 normal breathing cycles aimed at developing an algorithm capable of separating normal from abnormal breathing cycles, reporting 96.9% sensitivity and 63.7% specificity.

51.4 The Issue of Accuracy Versus Reliability

The accuracy of a machine learning algorithm is judged by its ability to correctly predict the unseen test dataset. Models are created and tested with instances culled from the same data population, and it is common to find reports of algorithms having very high accuracy scores in the machine learning literature. Given a judicious selection of features, a sufficiently large number of instances, and a wise choice of algorithm, the most likely outcome will be a highly accurate model. If the data are true and verifiable, the model's predictions are also bound to be reliable. On the other hand, when a model trained with untested or faulty data is presented with data drawn from the same population, the predictions are likely to be accurate but totally unreliable. As some have succinctly put it, rubbish in, rubbish out.

This begs the question of what are the limits of model reliability. Whereas AI is able to consider numerous variables and minimize human bias in data classification, it cannot insure model reliability. Therefore, the greatest challenge when creating a clinical machine learning model lies in identifying the gold standard to be used in the classification. A great deal of what we see and do in medicine is highly subjective, and unanimity of opinion is seldom found among intensivists. For example, a study [46] on interobserver reliability of clinicians in diagnosing ARDS according to the Berlin definition found only a moderate degree of reliability (kappa = 0.50). The main driver of the variability was the interpretation of chest radiographs. Similar findings were noted in clinicians evaluating optic disk photographs for glaucoma (kappa 0.40–0.52) [47]. It is therefore unlikely that model reliability in the ICU will ever exceed 60–70%, even in the best of hands.

51.5 Conclusion

Experienced intensivists excel at collecting, classifying, and analyzing snapshots of clinical information to expeditiously reach a diagnosis and decide on treatment options. In the data-intensive environment of today's ICUs, however, intensivists must cope with a relentless flow of information, some of it useful, most of it not. According to a thoughtful essay by Alan Morris [48], intensivists must contend with no less than 236 variables when caring for patients on ventilatory support. The ability to catalog, correlate, and classify these variables on a continuous basis lies well beyond the capabilities of even the most knowledgeable and perceptive of clinicians.

The judicious application of AI technology can be of assistance in helping us deal with information overload. Machine learning algorithms have been used to analyze data stored in electronic medical records to predict ICU mortality and length of stay. They also have furthered our understanding of populations who may be at risk of disease progression or likely to experience medical complications. These retrospective studies, useful as they may be in the early identification and stratification of patients, represent only the low-lying fruit in AI research.

A more difficult task, but perhaps one with far greater potential, is the development of intelligent machine learning monitors capable of continuously assessing the human response to critical illness with a high degree of certainty. The development of such monitors will provide the knowledge and experience needed for the creation of the semi-autonomous ICU, an environment where intelligent machines provide most of the care delivered today by humans.

The full potential of AI will be realized once it becomes a trustworthy clinical adjunct to intensivists. By helping us cope with information overload, AI endowed machines may allow our faculties of reflection, imagination, and compassion to come to the fore when caring for fellow humans in distress. The future of AI in the ICU is indeed bright. As with all new technologies, there will be zealots and pharisees, ups and downs, elations and disappointments, as well as thorny ethical quandaries. I have no doubt, however, that AI is here to stay, and it behooves us to become familiar with this technology for the betterment of our patients.

References

1. Proposed Regulatory Framework for Modifications to Artificial Intelligence/Machine Learning (AI/ML)-Based Software as a Medical Device (SaMD). https://www.fda.gov/media/122535/download. Accessed 20 Aug 2019.
2. Gottfredson LS. Mainstream science on intelligence: an editorial with 52 signatories, history, and bibliography. Intelligence. 1997;24:13–23.
3. Gobet F, Clarkson G. Chunks in expert memory: evidence for the magical number four ... Or is it two? Memory. 2004;12:732–47.
4. Gardner RM, Scoville OP, West BJ, Bateman B, Cundick RM Jr, Clemmer TP. Integrated computer systems for monitoring of the critically ill. Proc Annu Symp Comput Appl Med Care. 1977;1:301–7.
5. Grossman R, Hew E, Aberman A. Assessment of the ability to manage patients on mechanical ventilators using a computer model. Acute Care. 1983–1984;10:95–102.
6. Ohlson KB, Westenskow DR, Jordan WS. A microprocessor based feedback controller for mechanical ventilation. Ann Biomed Eng. 1982;10:35–48.
7. Sittig DF, Gardner RM, Pace NL, Morris AH, Beck E. Computerized management of patient care in a complex, controlled clinical trial in the intensive care unit. Comput Methods Prog Biomed. 1989;30:77–84.
8. Henderson S, Crapo RO, Wallace CJ, East TD, Morris AH, Gardner RM. Performance of computerized protocols for the management of arterial oxygenation in an intensive care unit. Int J Clin Monit Comput. 1991-1992;8:271–80.
9. Müller AC, Guido S. Introduction to machine learning with Python: a guide for data scientists. Sebastopol, CA: O'Reilly Media; 2017.
10. Escobar GJ, Turk BJ, Ragins A, et al. Piloting electronic medical record-based early detection of inpatient deterioration in community hospitals. J Hosp Med. 2016;11(Suppl 1):S18–24.
11. Beam AL, Kohane IS. Big data and machine learning in health care. JAMA. 2018;319:1317–8.
12. Hosny A, Parmar C, Quackenbush J, Schwartz LH, Aerts HJWL. Artificial intelligence in radiology. Nat Rev Cancer. 2018;18:500–10.
13. Litjens G, Sánchez CI, Timofeeva N, et al. Deep learning as a tool for increased accuracy and efficiency of histopathological diagnosis. Sci Rep. 2016;6:26286.
14. Kassahun Y, Yu B, Tibebu AT, et al. Surgical robotics beyond enhanced dexterity instrumentation: a survey of machine learning techniques and their role in intelligent and autonomous surgical actions. Int J Comput Assist Radiol Surg. 2016;11:553–68.
15. Johnson KW, Torres Soto J, Glicksberg BS, et al. Artificial intelligence in cardiology. J Am Coll Cardiol. 2018;71:2668–79.
16. Choi E, Schuetz A, Stweart WF, Sun J. Using recurrent neural network models for early detection of heart failure onset. J Am Med Inform Assoc. 2017;24:361–70.
17. Tang TT, Zawaski JA, Francis KN, Qutub AA, Gaber MW. Image-based classification of tumor type and growth rate using machine learning: a preclinical study. Sci Rep. 2019;9:12529.
18. Houthooft R, Ruyssinck J, van der Herten J, et al. Predictive modelling of survival and length of stay in critically ill patients using sequential organ failure scores. Artif Intell Med. 2015;63:191–207.
19. Nassar AP Jr, Caruso P. ICU physicians are unable to accurately predict length of stay at admission: a prospective study. Int J Quat Health Care. 2006;1:99–103.
20. Sotoodeh M, Ho JC. Improving length of stay prediction using a hidden Markov model. AMIA Jt Summits Transl Sci Proc. 2019;2019:425–34.
21. Lin YW, Zhou Y, Faghri F, Shaw MJ, Campbell RH. Analysis and prediction of unplanned intensive care unit readmission using recurrent neural networks with lon short term memory. PLoS One. 2019;14:e0218942.
22. Awad A, Bader-El-Den M, McNicholas J, Briggs J. Early hospital mortality prediction of intensive care unit patients using an ensemble learning approach. Int J Med Inform. 2017;108:185–95.

23. Awad A, Bader-El-Den M, McNicholas J, Briggs J, El-Sonbaty Y. Predicting hospital mortality for intensive care unit patients: time-series analysis. Health Informatics J. 2019; July 26, https://doi.org/10.1177/1460458219850323 [Epub ahead of print].
24. Holmgren G, Andersson P, Jakobsson A, Frigyesi A. Artificial neural networks improve and simplify intensive care mortality prognostication: a national cohort study of 217,289 first-time intensive care unit admissions. J Intensive Care. 2019;7:44.
25. Rau CS, Wu SC, Chuang JF, et al. Machine learning models of survival prediction in trauma patients. J Clin Med. 2019;8:799.
26. Kim SY, Kim S, Cho J, et al. A deep learning model for real-time mortality prediction in critically ill children. Crit Care. 2019;23:279.
27. Yoon JH, Mu L, Chen L, et al. Predicting tachycardia as a surrogate for instability in the intensive care unit. J Clin Monit Comput. 2019;33:973–98.
28. Vistisen ST, Johnson AEW, Scheeren TWL. Predicting vital sign deterioration with artificial intelligence or machine learning. J Clin Monit Comput. 2019;33:949–51.
29. Giannini HM, Ginestra JC, Chivers C, et al. A machine learning algorithm to predict severe sepsis and septic shock: development, implementation, and impact on clinical practice. Crit Care Med. 2019;47:1485–92.
30. Banerjee I, Sofela M, Yang J, et al. Development and performance of the pulmonary embolism result forecast model (PERFORM) for computed tomography clinical decision support. JAMA Netw Open. 2019;2:e198719.
31. Zeiberg D, Prahlad T, Nallamothu BK, Iwashyna TJ, Wiens J, Sjoding MW. Machine learning for patient risk stratification for acute respiratory distress syndrome. PLoS One. 2019;14:e0214465.
32. Tran NK, Sen S, Palmieri TL, Lima K, Falwell S, Wajda J, Rashidi HH. Artificial intelligence and machine learning for predicting acute kidney injury in severely burned patients: a proof of concept. Burns. 2019;45:1350–8.
33. Flechet M, Falini S, Bonetti C, et al. Machine learning versus physicians' prediction of acute kidney injury in critically ill adults: a prospective evaluation of the AKIpredictor. Crit Care. 2019;23:282.
34. Zhang Z, Ho KM, Hong Y. Machine learning for the prediction of volume responsiveness in patients with oliguric acute kidney injury in critical care. Crit Care. 2019;23:112.
35. Li BY, Oh J, Young VB, Rao K, Wiens J. Using machine learning and the electronic health record to predict complicated Clostridium difficile infection. Open Forum Infect Dis. 2019;6:ofz186.
36. Thille A, Rodriguez P, Cabello B, Lellouche F, Brochard L. Patient-ventilator asynchrony during assisted mechanical ventilation. Intensive Care Med. 2006;32:1515–22.
37. Chen CW, Lin WC, Hsu CH, Cheng KS, Lo CS. Detecting ineffective triggering in the expiratory phase in mechanically ventilated patients based on airway flow and pressure deflection: feasibility of using a computer algorithm. Crit Care Med. 2008;36:455–61.
38. Blanch L, Sales B, Montanya J, et al. Validation of the better care® system to detect ineffective efforts during expiration in mechanically ventilated patients: a pilot study. Intensive Care Med. 2012;38:772–80.
39. Marchuk Y, Magrans R, Sales B, et al. Predicting patient-ventilator asynchronies with hidden Markov models. Sci Rep. 2018;8:17614.
40. Rehm GB, Han J, Kuhn B, et al. Creation of a robust and generalizable machine learning classifier for patient ventilator asynchrony. Methods Inf Med. 2018;57:208–19.
41. Adams JY, Lieng MK, Kuhn BT, et al. Development and validation of a multi-algorithm analytic platform to detect off-target mechanical ventilation. Sci Rep. 2017;7:14980.
42. Sottile PD, Albers D, Higgins C, Mckeehan J, Moss MM. The association between ventilator dyssynchrony, delivered tidal volume, and sedation using a novel automated ventilator dyssynchrony detection algorithm. Crit Care Med. 2018;46:e151–7.
43. Gholami B, Phan TS, Haddad WM, et al. Replicating human expertise of mechanical ventilation waveform analysis in detecting patient-ventilator cycling asynchrony using machine learning. Comput Biol Med. 2018;97:137–44.

44. Mulqueeny Q, Redmond SJ, Tassaux D, et al. Automated detection of asynchrony in patient-ventilator interaction. Conf Proc IEEE Eng Med Biol Soc. 2009;2009:5324–7.
45. Loo NL, Chiew YS, Tan CP, Arunachalam G, Ralib AM, Mat-Nor MB. A machine learning model for real-time asynchronous breathing monitoring. IFAC-PapersOnLine. 2018;51:378–83.
46. Sjoding MW, Hofer TP, Co I, Courey A, Cooke CR, Iwashyna TJ. Interobserver reliability of the Berlin ARDS definition and strategies to improve the reliability of ARDS diagnosis. Chest. 2018;153:361–7.
47. Nicolela MT, Drance SM, Broadway DC, Chauhan BC, McCormick TA, LeBlanc RP. Agreement among clinicians in the recognition of patterns of optic disk damage in glaucoma. Am J Ophthalmol. 2001;132:836–44.
48. Morris AH. Human cognitive limitations. Broad, consistent, clinical application of physiological principles will require decision support. Ann Am Thorac Soc. 2018;15(Suppl 1):S53–6.

Index

A
Abdominal compartment syndrome (ACS), 546
Acetaminophen, 287
Acid base disorders, 352
Activities of daily living (ADL), 403
Acute brain injury, 428, 443
Acute cor pulmonale, 146
Acute hemorrhage, 332
Acute hypoxemic respiratory failure, 53
Acute kidney injury (AKI), 119, 345, 433, 531, 549
Acute phase reactant protein, 129, 130
Acute respiratory distress syndrome (ARDS), 25, 53, 67, 82, 91, 307, 442
Acute respiratory failure, 3, 32
Advance directives, 643
Air mobile stroke units, 388
Airway occlusion pressure, 12, 13, 29, 30
Airway resistance, 41
Alcohol withdrawal syndrome, 571
Alveolar macrophage-derived extracellular vesicles, 56
Alveolar macrophages, 62
Anakinra, 266
Analgesia, 474
Angiopoietin-2 (Ang-2), 92
Antidiabetic drugs, 218
Antimicrobial de-escalation therapy, 129
Antimicrobial therapy, 218
Anti-PD-1/anti-PD-L1 immunotherapy, 275
Apoptosis, 71, 94, 113, 274, 443, 494
Arterial gas embolism, 562, 563
Artificial intelligence (AI), 677
Asthma, 76
Atelectasis, 7, 25
Atelectrauma, 82
Atrial natriuretic peptide (ANP), 216, 254
Autologous transfusion, 318

B
Barotrauma, 81
Biomarker-based mortality risk model, 76
Blood pressure measurement, 195
Blood transfusions, 312, 370, 647, 661
Bone marrow biopsies, 265
Brain death, 491
Brain ultrasonography, 479
Bronchoalveolar lavage fluid (BALF), 94
Burnout syndrome, 634
Bush Francis Catatonia Rating Scale (BFCRS), 463

C
Capillary refill time (CRT), 250
Cardiac arrest, 76, 101, 491, 507, 649
Cardiac troponins (cTn), 114, 120
Cardiogenic shock, 223
Cardiopulmonary resuscitation (CPR), 471, 491, 649
Cardiovascular surgery, 336, 337
Cast nephropathy, 533
Catatonia, 463
Cationic antimicrobial protein, 130
Cell-free hemoglobin, 287
  acetaminophen, 287–289
Central chemoreceptors, 8
Central venous pressures (CVP), 176
Cerebral edema, 492, 493
Cerebral hypoperfusion, 494
Chimeric antigen receptor (CAR)-T-cell therapy, 536

Chronic critical illness, 615, 617
Citrate infusion rate, 349, 351
Citrate load, 349, 351–353
Coagulopathy, 332, 434
Coma, 457, 461, 562
Compensatory anti-inflammatory (CARS), 415
Continuous renal replacement therapy (CRRT), 125, 131, 346
Continuous veno-venous hemodialysis (CVVHD), 348
Continuous veno-venous hemofiltration (CVVH), 127
C-reactive protein (CRP), 101, 125
Critical Care Societies Collaborative, 634, 635
Critical illness polyneuromyopathy, 587

D

Damage-associated molecular patterns (DAMPs), 102, 214, 265
Damage control resuscitation, 367
Decompressive laparotomy, 546, 553
Dehydration, 162
Delirium tremens, 569, 572
Diaphragm atrophy, 587
Diaphragm dysfunction, 587
Diaphragm electrical activity (EA_{di}), 11, 12, 31, 86
Diaphragm injury, 589
Diaphragm proteolysis, 596
Diaphragm ultrasound technique, 14, 31
Direct thrombin inhibitor, 347, 348
Disability-adjusted life years (DALYs), 398
Distributive shock, 415
Donor warm ischemia time, 507
Do-not-attempt cardiopulmonary resuscitation (DNA-CPR), 649
Driving pressure (ΔP), 27, 68, 445
Dynamic arterial elastance (Ea_{dyn}), 199
Dynamic indices, 238
Dysbiosis, 294

E

Early mobilization, 590
Ebb phase, 166
Eccentric diaphragm contractions, 588
Eccentric loading, 25
Echocardiography, 145, 181
Effective arterial elastance (E_a), 206
Elastic mechanical power (MP_{ELAST}), 41
Electrical activity of diaphragm (EA_{di}), 31, 86
Electrocardiogram (EKG), 431

Emergency medical services (EMS) systems, 365, 371, 372
Emotional and behavioral feedback, 9
End-expiratory occlusion test, 166
Endocan, 129
End-organ dysfunction, 176
End-organ function, 224
Endothelial progenitor cells (EPCs), 61
End-stage liver disease, 337
Energy expenditure, 41
Ergotrauma, 40
Esophageal pressure (P_{es}) monitoring, 26, 27
Excessive concentric loading, 24
Excessive PEEP, 25
Exosomes, 54
Expiratory muscles, 8
Expiratory occlusion maneuver, 29
Extra-alveolar microvessels, 147
Extra-cardiac echocardiographic parameters, 183
Extracellular vesicles, 62, 320
Extracorporeal CO_2 removal ($ECCO_2R$), 16
Extracorporeal filter, 352
Extracorporeal membrane oxygenation (ECMO), 307, 341, 508

F

Fecal microbiota transplantation (FMT), 300
Ferritin, 265
Fibrinolysis, 334, 335
Firmicutes, 294
5-point ordinal scale, 241
Flow phase, 167
Fluid balance, 161
Fluid bolus, 164
Fluid challenge, 164
Fluid dynamics, 166, 167
Fluid loading, 215
Fluid overload, 167
Fluid responsiveness, 165, 660
Fluid resuscitation, 146
Fluid stewardship, 154
Freeze thawing of platelets, 320
Frozen platelets, 318
Functional capillary density, 236
Functional warm ischemia time, 507

G

Gas embolism, 559
Gilcher's rule, 164
Glasgow Coma Scale (GCS) score, 105, 460
Global Burden of Disease (GBD) study, 398

Global increased permeability syndrome, 168
Glycocalyx, 137, 214, 246
Golden hour, 623
Gut microbiota, 294

H
Handheld vital microscopes, 253
Haptoglobin, 286, 287
Heart transplantation, 513, 514
Helicopter-based mobile stroke units, 388, 389
Hematological malignancy, 522
Hemodilution, 142, 248
Hemodynamic algorithms, 199
Hemodynamic monitoring, 181, 197, 664
Hemodynamic optimization, 205
Hemodynamic resuscitation, 207, 235
Hemoglobin toxicity, 283, 284
Hemolysis, 282, 283
Hemopexin, 287
Hemophagocytic lymphohistiocytosis (HLH), 261, 266
Heparan sulfate, 138
Heparin binding protein (HBP), 130
Hepatic artery thrombosis, 337
Hering-Breuer reflexes, 9
Heterogeneity index, 236
High cutoff veno-venous hemodialysis (HC-CVVH), 108
High-frequency jet ventilation, 561
Highly sensitive C-reactive protein (hsCRP), 101
High mobility group 1 protein (HMGB-1), 128
Horizontal diastolic waveform, 176
Hyperbaric oxygen therapy, 564
Hypercatabolic metabolic state, 167
Hyperchloremic acidosis, 216
Hyperfibrinolysis, 334
Hyperlactatemia, 350, 626
Hyperoxia, 108
Hypervolemia, 164, 254
Hypotension, 195
Hypotension prediction index (HPI), 200
Hypovolemia, 162
Hypovolemic shock, 415
Hypoxia, 102
Hypoxic-ischemic brain injury, 492, 493

I
Immune checkpoint inhibitors, 272, 536
Incident dark-field (IDF), 225, 253
Inducible NO synthase (iNOS), 415
Information technology, 380

Inspiratory occlusion maneuvers, 27, 28
Intensive care unit (ICU), 194
Intercellular adhesion molecule-1 (ICAM-1), 56
Interleukin-6 (IL-6), 101
Interleukin-8 (IL-8), 72, 93
Interleukin-10, 442
Intra-abdominal hypertension (IAH), 167, 550
Intra-abdominal pressure (IAP), 544
Intra-alveolar microvessels, 147
Intracranial pressure (ICP), 478
Intraoperative hypotension, 190
Intrarenal hemodynamics, 184
Intravenous fluids, 137, 145, 153, 215, 228, 242, 254, 368
Ischemia-reperfusion syndrome, 214

K
Kidney transplantation, 513
Kunicki morphological scoring system, 319

L
Lactate, 252, 353, 624
Latent class analysis (LCA), 72
Lateral parafacial nucleus, 8
Left ventricular (LV) dysfunction, 175
Liver transplantation, 337, 511, 512
Low-molecular-weight heparin (LMWH), 218, 347
Lung mechanics, 42
Lung-protective ventilation strategy, 10
Lung transplantation, 512, 513
Lymphopenia, 276

M
Maastricht classification, 503
Machine learning, 669
Macrohemodynamic variables, 245
Macrophage activation syndrome, 266
Maintenance fluids, 157, 158
Marini method, 597
Massive transfusion protocol, 335
Mean arterial pressure (MAP), 190, 433, 478
Mean pulmonary artery pressure (MPAP), 150
Mechanical circulatory support, 223
Mechanical energy, 40, 41
Mechanical power, 42, 43
Mechanical ventilation, 15, 29, 38, 85, 441, 591
Medical Research Council (MRC) scale, 584
Mental Capacity Act, 644, 649

Mesenchymal stromal cells (MSCs), 60
Metabolic acidosis, 352
Microcirculation, 214, 223, 235, 248, 313
Microcirculatory targets, 249
Microvascular flow index (MFI), 236, 253–255
Microvascular perfusion, 253
Microvesicles, 54
Mobile stroke units, 383
Modified Rankin Scale (mRS), 443
Moore's Law, 667
Motor vehicle collision, 407
Multimodal monitoring systems, 443
Multiple organ dysfunction syndrome (MODS), 297, 549
Multiple organ failure (MOF), 227
Muscle atrophy, 585
Muscle dysfunction, 586
Myocardial depression, 147
Myocardial strain, 182
Myotrauma, 21, 24, 588

N

Neurally adjusted ventilatory assist (NAVA), 31
Neurogenic pulmonary edema, 57
Neuromechanical efficiency index, 12
Neuromuscular blocking agents (NMBAs), 16
Neuronal apoptosis, 494
Neutrophil chemotactic factor, 56
Neutrophil extracellular vesicles, 59, 62
Nitric oxide, 283, 494
Non-cerebral organ failure, 101
Non-heart-beating donation, 503
Noninvasive hemodynamic monitoring, 196
Noninvasive ventilation (NIV), 83
Non-mechanical bleeding control interventions, 367
Norepinephrine, 208, 414
Normothermic regional perfusion, 508

O

Occlusion maneuvers, 29
Oncologic therapies, 76
Oncotic pressure, 139
Organ donation, 491, 503
Organ perfusion, 169
Orthogonal polarized spectroscopy (OPS), 225, 254
Osteopontin, 128

Out-of-hospital cardiac arrest (OHCA), 103, 104, 491
Oxygen transport, 241

P

Pancreas transplantation, 513
Parenteral nutrition, 159
Passive leg raising (PLR), 150, 165
Patient self-inflicted lung injury (P-SILI), 9, 22–24
Pediatric septic shock, 76
Pendelluft, 26, 84, 85
Pentraxin-3 (PTX3), 101, 129, 130
Perfused vessel density (PVD), 236
Peripheral chemoreceptors, 8
Peripheral perfusion index, 252
Persistent inflammatory and catabolic syndrome, 415
Pharmacodynamics, 156
Pharmacokinetics, 155
Polycompartment syndrome, 549
Positive end-expiratory pressure (PEEP), 149, 150, 444
Post-cardiac arrest syndrome, 76
Posthepatic portal hypertension, 184
Post-intensive care syndrome (PICS), 617
Postoperative cognitive dysfunction (POCD), 192
Postpartum hemorrhage, 338, 339
Prebiotics, 298
Pre-Bötzinger complex (preBötC), 4, 7
Prediction of Alcohol Withdrawal Severity Scale (PAWSS), 577
Predictive enrichment, 68, 73, 281
Preload dependence, 238
Presepsin (sCD14-ST), 101, 103, 130
Pressure Muscle Index (PMI), 85
Proadrenomedullin (MR-proADM), 129
Probiotics, 298
Procalcitonin (PCT), 101, 103, 127, 128
Prognostic enrichment, 70
Protective ventilation, 82
P-selectin, 320
Pulmonary artery catheter (PAC), 176
Pulmonary artery occlusion pressure (PAOP), 150, 165, 181
Pulmonary artery pressure (PAP), 178, 227
Pulmonary artery pulsatility index (PAPi), 180
Pulmonary edema, 22, 84
Pulmonary embolism, 146

Index

Pulmonary hypertension, 175
Pulmonary vascular resistance (PVR), 145
Pulmonary venous pressure, 148
Pupillary dilation reflex, 474
Pupillometry, 470, 498

Q

Quality of life (QoL) measures, 526, 598, 617

R

Reactive oxygen species (ROS), 102
Red blood cell (RBC), 229, 310, 335
Regional citrate anticoagulation (RCA), 348, 349
Regional heparin–protamine anticoagulation, 356, 357
Regional stroke care systems, 382
Renal replacement therapy (RRT), 549
Renin-angiotensin-aldosterone system (RAAS), 164
Resistive mechanical power (MP_{RES}), 41
Respiratory control centers, 4, 6
Respiratory drive, 11
Respiratory muscle pressure, 26, 27
Respiratory muscle rehabilitation, 605, 606
Resuscitation fluids, 157
Return of spontaneous circulation (ROSC), 101
Richmond Agitation-Sedation Scale (RASS), 434, 461, 483, 574
Right-to-left filling pressure ratio, 177
Right ventricular afterload, 146, 149, 151
Right ventricular dysfunction, 145, 175, 176
Right ventricular ejection fraction (RVEF), 181
Right ventricular failure, 176
Right ventricular fractional area change (RVFAC), 181
Right ventricular function index (RVFI), 177, 178, 180
Right ventricular length-force index, 177
Right ventricular myocardial performance index (RVMPI), 181
Right ventricular pressure waveform, 176
Right ventricular stroke work index (RVSWI), 177, 180
Rotational thromboelastometry (ROTEM), 321, 332

S

Sepsis, 125, 214, 264, 340, 341, 624
Septic shock, 166, 167, 206, 246, 271, 340
Sequential organ failure assessment (SOFA), 106
Sidestream dark-field (SDF) imaging, 225, 235, 253
Skin mottling, 251
Sniff nasal inspiratory pressures (SNIP), 589
Soluble receptor for advanced glycation end-products (sRAGE), 92
Soluble suppression of tumorigenicity 2 (sST2), 101, 104
Speckle-tracking echocardiography, 182
Sphingosine-1-phosphate (S1P), 254
Splanchnic mesenteric vasculature, 164
Spontaneous breathing, 31
Standardized mortality ratios (SMR), 400
Starling principle, 140, 141
Statins, 218
ST-elevation myocardial infarction (STEMI), 658
Subarachnoid hemorrhage (SAH), 479
Sublingual microcirculation, 237
   See also Microcirculation
Surfactant protein-D (SP-D), 92
"Swirling" test, 319
Synbiotics, 298–300
Syndecan-1, 138
Systemic inflammatory response syndrome (SIRS), 214, 264, 415

T

Targeted temperature management (TTM), 108
T cell exhaustion, 272
Telemedicine, 380, 381
Thoracic receptors, 9
Thromboelastography (TEG), 321, 332
Thrombolux technology, 319
Thrombolytic therapy, 385
Tissue hypoxia, 229, 246
Transcutaneous electrical muscle stimulation (TEMS), 592
Transdiaphragmatic pressure (P_{di}), 27
Transfusion-associated lung injury (TRALI), 370
Transpulmonary pressure (P_L), 26, 148
Transvascular pressure, 22
Trauma-induced coagulopathy, 334

Trauma systems, 398, 404
Traumatic brain injury (TBI), 387, 428, 444, 472
Tricuspid annular plane systolic excursion (TAPSE), 181, 182
Troponitis, 114
Tumor lysis syndrome, 536

U
Ultrasound, 14, 31, 175, 474, 586, 662
Unassisted TeleStroke Scale (UTSS), 381
Unfractionated heparin (UFH), 217, 347
Urine output, 169

V
Vascular access, 357, 358
Vascular endothelium, 249
Vasodilatory shock, 415
Vasopressin, 414
Vasopressin 1R (V1R) receptors, 414
Vasopressors, 200, 413
Venous gas embolism, 561
Venous thromboembolism, 339, 340
Venous vasodilators, 255
Veno-venous extracorporeal membrane oxygenation (VV-ECMO), 451
    See also Extracorporeal membrane oxygenation
Ventilator-associated pneumonia (VAP), 430, 431
Ventilator asynchronies, 22
Ventilator-induced lung injury (VILI), 21, 37, 442
Ventriculoarterial coupling, 206
Viscoelastic tests, 321, 332–335
Vitamin C, 289
Volatile anesthetics, 216
Volume kinetics, 155
Volutrauma, 81
Von Willebrand factor (vWF), 81, 93

W
West zone 3, 148
Withdrawal of life sustaining therapies, 414, 507
Work of breathing (WOB), 14, 40

Critical Care

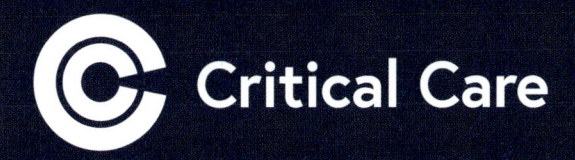

Thinking of publishing?
Choose *Critical Care*

- 2018 Impact Factor: 6.959
- Over 500,000 articles accesses per month
- Widest possible dissemination of your research: Fully Open Access - over 100,000 Altmetric mentions in 2019

Questions about submitting?
Contact **maritess.reyes@springernature.com**

Scan the QR code to visit the journal homepage:

BMC
Part of Springer Nature